Surgery of the Ear and Temporal Bone

2nd Edition

Surgery of the Ear and Temporal Bone

2nd Edition

Editors
Joseph B. Nadol, Jr., MD
Walter Augustus Lecompte Professor and Chairman
Department of Otology and Laryngology
Harvard Medical School
Chief, Department of Otolaryngology
Massachusetts Eye and Ear Infirmary
Boston, Massachusetts

Michael J. McKenna, MD
Associate Professor
Department of Otology and Laryngology
Harvard Medical School;
Surgeon, Department of Otolaryngology
Massachusetts Eye and Ear Infirmary
Boston, Massachusetts

Medical Illustrator
Robert J. Galla
Massachusetts Eye and Ear Infirmary
Boston, Massachusetts

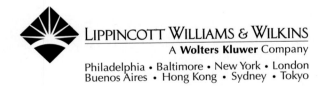
LIPPINCOTT WILLIAMS & WILKINS
A **Wolters Kluwer** Company
Philadelphia • Baltimore • New York • London
Buenos Aires • Hong Kong • Sydney • Tokyo

Acquisitions Editor: Robert Hurley
Developmental Editor: Eileen Wolfberg
Marketing Manager: Sara Bodison
Production Editor: Dave Murphy
Compositor: Graphic World, Inc.
Printer: Quebecor World Kingsport

Library of Congress Cataloging-in-Publication Data

Surgery of the ear and temporal bone / editors, Joseph B. Nadol Jr., Michael J. McKenna; medical illustrator, Robert J. Galla.—2nd ed.
    p. ; cm.
    Prev. ed.: New York : Raven press, c1993.
    Includes bibliographical references and index.
    ISBN 0-7817-2046-X
    1. Ear—Surgery. 2. Temporal bone—Surgery. I. Nadol, Joseph B. II. McKenna, Michael J.
    [DNLM: 1. Ear—surgery. 2. Temporal Bone—surgery. WV 200 S961 2004]
    RF126.S87 2004
    617.8'059—dc22

                       2004057749

Dedication

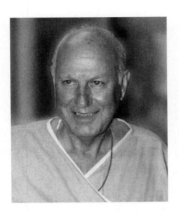

This second edition is dedicated to Harold Frederick Schuknecht, M.D., who served as co-editor for the first edition. He served as the Walter Augustus Lecompte Professor and Chair of the Department of Otology and Laryngology at the Harvard Medical School and the Chief of Otolaryngology at the Massachusetts Eye and Ear Infirmary between 1961 and 1987. Dr. Schuknecht was not only an accomplished otologist, but a world-recognized investigator in the anatomy and pathology of the ear. He was a willing and gifted teacher, mentor, and friend. The temporal bone collection at the Massachusetts Eye and Ear Infirmary, which he founded, and the tradition of insisting on scientific and histopathologic evidence in the process of clinical judgment which he fostered, serve as cornerstones of this text.

Contributors

Edward L. Applebaum, M.D. *Professor and Chairman, Department of Otolaryngology—Head and Neck Surgery, Northwestern University Feinberg School of Medicine, Chief of Otolaryngology, Northwestern Memorial Hospital, Chicago, Illinois*

Arlene Barr, M.D. *Associate Professor of Neurology and Rehabilitation, College of Medicine, University of Illinois at Chicago, Chicago, Illinois*

K. Paul Boyev, M.D. *Assistant Professor of Otolaryngology—Head and Neck Surgery, University of South Florida, College of Medicine, Tampa, Florida*

Mack L. Cheney, M.D. *Associate Professor of Otology and Laryngology, Harvard Medical School, Director, Facial Plastics & Reconstructive Surgery Service, Surgeon in Otolaryngology, Massachusetts Eye and Ear Infirmary, Boston, Massachusetts*

Michael J. Cunningham, M.D. *Associate Professor of Otology and Laryngology, Harvard Medical School, Surgeon in Otolaryngology, Massachusetts Eye and Ear Infirmary, Boston, Massachusetts*

Hugh D. Curtin, M.D. *Professor of Radiology, Harvard Medical School, Chief of Radiology, Massachusetts Eye and Ear Infirmary, Boston, Massachusetts*

David H. Darrow, M.D., D.D.S. *Associate Professor, Department of Otolaryngology, Eastern Virginia Medical School, Hospital Attending, Department of Otolaryngology, Children's Hospital of the King's Daughters, Norfolk, Virginia*

Antonio De la Cruz, M.D. *Clinical Professor of Otolaryngology, University of Southern California of Medicine, Director of Education, House Ear Institute, Inc., Los Angeles, California*

Marlene L. Durand, M.D. *Assistant Professor of Medicine, Harvard Medical School, Director, Infectious Disease Service, Massachusetts Eye and Ear Infirmary, Boston, Massachusetts*

Roland D. Eavey, M.D. *Associate Professor of Otology and Laryngology, Harvard Medical School, Director, Pediatric Otolaryngology Service, Surgeon in Otolaryngology, Massachusetts Eye and Ear Infirmary, Boston, Massachusetts*

Aaron Fay, M.D. *Instructor in Ophthalmology, Harvard Medical School, Instructor in Oculofacial Surgery, Massachusetts Eye and Ear Infirmary, Boston, Massachusetts*

Jose N. Fayad, M.D. *Clinical Associate Professor of Otolaryngology, University of Southern California, Associate, House Ear Clinic, Inc., Los Angeles, California*

Mark R. Gacek, M.D. *Premier Medical Group, Mobile, Alabama*

Richard R. Gacek, M.D. *Department of Otolaryngology–Head and Neck Surgery, University of Massachusetts Medical School, University of Massachusetts Medical Center, Worcester, Massachusetts*

Bruce J. Gantz, M.D. *Professor and Head, Department of Otolaryngology—Head and Neck Surgery, University of Iowa College of Medicine, Iowa City, Iowa*

Richard E. Gliklich, M.D. *Associate Professor of Otology and Laryngology, Harvard Medical School, Surgeon in Otolaryngology, Massachusetts Eye and Ear Infirmary, Boston, Massachusetts*

Tessa A. Hadlock, M.D. *Instructor in Otology and Laryngology, Harvard Medical School, Department of Otolaryngology, Massachusetts Eye and Ear Infirmary, Boston, Massachusetts*

Jeffrey P. Harris, M.D., Ph.D. *Professor and Chief of Otolaryngology—Head and Neck Surgery, University of California, San Diego, UCSD Medical Center–Hillcrest, San Diego, California*

Robert W. Jyung, M.D. *Assistant Professor of Surgery–Division of Otolaryngology, University of Medicine and Dentistry of New Jersey, Director of Otology/Neurotology, The University Hospital/UMDNJ, Newark, New Jersey*

Avinash Khanna, M.D. *Cardiology Fellow, University of Missouri-Kansas City at Mid America Heart Institute, Kansas City, Missouri*

David W. Kim, M.D.

Arvind Kumar, M.D. *Professor of Otolaryngology—Head and Neck Surgery, University of Illinois at Chicago, Adjunct Professor, Department of Otolaryngology—Head and Neck Surgery, Northwestern University, Hinsdale, Illinois*

Robert A. Levine, M.D. *Assistant Professor of Neurology, Harvard Medical School, Assistant in Otolaryngology, Massachusetts Eye and Ear Infirmary, Boston, Massachusetts*

Richard M. Levinson, M.D. *Assistant Clinical Professor, Department of Otolaryngology, University of Minnesota, Staff Surgeon, ENT Specialty Care of Minnesota, Minneapolis, Minnesota*

Richard F. Lewis, M.D. *Assistant Professor of Otology and Laryngology, Harvard Medical School, Consultant in Otoneurology, Massachusetts Eye and Ear Infirmary, Boston, Massachusetts*

Robert L. Martuza, M.D. *Higgins Professor of Neurosurgery, Harvard Medical School, Chief of Neurosurgery, Massachusetts General Hospital, Boston, Massachusetts*

Trevor J. McGill, M.D. *Professor of Otology and Laryngology, Harvard Medical School, Associate Chief of Otolaryngology, Department of Otolaryngology, Children's Hospital, Boston, Massachusetts*

Michael J. McKenna, M.D. *Associate Professor of Otology and Laryngology, Harvard Medical School, Surgeon in Otolaryngology, Massachusetts Eye and Ear Infirmary, Boston, Massachusetts*

Saumil N. Merchant, M.D. *Associate Professor of Otology and Laryngology, Harvard Medical School, Surgeon in Otolaryngology, Massachusetts Eye and Ear Infirmary, Boston, Massachusetts*

Dianne H. Meyer, Ph.D. *Chairperson, Department of Communication Disorders and Sciences, Director, Section of Communicative Disorders, Otolaryngology and Bronchoesophagology, Rush University, Chicago, Illinois*

William W. Montgomery, M.D. Deceased. *John W. Merriam Professor of Otology and Laryngology, Harvard Medical School, Senior Surgeon in Otolaryngology, Massachusetts Eye and Ear Infirmary, Boston, Massachusetts*

Joseph B. Nadol, Jr., M.D. *Walter Augustus Lecompte Professor and Chairman, Department of Otology and Laryngology, Harvard Medical School, Chief of Otolaryngology, Massachusetts Eye and Ear Infirmary, Boston, Massachusetts*

Aftab Patni, M.D.   *Neurotologist, Department of Otolaryngology, Ear, Nose, Throat, and Plastic Surgery Associates, Winter Park, Florida*

Brian P. Perry, M.D., F.A.C.S.   *Clinical Assistant Professor of Otolaryngology, University of Texas Health Science Center, Chief of Otolaryngology, Southwest Texas Methodist Hospital, San Antonio, Texas*

Dennis S. Poe, M.D.   *Assistant Clinical Professor of Otology and Laryngology, Harvard Medical School, Surgeon, Department of Otolaryngology, Children's Hospital, Boston, Massachusetts*

Reza Rahbar, D.M.D., M.D.   *Assistant Professor, Department of Otology and Laryngology, Harvard Medical School, Associate in Otolaryngology, Children's Hospital, Boston, Massachusetts*

Mitchell J. Ramsey, M.D.   *Staff Physician in Otolaryngology, Tripler Army Medical Center, Tripler AMC, Hawaii*

Jamie M. Rappaport, M.D., C.M., F.R.C.S.(C)   *Assistant Professor of Otolaryngology, McGill University, Director of Otology and Neurotology, Sir Morimer B. Davis Jewish General Hospital, Montreal, Quebec, Canada*

Steven D. Rauch, M.D.   *Associate Professor of Otology and Laryngology, Harvard Medical School, Surgeon in Otolaryngology, Massachusetts Eye and Ear Infirmary, Boston, Massachusetts*

Steven F. Ronner, Ph.D.   **Deceased.** *Department of Neurosurgery, Massachusetts General Hospital, Boston, Massachusetts*

Peter A.D. Rubin, M.D.   *Associate Professor of Ophthalmology, Harvard Medical School, Director, Eye Plastic, Orbital and Cosmetic Surgery Service, Department of Ophthalmology, Massachusetts Eye and Ear Infirmary, Boston, Massachusetts*

Osamu Sakai, M.D.   *Assistant Professor of Radiology, Boston University School of Medicine, Staff Neuroradiologist, Department of Radiology, Boston Medical Center, Boston, Massachusetts*

Harold F. Schuknecht, M.D.   **Deceased.** *Professor Emeritus and Chairman Emeritus of Otology and Laryngology, Harvard Medical School, Emeritus Chief of Otolaryngology, Massachusetts Eye and Ear Infirmary, Boston, Massachusetts*

Herbert Silverstein, M.D.   *Clinical Professor of Surgery, Division of Otolaryngology, University of South Florida, Tampa, Florida, President, Ear Research Foundation, Sarasota, Florida*

Robert A. Sofferman, M.D.   *Professor of Surgery, Chairman, Division of Otolaryngology, University of Vermont School of Medicine, Burlington, Vermont*

Jeffrey H. Spiegel, M.D., F.A.C.S.   *Assistant Professor, Department of Otolaryngology—Head and Neck Surgery, Department of Plastic Surgery, Boston University School of Medicine, Attending Physician, Boston Medical Center, Boston, Massachusetts*

Hinrich Staecker, M.D.   *Assistant Professor, Department of Otolaryngology, University of Maryland School of Medicine, Baltimore, Maryland*

Aaron R. Thornton, Ph.D.   *Retired, West Des Moines, Iowa*

Conrad Wall, III, M.D.   *Associate Professor of Otology and Laryngology, Harvard Medical School, Director, Jenks Vestibular Diagnostic Laboratory, Massachusetts Eye and Ear Infirmary, Boston, Massachusetts*

Pa-Chun Wang, M.D., M.Sc.   *Associate Professor, Department of Public Health, College of Public Health, China Medical University, Taichung, Taiwan, Staff Otolaryngologist, Department of Otolaryngology, Cathay General Hospital, Taipei, Taiwan*

Preface

As in the first edition, in *Surgery of the Ear and Temporal Bone* we have attempted to document a tradition and school of otologic surgical management that has evolved at the Massachusetts Eye and Ear Infirmary. To this end, the text is organized on the basis of clinical problems presented by our otologic patients rather than organized by category of surgical procedure. In this edition, new sections have been added, including intraoperative monitoring of cranial nerves, outcome studies in ear surgery, the management of congenital cholesteatoma of the middle ear and mastoid, tumors of the facial nerve, superior canal dehiscence syndrome, and transtemporal transpetrous osseous approaches to the cranial base. In addition, many chapters have been significantly updated, in particular that on cochlear implantation. Treatment of disorders of the facial nerve has been significantly reorganized to segregate management of injury from that of Bell's palsy and Herpes zoster, and a chapter on facial reanimation surgery has been added.

The chapters in general are organized around the needs for surgical decision making, providing discussion of indications, contraindications, complications and therapeutic alternatives. As in the first edition, the chapters have been written largely by those who have been directly involved in the residency, fellowship training, and continuing medical education programs at the Infirmary.

Where possible, we have documented histopathology of the human temporal bone, including histopathology following surgical intervention, from our collection at the Massachusetts Eye and Ear Infirmary. It is our conviction that the incorporation of knowledge derived from histopathologic study and from laboratory investigation provides a unique vantage point to judge the likely medical needs of patients and relative merits of surgical interventions. For example, the chapter on ossiculoplasty and tympanoplasty has been extensively revised to include recent knowledge generated in our basic science laboratories. In addition, our concepts for management of otosclerosis, acoustic neuromas, and facial nerve monitoring have been heavily influenced by data from the laboratory. It is the authors' sincere hope that this text will provide a rational basis for diagnosis and management, both medical and surgical, of disorders of the ear, and that this knowledge will, in the final analysis, accrue to the benefit of our patients.

Joseph B. Nadol, Jr., M.D.
Michael J. McKenna, M.D.

Acknowledgments

We wish to thank our contributors for their scholarly efforts and Bob Galla for his medical illustrations in which he continually strives to provide anatomic detail, accuracy and clarity. We are also very grateful for the assistance of Carol Ota, Eileen Nims, and Richard Cortese for their valuable help in producing this second edition.

Contents

Part. I. EXAMINATION OF THE EAR

Part II. SOFT TISSUE APPROACHES AND MANAGEMENT

Part III. OSSEOUS APPROACHES TO THE TEMPORAL BONE

Part VII. SURGERY FOR VERTIGO

Part VIII. SURGERY FOR TRAUMA TO THE TEMPORAL BONE AND DYSFUNCTION OF THE FACIAL NERVE

Part IX. SURGERY FOR TUMORS OF THE TEMPORAL BONE

Part X. PLASTIC AND RECONSTRUCTIVE SURGERY OF THE AURICLE

Examination of the Ear

CHAPTER 1

Office Examination of the Ear

Joseph B. Nadol, Jr., and Harold F. Schuknecht

Although examination of the ear is relatively free of discomfort and is less demanding of time than most medical examinations, special equipment is needed and a meticulous routine should be followed. The wide array of ear diseases that are seen by the otologist may range from a patient with impacted cerumen to a patient in coma from otogenic meningitis. The following discussion relates to the nonemergent visit to the otologist's office.

The office of a practicing otologist needs at least two rooms equipped for standard examination of the ear, nose, and throat. In addition, there should be a room known informally as the "scope room," where examinations and minor procedures can be performed using a binocular microscope and an ear irrigating station. Conventional audiometry, tympanometry, brainstem evoked response (BSER), and electronystagmography (ENG) should also be incorporated into the office practice or be conveniently available.

Any medical practice benefits from the immediate availability of support facilities, such as an emergency unit, clinical laboratory, radiology, and medical consultation.

MEDICAL HISTORY

In no other specialty than otology is it more true that the right questions need to be asked to aid in the process of diagnosis. For simple problems (e.g., wax impaction), there is no diagnostic challenge, but for more complicated problems, the time of onset, rate of progression, associated symptoms, magnitude of discomfort and disability, precipitating events, previous therapy, family history, and effect on quality of life must be considered. The medical history, including review of systems and current use of medications, may reveal pertinent information.

When confronted by a patient with an ear disorder, the otologist should not make a hasty decision regarding the validity or seriousness of the complaints. Allow the patient time to present the case as he or she sees it and then proceed with questions necessary to elicit further information.

INSPECTION AND OTOSCOPY

Gross inspection and digital palpation may reveal the presence of congenital malformations, inflammatory conditions, and neoplastic disorders of the auricle, external meatus, and periauricular area.

Examination of the external canal and tympanic membrane may begin with a handheld otologic speculum and illumination with a head mirror or head light. A handheld otoscope with a magnification of 2.5X and its own light source is an adequate screening tool to determine normalcy or pathology of the tympanic membrane. If a pathologic condition is detected or suspected, a binocular microscope with a magnification of 6X to 40X is essential. This can be wall mounted for examination with the patient in a sitting position or floor mounted for examination with the patient in a recumbent position (Fig. 1.1). Other handheld equipment essential for the otologic examination include no. 5 and no. 20 French suction tips, forceps (Hartmann and alligator), and wax curettes (Fig. 1.2).

Depending on the symptoms and initial otologic findings, further examination may include pressure otoscopy (Fig. 1.3), instrumental manipulation of the manubrium and tympanic membrane, and occasionally incisions done under local anesthesia to determine the status of middle ear pathology.

Examining and recording the findings of otoscopy should be a systematic endeavor. The appropriate size of the speculum will be determined by the age of the patient, the tortuosity of both the fibrocartilaginous and bony parts of the ear canal, and the obstruction to view by hair in the meatus of male patients' ears. It is advantageous to use the largest possible speculum. Any manipulations, such as removal of wax,

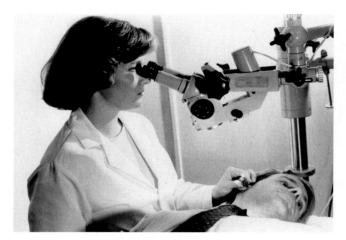

FIG. 1.1 The otologist's office must have a "scope room" equipped with a binocular operation microscope and suitable instruments. This microscope provides fiberoptic illuminated views with magnification selections (using 10X oculars) of 6X, 10X, 25X, and 40X. In the office setting it is used for examinations, minor procedures, and postoperative care.

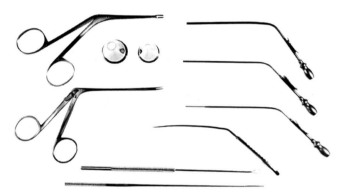

FIG. 1.2 Photograph of standard otologic examination equipment.

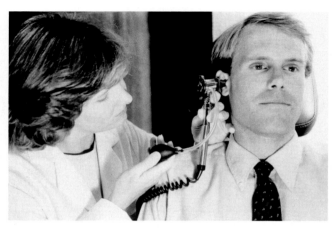

FIG. 1.3 Pressure otoscopy is done by alternately increasing and decreasing the pressure in the external auditory canal while observing the tympanic membrane, manubrium, and middle ear under magnification. The maneuver may be done with the aid of either a binocular or monocular microscope. A Siegle otoscope, with its 2.5X magnification, is usually not adequate for this evaluation. The speculum must form a tight seal in the ear canal. The test is useful in evaluating the mobility of the tympanic membrane and manubrium, identifying effusions of the middle ear, and differentiating perforations from transparent dimeric membranes.

keratin, dried exudate, or other debris, and fluid discharge are best accomplished with 6X or higher magnification to prevent trauma and pain. It is essential that this be accomplished because epithelial debris, cerumen, and hardened exudate often obscure an underlying pathologic process.

The external auditory canals are inspected for congenital anomalies, ulceration, granulation, stenosis, bony osteoma, or exostoses. The quality of the epidermis should be noted. The firmness of smooth outgrowths may be tested by instrumental palpation but with gentleness to prevent lacerations or hematomas. If surgery is contemplated, the extent of convexity of the anterior canal wall is recorded.

Examination of the tympanic membrane and middle ear involves the assessment of two principal anatomic areas: (i) the pars tensa and middle ear and (ii) the pars flaccida and epitympanum. Positive findings should be recorded in narrative form accompanied by a sketch. A convention for diagrammatic representation of pathology of the tympanic membrane should be adopted. For example, in our office a retraction pocket or replacement membrane is outlined in

blue, a perforation outlined in red, and granulation represented as a red area (Fig. 1.4).

A patulous eustachian tube is an often overlooked disorder. The history is often adequate to make the diagnosis and consists of autophony, which disappears in the recumbent position. Examination will reveal respiratory movements of the tympanic membrane. These movements can be accentuated by having the patient block one nostril by digital pressure on the nose and breathe forcefully through the open nostril.

An intact pars tensa is not necessarily an indication of a healthy middle ear. Variations in texture and color and response to pressure otoscopy will convey to the experienced otoscopist the presence of middle ear disease such as serous effusion, acute otitis, neoplastic disease, fibrocystic sclerosis of the middle ear, and vascular anomalies (e.g., aberrant carotid, high jugular bulb). Diffuse or focal areas of retraction of the pars tensa should be identified and recorded, and if a conductive hearing loss is present, malleus mobility should be evaluated by pressure otoscopy. If the tympanic membrane shows areas of dimeric membrane (thin replacement membrane), these should be noted; retractions attached to the incus (myringoincudopexy) or stapes (myringostapediopexy) should also be identified and recorded.

Perforations of the pars tensa are characterized in terms of size and location, as well as in the appearance of their margins. Thickened margins are usually associated with fibrous thickening of the pars tensa and indicate previous chronic or recurring inflammatory disease. Keratin accumulation at the margins of the perforation is suggestive that the squamous epithelium has extended onto the medial surface of the tympanic membrane. The mucosa of the middle ear can be inspected

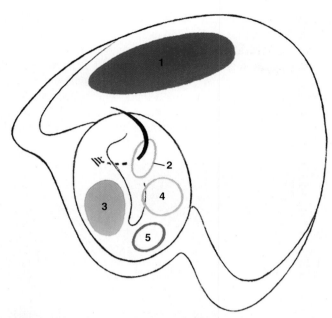

FIG. 1.4 Conventions for documentation of otologic pathology: *(1)* Granulation or deepithelialization, *(2)* retraction pocket, *(3)* tympanosclerotic plaque, *(4)* monomeric replacement membrane, *(5)* perforation.

through the perforation and evaluated for evidence of acute or chronic pathologic change such as inflammatory or fibrous thickening, polypoid hypertrophy, ulceration, granulations, and epidermization. Exuberant tissue may be suggestive of neoplastic disease and require biopsy, but the surgeon should keep in mind the possibility of an aberrant carotid, high jugular bulb, or aberrant facial nerve. Also, biopsies and removal of polyps, which may be an essential part of a thorough evaluation of the ear, should be done without disturbing the ossicles, particularly the stapes.

Ossicular pathology can often be identified by inspection, particularly if there is a large perforation or a retracted dimeric membrane in the posterosuperior quadrant of the pars tensa. Common areas of resorptive osteitis are the long process of the incus, the crural arch, and the manubrium. Gentle instrumental manipulations may be helpful in differentiating ossicular mobility or fixation. With large perforations of the pars tensa, the unopposed pull of the tensor tympani muscle often results in medial displacement of the inferior end of the manubrium and occasionally fibrous adhesion to the promontory.

Cholesteatoma of the middle ear may occur alone or in association with cholesteatoma of the epitympanum or mastoid. Cholesteatoma implies the retention of keratin and often mandates surgical correction. It must be differentiated from epidermization, which is also an epidermis-lined region of the middle ear but without retention of keratin and therefore not progressive and in itself not an indication for surgery. Cholesteatoma is often associated with erosion of ossicles, as well as the posterior bony tympanic annulus and the scutum (lateral wall of the epitympanum). Occasionally an attic cholesteatoma may cause erosion of the scutum, re-

sulting in an "autoatticotomy." Rarely, after invading the mastoid, cholesteatoma will cause resorption of the posterior wall of the external auditory canal, thus exteriorizing itself in what is known as "nature's radical."

Attic retraction pockets are retractions of the pars flaccida (Shrapnel's membrane) into the lateral epitympanic compartment and are caused by chronic or recurring negative pressure in the middle ear. The retraction may consist of a slight medial bowing of the membrane or a deep pocket extending onto the lateral surfaces of the body of incus and head of malleus with varying degrees of resorption of the scutum. If the pocket is clean and dry, it is usually nonprogressive and of no clinical significance. Deeper retractions that collect keratin are so-called symptomatic retraction pockets. Particularly if granulations or suppuration occur, such retractions are often progressive, causing erosion of ossicles and extension into the medial epitympanic compartment, antrum, and mastoid. This condition mandates surgical correction. It is usually not difficult to differentiate a benign nonprogressive retraction pocket from an attic cholesteatoma.

CERUMEN REMOVAL

Cerumen often obstructs the otoscopic view and therefore must be removed before otoscopy can be performed. In some patients, recurring wax impactions are a cause for conductive hearing loss. In male patients, hair in the ear canal may be a contributing factor to wax impaction. Minor cerumen accumulations can be removed with loops under appropriate magnification, whereas larger accumulations may additionally require irrigation. The standard ear wash syringes may be satisfactory for an office setting, but for an otologic clinic, a thermally controlled ear wash station is a great convenience (Fig. 1.5).

HEARING ASSESSMENT

The Rinne and Weber tests are a standard part of any otologic evaluation and are used to differentiate conductive from sensorineural hearing loss. There is little to be gained by using several tuning forks of different frequencies; the 512-Hz aluminum alloy fork, with its prolonged decay time, is most suited for these tests. The fork is struck firmly on a semisolid surface (e.g., patella, elbow, knuckle) and the overtones are damped by momentarily placing a finger on the base of the vibrating tines.

The Rinne test is done by determining whether the patient senses the tone to be louder when the activated fork is held near the auricle (Fig. 1.6) or when the stem of the fork is firmly pressed on the mastoid in an area where the scalp is thinnest, which is immediately posterior to the auricle (Fig. 1.7). By convention, the Rinne test is positive if the tone is louder by air and negative when it is louder on bone. When there is no perceptible difference in loudness, the test is said to be equivocal. A negative Rinne test signals a 20-dB or greater conductive hearing loss.

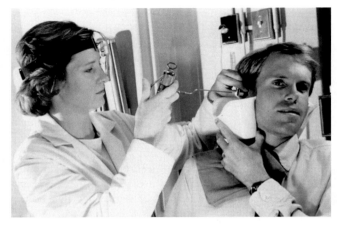

FIG. 1.5 Irrigation for wax removal is facilitated by an ear wash station. A convenient instrument for this purpose is the "warm water spurter," which is connected to the building's water and electrical systems. Its components consist of a wall-mounted heating tank that keeps a reservoir of water at a constant temperature, a flexible hose that leads from the tank to a handheld dispenser that is also electrically heated, and several detachable irrigation tubes. (Warmwasserdruckspritze, available from Haeberle and Company, 7 Stuttgart 80, Breitweineustrasse 15, Postfache 80 0524, Germany.)

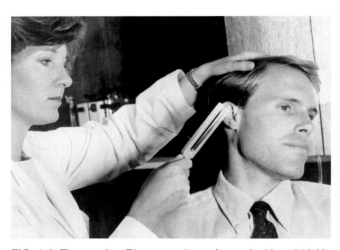

FIG. 1.6 The routine Rinne test is performed with a 512-Hz aluminum alloy tuning fork. Because of its long amplitude decay time, the test can be performed simply by asking the patient to judge whether the loudness of the tone is greater at the ear (air conduction) or on the bone (bone conduction) or sensed to be of equal or the same loudness (equivocal). An alternative method is to hold the fork at the ear and, when the tone is no longer heard, to immediately test the bone conduction without reactivating the fork.

The Weber test requires that the patient make a determination as to whether the tone is sensed to be louder on one side when the stem of the activated fork is placed firmly against the skull (Fig. 1.8). Because there is virtually no attenuation across the skull, the fork can be placed on it anywhere; the forehead is the most convenient site. The Weber test lateralizes to the ear with a conductive hearing loss or, in the case of bilateral disease, to the ear with the greatest con-

ductive hearing loss. The Weber test is of no value in the assessment of pure sensorineural hearing losses; even in cases of total unilateral hearing loss, there is no sense of lateralization. Because patients with a unilateral conductive hearing loss may not wish to risk their credibility with the examiner by admitting that the tone is loudest in the diseased ear, it may be wise to advise them that this is a possibility. The Weber test can be recorded as lateralizing to the right or left or not lateralizing.

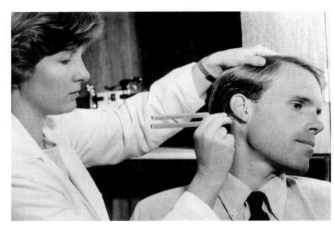

FIG. 1.7 After the patient has had a few seconds to experience the air conduction loudness level, the stem of the tuning fork is immediately placed on the mastoid with firm pressure.

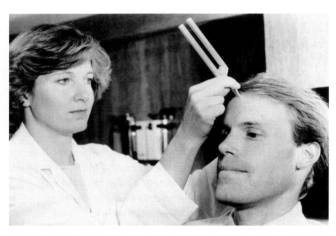

FIG. 1.8 The Weber test is also performed with a 512-Hz tuning fork. After activating the fork, the stem is placed on the forehead and the patient makes a judgment as to whether the tone is louder in one ear or the other or sensed to be of equal loudness.

Before sending the patient for audiometric tests, the otologist should make a rough assessment of the hearing capability of both ears. This is readily accomplished by masking the nontest ear with a Bárány noise box while the patient is asked to repeat spoken spondee words or numbers delivered to the test ear at different loudness levels (Fig. 1.9). This minimizes the risk of operating on a nonhearing ear or an only hearing ear in the unlikely event of flawed audiometric tests.

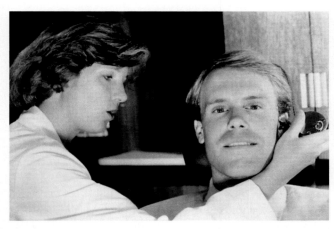

FIG. 1.9 The Bárány noise box is an excellent masking device for the office examination. To be effective, the adapter of the noise box must seal the ear canal. It generates a broad spectrum of sound levels from 90 to 105 dB and is not harmful to hearing because of the short stimulus periods used. There are adapters for the normal ear canal and for the surgically enlarged meatus. The noise box is used to mask hearing in one ear while testing the opposite ear. Live voice, monitored for loudness, is used to determine gross levels of hearing loss. The noise box is also effective in activating the crossed stapedial reflex and evoking the Tullio phenomenon.

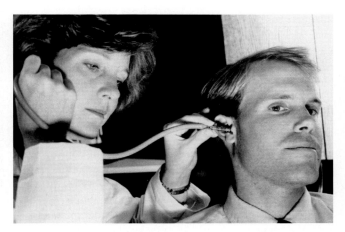

FIG. 1.10 The auscultation tube is used to detect objective tinnitus and must be performed in a room with a low ambient noise level. The ear canal adapters at one end are provided in graded sizes that are removable for sterilization.

OTHER TESTS

Auscultation

Constant high-pitched or low-pitched tinnitus is subjective and cannot be heard by an examiner. However, objective tinnitus may occur as an intermittent clicking sensation in association with palatal myoclonus or a pulsating hum synchronous with heartbeat caused by internal carotid, jugular bulb anomalies, or vascular lesions. An auscultation tube facilitates the detection of objective tinnitus. This simple device is a short rubber tube having inserts at opposite ends for the ear canals of the examiner and patient (Fig. 1.10). Auscultation with the stethoscope over the ear canal, mastoid, and neck may also be helpful.

Paper Patch

The paper patch maneuver is used principally to predict the probable hearing level that can be achieved by surgical closure of a perforation of the tympanic membrane. A patch of thin paper of appropriate size is coated on one surface with ointment and placed over the perforation. Results of hearing tests before and after application of the paper patch provide a prediction of the functional outcome of surgical repair of the tympanic membrane perforation. It may also provide evidence for ossicular pathology and the potential need for ossicular reconstruction.

Stapedial Reflex

When the stapes is visible through a perforation and the hearing is good in the opposite ear, the crossed stapedial re-

flex test can be used to assess mobility of the stapes. This test is accomplished by observing the stapes and stapedius tendon under magnification while stimulating the opposite ear with bursts of noise from a Bárány noise box.

Inflation

In selected patients, inflation can be of diagnostic value. For example, (i) the extent of retraction and mobility of the tympanic membrane or retraction pockets can be determined; (ii) the appearance of fluid lines after inflation confirms the presence of serous effusion; (iii) the presence of a small perforation that escapes visual detection may be confirmed by simultaneous inflation and auscultation, and its location can be determined by placing a small amount of fluid in the ear and observing the site where bubbles are generated; (iv) when there is a dry perforation of the tympanic membrane, simultaneous inflation and auscultation provide a measure of the capability of the eustachian tube to pass air. Any form of forced inflation, however, is unphysiologic and therefore is not a valid test of eustachian tube function.

Inflation can be accomplished by three methods: (i) the Valsalva maneuver, in which the patient pinches the nostrils and then with lips tightly closed blows out the cheeks as if playing a trumpet; (ii) the politzerization maneuver, in which the examiner forces air into one nostril with a Politzer bag with nasal tip while the other nostril is pinched shut and the patient simultaneously swallows or repeatedly vocalizes "Coca-Cola" or "K,K,K" as the Politzer bag is squeezed; and (iii) use of the calibrated Senturia inflator attached to an air pressure outlet and having a bypass valve that can be adjusted to control the amount of pressure that is delivered to the nasopharynx via the nostril as the patient swallows.

The effectiveness of inflation can be monitored by inspection of the tympanic membrane during or after inflation or by auscultation. The magnitude of pressure should be just adequate to accomplish inflation; there are reports of excessive pressures causing extension of air into the intracranial cavity. Inflation is of doubtful therapeutic value except possibly in the early stage of acute barotrauma or chronic mild eustachian tube hypofunction.

ASSESSING THE VESTIBULAR SYSTEM

The otologic history and the results of assessment of hearing in the office serve as guides as to what extent the vestibular system should be examined. Even when the patient denies having had any form of disequilibrium, past or present, there are conditions when examination of the vestibular system is indicated. For example, unilateral partial or complete loss of vestibular function in one ear can take place without causing vertigo if the underlying pathologic change occurs gradually over a long period. Any patient who complains of disequilibrium (current, recent, or past) should have several simple vestibular tests performed in the office. Vestibular tests are based on measurements of abnormality in the vestibuloocular and vestibulospinal reflexes.

SPONTANEOUS NYSTAGMUS

Most ear, nose, and throat (ENT) consoles have outlets that accommodate illuminated Frenzel glasses (Fig. 1.11). The examining room should be equipped with a single switch that will extinguish all other lights. The Frenzel glasses have 20-diopter lenses that magnify the eyes and eliminate ocular fixation. If nystagmus is present, it is recorded as mild, moderate, or severe and the direction of the quick component is noted. If nystagmus is absent or mild and the tympanic membranes are intact, the examination can proceed to the caloric test.

Caloric Tests

The finding of a unilateral suppressed caloric response is often of diagnostic significance (e.g., Ménière's disease, acoustic tumor, vestibular neuritis). A quick, simple, cold-water caloric test that is not productive of vegetative symptoms should be available in every otolaryngologist's office practice; preferably the test should be done by the physician. Bithermal Hallpike caloric tests are too time-consuming to be compatible with a busy office practice and should be reserved for the ENG evaluation. An office caloric test may obviate the need for an ENG evaluation.

The Kobrak minimal caloric test is suitable for the office setting and is done as follows: With the Frenzel glasses in place and the head tilted backward at an angle of 60 degrees, 5 ml of water at a temperature of 80°F (23°C) is injected through a 20-gauge needle against the tympanic membrane over a period of 10 seconds (Fig. 1.12). Although the duration of the nystagmus is not the most sensitive parameter of the vestibuloocular reflex, it is a useful measurement (normal: 1 to $2\frac{1}{2}$ minutes). The opposite ear can be tested immediately in an identical manner; a waiting time between the tests is unnecessary. Although the normal response times vary among patients, they should be bilaterally symmetrical provided that the stimulus has been delivered in an identical manner. Therefore an asymmetry of response is abnormal, with the longer response representing normal, unless one is dealing with bilateral ear disease or directional preponderance. This method does not permit a measurement of the speed of the slow component of the nystagmus; however, a sophisticated examiner can readily detect gross asymmetries in amplitude and speed of the responses in the two ears. This test will not produce

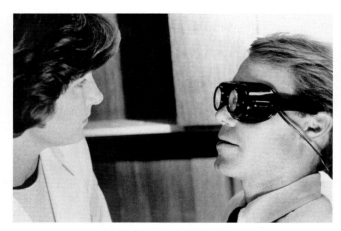

FIG. 1.11 Frenzel glasses are internally illuminated and contain 20-diopter lenses. When used in subdued light, they effectively eliminate ocular fixation. They are indispensable as an aid in detecting small magnitudes of spontaneous and induced nystagmus or ocular deviation.

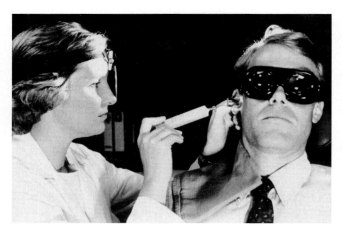

FIG. 1.12 The Kobrak minimal caloric test is a useful procedure that can be incorporated into a busy office schedule. If equipment and assistance are readily available, the entire test procedure can be performed in 6 to 10 minutes. The irrigation is done with a 10-ml syringe via a 20-gauge needle that has been soldered onto a standard ear speculum.

vegetative symptoms (nausea, sweating, vomiting, diarrhea) and can be repeated at future appointments as necessary without objections from the patient. When no response is generated by the 80°F test, a 5-ml ice water test is administered. (The ice water test should not be used unless it has been determined that there is no response to an 80°F stimulus.)

Fistula Test

The fistula test is performed by alternately increasing and decreasing the pressure in the external auditory canal with a Politzer bag in connection with an ear canal adapter (Fig. 1.13), with a Siegle otoscope, or simply by digital pressure on the ear canal. There are three mechanisms by which manipulation of pressures in the middle ear can activate the vestibuloocular and vestibulospinal reflex arcs:

1. In the case of a bony fistula in a semicircular canal (usually the lateral canal in chronic otitis media with cholesteatoma), the pressure changes are transmitted to the fistula, which causes endolymph movement and cupular displacement with nystagmus and subjective vertigo. In the case of a fistula of the lateral canal, the slow component of the nystagmus is to the opposite side with positive pressure and to the same side with negative pressure, and the nystagmoid movements are large. The fistula test maneuver may elicit ocular deviation in some cases with a dehiscent superior semicircular canal syndrome.
2. In the event of vestibulofibrosis, as occurs in endolymphatic hydrops, fibrous bands may connect the foot-

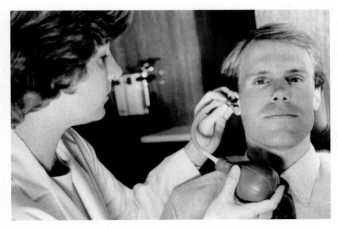

FIG. 1.13 In the fistula test, a Politzer bag is used to apply positive or negative pressure at the ear canal. If the examiner wishes to use both positive and negative pressure, he or she simply places a thumb on the ball valve and squeezes the bag to partially collapse it before proceeding with the test. Adapters must seal the ear canal to prevent escape of air, which may induce a caloric response.

plate of the stapes to the utricular macula; therefore footplate movements generated by the fistula tests cause movement of the utricular macula. The objective vestibuloocular manifestation is two or three short eye jerks on both positive and negative pressure, but greater on negative pressure. This response is known as a positive Hennebert's sign—that is, a positive fistula test in the presence of an intact tympanic membrane. The sign is present in more than 25% of Ménière's patients. It is even more common in congenital syphilis, though not pathognomonic as was previously thought (1).

3. When a positive fistula test is elicited in a patient with a perilymph fistula of the oval or round window, it is probably caused by the movement of an air bubble within the labyrinth (pneumolabyrinth) (2). The vertigo is transient and the nystagmus is often minimal and variable, yet they can be important diagnostic findings when correlated with medical history and other otologic findings.

Positional Tests

The otologic history is important in determining whether positional tests should be done. Motion-induced vertigo is a common manifestation of trauma or degenerative changes of aging. Severe spinning and disorienting vertigo induced by positional changes are often caused by high-density deposits on the cupula of the posterior semicircular canal (cupulolithiasis) (3–5) or within the lumen of the semicircular canals.

The test method for the elucidation of cupulolithiasis has been clearly described by Citron and Hallpike (5). The patient is seated on an examination table and the examiner places the patient sequentially in right ear–down and left ear–down positions and records the nystagmus in terms of time delay of onset, duration, and the characteristics of the eye movements, as well as fatigability on repeated positioning (Figs. 1.14 and 1.15).

Other Vestibular Tests

Abnormalities that are reflected in the vestibulospinal pathways are ataxia, a positive Romberg test, abnormalities in tandem walking, and walking in a circle. Simple tests of cerebellar function include the finger-to-nose maneuver and rapid alternating movements.

COMPLETE ENT EXAMINATION

A complete ENT examination is an essential part of the initial office visit. The nose, mouth, throat, nasopharynx, larynx, and neck are examined by direct vision, mirror, or fiberoptic methods. The status of the facial nerve function on both sides should be documented.

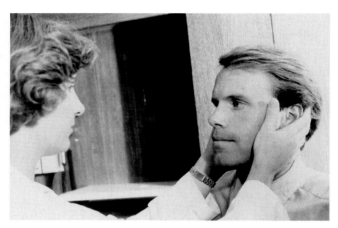

FIG. 1.14 The Hallpike maneuver for positional vertigo is to place the patient alternately from the sitting position to right and subsequently left head-hanging positions.

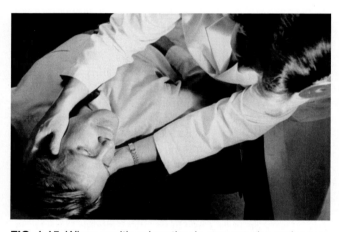

FIG. 1.15 When positional vertigo is present, the patient experiences vertigo and demonstrates nystagmus when the involved ear is in the undermost position (see text).

CONCLUDING THE OFFICE VISIT

Assuming that the entire office routine is necessary, including caloric testing, the examination can usually be accomplished within 30 minutes, and for many patients less time is needed. It is expedient to have conventional audiometric evaluation as a component of the initial office visit, and this evaluation, of course, requires additional time.

The examiner now decides what additional test data, if any, are needed to confirm a diagnosis and formulate a plan of treatment. In the interest of controlling health care costs, requests for further laboratory tests should be selective. Many patients will provide medical records and test data from recent evaluations that need not be repeated. Among the additional procedures that may be necessary are evoked response audiometry, electronystagmography, and other vestibular tests; computerized axial tomography; magnetic resonance imaging; hearing aid evaluation; and electrical tests of facial nerve function. If surgery is contemplated, it may be prudent to acquire clearance for general anesthesia from a medical consultant.

The office visit is concluded by a discussion with the patient and accompanying persons of the findings, diagnosis, therapeutic options, and prognosis. If a diagnosis is not apparent and further tests are necessary, the final opinion will have to be postponed.

REFERENCES

1. Nadol JB Jr. Positive "fistula sign" with an intact tympanic membrane. Clinical report of three cases and histopathological description of vestibulofibrosis as the probable cause. *Arch Otolaryngol* 1974;100: 273–278.
2. Yanagihara N, Nishioka I. Pneumolabyrinth in perilymphatic fistula: report of three cases. *Am J Otol* 1987;8:313–318.
3. Dix MR, Hallpike CS. The pathology, symptomatology and diagnosis of certain common disorders of the vestibular system. *Ann Otol Rhinol Laryngol* 1952;61:987–1016.
4. Schuknecht HF. Cupulolithiasis. *Arch Otolaryngol* 1969;90:765–778.
5. Citron L, Hallpike CS. Observations upon the mechanism of positional nystagmus of the so-called "benign paroxysmal type." *J Laryngol Otol* 1956;70:253–259.

CHAPTER 2

Photography and Documentation of Pathologic Findings

Steven D. Rauch and Jeffrey H. Spiegel

Continuing advances in imaging technology enable the physician to supplement medical record narratives and sketches with conventional and digital photographs, slides, and video recordings of physical findings. This chapter will present and discuss the rationale, principles, and techniques of photo documentation as they apply to otology. For a more detailed tutorial on many topics in standard medical photography, the reader is referred to general texts on the subject, such as that by Hansell (1).

REASONS FOR PHOTODOCUMENTATION

Photo documentation provides a visual record of physical findings at the time of patient examination. Regardless of the medium—still photograph, slide, or video—it is an eloquent record rarely equaled by narrative description. Patient care is undeniably improved by such objective documentation. Issues of interval assessment of change, as well as communication between doctor and patient or between physicians are facilitated. Furthermore, this record is available for research and teaching purposes even when the patient is not. There are also obvious medicolegal benefits that accrue from careful record keeping in general and from photographic records specifically, because once the physical appearance of the patient is altered by time, pathology, or surgical intervention, there is no other means of demonstrating interval change. These three uses of photodocumentation—patient care, education and research, and medicolegal—are compelling reasons to include patient imaging as one of the standards of care.

GENERAL PRINCIPLES OF MEDICAL PHOTOGRAPHY

Patient Consent

There are certain general principles of photodocumentation in the medical record that apply regardless of specialty or subject matter. As part of the medical record, the patient's

photograph is subject to the same considerations of confidentiality as any other personal medical document. This includes accuracy of labeling (patient's name, medical record number, and date) and restriction of access to only those individuals with a legitimate need to review the data to provide patient care. Any other use of the photographic record, such as for teaching or publication, requires the patient's consent. Obviously, if there are any features of the clinical photograph permitting identification of the patient, written consent is mandatory and masking of identifying features is appropriate prior to presentation or publication. Adoption of a simple, standardized photographic consent form for office use is an excellent idea. These forms are readily available from any hospital audiovisual department, as are general guidelines regarding issues of consent as they relate to photographic records. The clinician can consider incorporating an imaging consent form into the standard paperwork completed by each patient.

Standardization of Composition

Because one of the major applications of photodocumentation is for interval assessment of physical findings, it is imperative that variables of lighting, magnification, and angle of view be consistent between images. This is accomplished simply by adoption of office standards for photographic equipment, setting, and conditions. Standards should include a designated format (standard, digital, or both), choice of film or camera settings, light source, lenses, and distance from subject for each common subject photographed. For instance, all external ear (pinna) photographs should be taken using a macro lens at a 1:4 view ratio (as read from the lens barrel or a film-based camera), direct flash lighting, and automatic shutter speed and f-stop exposure settings for the particular film type chosen. Similarly, endoscopic photographs of the ear canal and tympanic membrane should be obtained at a standard zoom setting of 90 to 120 mm (depending on physician preference [Fig. 2.1]) using an auto-

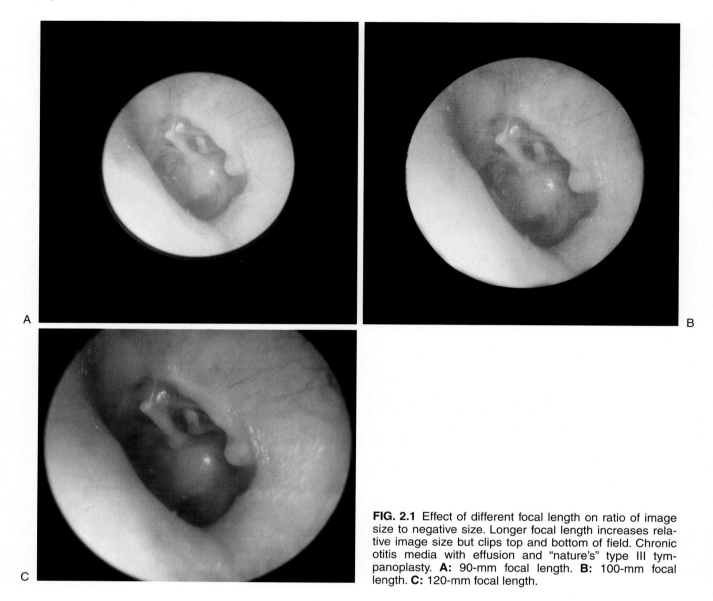

FIG. 2.1 Effect of different focal length on ratio of image size to negative size. Longer focal length increases relative image size but clips top and bottom of field. Chronic otitis media with effusion and "nature's" type III tympanoplasty. **A:** 90-mm focal length. **B:** 100-mm focal length. **C:** 120-mm focal length.

matic exposure setting coupled to stroboscopic flash illumination generated by the light source. For digital imaging, a standard composition and focal length, along with uniform settings and resolution, are necessary. The key here is internal consistency among photographs within the office. It is not strictly necessary to adopt the same routine as that used in another setting. It is advisable to record camera equipment and setting information, however, to permit duplication of results by others if necessary. Exposure settings and equipment information should also be recorded in those cases in which photographs are taken of unusual subject matter. For example, in a patient with a genetic syndrome, photographs of associated skeletal or ophthalmic anomalies might be desirable but have not been standardized in an otology office.

PHOTOGRAPHIC STUDIO

Although a room dedicated to photography may not be feasible, it is advantageous to have some dedicated space (even in the form of a locking, rolling cabinet) for picture taking and for equipment storage. Equipment maintenance is critical for protecting the investment in hardware and for sustaining optimum picture quality. Dedicated space ensures minimum wear and tear on equipment from setup and breakdown time, transportation, and rough handling. An office studio space also facilitates standardization of patient positioning and lighting. In many cases an adequate "studio" can consist of a blue backdrop against a wall in an area of the office with appropriate lighting. A smooth, organized, and efficient photography routine lends an air of professionalism that is reassuring to patients.

PRINCIPLES OF PHOTOGRAPHIC COMPOSITION

Appreciation of the general effects of lighting, film, color, and composition on the photographic record is essential. Lighting may be provided by ambient room light, an assortment of camera-mounted or freestanding flash devices, fiber-optic cable (in the case of endoscopic photography), or studio lights. Most film is color-balanced for daylight, a true white light compared with the yellow of incandescent (tungsten) light or green of fluorescent lights. Ambient light rarely provides adequate illumination and often introduces unpleasant color distortion because of mismatch between the color temperature of the light and the color balance of the film. Aside from the obvious need for adequate illumination for the subject, the major consideration in choice of lighting is shadow. The nearer the light source to the axis of view from subject to camera lens, the less shadow is thrown across the field of view. The more oblique the incident light upon the subject, the longer the shadow (Fig. 2.2). In a two-dimensional photograph, the major source of depth cuing is shadow. A long shadow from oblique lighting tends to enhance surface textural detail while obscuring or distorting color. Coaxial illumination (as provided by a "ring flash" or through an endoscope) results in a uniformly lighted subject and elimination of shadows, which provides excellent color detail but "flattens" all surface texture. Coaxial illumination is best used for objects within an orifice, such as the mouth or ear canal. Oblique lighting is excellent for demonstrating surface detail, as in rashes or other skin lesions. General surface photography of surgical fields, body parts, or portraiture is best achieved by a compromise using diffused lighting located 30 to 60 degrees above the subject and slightly to one side (so-called $^3/_4$ lighting), simulating midmorning sunlight.

Photo composition has both aesthetic and practical aspects. The inclusion of some object or structure to provide a sense of scale or relative size and to provide anatomic orientation for the viewer is particularly important when photographing a surgical field (Fig. 2.3). Much of the region is beneath the drapes and the viewer may literally not know which end is up. The simple inclusion of a chin, nose, or ear lobe may be all that is necessary to orient the viewer. Another practical objective of photographic composition is to lead the viewer's eye to the important aspects of the subject. Aside from including the subject of interest and features for scale

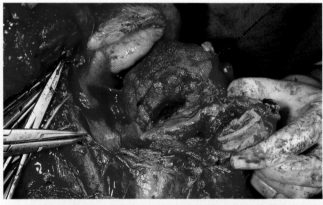
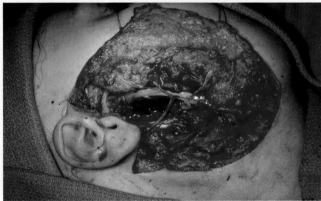

FIG. 2.3 Composition greatly influences the effectiveness with which the photograph communicates information. **A:** Poor composition. Composite resection of right mandible and neck. Note lack of landmarks to orient viewer to relevant anatomy, as well as distracting instruments and bloody glove. **B:** Picture is visually simple, provides landmarks for orientation and scale, and avoids distracting objects or panoramic view.

FIG. 2.2 Effect of angle of incidence of illumination on shadow length. As the angle of incidence of illumination becomes progressively more oblique, the shadow length *(S)* becomes progressively longer. Longer shadows enhance surface textural detail, whereas shorter shadows provide more even illumination.

and orientation, all other extraneous items are distracting and should be excluded. Surgical instruments, sponges, and surgeon's fingers should be excluded from photographs of surgical fields or specimens. Panoramic views are inappropriate when the area of interest is small, such as showing the entire side of the head if the pinna is the subject of interest.

Aesthetic aspects of photographic composition are harder to define. In portrait views, one should try to capture a pleasant facial expression with a slight smile and both eyes open. Intraoperative photographs should avoid depiction of excessively bloody surgical fields by covering the perioperative site with clean towels, cleaning any visible surgical instruments, and putting clean gloves on hands that will remain in the picture. Gratuitously grotesque photographs of injuries, lesions, or intraoperative defects are to be discouraged unless they specifically make a point or document an important feature of the case, such as tumor margins or anatomic variation. Adherence to a general effort to obtain visual simplicity with the minimum subject size that clearly portrays the field of interest and adequately orients the viewer will usually result in good photodocumentation.

Choice of Film

Many options for choice of film are available. Film for color prints or slides are available in a variety of speeds (ASA rating). The "faster" the film, the more light sensitive it is and therefore the less light or exposure time necessary to obtain the picture. However, faster film tends to be slightly lower resolution or "grainier" and also have less color saturation. Film in the ASA 100 or 200 range is a good compromise between the features of speed, resolution, and color saturation. Different films also have different color balance. In other words, the apparent color saturation will vary in different parts of the color spectrum. Generally, Kodachrome (Eastman Kodak Co., Rochester, NY) tends to have very rich reds, whereas Ektachrome (Eastman Kodak Co., Rochester, NY) has a bluish cast and Fujichrome (Fuji Photo Film Co., Ltd., Tokyo) emphasizes greens and yellows. If there is a lot of red color in the subject, a film rich in red (such as Kodachrome) may fail to show good differentiation of subtle color differences, whereas a "cooler" bluish Ektachrome film may resolve subtle red shadings better. Kodachrome is the gold standard for archival storage of photographic records. It is known to be color stable for decades. Ektachrome is less stable and, even under ideal storage conditions, will fade over many years. Kodachrome and Ektachrome have different processing requirements as well. Kodachrome uses a chemical sequence known as C41 that is time-consuming and available only at larger processing laboratories. Ektachrome uses E6 processing, which is rapid and widely available in many small photofinishing operations and often on site in hospital audiovisual departments. As a result, Ektachrome slides are usually available within 24 hours or less, whereas Kodachrome slides typically have a 5- to 10-day turnaround time from shooting to viewing.

Choosing among the different films is ultimately a personal choice based on these considerations of color balance, longevity, and rapidity of processing.

The decision to use print or slide transparency film is based on planned use of the photographs. Generally it is rather simple to make prints from slides using one of several instant film slide printers available. On the other hand, there is no simple way to make transparencies from prints. Thus if there is any consideration of using the pictures for presentation or teaching, slides are preferable and instant prints can be made from them for inclusion in the medical record or for providing copies to other physicians.

Equipment and Techniques

All photographic equipment exists to capture light and store the associated image for viewing at a later time. Traditional film-based cameras gather light through a lens, which is focused to allow a clear image to strike a photosensitive plane (the film). This film must then be processed (developed) into a positive or negative image. Once developed, the film can be displayed as a projected slide or converted into a print by projecting a negative image onto photographic paper, which itself must then be developed.

Among the advantages of film-based photography are familiar equipment, high-quality images, and permanence of the photograph. Disadvantages include the need to wait for the photographs while the film is processed, storage of the photographs, relatively high cost per image following initial equipment purchase, and relative difficulty with editing, cropping, and duplicating the images for use in medical publications or other academic pursuits. Computer scanners are available that use a special sensor to react to light from the photograph to create a digital file. This digital file is then available to edit with a computer.

Digital cameras are similar to traditional cameras in that light is captured by a lens and focused onto a photosensitive plane. However, rather than film, the photosensitive plane is a charged-coupled device (CCD). Each CCD breaks the photographic subject into a number of small frames termed pixels; each pixel is assessed for color and intensity, then stored as a numerical value. Computer software within the camera combines all the pixels into a single image file, which is then stored in any of a number of available formats (e.g., JPEG, PICT, TIFF, GIF) on an internal memory chip or card. The number of pixels on the CCD, processing time to store the image, image storage capacity, and storage format contribute to determine the ultimate image quality and in most cases the camera price. Once stored, the digital image file is immediately available for review, display, and editing. Advantages of digital photography include the ability to immediately review the image and determine if it is suitable, versatile editing and storage, and low cost per image following initial equipment investment. Additionally, the rapidity with which a digital image is available allows for many creative uses within medical practice (2). For example, a patient is able to see his or her ear with the physician while an area of concern is discussed. Disadvantages include new equipment and software to learn, lower-quality images (with many storage formats and equipment, although the images are typically adequate for most uses), and ethical considerations due to the ease of image manipulation. With improvements in digital camera image processing and databasing, it is likely that digital technology will soon replace film-based photography for most clinical applications.

Still Photography

Three common subjects for still photography in the otologist's office are portraits, pinna, and endoscopic views of the tympanic membrane and ear canal.

Portraits

Portraits are useful to document facial nerve function by utilizing a standard series of photographs of various facial movements, including face in repose, eyebrows raised, eyes closed tightly, puffed cheeks, big smile, and tightening neck muscles (Fig. 2.4), or for demonstrating craniofacial anomalies, such as Treacher Collins syndrome, hemifacial microsomia, or microtia. For standard photography, portraits should be taken with a 35-mm camera using a lens of 85- to 115-mm focal length to avoid "fisheye" distortion of shorter focal length lenses, which artifactually expand the proportions of the center of the photograph relative to the periphery. A macro lens is preferable because it may also be used

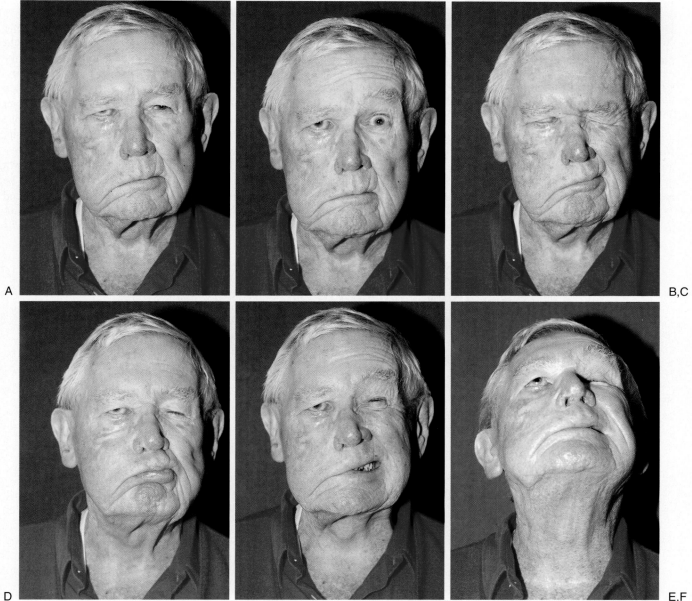

FIG. 2.4 Standard views of facial paralysis with camera at patient's eye level. **A:** Face in repose. **B:** Eyebrows raised. **C:** Eyes closed tight. **D:** Puffed cheeks. **E:** Big smile. **F:** Tightened neck.

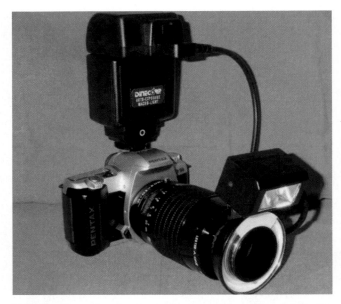

FIG. 2.5 Portraiture/surface photographic equipment. A 35-mm camera body with autowind film advance, 90-mm macro lens, and DineCorp macro flash. The combination of ring flash and front-mounted spot flash that can be fired singly or simultaneously allows for excellent control of shadow effects.

for close-up work. A macro lens capable of a 1:1 or 1:2 negative size-to-subject field size ratio (read off the lens barrel) at closest focal length is optimal (Fig. 2.5). Typically, several different negative size-to-subject field size ratios from 1:1 up to 1:10 are marked on the lens barrel and may be used as a convenient way of standardizing photographic format by setting the focus ring at the desired ratio mark and moving the camera closer and farther from the subject until the field is in focus. A 1:10 ratio, showing a full face with a small amount of space surrounding it, is ideal for portrait work (Fig. 2.6).

For digital image portrait photography, the physician should select a camera with a lens that provides the equivalent of a 35-mm SLR 85- to 115-mm focal length. High-end digital cameras accept the same lenses as used on 35-mm SLR cameras, but the CCD effectively multiplies the focal length. It is thus important to ascertain the multiplication factor for the camera you are using. Less expensive digital cameras utilize a built-in, noninterchangeable zoom lens (Fig 2.7). Again, the physician should determine the 35-mm focal length equivalent of the built-in lens to choose the proper camera and settings. Many camera retailers have this information readily available.

Next, proper image quality is important. Ektachrome slide film is considered by many to have a pixel equivalent of 4500 × 3000 (2). However, for most applications, an image with fewer pixels will be considered of equal quality. Only when an image is greatly enlarged do the increased pixels provide noticeable enhanced quality. In general, an image of 2 million pixels provides a picture suitable for use in a medical journal or slide show or to print from an ink-jet printer.

Lighting may be by diffused off-axis studio light or by a camera-mounted flash. A coaxial ring flash should be avoided for portrait work because it eliminates shadow and tends to produce an ocular red reflex that is aesthetically unpleasant. Facial detail is best seen if the patient's hair is

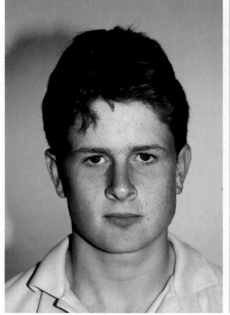 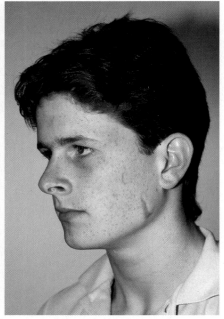

A   B

FIG. 2.6 A 1:10 ratio (read from the lens barrel) of negative size-to-subject field size is ideal for full-face portraiture, as in facial paralysis documentation (see Fig. 2.4) or in 18-month follow-up photographs **(A, B)** of a razor laceration of the left face. A 1:10 ratio encompasses the entire head and upper neck with an aesthetically pleasing empty border around the subject.

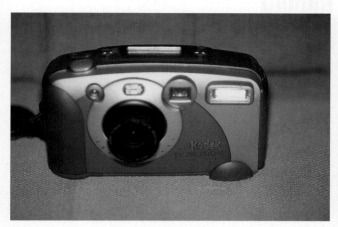

FIG. 2.7 Select a digital camera with appropriate image focal lengths (zoom) and number of pixels, macro-mode capability, in-camera screen for image review, and adequate storage capability.

pushed back from the forehead and ears, and all jewelry removed. The same lens and camera-mounted flash is appropriate for pinna photographs. The view ratio mark on the lens barrel should be set at 1:4 (Fig. 2.8). Additional close-up views of small skin lesions may be obtained at 1:3, 1:2, or 1:1 settings. Focal lengths less than 18 inches from the subject require a near-coaxial light source (a small-point light source attached to the edge of the lens barrel) to provide slight shadowing for depth cues without the excessive obliquity produced by a flash mounted on top of the camera. Alternatively, a ring flash may be used but will wash out shadows.

Standardization of portrait views require that the patient have uniform head position in all photographs. This can be obtained by asking subjects to hold their head such that the Frankfort plane is parallel to the floor.

Endoscopic Photography of the Tympanic Membrane

Endoscopic photography uses different equipment from that described earlier (Fig. 2.9). Rod lenses, originally developed by Hopkins, utilize highly innovative optics to provide a wide-angle view with a focal length from a few millimeters to infinity (3) and have been used to advantage in photography of the ear canal, tympanic membrane, and middle ear (4–7). A short rod lens of 3- to 6-mm diameter, with a straight-ahead angle of view and coaxial fiber-optic light cable, is mandatory. A coupling ring is used to attach the rod lens to the macro lens used for portrait and surface work, or the rod lens may be attached to a special 70- to 140-mm endoscopic zoom lens (Karl Storz Instrument Co.). This latter arrangement has the advantage of greater flexibility in enlarging the subject to fill the field of view of the slide. The fiber-optic light cable is best connected to a xenon light source, which is brighter and offers a better color balance than other types of lights. A simple xenon light source may be used with the camera's own automatic light metering sys-

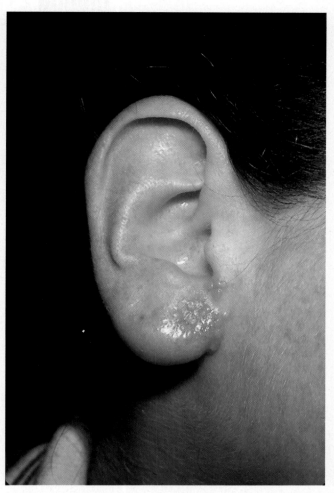

FIG. 2.8 A 1:4 ratio (read from the lens barrel) of negative size-to-subject field size is ideal for a full lateral view of the pinna, as in this case of herpes zoster oticus. A 1:4 ratio encompasses the entire subject with adequate inclusion of surrounding anatomy to provide orientation for the viewer.

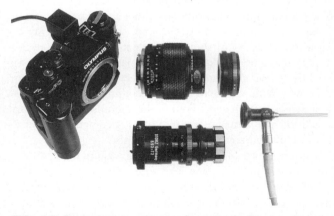

FIG. 2.9 Endophotography equipment. A 35-mm camera body with motor winder and endoscopic light source flash coupler cable, a 90-mm macro lens (as used for surface photography) and endoscopic rod lens coupler or a specialized endophotography 70- to 140-mm zoom lens, and a 4-mm diameter endoscopic rod lens with straight-ahead view angle and coaxial fiber-optic light cable to connect to xenon light source with built-in flash generator.

tem for correct exposure. A superior but costlier arrangement utilizes one of several xenon light sources available with a built-in stroboscopic flash generator. A special cable, available from the manufacturer of the light source, couples the flash generator directly to the light metering system of the camera and automatically controls the flash duration to obtain correct exposure.

Still photography of the ear canal and tympanic membrane can also be accomplished by attaching a camera to a beam splitter and adapter on an operation microscope. This technique eliminates the need to insert a long, thin, rod lens into the patient's ear canal and is more practical for intraoperative middle ear photography. However, it does not provide the panoramic view available through the rod lens and also has more difficulty providing uniform bright lighting to the subject.

Video Photography

Video photography offers both advantages and disadvantages as compared with still photography. Video recordings are the only practical way of capturing motion and sound, as needed to document facial paralysis or a voice disorder. Real-time video display enables the otologist to immediately show a patient his or her own pathologic physical findings, such as a tympanic membrane perforation, cholesteatoma, or child's ventilating tube (Fig. 2.10). The patient's understanding of his or her problems and compliance with therapy are thereby enhanced. Intraoperative video monitoring and recording allows the other members of the surgical team to watch and better understand the surgery and permits the acquisition of a record of intraoperative events.

Video recordings of full-face views of a patient are best achieved with a tripod-mounted standard camcorder and are particularly valuable in documentation of altered facial function. The camera should be at the patient's eye level. The patient should be positioned either sitting or standing in front of a neutral color background, such as light gray or light blue. The room should be brightly lit, with a studio-quality photo floodlight aimed at the patient from above and slightly to one side and a silver reflector diffuser to soften shadows. With sound, the video recording offers an excellent demonstration and record of the alteration of speech articulation and patient affect that often accompany the more obvious disfigurement of facial paralysis.

Current state-of-the-art recording equipment utilizes high-resolution 8-mm tape. This format has as high a resolution as older professional broadcast-quality $^3\!/_4$-inch tape and has the added benefit of much smaller size that facilitates storage. Depending on the need for compatibility with existing video recording and/or editing equipment, use of $^3\!/_4$-inch tape format may still be preferable to some. Endoscopic and intraoperative recordings are done using the xenon light source, rod lens, or microscope beam splitter mount described earlier for still photography. Video connec-

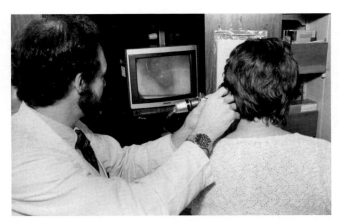

FIG. 2.10 Handheld office video endoscopy setup. A CCD chip camera attached to a 4-mm endoscopic rod lens with straight-ahead view angle, xenon light source, and video recorder and monitor provides a simple and flexible setup for helping patients to see and understand the pathologic findings. Findings can be viewed in real time or recordings can be made and shown moving, in slow motion, or as freeze-frame stills for presenting to the patient. Using a "screen shooter" hood attached to a Polaroid instant camera, still prints of freeze-frame screen images can be given to the patient or sent to the referring physician.

tors for microscope use are available in several different focal lengths, resulting in different degrees of magnification of the field of view. The 74-mm and 137-mm sizes available from Zeiss are most appropriate for otologic surgery. Tiny solid-state cameras utilizing CCD chips that are extremely light sensitive and have high resolution and color accuracy are ideal for video endoscopy and video microscopy. Several such cameras are currently available, either as freestanding equipment or as photodocumentation equipment packages sold bundled with the operating microscope or endoscopic rod lenses.

Prior to draping the video microscope at the beginning of surgery, the microscope-mounted video camera should be activated and the image on the monitor brought into sharp focus at high magnification. The ocular lenses of the microscope can then be adjusted so the surgeon's view is parfocal with the video camera. A useful general practice during intraoperative video recording is to start the recording when the field of view is properly focused and aimed at the subject of interest with no instruments in the field. Instruments are then slowly introduced and a portion of the surgery filmed. The instruments are slowly withdrawn, and the film is paused until the next phase of the procedure is ready for filming. This routine provides the effect of the operation unfolding before the viewer and eliminates the distracting effect of instruments appearing and disappearing from the field of view during the replay of the tape. It also minimizes the need for postproduction video editing to create presentation-quality films. Recently several manufacturers have developed video printers that permit generation of an instant still print from a single frame of a video recording. A less expensive alternative is to use a Polaroid camera with a "screen shooter" hood to produce an instant print of a freeze-frame video image by photographing the monitor screen.

STORAGE OF PHOTOGRAPHIC RECORDS

Photodocumentation constitutes an invaluable and irreplaceable part of the medical record and is subject to the same requirements of confidentiality. As such, the slides, photographs, and tapes must be stored safely and securely. They must either be appended to the remainder of the medical record or be stored with relevant identifying information to permit retrieval. Depending on personal preference and need, photographic records can be stored according to a case- or patient-based filing system or by a topic-based filing system, with or without cross-referencing. Hospital medical records departments and medical library personnel can provide valuable assistance in designing and implementing a suitable file system. Audiovisual department personnel will also be helpful in providing guidance in obtaining slide storage folders and racks of archival quality. Low-cost, low-quality slide folders are often made of plastics that give off volatile fumes that can distort or destroy transparencies. Videotapes are vulnerable to magnetic or electromagnetic damage and moisture and must therefore be stored in a safe, magnetically and electrically shielded area.

Digital images provide unparalleled ease of storage. Once transferred into a computer, images can be stored on the hard disk or on any of a number of external storage devices. For those who plan to regularly utilize this medium, the hard disk will soon prove to be of inadequate size for permanent image storage. Tape and disk drives are available for high-capacity image storage, but perhaps the best current option is the use of a read/write compact disk (CD). CDs have high capacity (more than 600 MB), are low cost, and have very high durability and longevity. Additionally, they are not easily accidentally erased and require minimal storage space.

Digital images are best catalogued with a digital image database software program. These programs allow the physician to enter relevant patient information to be stored with each photograph. At a later date, the physician can enter the patient's name, number, diagnosis, date seen, or any other selected variable and have the images quickly available. Searching for images with conventional slide storage is considerably less facile and flexible.

ETHICS

With improved image processing technology comes an increased responsibility to not abuse image editing software. Photographs can be placed into a computer, edited, printed, and feigned as an original. Although certain forms of editing are valuable and usually harmless (e.g., cropping borders, adding text or arrows), others can have significant impact (e.g., changing colors and shapes, adding to or removing from the original image). In some situations, standard film-based photography can have more value than the more easily modified digital images. Physicians are encouraged to obtain image processing software that provides image authentication. This allows the software to record any changes from the original image and determine when a photograph has been modified.

REFERENCES

1. Hansell P, ed. A *Guide to Medical Photography*. Lancaster, England: MTP Press Limited, 1979.
2. Spiegel JH, Singer MI. Practical approach to digital photography and its applications. *Otolaryngol Head Neck Surg* 2000;123:152–156.
3. Hopkins HH. Optical principles of the endoscope. In: Berci G, ed. *Endoscopy*. New York: Appleton-Century-Crofts, 1976:3.
4. Konrad HR, Berci G, Ward P. Pediatric otoscopy and photography of the tympanic membrane. *Arch Otolaryngol* 1979;105:431–433.
5. Chole RA. Photography of the tympanic membrane. *Arch Otolaryngol* 1980;106:230–231.
6. Hawke M. Telescopic otoscopy and photography of the tympanic membrane. *J Otolaryngol* 1982;11:35–39.
7. Yanagisawa E. Effective photography in otolaryngology-head and neck surgery: tympanic membrane photography. *Otolaryngol Head Neck Surg* 1982;90:399–407.

CHAPTER 3

Audiologic Tests for Otologic Surgery

Dianne H. Meyer and Edward L. Applebaum

This chapter describes audiologic tests used in the diagnosis and measurement of hearing disorders. The first section reviews basic audiologic procedures, including pure-tone and speech audiometry, acoustic immittance, auditory brainstem response (ABR), and evoked otoacoustic emissions (EOAEs). The following sections discuss the application of these basic procedures, as well as other specialized tests, in the evaluation of conductive, sensorineural, and central auditory disorders. Two patient groups, young children and patients with nonorganic hearing loss, require modified procedures, and these are discussed in the last sections. An effective audiologic evaluation depends on careful test selection and knowledgeable interpretation of the results.

BASIC AUDIOLOGIC PROCEDURES

Pure-tone and Speech Audiometry

The evaluation of all complaints of hearing loss begins with the determination of air- and bone-conduction pure-tone thresholds, the speech recognition threshold (SRT), and word recognition scores. These basic measurements reveal the severity of hearing loss within the tested frequencies and indicate whether the loss is conductive, sensorineural, or mixed. By convention, routine audiometric measurements are made only for the frequencies in the range of 250 to 8,000 Hz, even though normal hearing may encompass a far greater spectrum (20 to 20,000 Hz). Some patients' complaints of hearing problems and tinnitus may not be diagnosed if the losses occur in frequencies not routinely tested. It is possible to obtain thresholds at frequencies above 8,000 Hz, but specialized equipment and calibration procedures are required.

Speech audiometry refers to measurements of the SRT and word recognition ability. Taken together, these two measures serve as a check on the pure-tone results, help in the diagnosis of retrocochlear problems, and indicate how the hearing loss impacts on the patient's day-to-day communication. The SRT is the patient's threshold for spondee

words, and it should agree closely with pure-tone thresholds at 500, 1,000, and 2,000 Hz. Word recognition is a suprathreshold test that indicates how well the patient is able to understand speech when it is made loud enough to hear easily. Word recognition is expressed as the percentage of phonetically balanced words correctly recognized at a specified level above the SRT (usually 40 to 50 dB above the SRT). In general, better pure-tone thresholds result in higher word recognition scores.

An essential part of audiometric testing is masking. As a general rule, masking must be used whenever it is possible for the test signal to cross the skull and be heard in the nontest ear. For air-conduction thresholds, this possibility exists when the signal to the test ear exceeds bone conduction sensitivity in the nontest ear by an amount equal to or greater than interaural attenuation. With standard audiometric earphones, attenuation across the skull is 40 dB; with insert phones, the attenuation is 70 to 90 dB, depending on the depth of insertion (1,2). For bone conduction testing, interaural attenuation is essentially nonexistent. Therefore the nontest ear must be masked whenever an air bone gap is present. These masking principles apply for both pure-tone and speech audiometry.

Some hearing disorders are characterized by distinctive audiometric configurations, such as the high-frequency notch associated with noise exposure. Other audiometric patterns, such as the degree of symmetry between ears, may determine if additional evaluation of the hearing loss is needed.

Pure-tone and speech audiometry should be done for all patients before and after otologic surgery, unless the patient is unable to cooperate. To allow for adequate healing after surgery, the first postoperative test usually is deferred until about 6 weeks after the operation. If a postoperative complication is suspected, testing is done sooner. Follow-up audiometry may be done as early as 1 to 2 weeks after myringotomy with placement of ventilating tubes and still be indicative of the hearing improvement resulting from the surgery.

Acoustic Immittance Measurements

Acoustic immittance measurements evaluate how well energy flows through the outer and middle ear systems. The basic measurements include tympanometry and acoustic reflexes, both of which are often considered routine parts of an audiologic evaluation. Immittance measurements are sensitive to middle ear problems, and they help to differentiate cochlear from retrocochlear disorders. The measurements are made by delivering a pure-tone signal through a probe that fits snugly in the ear canal. The sound pressure level (SPL) of this "probe tone" is monitored while the air pressure is varied in the external ear canal. Any changes from the normal SPL patterns are related to the functional integrity of the ear.

Several classification systems have been proposed for tympanograms, some descriptive in nature and others that analyze shapes based on multiple probe tone frequencies and resistance and reactance components. Figure 3.1 shows a commonly used classification that categorizes tympanograms on the basis of shape and tympanometric pressure peak (3). These basic types are based on adult ears and are associated with a low-frequency probe tone, usually 226 Hz. Type A is a normal tympanogram with peak immittance at or near 0 decaPascals (daPa). Variations of type A include type A_S, in which the peak is shallower than normal, and type A_D, in which the peak is higher than normal. Type A_S may be found in cases of ossicular fixation, whereas type A_D may be found with ossicular discontinuity or tympanic membrane abnormality. The type B, or "flat," tympanogram depicts very little or no change in immittance with variation in air pressure and is found in cases of middle ear effusion. The type C tympanogram has a negative peak, indicating negative air pressure in the middle ear space.

Tympanometry is ordered when there is a question about the mobility of the tympanic membrane, the air pressure within the middle ear space, or the status of the ossicular chain. It provides useful information about middle ear effusions that may not be obvious clinically, such as an effusion

behind a thick or opacified tympanic membrane that impairs otoscopic evaluation of the middle ear. Tympanometry is done to determine the presence of persistent, abnormally high or low middle ear pressures in patients with complaints of aural fullness. It is valuable in differentiating between abnormally fixed or interrupted ossicular chains behind an intact tympanic membrane. In patients with rhythmic tinnitus or clicking sensations in their ears, tympanometry is used to determine if the tympanic membrane is being contracted abnormally by clonic middle ear muscle contractions.

The acoustic reflex, or stapedius muscle reflex, is a bilateral response that occurs in response to loud sounds. In normal ears the reflex occurs at 70- to 100-dB hearing level (HL) for pure-tone signals (4). Clinical measurements include reflex threshold, the lowest sound level that elicits the reflex, and reflex decay. Both contralateral and ipsilateral reflexes can be measured, thereby testing the entire reflex arc, including eighth nerve, low brainstem, and facial nerve pathways. Acoustic reflex testing is ordered when lesions of these structures are suspected, such as in acoustic neuromas and brainstem infarctions, and to help determine the site of involvement of facial nerve disorders.

Auditory Brainstem Response

As one of several groups of auditory evoked potentials, the auditory brainstem response does not directly measure hearing but does measure a process that is highly related to hearing sensitivity. The ABR measures electrical activity of the auditory nerve and auditory pathway to the mid-brainstem level. The ABR offers the advantages of being easy to measure in children and adults. It is sensitive to both auditory and neurologic disorders but does not require a behavioral response from the patient.

The ABR consists of a series of five to seven waves with latencies between 1 and 10 msec following stimulus presentation (Fig. 3.2). Waves I and II are generated by the peripheral auditory nerve, and waves III, IV, and V are generally related to the cochlear nucleus, superior olivary complex, and nuclei of the lateral lemniscus, respectively (5). Clicks are the best stimuli to elicit the ABR because of their abrupt onset and broad frequency spectrum. The click-evoked ABR provides information about the basal end of the cochlea and is associated with hearing sensitivity in the 2,000 to 4,000 Hz region. More frequency-specific information may be obtained with tone bursts, filtered clicks, and masking techniques.

Clinical interpretation of the ABR is based on measurements of wave latencies, interpeak intervals (IPI), and wave V threshold (see Fig. 3.2). The *wave V latency-intensity function* refers to the increase in wave V latency as stimulus intensity decreases. Changes in the shape of the latency-intensity function and in the amount that it deviates from the expected normal function are used to predict type and degree of hearing losses. Patterns associated with conductive

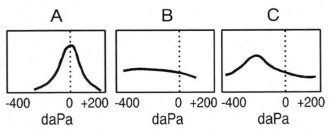

FIG. 3.1 A commonly used classification system for tympanograms. *Type A* is a normal tympanogram with peak immittance at or near 0 daPa. The *type B* tympanogram indicates little or no change in immittance with variation in air pressure. The *type C* tympanogram indicates the presence of negative air pressure in the middle ear space. daPa, decaPascals.

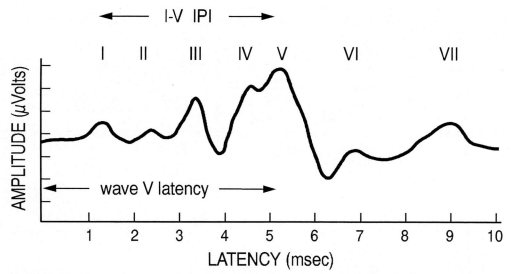

FIG. 3.2 An ABR waveform from a normal-hearing adult subject. The *arrow* illustrates measurement of the I to V interpeak interval (IPI).

hearing loss and with high-frequency cochlear hearing loss are shown in Figure 3.3.

The clinical applications of the ABR are varied. The procedure plays an important role in determining auditory thresholds of young infants and other difficult-to-test patients. It is useful in detecting the presence of lesions in the auditory pathway, such as in acoustic neuroma or multiple sclerosis. It also is valuable for intraoperative monitoring of the integrity of the ear and auditory pathway during intracra-

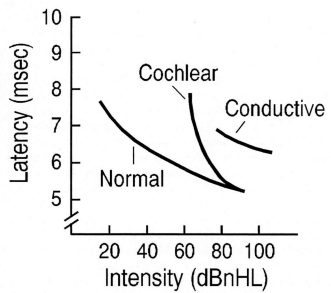

FIG. 3.3 Wave V latency-intensity functions. General patterns are shown for normal hearing, high-frequency cochlear hearing loss, and conductive hearing loss.

nial surgery near these structures. Automated versions of the ABR are used in newborn hearing screening.

Evoked Otoacoustic Emissions

Evoked otoacoustic emissions are sounds recorded in the ear canal that are associated with normal cochlear function. They do not measure hearing sensitivity directly, but their presence is highly related to normal outer hair cell activity. Although they may occur spontaneously, the most common clinical application is to measure the emissions in response to an evoking stimulus. Transient evoked otoacoustic emissions (TEOAEs), which occur after the presentation of a brief stimulus such as a click, typically are measured if hearing thresholds do not exceed 30-dB HL. Distortion product otoacoustic emissions (DPOAEs) are produced by the ear in response to two simultaneous pure-tones. They are present if hearing thresholds do not exceed 50 dB HL (6). The middle ear system must be normal in order for EOAEs to be measured.

Clinical interpretation of EOAEs is based on amplitude of the emission at a specific frequency or across a frequency range. To be accepted as a response, the EOAE must have good replicability and must exceed the noise floor measured at the time of testing. Figure 3.4 shows a normal TEOAE response from an adult.

The measurement of EOAEs has many clinical applications, including differentiation between sensory and neural hearing loss, monitoring of cochlear function of patients treated with ototoxic drugs, tinnitus evaluation, and monitoring of noise-induced hearing loss. EOAEs are essential to the audiologic evaluation of young infants and other difficult-to-test patients. They are used extensively in newborn hearing screening.

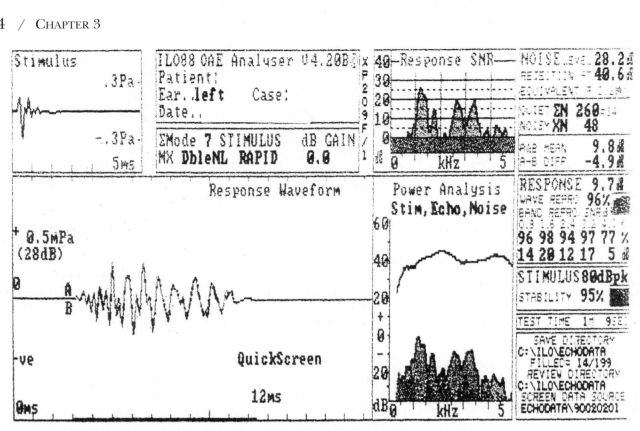

FIG. 3.4 A transient evoked otoacoustic emission result for a normal-hearing adult patient. The response waveforms (*A* and *B*) are superimposed, reflecting high reproducibility (96%). The signal-to-noise ratio (SNR) shows a strong emission response from 800 to 3,200 Hz.

AUDIOLOGIC EVALUATION OF CONDUCTIVE HEARING LOSS

An audiologic evaluation for conductive hearing losses should include pure-tone air- and bone-conduction thresholds, speech audiometry, and immittance measurements. Careful masking must be used in all cases. The ABR may be used to estimate conductive hearing losses when patients are unable to give reliable behavioral responses. Patterns of air-conduction thresholds alone are not sufficient to diagnose conductive hearing losses, as was once thought.

Clinical indicators published by the American Academy of Otolaryngology–Head & Neck Surgery recommended pure-tone and speech audiometry be completed preoperatively and postoperatively for mastoidectomy, myringotomy and tympanostomy tubes, stapedectomy, and tympanoplasty procedures (7). In addition, the guidelines recommended tympanometry prior to myringotomy and tympanostomy tubes, and tympanometry plus acoustic reflex testing prior to stapedectomy surgery.

Pure-tone and Speech Audiometry

The expected finding on the pure-tone audiogram is the air-bone gap, indicated by better thresholds by bone conduction than by air conduction. Although air- and bone-conduction thresholds alone cannot identify a specific ear disease, they may reflect changes that have occurred in the middle ear transmission properties. A greater loss at the low frequencies suggests an increase in the stiffness of the middle ear system, whereas a greater loss at the high frequencies is associated with an increase in the mass of the system. An example of these relationships can be seen in the course of otitis media (8). In the early stages of the disease, as middle ear air pressure is reduced, the tympanic membrane and ossicular chain may become increasingly stiff, resulting in a rising air conduction audiometric configuration with normal bone conduction. Later, high-frequency thresholds may be affected as fluid accumulates and causes mass loading of the ossicular chain. The additional loss in sensitivity at the high frequencies results in a flat audiometric configuration.

Middle ear disorders also may influence bone-conduction thresholds. Changes in bone conduction can occur when the disease process alters the resonant characteristics of the ossicular system or middle ear space. For example, the "Carhart notch" associated with otosclerosis is a slight loss in bone-conduction threshold maximal in the frequency region around 2,000 Hz (9). The phenomenon occurs because otosclerotic stapes fixation eliminates the influence of normal ossicular resonance on bone-conduction thresholds at 1,500 to 2,000 Hz. Following surgery, this mild depression in bone-conduction thresholds is not seen, explaining why there is sometimes an apparent improvement in bone-conduction thresholds ("overclosure" of the air-bone gap).

Speech audiometry with conductive hearing loss should result in SRTs that are in agreement with air-conduction thresholds in the most important speech frequencies (500 to 2,000 Hz). If bone-conduction responses are normal, word recognition scores should be 90% or better when test words are delivered at a sufficiently high sensation level, usually about 40 dB above the SRT. It also is possible to administer speech audiometry via bone conduction if the audiometer is calibrated for speech delivered through the bone receiver. This technique is especially useful with patients who show poor reliability in air- and bone-conduction pure-tone testing.

Expected audiometric results for conductive disorders are described in Table 3.1. It is apparent that different types of middle ear disease may have similar effects on the sound conductive system and therefore may result in similar audiometric configurations.

Audiometric Masking

Appropriate masking is important in the evaluation of all hearing losses, but it is critical with conductive hearing loss. Unrecognized errors can lead to useless and perhaps even harmful surgery on a nonhearing ear. Bilateral conductive loss presents a special audiometric testing problem referred to as the masking dilemma. In this situation the intensity level of the masking noise needed to mask the nontest ear is so high (due to the degree of air-conduction loss in that ear) that the masking noise itself may cross over via bone conduction and elevate the threshold in the test ear. The use of insert phones, rather than supra-aural earphones, often eliminates the need for masking and avoids many masking dilemmas.

Acoustic Immittance Measurements

Tympanometric and acoustic reflex findings in combination with a complete audiogram can confirm the presence of

TABLE 3.1. *Summary of audiometric and immittance findings for selected conductive hearing losses*

Disease	Audiometric findings	Tympanogram	Acoustic reflex
Aural atresia	Maximum conductive loss	Cannot evaluate	Cannot evaluate
Cholesteatoma	Hearing loss varies, depending on the location and size of the cholesteatoma; occasionally hearing is normal (10)	Type A_S, A_D, or B, depending on ossicular chain involvement	Usually elevated or absent with probe and tone to the involved ear
Discontinuity of the ossicular chain	Flat configuration, 50–60 dB (11)	Type A_D (low-frequency probe)	Usually absent with probe and tone to the involved ear
Glomus tumors	Conductive, mixed, or sensorineural loss; degree of loss ranges from normal to severe (12)	Variable, depending on ossicular chain involvement; may show vascular perturbations	With probe to involved ear, reflexes may be absent or impossible to measure due to pulsations
Malleus fixation	Usually a rising configuration due to increased stiffness; 40–60 dB; sensorineural component may be present (13)	Type B or A_S	Absent with sound and probe to the involved ear
Otitis media with effusion	Audiometric contour depends on the stage of the disease and the relative stiffness and mass effects; usually ranges between 10 and 40 dB (14)	In early stages, type C, and then progresses to type B	Absent with sound and probe to the involved ear
Otosclerosis	Initially a rising configuration; as stapes fixation increases, the configuration flattens; maximum air-bone gap about 50 dB; bone conduction may show Carhart notch at 2 kHz (15)	Type A or A_S	Usually absent with sound and probe to the involved ear; in early stages, reflexes may be present and characterized by negative deflections and an on-off effect
Perforation of the tympanic membrane (TM)	Hearing loss depends on size and location of the perforation; small perforations in the posterior half of the TM affect low-frequency hearing; perforations in the anterior area affect high-frequency hearing (16)	Type B	Absent with probe to the involved ear
Atelectasis	Variable, depending on extent of tympanic membrane collapse	Type C or B	Often absent
Tympanosclerosis	Mild to moderate loss, depending on amount and location of plaque deposits (17)	Type C or A_S; type A if tympanic membrane is not involved	May be absent with probe to the involved ear

conductive hearing loss and differentiate among types of conductive pathology. Table 3.1 includes the tympanogram type and acoustic reflex pattern typically found for selected conductive hearing disorders.

When interpreting tympanogram shapes, it must be remembered that in the presence of more than one middle ear lesion, the more lateral pathology will dominate. For example, the combination of otosclerosis and a monomeric tympanic membrane will likely result in a tympanogram with high compliance, reflecting the thin and flaccid tympanic membrane.

The acoustic reflex is extremely sensitive to middle ear pathology, even when conductive hearing loss is not apparent on the pure-tone audiogram. An air-bone gap of only 5 dB in the probe ear is enough to obscure measurement of the reflex, and an air-bone gap of greater than 30 dB in the stimulated ear will prevent measurement of the reflex in a normal hearing probe ear (18). A distinctive pattern occurs with early otosclerosis in that reflexes may show a negative, biphasic pattern known as the on-off effect (19).

Auditory Brainstem Response

The ABR may be needed to identify and quantify conductive hearing loss in patients unable to be evaluated by behavioral methods, such as newborns, infants, young children, and developmentally delayed or cognitively impaired patients. The effect of conductive pathology on the click-evoked ABR is to prolong the latencies of the component waves. As shown in Figure 3.3, the slope of the latency-intensity function with conductive hearing loss is parallel to the normal slope. The amount in decibels that the wave V latency-intensity function is shifted approximates the degree of conductive hearing loss. All the ABR waves are shifted approximately equally, so the interpeak intervals remain within normal limits.

The bone-conduction ABR provides a more direct estimate of cochlear function. Bone-conduction ABR is especially valuable in infants with aural malformations in whom air-conduction and immittance measurements may be difficult or impossible to do. In newborns who fail hearing screening, ABR may help to identify conductive involvement.

Figure 3.5 shows air conduction and bone conduction for a 23-month-old infant with bilateral microtia, complete atresia of the right external auditory canal, and partial atresia of the left external auditory canal. Inner ear structures appeared normal on computerized tomography. There was a shift in the ABR latency-intensity function for air conduction, but the bone-conduction responses fell within the expected normal range. The ABR results supported the behavioral responses that indicated a 60-dB conductive hearing loss. This case also demonstrates how contralateral masking may be needed with ABR and that masking dilemmas may exist. Because of the patient's absent or malformed external auditory canals, insert receivers could not be used to increase the interaural attenuation. The ABR results therefore reflected function of the better cochlea if a difference in hearing existed between the two ears. Bone-conduction ABR has a number of calibration and interpretive considerations, but it is invaluable as a procedure to identify or confirm conductive involvement in difficult-to-test patients.

AUDIOLOGIC EVALUATION OF SENSORINEURAL HEARING LOSS

Pure-tone and speech audiometry and immittance measurements are obtained for all patients with suspected pathology of the cochlea and/or eighth nerve. The ABR is included when a lesion of the eighth nerve is suspected and when behavioral thresholds are in question or cannot be done. An-

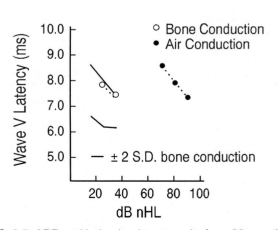
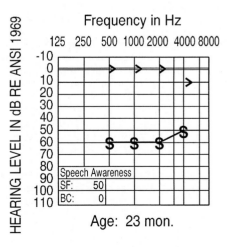

FIG. 3.5 ABR and behavioral test results for a 23-month-old infant with bilateral microtia, complete atresia of the right external auditory canal, and partial atresia of the left external auditory canal. ABR results are shown for the left ear. Responses to bone conduction ABR were in the expected normal range and were consistent with behavioral bone conduction results. Responses to bone conduction ABR showed an expected shift in the latency-intensity function.

other auditory evoked potential, electrocochleography (EcochG), is useful in the diagnosis of Ménière's disease. Table 3.2 summarizes the audiometric results for selected sensorineural hearing losses.

Pure-tone and Speech Audiometry

If otoscopic findings and all immittance results are normal, it may not be necessary to obtain bone-conduction thresholds. Because outer and middle ear function are normal, air-conduction thresholds alone will reveal the severity and symmetry of the hearing loss. For SNHL such as endolymphatic hydrops, periodic pure-tone threshold testing is helpful in evaluating the benefits of treatment or progression of the disease.

The SRT validates the air-conduction thresholds, and word recognition scores reveal the impact of the sensorineural hearing loss on speech understanding. In the case of cochlear hearing loss, it is expected that the amount of difficulty with word recognition is proportionate to the severity of the loss. If word recognition is poorer than expected, then the possibility of retrocochlear involvement should be considered. The word recognition score alone does not differentiate cochlear from retrocochlear pathology, but it may lead to suspicion of a retrocochlear disorder (37).

A variant of routine word recognition testing is to obtain a performance-intensity function. In this procedure, word recognition scores are obtained at both low and high intensity levels. An abnormal amount of "rollover" in the function

TABLE 3.2. *Summary of site of disorder and audiometric findings for selected sensorineural hearing losses*

Disease	Site of Disorder	Audiologic findings
Acoustic tumor	Cranial nerve (CN) VIII	Usually, unilateral hearing loss with a sloping configuration; mild to profound; occasionally presents as sudden loss; word recognition may be disproportionate to pure-tone loss (20); presence of normal OAEs indicate cochlear integrity
Auditory neuropathy	CN VIII or inner hair cells	Mild to moderate hearing loss; abnormal ABR; OAEs present that do not suppress with contralateral noise; absent acoustic reflexes (21)
Autoimmune	Cochlea	Bilateral hearing loss; asymmetric; progressive over weeks or months (22)
Diabetes mellitus	Cochlea or CN VIII	Hearing may be normal; when loss is present, is usually bilateral, sloping, mild to profound (23)
Herpes zoster oticus (Ramsay Hunt syndrome)	Cochlea or CN VIII	Unilateral hearing loss; usually sloping; mild to profound; milder losses may show complete recovery (24)
Ménière's disease	Cochlea	Usually unilateral hearing loss; rising, flat, or sloping configuration; loss fluctuates initially; eventually, moderate to severe permanent loss (25); OAEs usually absent, but may be normal (26)
Meningitis	Cochlea	Usually bilateral, profound hearing loss; mild to severe losses have been reported, as well as unilateral and asymmetric loss; initial thresholds may later improve or show further decline (27)
Multiple sclerosis	CN VIII and brainstem auditory pathways	Usually normal or mild hearing loss; when loss is present, may be unilateral or bilateral, often sloping (28)
Noise-induced	Cochlea	Bilateral, symmetric hearing loss; unilateral occurs less often; initially a mild loss at the 3- to 6-kHz region; stabilizes at 60–70 dB; eventually, other frequencies become impaired (29); abnormal OAEs (26)
Ototoxicity	Cochlea	Bilateral hearing loss; rarely unilateral; may be asymmetric; initially high-frequency loss; with advanced toxicity, additional frequencies are involved; mild to profound (30); OAE abnormalities may precede audiometric changes (26)
Perilymphatic fistula	Cochlea	Normal or mild to moderate hearing loss; may fluctuate (31)
Presbycusis	Cochlea or CN VIII	Bilateral, symmetric, progressive hearing loss; sloping or flat configuration; mild to severe (32); absent OAE or decreased amplitude (26)
Sudden hearing loss	Varies, depending on etiology	Unilateral hearing loss; sloping, flat, or rising configuration; usually moderate to severe (33)
Syphilis (congenital)	Cochlea; CN VIII and central auditory pathways may be involved	*Onset in childhood:* bilateral, symmetric, profound hearing loss. *Onset in adulthood:* asymmetric hearing loss, often fluctuates; typically a flat configuration; occasionally conductive involvement; poor word recognition (34)
Temporal bone fracture	Cochlea or external ear, middle ear	Usually unilateral hearing loss; audiometric configuration varies; mild to profound; hearing may show fluctuation, recovery, or deterioration; longitudinal fracture results in conductive or mixed loss; transverse fracture in sensorineural loss (35)
Vascular loop	Cochlea or CN VIII	Unilateral hearing loss; mild to moderate; usually, sloping configuration, but may be flat (36)

occurs when the word recognition score becomes poorer as the intensity level is increased. The presence of significant rollover raises suspicion of a retrocochlear disorder, although the absence of rollover does not rule out the possibility of retrocochlear involvement (37).

Acoustic Immittance Measurements

The acoustic reflex is used to help differentiate cochlear from retrocochlear pathology. Reflex threshold levels, reflex decay, and the pattern of ipsilateral and contralateral reflexes are all important in the diagnostic evaluation. Cochlear pathology is indicated when the acoustic reflex is present at a sensation level less than 60-dB HL. That is, the difference between the behavioral threshold and the acoustic reflex threshold at the same frequency is less than 60 dB. As the degree of cochlear hearing loss increases, the reflex sensation level decreases. Thus with cochlear hearing losses of 85-dB HL, the expected reflex sensation level is approximately 25 dB.

With retrocochlear pathology, the reflex threshold and/or the time course of the reflex may be affected. Unexplained absence of the reflex or elevated reflex thresholds, especially in the presence of normal or near-normal hearing, are signs of eighth nerve pathology. This general rule applies to testing done at 500, 1,000, and 2,000 Hz but not at 4,000 Hz, where the reflex may be absent even in normal hearing patients.

Decay of the acoustic reflex is measured at 10 dB above the reflex threshold. If the reflex amplitude declines more than 50% over a 10-second period, eighth nerve pathology is suspected.

Auditory Brainstem Response

The ABR is needed in the evaluation of sensorineural hearing loss when behavioral thresholds cannot be obtained (e.g., with young infants) and when an eighth nerve or brainstem lesion is suspected. This section will consider the use of ABR to differentiate cochlear from retrocochlear lesions. The application of ABR in pediatric evaluations is discussed later in the chapter.

Many studies have looked at the effects of cochlear hearing loss and eighth nerve tumors on the ABR. *Cochlear* hearing loss usually shows a delayed or absent wave I, which may result in a shortened I to III or I to V interpeak interval. Wave V typically shows normal or near-normal latency at high intensity levels and prolonged latency at lower intensity levels, often giving the latency-intensity function for cochlear hearing loss an L shape, as shown in Figure 3.3.

The ABR in *retrocochlear* hearing loss usually is characterized by delayed or absent later waves, prolonged interpeak intervals, and significant interaural latency differences. The strongest indicators of retrocochlear pathology are a prolonged I to V interpeak interval and abnormal wave V interaural latency difference. Based on a series of 75

eighth nerve tumor ears and 684 nontumor ears, the use of these combined criteria resulted in overall 92% sensitivity and 88% specificity. Sensitivity was highest for tumors 2 cm or larger (100%) and lowest for tumors 1 cm or smaller (82%) (38).

In some clinics, wave V latencies are first adjusted to account for degree of high-frequency hearing loss before comparisons are made to normative data or between ears. This is thought to correct for the amount of delay caused solely by the degree of hearing loss. A frequent approach is to adjust the measured wave V latency by subtracting 0.10 msec for every 10 dB of hearing loss greater than 50 dB HL at 4,000 Hz (39). Some investigators have challenged this approach, pointing out that latency measurements show variability even among patients with similar hearing losses (40). An alternative approach is to apply a standard upper limit for latency values, such as 0.4 msec for interaural latency difference and 4.5 msec for I to V interpeak interval. In addition to measurements of interwave and interaural latencies, analysis of ABR morphology and other more complex algorithms for ABR analysis have been applied (41). Combined with standard analysis, these methods may increase the sensitivity for the detection of smaller lesions, which result in more subtle ABR changes.

With recent advances in medical imaging, the question arises as to whether the ABR should even be used when patients are suspected of a retrocochlear lesion, specifically acoustic nerve tumors. Although the detection capabilities of computerized tomography (CT) and magnetic resonance imaging (MRI) are extremely good, they are costly and, in the case of CT, expose the patient to radiation. Scheduling these imaging studies in another office results in diagnostic delay and patient inconvenience. The ABR has proved to be a powerful predictor of acoustic nerve tumors, yet is noninvasive and relatively inexpensive. The ABR, as well as acoustic reflex testing, are excellent screening tests to rule out tumors, especially in communities in which MRI and CT are not readily available. The American Academy of Otolaryngology–Head & Neck Surgery has recommended that ABR be included as a preoperative test for acoustic neuroma surgery (7).

Electrocochleography

Electrocochleography refers to the recording of the cochlear microphonic (CM), summating potential (SP), and action potential (AP). These stimulus-related electrical potentials reflect function of the inner ear and auditory nerve. The ECochG is used to evaluate patients suspected of having Ménière's disease, to help identify wave I of the ABR, and to monitor cochlear function during acoustic tumor surgery.

The SP and AP are the most important components of the EcochG, because the CM is variable and often difficult to differentiate from stimulus artifact. The EcochG response is usually recorded to click stimuli, either separate rarefaction and condensation clicks that are added together off-line or alternating polarity clicks. This technique cancels the CM, leaving the SP and AP. A normal EcochG response is shown in Figure 3.6.

Improved technology and more acceptable recording electrodes have contributed to the interest in and the ease of recording the EcochG. Without doubt, EcochG is best recorded with transtympanic electrodes that penetrate the tympanic membrane (TM) and contact the promontory directly, but the invasive nature of these electrodes limits their clinical applicability. Fortunately, TM electrodes and extratympanic electrodes have been improved and offer the combined advantage of acceptable recordings and ease of application.

In the diagnosis of Ménière's disease and other causes of endolymphatic hydrops, EcochG is interpreted by comparing the patient's SP:AP amplitude ratio either with normative data or with a generally accepted ratio of about 0.45 (42,43). A ratio that exceeds the expected level occurs in about 60% of patients with Ménière's disease. Furthermore, the enlarged SP:AP ratio is more likely to be present if patients are experiencing symptoms at the time of testing, especially aural fullness or pressure and some degree of hearing loss (44,45).

The EcochG technique is useful in the identification of wave I of the ABR because it is assumed that wave I of the ABR and the AP response of EcochG have the same generator site. The EcochG electrode arrangement can help to identify a wave I that may not be apparent on the conventionally recorded ABR. During intraoperative monitoring, combined EcochG and ABR may provide clearer tracings in less time (43).

Evoked Otoacoustic Emissions

Otoacoustic emissions play a role in the identification and differential diagnosis of SNHL. Their most common application is to identify SNHL with newborns and infants,

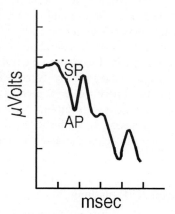

FIG. 3.6 An EcochG waveform from a normal-hearing subject, illustrating identification of the SP and AP. (Waveform courtesy of Jaynee H. Calder, Ph.D.)

which is discussed later in the chapter. In the adult population they are used to differentiate cochlear from retrocochlear hearing loss and to monitor cochlear function in cases such as ototoxicity and noise exposure. The EOAEs are not present if outer hair cell function has been compromised. The EOAEs may even be affected before hearing loss is apparent on the audiogram.

In the presence of retrocochlear hearing loss, such as an acoustic tumor, normal EOAEs would indicate that outer hair cell function is normal. Concomitant cochlear involvement would be assumed if the EOAEs were absent.

EVALUATION OF CENTRAL AUDITORY PROCESSING DISORDERS

The pioneering work of Bocca and his colleagues in the 1950s demonstrated how special procedures could be used to evaluate the auditory pathways of the brain and brainstem (46,47). During the pre-MRI era, these central auditory tests played an important role in aiding the diagnosis of neurologic lesions and in understanding central auditory function. Similar and more refined procedures are used today to evaluate patients who have complaints of hearing difficulty in the presence of a normal audiogram, patients with central nervous system disorders that affect the central auditory system, and patients with learning problems possibly related to auditory processes (48).

Central auditory processes refer to the mechanisms and manner by which the auditory system achieves the following: sound localization and lateralization; auditory discrimination; auditory pattern recognition; temporal aspects of audition, including temporal resolution, temporal masking, temporal integration, temporal ordering; and decreased auditory performance with competing or degraded acoustic signals. A patient with a deficiency in one or more of these areas is considered to have a central auditory processing disorder (CAPD) (49). Three groups of patients account for most CAPD: *children,* often in association with a learning disability, attention-deficit disorder, or language disorder; *adults,* related to an identified lesion of the central auditory system; and *older adults,* resulting from the effects of aging and/or neurodegenerative disease.

The assessment of CAPD is best accomplished by a team that includes the otologist, audiologist, and speech-language pathologist. The purpose of the assessment is to determine the presence of the CAPD, describe its parameters, and plan an appropriate intervention program (49).

Pure-tone and Speech Audiometry

Processing of the relatively simple signals used in routine audiometry is usually not affected by CAPD. Because of the redundancy present in the central auditory system, even severe lesions may have little effect on pure-tone and speech audiometry. Routine audiometry remains an essential part of the evaluation, however, because peripheral hearing loss can influence the results of central auditory tests. In addition, disorders such as ablation of the cochlea and/or auditory nerve, noise-induced hearing loss, and presbycusis may lead to atrophy and degeneration of auditory areas in the brainstem and cortex (50). Thus the sensory deficit shown by the audiogram may be related to changes in the central auditory system.

Behavioral Tests for Central Auditory Processing

Many tests for CAPD are available commercially. Several categories of measurements are recommended, including the following:

- Temporal processes—ordering, discrimination, resolution, and integration
- Localization and lateralization
- Low-redundancy monaural speech (time compressed, filtered, interrupted, competing, etc.)
- Dichotic stimuli, including competing nonsense syllables, digits, words, and sentences
- Binaural interaction procedures (e.g., masking level difference)

Tests selected should be driven by the referring complaint and should generally include both verbal and nonverbal stimuli. The battery of tests must be age appropriate and within the patient's attention and motivation capability (49).

Auditory Evoked Potentials

Auditory evoked potentials (AEPs) assess different functions of the central auditory system compared with behavioral test methods, and therefore they may increase the sensitivity of the CAPD battery. The AEPs become especially important if the patient is unable to be tested behaviorally. The central AEPs include ABR, middle latency evoked response (MLR), late potentials, P300, and mismatched negativity (MMN).

In the ABR, waves III, IV, and V are related to auditory function at the low- to mid-brainstem level. In particular, a prolonged III to V interpeak interval may indicate brainstem or central disorders. The ABR's sensitivity to brainstem lesions, however, is not as high as its sensitivity to acoustic tumors (51).

The MLR refers to the electrical response occurring between 8 and 50 msec following onset of an auditory stimulus (52). In normal subjects, the recording is characterized by a positive peak (Pa) at about 30 msec. Generator sites of the middle latency response include the auditory thalamocortical pathway, the mesencephalic reticular formation, and the inferior colliculus. Clinical studies have demonstrated the effects of cortical lesions on the middle latency response and maturational effects on the response in children (53,54).

The auditory late response occurs between 50 and 250 msec following an effective stimulus (55). It is characterized by a negative peak (N1) at about 100 msec and a positive peak (P2) at about 180 msec. The primary generator site for the late response is the auditory cortex. For both children and adults, an abnormal late response in the presence of normal peripheral hearing can indicate central auditory involvement. The late response is affected by sleep state and by maturation.

The MMN is an evoked potential with a latency of about 200 msec that is thought to originate in the thalamocortical areas of the central auditory system. It is called "mismatch" because it occurs when there is a change or mismatch in a series of acoustic events and "negative" because the response is a negative-polarity waveform (56). An "oddball" paradigm is used to elicit the MMN. That is, two different stimuli are presented in a random sequence, one of which is presented more frequently than the other. The MMN results from the auditory system's ability to respond to the change in stimuli, and even very small differences between the stimuli will evoke the response. Patients do not need to attend to the stimuli for the response to occur, indicating that the MMN provides a measure of cortical sensory discrimination rather than cognitive processing. The MMN is elicited only by auditory stimuli. It is used to identify neurophysiologic correlates for CAPD and to help differentiate auditory problems from attention deficits or more pervasive cognitive problems (57).

The P300 response is characterized by a large positive-polarity waveform in the 300 msec region, and its generator site is the auditory association cortex. The oddball paradigm, described earlier, is also used to elicit this response. With the P300 response, however, the patient is instructed to attend to the stimuli, usually by counting the number of infrequent signals. The P300 provides a broad measure of cognitive processing of stimulus differences. It is affected by lesions of the auditory cortex but may also be influenced by nonauditory disorders (58).

Acoustic Immittance Measurements

The presence of a normal tympanogram and normal acoustic reflexes confirm the absence of middle ear involvement, which may be helpful in the evaluation of CAPD. Because the acoustic reflex depends on the integrity of the entire reflex pathway, the pattern of ipsilateral and contralateral responses can help identify disorders in the afferent, efferent, or brainstem portion of the pathway. A brainstem lesion below the level of the superior olivary complex is suspected when contralateral reflexes are absent, with ipsilateral reflexes present. If a lesion is at the level of the cortex or high brainstem, no effect on the acoustic reflex would be expected.

Evoked Otoacoustic Emissions

In the normal ear, the amplitude of EOAEs is reduced when noise is presented to the contralateral ear. This normal suppression of the EOAE is mediated by the olivocochlear system of the efferent auditory pathway. Some patients with central or neural involvement do not show this normal suppression (59). In addition, integrity of the olivocochlear bundle has been linked to the ability to hear well in noise. Because difficulty hearing in the presence of competing signals is associated with CAPD, it may be useful to assess suppression of the EOAE (58).

AUDIOLOGIC EVALUATION OF INFANTS AND YOUNG CHILDREN

With today's armamentarium of physiologic and behavioral tests, it is possible to accurately assess the hearing ability of any child, regardless of age or ability to cooperate. Even with very young infants, it is possible to obtain separate-ear threshold data and information on the middle ear and sensorineural system. The best approach is to combine the use of behavioral and physiologic tests, both to improve the precision of the evaluation and as a "cross-check" (60). Accurate assessment and management of hearing loss and ear disease in children is important to ensure normal speech and language, educational, social, psychologic, and vocational development. This section describes audiologic procedures that are appropriate for infants and young children.

Newborn Screening

Universal newborn hearing screening has become widely accepted in the United States during the past decade. Following the National Institutes of Health (NIH) recommendation in 1993 that EOAEs and ABR be used to screen all newborns, these procedures have been incorporated into portable, automated screening devices (61). Data from large-scale screening programs using EOAEs and/or ABR suggest that it is reasonable to expect experienced programs to screen at least 90% of births, to maintain low follow-up rates, and to achieve follow-up testing on at least half the infants referred (62,63).

The Joint Committee on Infant Hearing (JCIH), a multidisciplinary committee, has guided national policy on newborn hearing screening for more than 30 years. In its 2000 Position Statement, the JCIH called for screening of all newborns, followed by audiologic and medical evaluations by 3 months of age and referral to appropriate intervention by 6 months of age. It endorsed the development of family-centered, community-based early hearing detection and intervention (EHDI) systems. The JCIH presented risk factors for use in neonates where universal hearing screening is not yet available (Table 3.3) (64).

Infants Less Than 6 Months of Age

Infants at this age who are referred because they failed a newborn hearing screening usually need a rescreening. If an infant fails the rescreening, or if other concerns about hearing are raised, a complete audiologic evaluation is needed. The evaluation should include ABR, EOAEs, behavioral observation audiometry, and acoustic immittance measurements. At this age, the ABR and EOAE are the most important predictors of auditory sensitivity. It is important to remember, however, that neither of these tests evaluates hearing in the perceptual sense. Information about how the infant responds behaviorally to sound is needed to complete the evaluation and to help interpret the physiologic test results.

TABLE 3.3. *Joint committee on infant hearing risk indicators*

Birth through 28 days where universal hearing screening is not yet available:
- An illness or condition requiring admission of 48 hours or greater to a neonatal intensive care unit
- Stigmata or other findings associated with a syndrome known to include a sensorineural and/or conductive hearing loss
- Family history of permanent childhood sensorineural hearing loss
- Craniofacial anomalies, including those with morphological abnormalities of the pinna and ear canal
- *In-utero* infections such as cytomegalovirus, herpes, toxoplasmosis, or rubella

29 days through 2 years—place an infant at risk or progressive or delayed-onset hearing loss:
- Parental or caregiver concern regarding hearing, speech, language, and/or developmental delay
- Stigmata or other findings associated with a syndrome known to include a sensorineural or conductive hearing loss or eustachian tube dysfunction
- Postnatal infections associated with sensorineural hearing loss, including bacterial meningitis
- *In-utero* infections such as cytomegalovirus, herpes, rubella, syphilis, and toxoplasmosis
- Neonatal indicators—specifically hyperbilirubinemia at a serum level requiring exchange transfusion, persistent pulmonary hypertension of the newborn associated with mechanical ventilation, and conditions requiring the use of extracorporeal membrane oxygenation (ECMO)
- Syndromes associated with progressive hearing loss such as neurofibromatosis, osteopetrosis, and Usher's syndrome
- Neurodegenerative disorders, such as Hunter syndrome, or sensory motor neuropathies, such as Friedreich's ataxia and Charcot-Marie-Tooth syndrome
- Head trauma
- Recurrent or persistent otitis media with effusion for at least 3 months

From American Academy of Audiology. Joint Committee on Infant Hearing Year 2000 Position Statement. *Audiol Today* 2000;[Special Issue]:6–27, with permission.

The infant ABR, compared with the adult response, shows prolonged wave latencies. The latencies decrease as the infant matures, with Wave I reaching the adult value at about 2 to 3 months of age and wave V at 1 to 2 years of age. Because of these maturational changes, ABR latencies for an infant must be compared with normative data established with infants of the same gestational age.

Infant ABR measurements should utilize stimuli that will provide information across the frequency spectrum. A common practice is to obtain recordings for the conventional click stimulus, which reflects activity at the 2- to 4-KHz range, and for a low-frequency tone burst such as 250 or 500 Hz. By using ABR data from these two frequency regions, the degree and configuration of hearing loss can be estimated. The ABR wave V threshold for a click is usually within 10 to 15 dB of behavioral threshold at 2,000 to 4,000 Hz. If the ABR air-conduction threshold is elevated, a bone-conduction ABR will help identify possible conductive involvement and assess cochlear reserve. Infants age 0 to 3 months can often be tested in natural sleep, but older infants may require sedation for the ABR.

Like the ABR, EOAEs are well suited for evaluating the infant's auditory function because they do not require a behavioral response. As noted previously, EOAEs are highly sensitive to mild degrees of hearing loss and they are very specific to outer hair cell dysfunction. They provide information across a range of frequencies, which helps to determine the configuration of the hearing loss. If EOAEs are normal, middle ear function is also normal.

Evoked otoacoustic emissions are critical for the identification of auditory neuropathy, a recently recognized disorder in infants and children. Auditory neuropathy is characterized by normal outer hair cell function, in conjunction with elevated thresholds, abnormal ABR, and abnormal middle ear reflexes (65). Without EOAE results, these infants may easily be misdiagnosed with sensorineural hearing loss. It is important to identify auditory neuropathy because these infants may later show other neurologic dysfunction and because their audiologic management is different than that for SNHL (21).

Behavioral observation audiometry (BOA) refers to observation of the infant's overt behavioral responses to live voice and frequency-specific stimuli. Minimum response levels are obtained to signals across a range of frequencies. At this age, responses consist primarily of arousal, limb movement, eye blinks, and changes in sucking and respiration. They are most easily elicited with moderate- to high-intensity signals. Carefully applied BOA can yield valuable information on how the infant responds to sound, but it is limited in its precision for estimating auditory thresholds. It also reflects response levels of the better ear if an ear difference exists.

Acoustic immittance measurements may identify middle ear problems not apparent by otoscopy, although there has been some controversy about the use of immittance with infants at this age (66). Use of a high-frequency probe tone (> 660Hz) provides more valid results in young infants be-

cause of the differences in the size and resonance characteristics of their ears. Nonetheless, caution should be used when interpreting results for infants less than 6 months of age.

Infants 6 to 30 Months of Age

Behavioral measurements play a major role in audiologic evaluation at this age. By 5 to 6 months, normally developing infants are able to make head-turn responses to sound. Visual reinforcement audiometry (VRA) capitalizes on this skill by reinforcing a head-turn response toward a known signal with an interesting visual reinforcer, such as an animated toy. In this way, minimum response levels are obtained for frequency-specific signals, either via sound field or, preferably, for each ear separately. Normal-hearing infants show response levels better than 20 dB between 500 and 4,000 Hz. Bone-conduction levels are similarly obtained, often with masking. The SRT and word recognition are evaluated with materials appropriate for the child's speech and language skills.

The EOAE testing provides a cross-check for the VRA results. In the presence of SNHL, EOAE testing helps to identify auditory neuropathy, as described earlier. As with younger infants, a normal EOAE result also indicates normal middle ear function.

Immittance measurements at this age level are interpreted as they would be for older children and adults. ABR testing is needed when behavioral results are questionable or to confirm SNHL that is found behaviorally. The same ABR procedure described for younger infants applies for this age.

Children 30 to 48 Months of Age

Once children reach a cognitive age of 2 to 3 years, they can be tested by means of conditioned play audiometry. The child is taught to respond to a sound by placing a peg in a peg board, dropping a block in a pail, or a similar task. Use of insert phones or supra-aural earphones enables separate-ear responses to be obtained. With a cooperative child, reliable responses can be obtained down to threshold levels for both air and bone conduction. The results are interpreted as they would be for an older child or adult. As with younger infants, age-appropriate materials are used for SRT and word recognition testing.

With young children, it is not always possible to obtain complete air- and bone-conduction thresholds, due to fatigue or inattentiveness. Immittance testing will give information about the middle ear system without relying on the child's attention. Similarly, EOAE and ABR testing are used to confirm the behavioral results, especially if test reliability is questionable or if results are incomplete. The EOAE testing is essential if auditory neuropathy is a consideration.

EVALUATION OF NONORGANIC HEARING LOSS

Hearing loss that cannot be explained by an auditory pathology is referred to as nonorganic hearing loss, functional hearing loss, or pseudohypacusis. Nonorganic hearing loss has been described in both adults and children. Financial or psychologic gain is usually an underlying factor. This section describes procedures that identify and confirm the presence of nonorganic hearing loss. To some extent, these tests also may estimate true auditory thresholds. Often the determination of true threshold is more difficult than verifying a nonorganic hearing loss.

Pure-tone and Speech Audiometry

The patient with nonorganic hearing loss often responds inconsistently to repeated pure-tone testing and often indicates an equal amount of hearing loss across the test frequencies. Two findings on pure-tone and speech audiometry are highly indicative of nonorganic hearing loss:

- Absence of a shadow curve in the presence of severe to profound unilateral hearing loss. This outcome is most easily seen when supra-aural earphones are used in testing. Once the test signal in the ear under question exceeds interaural attenuation, the patient should begin to respond because of crossover to the better ear. Failure to respond suggests nonorganic involvement.
- Disagreement between the SRT and the average of the two best thresholds obtained at 500, 1,000, and 2,000 Hz. If the SRT is more than 10 dB better than the pure-tone average, response validity should be questioned.

Stenger Test

Many special tests have been developed to identify nonorganic hearing loss, some of which require special tape-recorded material or modification of audiometric equipment. Probably the best known of these procedures is the Stenger, a test for unilateral nonorganic hearing loss (67). The test is based on the principle that when both ears simultaneously hear a tone of the same frequency, the tone will be perceived only in the ear in which it is louder. During testing, the tone is delivered slightly above threshold in the normal ear and slightly below the admitted threshold of the poor ear. Patients with nonorganic hearing loss will indicate that they no longer hear a tone because it is below their admitted threshold in the poor ear. If a hearing loss actually existed, however, the patient would still hear a tone because it is present at a suprathreshold level in the normal ear. A positive Stenger results when the patient fails to respond. The Stenger can be done as a screening test or as a threshold-seeking test. Tone or speech can be used as signals.

Evoked Otoacoustic Emissions, Acoustic Reflex, and Auditory Brainstem Response

The EOAEs are a quick check of the validity of threshold testing, because they are present only with normal or near-normal hearing. They are an appropriate check for nonor-

ganic hearing loss if no middle ear disorder is present. The acoustic reflex is helpful because of the predictable relationship between pure-tone threshold and the reflex threshold at the same frequency. A reflex sensation level less than 10 dB is highly unusual and should raise suspicion of nonorganicity. Another indication is a reflex threshold that is better than the admitted pure-tone or speech recognition threshold.

ABR testing is indicated if the results of more routine tests are conflicting or if additional confirmation of the nonorganic nature of the hearing loss is needed. In such cases, wave V threshold and wave V latencies for clicks or tone pips are used to estimate true auditory threshold.

REFERENCES

1. Zwislocki J. Acoustic attenuation between the ears. *J Acoust Soc Am* 1953;25:752–759.
2. Killion MC, Wilber LA, Gudmundsen GI. Insert earphones for more interaural attenuation. *Hear Instruments* 1985;36:34–36.
3. Jerger J. Clinical experience with impedance audiometry. *Arch Otolaryngol* 1970;92:311–324.
4. Metz O. The acoustic impedance measured on normal and pathological ears. *Acta Otolaryngol (Stockh)* 1946;Suppl 63.
5. Moller AR, Jannetta PJ, Sekhar LN. Contributions from the auditory nerve to the brain-stem auditory evoked potentials (BAEPs): results of intracranial recording in man. *Electroencephalogr Clin Neurophysiol* 1988;71:198–211.
6. Lonsbury-Martin BL, Martin GK. The clinical utility of distortion-product otoacoustic emissions. *Ear Hear* 1990;11:144–154.
7. American Academy of Otolaryngology—Head & Neck Surgery (AAO-HNS). 1999 Clinical Indicators Compendium. *AAO-HNS Bull* 1999; October.
8. Jerger S, Jerger J. Otitis media. In: *Auditory Disorders: A Manual for Clinical Evaluation.* Boston: Little, Brown, 1981:125–130.
9. Carhart R. Effect of stapes fixation on bone conduction response. In: Schuknecht HF, ed. *Otosclerosis.* Boston: Little, Brown, 1962:175–197.
10. Paparella MM, Rybak L. Congenital cholesteatoma. *Otolaryngol Clin North Am* 1978;11:113–120.
11. Kirikae I. Physiology of the middle ear including eustachian tube. In: Paparella MM, Shumrick DA, eds. *Otolaryngology,* vol 1, 2nd ed. Philadelphia: WB Saunders, 1980:199–215.
12. Cole JM. Glomus jugulare tumor. *Laryngoscope* 1977;87:1244–1258.
13. Tos M. Bony fixation of the malleus and incus. *Acta Otolaryngol (Stockh)* 1970;70:95–104.
14. Paparella MM. The middle ear effusions. In: Paparella MM, Shumrick DA, eds. *Otolaryngology,* vol 2, 2nd ed. Philadelphia: WB Saunders, 1980:1422–1444.
15. Pinsker OT. Otological correlates of audiology. In: Katz J, ed. *Handbook of Clinical Audiology.* Baltimore: Williams & Wilkins, 1972:36–59.
16. Terkildsen K. Pathologies and their effect on middle ear function. In: Feldman AS, Wilber LA, eds. *Acoustic Impedance and Admittance—the Measurement of Middle Ear Function.* Baltimore: Williams & Wilkins, 1976:78–102.
17. Gibb AG. Non-suppurative otitis media. In: Ballantyne J, Groves J, eds. *Diseases of the Ear, Nose and Throat,* vol 2, 4th ed. London: Butterworth, 1979.
18. Jerger J, Anthony L, Jerger S, Mauldin L. Studies in impedance audiometry. III. Middle ear disorders. *Arch Otolaryngol* 1974;99:165–171.
19. Forquer BD, Sheehy JL. The negative on/off effect in cochlear and early stapedial otosclerosis. *Ear Hear* 1981;2:256–259.
20. Brackmann DE. A review of acoustic tumors: 1979–1982. *Am J Otol* 1984;5:233–244.
21. Hall JW. Clinical applications of otoacoustic emissions in children. *Handbook of Otoacoustic Emissions.* San Diego: Singular Publishing, 2000:389–490.
22. McCabe BF. Autoimmune sensorineural hearing loss. *Ann Otol Rhinol Laryngol* 1979;88:585–589.
23. Axelsson A, Sigroth K, Vertes D. Hearing in diabetics. *Acta Otolaryngol (Stockh)* 1978;[Suppl 356].

24. Harbert F, Young IM. Audiologic findings in Ramsay Hunt syndrome. *Arch Otolaryngol* 1967;85:632–639.
25. Dayal VS, Kane N, Mendelsohn M. Patterns of pure tone hearing loss. A comparative study of presbyacusis, multiple sclerosis, Menière's and acoustic neuroma. *Acta Otolaryngol (Stockh)* 1970;69:329–332.
26. Hall JW. Clinical applications of otoacoustic emissions in adults. *Handbook of Otoacoustic Emissions.* San Diego: Singular Publishing, 2000:481–544.
27. Berlow SJ, Caldarelli DD, Matz GJ, et al. Bacterial meningitis and sensorineural hearing loss: a prospective investigation. *Laryngoscope* 1980;90:1445–1452.
28. Mustillo P. Auditory deficits in multiple sclerosis: a review. *Audiology* 1984;23:145–164.
29. Cooper JC, Owen JH. Audiologic profile of noise-induced hearing loss. *Arch Otolaryngol* 1976;102:148–150.
30. Matz GJ, Lerner SA. Drug ototoxicity. In: Beagley HA, ed. *Audiology and Audiological Medicine,* vol 1. New York: Oxford University Press, 1981:573–592.
31. Seltzer S, McCabe BF. Perilymph fistula: the Iowa experience. *Laryngoscope* 1986;96:37–49.
32. Schuknecht HF. *Pathology of the Ear.* Cambridge, MA: Harvard University Press, 1974:351–414.
33. Mattox DE, Simmons FB. Natural history of sudden sensorineural hearing loss. *Ann Otol Rhinol Laryngol* 1977;86:463–480.
34. Karmody CS, Schuknecht HF. Deafness in congenital syphilis. *Arch Otolaryngol* 1966;83:18–27.
35. Wiet RJ, Valvassori GE, Kotsanis CA, et al. Temporal bone fractures. State of the art review. *Am J Otol* 1985;6:207–215.
36. Applebaum EL, Valvassori GE. Auditory and vestibular system findings in patients with vascular loops in the internal auditory canal. *Ann Otol Rhinol Laryngol* 1984;93[Suppl 112]:63–70.
37. Meyer DH, Mishler ET. Rollover measurements with Auditec NU-6 word lists. *J Speech Hear Disord* 1985;50:356–360.
38. Bauch CD, Olsen WO, Pool AF. ABR indices: sensitivity, specificity, and tumor size. *Am J Audiol* 1996;5:97–104.
39. Selters WA, Brackmann DE. Brainstem electric response audiometry in acoustic tumor detection. In: House WF, Luetje CM, eds. *Acoustic tumors,* vol 1. Baltimore: University Park Press, 1979:225–235.
40. Fowler CG, Durrant JD. The effects of peripheral hearing loss on the auditory brainstem response. In: Jacobson JT, ed. *Principles and Applications in Auditory Evoked Potentials,* Boston: Allyn & Bacon, 1994:237–250.
41. Don M, Masuda A, Nelson R, et al. Successful detection of small acoustic tumors using the stacked derived-band auditory brain stem response amplitude. *Am J Otol* 1997;18:608–621.
42. Coats AC. Electrocochleography: recording technique and clinical applications. *Semin Hear* 1986;7:247–266.
43. Ferraro JA, Ruth RA. Electrocochleography. In: Jacobson JT, ed. *Principles and Applications in Auditory Evoked Potentials,* Boston: Allyn & Bacon, 1994:100–122.
44. Ferraro JA, Arenberg IK, Hassanein RS. Electrocochleography and symptoms of inner ear dysfunction. *Arch Otolaryngol* 1985;111:71–74.
45. Staller S. Electrocochleography in the diagnosis and management of Meniere's disease. *Semin Hear* 1986;7:267–277.
46. Bocca E, Calearo C, Cassinari V. A new method for testing hearing in temporal lobe tumours. *Acta Otolaryngol (Stockh)* 1954;44:219–221.
47. Bocca E, Calearo C, Cassinari V, Migliavacca F. Testing "cortical" hearing in temporal lobe tumours. *Acta Otolaryngol (Stockh)* 1955;45:289–304.
48. American Speech-Language-Hearing Association. Assessment of central auditory processing disorders (CAPD) (Adults and Children). In: *Preferred Practice Patterns for the Profession of Audiology.* Rockville, MD, 1997.
49. American Speech-Language-Hearing Association Task Force on Central Auditory Processing Consensus Development. Central auditory processing: current status of research and implications for clinical practice. *Am J Audiol* 1996;2:41–54.
50. Musiek FE, Lamb L. Central auditory assessment: an overview. In: Katz J, ed. *Handbook of Clinical Audiology,* 4th ed. Baltimore: Williams & Wilkins, 1994:197–211.
51. Musiek FE, Josey A, Glasscock M. Auditory brainstem response interwave measurements in acoustic neuromas. *Ear Hear* 1986;7:100–105.
52. Kraus N, McGee T, Stein L. The auditory middle latency response. In: Jacobson JT, ed. *Principles and Applications in Auditory Evoked Potentials.* Boston: Allyn & Bacon, 1994:155–178.
53. Kraus N, Ozdamar O, Hier D, et al. Auditory middle latency responses (MLRs) in patients with cortical lesions. *Electroencephalogr Clin Neurophysiol* 1982;54:275–287.
54. Kraus N, Smith DI, Reed NL, et al. Auditory middle latency response in children: effects of age and diagnostic category. *Electroencephalogr Clin Neurophysiol* 1985;62:343–351.
55. Hall JW. Overview of auditory evoked responses: past, present, and future. *Handbook of Auditory Evoked Responses.* Boston: Allyn and Bacon, 1992:3–40.
56. Kraus N. The discriminating brain: MMN and acoustic change. *Hear J* 1996;5:10,41–43.
57. Kraus N, McGee T. Mismatch negativity in the assessment of central auditory function. *Am J Audiol* 1994;2:39–51.
58. Chermak D, Musiek F. Electrophysiologic assessment of central auditory processing disorders. *Central Auditory Processing Disorders.* San Diego: Singular Publishing, 1997;129–150.
59. Berlin CI, Hood LJ, Cecola P, et al. Does type I afferent neuron dysfunction reveal itself through lack of efferent suppression? *Hear Res* 1993;65:40–50.
60. Jerger JF, Hayes D. The cross-check principle in pediatric audiometry. *Arch Otolaryngol* 1976;102:614–620.
61. National Institutes of Health. Early identification of hearing impairment in infants and young children. *NIH Consensus Statement* 1993;11:1–24.
62. Finitzo T, Albright K, O'Neal J. The newborn with hearing loss: detection in the nursery. *Pediatrics* 1998;102:1452–1460.
63. Thomson V. The Colorado newborn hearing screening project. In: Finitzo T, Roizen N, Sininger Y, eds. Joint Committee on Infant Hearing Forum. *Am J Audiol* 1997;6[Suppl]:74–77.
64. American Academy of Audiology. Joint Committee on Infant Hearing Year 2000 Position Statement. *Audiol Today* 2000;[Special Issue]:6–27.
65. Starr A, Picton TW, Sininger Y, et al. Auditory neuropathy. *Brain* 1996;119:741–753.
66. Northern JL, Downs MP. Physiological hearing tests. In: *Hearing in Children,* 4th ed. Baltimore: Williams & Wilkins, 1991:189–230.
67. Martin FN. Pseudohypacusis. In: Katz J, ed. *Handbook of Clinical Audiology,* 4th ed. Baltimore: Williams & Wilkins, 1994:553–567.

CHAPTER 4

Imaging of the Temporal Bone

Hugh D. Curtin and Osamu Sakai

Imaging has become an integral part of the evaluation of many otologic problems (1–3). Computed tomography (CT) and magnetic resonance imaging (MRI) are the primary tools of modern imaging of the temporal bone. The appropriate modality depends on the clinical problem because these imaging systems provide very different information. Because the anatomy and pathology clearly shown by one modality may be completely invisible in the other, design of the imaging plan is of obvious importance.

This chapter is not a complete description of lesions involving the temporal bone. Rather, we will provide a strategy for imaging in various clinical situations and show the landmarks and findings that are most important in making decisions. Radiologists may vary in the selection of an approach to arrive at the information considered most important. Ongoing consultation and interaction between clinician and radiologist contribute significantly to the evolution of an appropriate imaging strategy.

COMPUTED TOMOGRAPHY AND MAGNETIC RESONANCE IMAGING

Although the technical details of MRI and CT imaging are inappropriate in this review, a few key terms and concepts will help the otolaryngologist to appreciate the strengths and limitations of each approach.

Computed tomography is based on electron density and follows the same principles as plain film radiography. Denser structures such as metal and bone stop more X-rays and therefore are white on the image, whereas less dense structures stop fewer and are darker or black. Most soft tissues are intermediate in density and are shown as various shades of gray. Muscle, tumor, and fluids all approximate the same density. Fat is substantially lower density and is darker than other soft tissues on CT. Iodinated contrast has a very high electron density and so makes any tissue or space that can be reached by the contrast more opaque or "whiter" than before the contrast is administered. Thus a tumor that has a blood supply will be whiter after injection of intra-

venous contrast than before. Contrast injected intrathecally opacifies the cerebrospinal fluid (CSF), which therefore appears white.

Bone and soft tissue algorithms are computer programs applied to the raw data obtained from the actual scan. These computer manipulations give additional information without additional radiation.

One of the most recent innovations in CT technology is the multidetector spiral CT machine. The use of multiple detectors allows extremely thin, direct scan images and the production of excellent multiplanar reformatted images. For instance, the computer takes the information from a direct axial image set and produces high resolution images in the coronal or sagittal plane. The resolution is the same in the reformatted image as in a directly acquired image. This technique gives the capability of high resolution reformatted images in any plane without the need for additional radiation to the patient.

Magnetic resonance imaging, as currently practiced, relies on the magnetic properties of hydrogen nuclei. A radio frequency is used to stimulate the nuclei and a sensitive antenna detects the signal emitted as the nuclei "relax"—that is, return to their normal state. The terms T_1 and T_2 refer to different types of relaxation of the nuclei. One of the most obvious findings of a T_1-weighted image is that fat has a very high signal and is therefore white on the image. Fluid such as CSF has a low signal and is dark but not black. Cortical bone and air have virtually no signal and so typically appear as true black. Various soft tissues appear as shades of gray. Intravenous gadolinium increases the signal, or brightness, of any vascularized tissue. Thus tissue (e.g., many solid tumors) is "brighter" on the postcontrast T_1-weighted image than on a similar sequence performed prior to contrast.

T_2-weighted images show low protein fluids such as CSF as a high signal (bright). Fat is usually dark. Newer, fast spin echo T_2-weighted sequences, however, show fat as bright unless fat suppression is used, which results in a dark T_2 appearance.

35

One of the advantages of MRI is the seemingly unending nuances that can be applied in modern sequence design. For example, fast flowing blood causes a black "signal void" on many sequences. However, other sequences can be made very sensitive to any type of movement and can show flow as bright. These specialized sequences are the basis of MR angiography. The fat signal is a key part of evaluating head and neck tumors. However, the high signal of fat can interfere with appreciation of subtle enhancement of various tumors and inflammation. Special fat suppression techniques can be added, allowing better visualization of even minimal enhancement adjacent to fat.

Although the great variety of available sequences provide more information, the varying appearances can be quite confusing when one first tries to work with MRI. Most imaging centers develop relatively standard protocols.

In otologic imaging the preferred modality depends on the region to be assessed. Cortical bone and air have the same appearance on MRI. Because neither gives signal, both appear black in the image. The ossicles are invisible in a normally aerated middle ear. With CT, bone and air are almost at the opposite ends of the density spectrum and so clear delineation of these structures is possible. With CT, soft tissue and fluid are different from bone and from air and so one can identify small amounts of fluid and soft tissue in the middle ear and mastoid region. For these reasons CT is usually the first study done for evaluation of the external auditory canal, middle ear, and mastoid.

Computed tomography and MR can both be used for imaging of the inner ear. Computed tomography emphasizes bone, showing the contours of the otic capsule and demonstrating the fluid-filled spaces as lucencies. Magnetic resonance imaging demonstrates the fluid directly with the bone represented by a signal void. In the internal auditory canal, MRI becomes the clear choice. High resolution MRI can show the actual nerves crossing the fluid of the internal auditory canal or can demonstrate subtle enhancement of a small tumor. The densities, even with enhancement, are not great enough for CT to reliably separate the structures in the canal.

CLINICAL AND REGIONAL EVALUATION

The radiologist must tailor the examination to the clinical presentation and expected diagnosis. Although there is overlap, an initial approach divides the temporal bone into several major regions. Imaging then is refined depending on the clinical question.

External Auditory Canal

The external auditory canal is easily accessible to direct inspection and so the diagnosis is frequently known prior to imaging. Most imaging is done for staging of congenital anomalies or to identify possible deeper extension of a lesion arising in the canal. Computed tomography is usually the first approach.

Congenital Lesions

Atresia of the external auditory canal is evaluated in axial and coronal planes using a bone algorithm CT. No contrast is used. The thickness of the atretic plate is best appreciated in the coronal plane (Fig. 4.1) (4,5). In a complete atresia the malleus may be fused to the atresia plate. Other fusions and abnormalities of ossicles are often appreciated.

The development of the middle ear and pneumatization of the mastoid are important for surgical planning (6). The width of the middle ear at the oval window and of the air space at the level of the horizontal semicircular canal give a good estimation of the development of the middle ear and can be appreciated in either axial or coronal plane. When atresia of the external auditory canal is associated with a severely atretic middle ear, bone is seen abutting the horizontal canal without an aerated antrum or mastoid (Fig. 4.2). The status of the stapes is assessed on axial and coronal images. The presence and integrity of the oval and round windows is assessed.

In patients with atresia of the external auditory canal the facial nerve usually is in an abnormal location. The mastoid segment appears to "migrate" anteriorly into the location usually taken by the external auditory canal. This is appreciated on either axial or coronal CT. Normally the mastoid segment of the facial nerve canal is located posteriorly in the same coronal plane as the posterior semicircular canal. In atresia of the external auditory canal, that segment of the canal is seen more anteriorly in the same plane as the round window niche. This finding is almost always present with significant atresias. The tympanic segment of the nerve can also be aberrant. The nerve can migrate inferiorly to be posi-

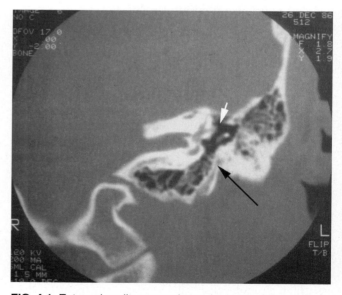

FIG. 4.1 External auditory canal atresia, coronal CT. There is a relatively thick atretic plate *(black arrow)*. The width of the air space at the level of the horizontal semicircular canal *(white arrow)* is normal. This plane is taken through the level of the oval window.

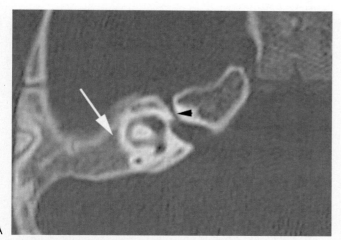

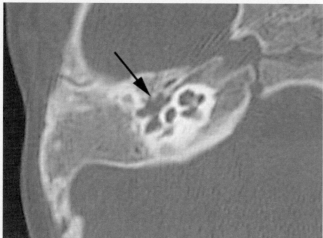

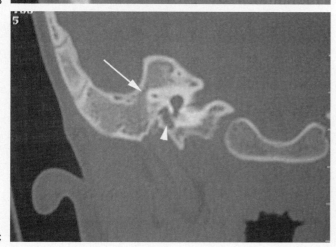

FIG. 4.2 Severe external auditory canal atresia, CT. **A:** Axial image through the level of the horizontal semicircular canal. There is no development of the mastoid or upper middle ear. Bone *(white arrow)* abuts the cortex of the otic capsule at the level of the horizontal canal. No air space is visualized. Labyrinthine segment of the facial nerve canal *(black arrowhead)*. **B:** Axial image of lower middle ear. The middle ear space *(arrow)* is narrow and opacified. **C:** Coronal image through the level of the round window. Bone *(arrow)* is seen immediately adjacent to the horizontal canal. There is a very small middle ear space *(arrowhead)*.

tioned in or near the oval window or even over the promontory (see Facial Nerve section in this chapter).

Finally the status of the labyrinth is documented. Though uncommon, an inner ear anomaly should be excluded to the extent possible by imaging.

Mass Lesions and Infection

Other than atresias, most lesions of the ear are evaluated in a similar way. The location and extent of the lesion are of primary concern. For example, does the lesion extend into the mastoid or through the tympanic membrane into the middle ear (Fig. 4.3)? Is there extension inferior or anterior to the external auditory canal (Fig. 4.4)? Does a lesion extend into the temporomandibular joint or the parotid gland?

Smooth expansion with an intact cortex is seen in keratosis obturans or cholesteatoma. The cortex of the external auditory canal is rounded but not infiltrated or destroyed. There is no deep invasion of the contiguous tissues without coexistent additional infection.

Exostoses produce cortical thickening protruding into and narrowing the canal. Often, centrifugal expansion will involve several walls of the canal. An osteoma tends to have a smaller attachment, presenting more commonly as a single mass. In each case the radiologist documents the proximity to the attachment of the tympanic membrane (Fig. 4.3). Is there a clear area of normal bone separating the lesion from the tympanic annulus?

Carcinoma of the external auditory canal and malignant or necrotizing otitis externa share many findings on imaging and may be evaluated with CT or MRI. Computed tomography has the advantage of showing subtle erosion of cortical bone because these pathologies destroy the cortex of the external auditory canal. There is enough fat in the parotid

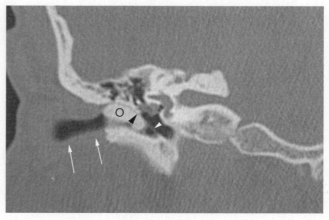

FIG. 4.3 Osteoma of the external auditory canal, coronal CT. The osteoma *(O)* fills much of the medial external auditory canal. It does not extend beyond the tympanic membrane *(white arrowhead)* into the middle ear. Note its relationship to the scutum *(black arrowhead)*. The cartilaginous portion of the external auditory canal *(white arrows)* is faintly visualized on this bone algorithm. The cortex of the osseous external auditory canal is intact.

gland and along the underside of the external auditory canal that CT is very effective in determining extension into the contiguous soft tissues (Fig. 4.4). Invasion through the cortex of bone or tympanic membrane into the middle ear is seen as obliteration of the air space on CT or as signal where there should be none on MRI. In MRI, both malignant or necrotizing otitis externa and carcinoma tend to be darker on T_2 than fluid caused by inflammation or obstruction in the mastoid. Magnetic resonance imaging may more easily define the margin of the pathology within the air spaces. The enhancement of tumors also may be slightly different. Inflamed mucosa tends to enhance slightly more than tumor or malignant or necrotizing otitis externa.

Malignant or necrotizing otitis externa tends to pass inferiorly through the fissures of Santorini between the bony and cartilaginous segments of the external auditory canal. This area is well seen in the coronal plane (Fig. 4.4). If there is invasion at this point, the lesion can extend medially, invading the fat in the stylomastoid foramen and extending across the soft tissues beneath the skull base. This may be detected with CT or MRI (7,8). The lesion can invade into the skull base at the petroclival synchondrosis, eventually extending intracranially. This extension is much less common with the advent of newer, more effective antibiotics.

Computed tomography shows the invasion of the cortex of the external auditory canal and extension into the mastoid as well as early extension into the subcranial soft tissues.

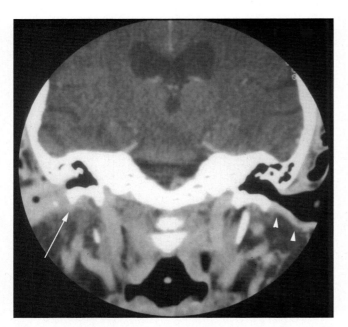

FIG. 4.4 Possible early malignant external otitis, coronal CT soft tissue algorithm. There is thickening of the cartilaginous external auditory canal on the right. A small amount of tissue *(arrow)* extends into the fatty tissue just beneath the external auditory canal. This is the approximate position of the fissures of Santorini at the junction of the cartilaginous and bony external canal. Compare with the intact fat and parotid just beneath the cartilaginous portion of the external canal *(arrowheads)* on the left side.

When a lesion traverses the mastoid or invades other parts of the skull base, MRI is preferred for showing involvement of the dura or the brain. Magnetic resonance imaging is also more sensitive for invasion of muscular structures such as the retropharyngeal or masticator muscles. One must analyze the margin of the tumor to determine if an additional examination is necessary. For instance, if the lesion is first evaluated with CT and is separated from muscle and from dura by intact fat or bone, MRI adds little to the evaluation.

Middle Ear

The middle ear is evaluated primarily with CT. The key landmarks are small cortical bony structures, ideal for CT imaging.

Chronic Otitis Media and Cholesteatoma

The most common indication for imaging in the middle ear is assessment of chronic otitis media and possible cholesteatoma. Opacification or fluid in the middle ear is obvious on either CT or MR. The advantage of CT is that subtle erosion of bone can be detected and the ossicles can be visualized. Cholesteatoma will erode the lateral wall of the attic and the scutum (junction of lateral wall of the attic and the roof of the external auditory canal), and this may be the earliest finding suggesting the presence of such a lesion (Fig. 4.5). The ossicles may be eroded or displaced. However, the findings may also occur in chronic granulomatous otitis media and are not specific for cholesteatoma.

Often the cholesteatoma has already been diagnosed otoscopically. Indeed, even when the diagnosis has not been confirmed, the most important goal of CT is not necessarily to make the diagnosis but rather to define abnormalities that may lead to complications during surgery. Three major landmarks are critical: the horizontal semicircular canal, the tegmen, and the canal of the facial nerve (Fig. 4.5). Each of these landmarks is represented by a cortical bony wall.

The horizontal semicircular canal protrudes into the antrum. As a cholesteatoma enlarges in the antrum, the lateral bony wall of the horizontal semicircular canal may be eroded (Fig. 4.6). This can be appreciated in axial or coronal imaging as a small lucent defect in the bone. An axial image is taken at an angle to show the entire circumference of the horizontal semicircular canal. The integrity of the bone on this image is very reassuring. Other semicircular canals can be eroded as well, but the horizontal semicircular canal is most commonly involved.

The tegmen tympani may be eroded or displaced by cholesteatoma. Search for a defect or dehiscence is particularly important in postoperative cases. An erosion or surgical defect may result in herniation of dura or even temporal lobe. Unfortunately, the tegmen presents a significant problem for imaging. The bone may normally be thin and lies in a sloping plane at an angle to both standard coronal and axial imaging. Pseudodefects are common because of partial

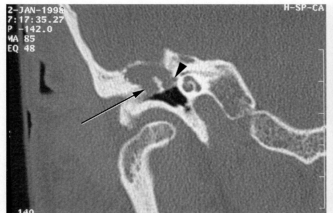
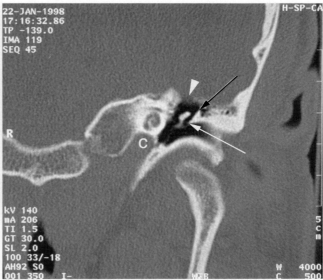

FIG. 4.5 Cholesteatoma of the attic and antrum. **A:** Coronal CT shows the cholesteatoma opacifying the attic and extending into the antrum. There is erosion of the scutum *(arrow)*. Note the relationship of the lesion to the tympanic segment of the facial nerve canal *(arrowhead)*. **B:** Coronal CT, opposite, normal side. The middle ear is well aerated and the bony landmarks intact. Note that the tegmen *(white arrowhead)* is very indistinct due to partial volume artifact. Scutum *(white arrow)*, upper spur of the lateral wall of the attic *(black arrow)*, and carotid canal *(C)* are also shown.

volume artifact (Fig. 4.5). Because the bone is thinner than the voxel (smallest digital imaging volume), the voxel contains both thin bone and soft tissue. The high density of the bone is averaged with the lower density of the adjacent soft tissue. Because only high densities are displayed as white, the averaged value gives the appearance of soft tissue and thus the bone is not apparent. A very small defect can theoretically be missed. Computed tomography demonstration of a thick intact bone, on the other hand, is a reliable finding. In questionable cases, MRI may be helpful. Magnetic resonance imaging will not show the bone but can show the inferior surface of the temporal lobe and document that there is no herniation of brain into the defect.

The position of the facial nerve and integrity of the fallopian canal are documented. One may not actually see the complete bone covering of the canal. There are common natural dehiscences and, again, partial volume plays a significant role. Erosion by cholesteatoma is unusual, but the radiologist should document the presence of disease adjacent to the canal of the facial nerve.

Finally, imaging can assess the pneumatization of the mastoid and involvement of small recesses of the middle ear, such as the round window niche and the sinus tympani, thus providing to the surgeon details to plan a surgical approach.

Vascular Lesions of the Middle Ear (Red Mass)

At our institution, CT is also the preferred imaging modality when a "red mass" is seen through the tympanic membrane (9). Though MRI can give significant information and can

often help make the diagnosis, many radiologists feel that CT provides additional information that can make the initial diagnosis more reliable (10,11). Magnetic resonance imaging or angiography may be done once the initial diagnosis is made.

There are two important landmarks: the lateral bony plate of the carotid canal and the lateral bony plate of the jugular foramen (Fig. 4.7). The position and appearance of these two structures allow the differentiation of the aberrant carotid artery, glomus tympanicum, and glomus jugulare tumors.

The first step in evaluation of the "red mass" is to exclude an aberrant carotid artery. The key landmark is the white line representing the lateral bony wall of the carotid canal. This bony plate is normally just anterior to the cochlea and should be intact. An aberrant artery extends further laterally in the middle ear (Fig. 4.8). The bony wall is usually incomplete, and the vessel is visible along the curve of the promontory of the cochlea. Often a persistent stapedial artery accompanies the aberrant carotid. The foramen spinosum will be absent because the middle meningeal artery arises from the aberrant carotid artery. On MRI an aberrant carotid is recognized by the lateral bend seen as the vessel enters the middle ear. This can also be diagnosed by the characteristic configuration on arteriography, using the frontal projection.

Once an aberrant carotid artery is excluded, attention moves to the bony plate of the lateral wall of the jugular foramen. The appearance of this plate is the most important finding in differentiating glomus tympanicum from glomus jugulare tumors. In the tympanicum the plate of bone is

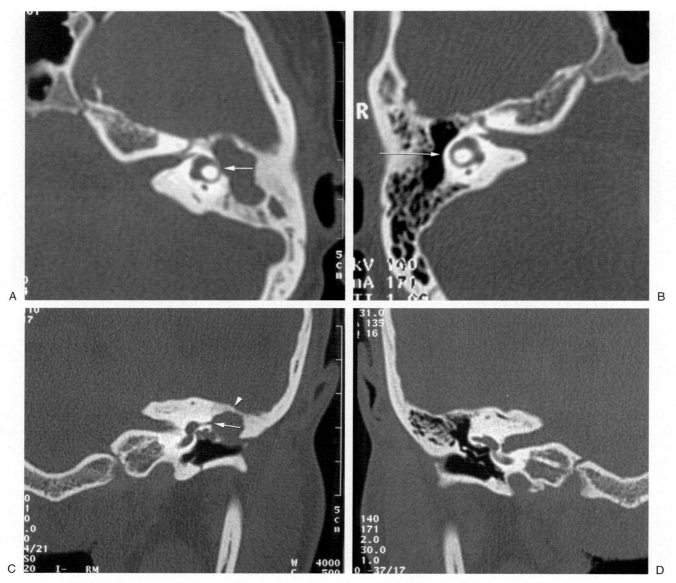

FIG. 4.6 Cholesteatoma eroding the horizontal semicircular canal, CT. **A:** Cholesteatoma opacifies the upper attic and antrum. Note the rounded, smooth margins. There is erosive scalloping of the bone covering the horizontal semicircular canal *(arrow)*. The cholesteatoma has reached the lumen of the canal, causing a fistula. **B:** Normal right side shows the intact cortex with a normal thickness *(arrow)*. **C:** Coronal CT shows the cholesteatoma eroding the horizontal canal *(arrow)*. Note the intact tegmen **(arrowhead).** The scutum and ossicular chain are also eroded. **D:** Normal coronal scan of opposite side.

sharp and intact. A glomus jugulare (jugulotympanicum) gives a subtle but distinct demineralization (Fig. 4.9). These findings are evident without intravenous contrast.

If the plate of the jugular fossa is intact, the diagnosis of glomus tympanicum is made. A hemangioma or other rare lesion of the middle ear can have a similar appearance. The key information needed from imaging is not the exact diagnosis but rather the determination that the lesion is confined to the middle ear. If, however, the plate is eroded and glomus jugulare is diagnosed, then MRI is often done to provide information about the medial extent and possible intracranial and infracranial extension (Fig. 4.10). Invasion of the jugular vein and sigmoid sinus, as well as residual flow within the vein, is

better evaluated on MRI. The relationship to the carotid artery, both vertical and transverse temporal segments, is assessed by either modality. Angiography is not usually needed to make the diagnosis but is done just prior to surgery in conjunction with embolization to decrease the vascularity.

Inner Ear and Otic Capsule

Otosclerosis

Otosclerosis is usually diagnosed clinically. Imaging may be done to confirm the diagnosis or to exclude other disease. The earliest finding is subtle demineralization of the anterior

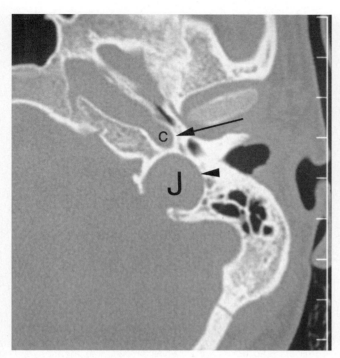

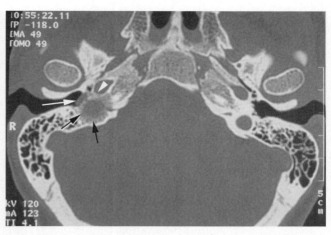

FIG. 4.9 Glomus jugulare, axial CT. The lesion *(white arrow)* was visualized through the tympanic membrane. There is demineralization *(black arrows)* around the jugular foramen. The white cortical line is indistinct and poorly visualized. A small amount of demineralized bone *(white arrowhead)* on the posterior cortex of the carotid canal indicates tumor. Compare the demineralized bone with the intact cortex and bone on the opposite side.

FIG. 4.7 Normal CT through the lower middle ear. The carotid artery *(C)* and jugular vein *(J)* are visualized in their respective canals. Note the white lines representing the lateral cortical plate of the carotid canal *(arrow)* and the lateral cortical plate of the jugular foramen *(arrowhead)*.

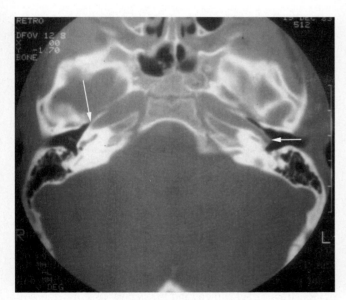

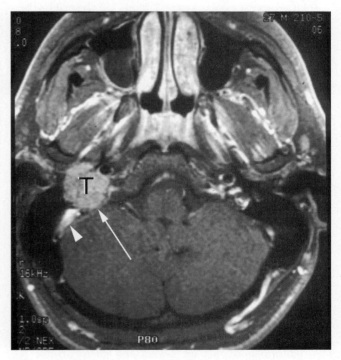

FIG. 4.8 Aberrant carotid artery, axial CT. The carotid artery on the left side *(short white arrow)* extends into the middle ear lateral to the cochlea. At this point it would be visualized through the tympanic membrane as a red mass. Note the position of the carotid canal on the opposite side *(long arrow)*.

FIG. 4.10 Glomus jugulare, MR T$_1$-weighted image after intravenous contrast. The tumor *(T)* is visualized in the region of the jugular foramen. Its interface *(arrow)* with the posterior fossa is clearly defined. The bright signal *(arrowhead)* in the sigmoid sinus represents slow flow of blood with gadolinium. The margins of the lesion can be clearly seen, though the bony landmarks cannot.

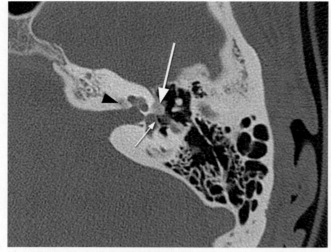

A

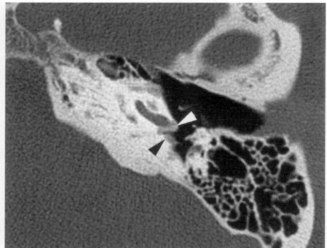

B

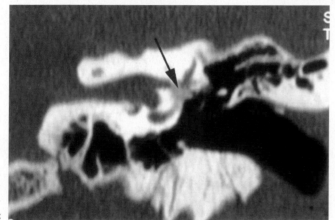

C

FIG. 4.11 Otosclerosis, multidetector CT. **A:** Axial scan at the level of the oval window shows the typical focus of demineralized bone *(large white arrow)*. The location is immediately anterior to the oval window. The bone is slightly enlarged and impinges on the stapes footplate *(small white arrow)*. Note the small area of demineralized bone *(black arrowhead)* just medial to the basal turn of the cochlea. **B:** Axial scan just inferior to **(A)** (level of the oval window). The bone along the margins *(arrowheads)* of the round window niche is demineralized and narrows the niche. **C:** Coronal reformatted image shows the demineralized focus of bone *(arrow)* just anterior to the oval window.

margin of the oval window (Fig. 4.11). On CT this area should be the same density as the remainder of the otic capsule. With fenestral otosclerosis, this area is slightly gray rather than the normal white of the otic capsule. Slight enlargement of the bone may impinge on the oval window. In retrofenestral or cochlear otosclerosis, the "graying" of the otic capsule is seen surrounding all or a portion of the cochlea (Fig. 4.12). The lucent area may abut the lumen or may be separated from it by a remaining thin, dense line.

Congenital Malformation

Congenital malformations of the ear are usually assessed using a bone algorithm CT (4). Computed tomography can detect malformations that are severe enough to involve the bone. Malformations that only affect the membranous labyrinth are not detected.

Cochlear malformations detectable by CT include segmentation anomalies and microcochlea (dwarf cochlea). Segmentation anomalies include the classic Mondini, in which the basilar turn is normal but the upper turns are represented by a single open sac (Fig. 4.13). Other variations include a small budlike diverticulum arising from the vestibule with an abnormal basal turn. A good landmark for

identifying these anomalies is the separation of the second and apical turn in the axial plane (Fig. 4.14). If this thin crest of bone is present, then these dilational anomalies are not present. Recently, more minor modiolar deficiencies have been described, with slight dilation of the second turn of the cochlea (12–14). In the microcochlea the segmentation is complete but all structures or turns are small.

Identification of a normal horizontal semicircular canal is good evidence that there is no severe anomaly of the vestibule or semicircular canals. The horizontal canal is the last formed and therefore is the most likely to be abnormal in congenital malformations of the peripheral vestibular system. The width of the lumen and the bone core or hub of the canal provide important information. Most anomalies will demonstrate larger lumen, and the central osseous hub will be smaller or absent. The canal may be represented by a saccular remnant or pouch (Fig. 4.15).

An enlarged vestibular aqueduct is one of the more common anomalies of the labyrinth. In the axial plane the aqueduct should be the same size or smaller than the contiguous posterior semicircular canal (Fig. 4.16).

Computed tomography has been the usual method of assessment of patients with a potential anomaly of the inner ear. As MRI achieves higher resolution, some doctors have

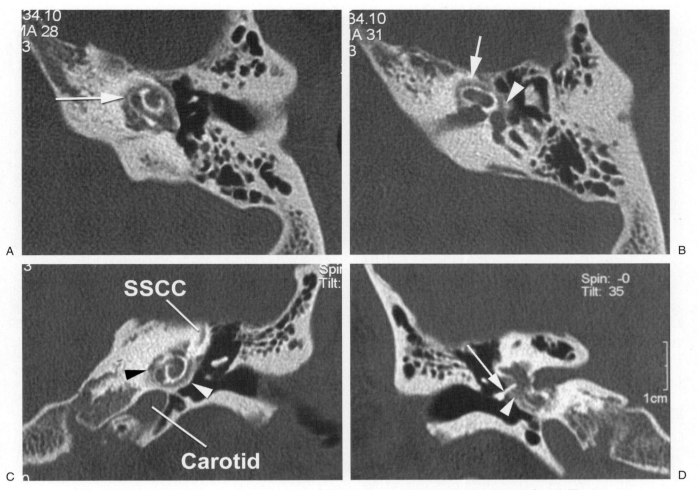

FIG. 4.12 Otosclerosis (severe), multidetector CT. **A:** Axial scan through the cochlea (left ear). The bone of the otic capsule bordering the cochlea is severely demineralized *(arrow)*. **B:** Axial scan slightly more superior than **(A)**. There is demineralization *(arrow)* of the otic capsule. Demineralization is also present *(arrowhead)* just anterior to the oval window. **C:** Coronal reformatted image *(left ear)* shows the demineralized bone *(arrowheads)* surrounding the cochlea. SSCC, superior semicircular canal. **D:** Coronal reformatted image of the opposite *(right)* side shows the position of a stapes prosthesis *(arrow)* projecting into the oval window. Note the enlarged demineralized bone *(arrowhead)* impinging on the window.

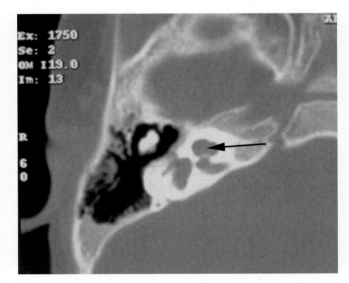

FIG. 4.13 Mondini malformation, axial CT. There is a cystic dilation of the cochlear turns with no obvious modiolus in the central area *(arrow)*. Compare with Figure 4.14.

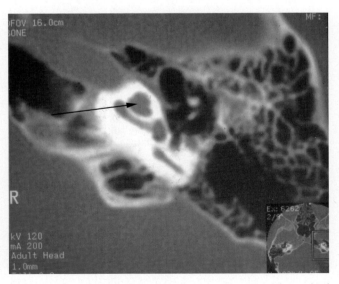

FIG. 4.14 Axial CT shows the bony separation *(arrow)* of second and third turns in the cochlea.

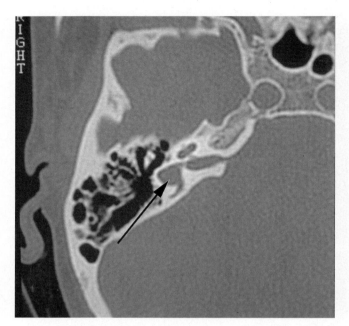

FIG. 4.15 Dilation abnormality of the horizontal semicircular canal. The horizontal semicircular canal is represented by a saclike dilation without evidence of a central core *(arrow)*. Compare with Figure 4.16.

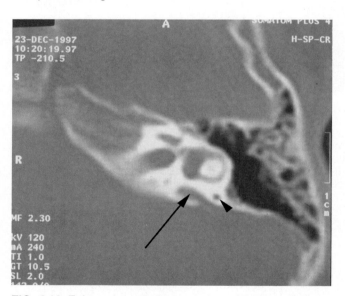

FIG. 4.16 Enlarged vestibular aqueduct, CT. The vestibular aqueduct *(arrow)* is widened. It is larger than the posterior semicircular canal *(arrowhead)*. Note the central core of the normal horizontal semicircular canal.

been using newer sequences to assess these patients (15). Magnetic resonance imaging can visualize the fluid spaces of the inner ear. Subtle changes in the configuration of the modiolus have been described (14). The ability to visualize the actual fluid spaces instead of the bony walls allows visualization of the endolymphatic sac rather than the vestibular aqueduct. Much of the enlargement of the sac may be extraosseous, lying between the leaves of the dura and thus not seen as completely on CT (Fig. 4.17). As further improve-

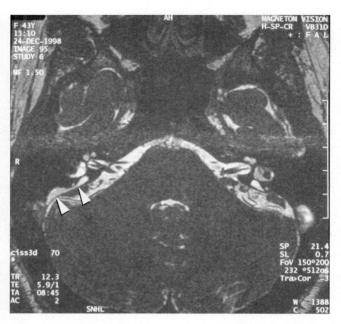

FIG. 4.17 Dilated vestibular aqueduct on MR. Heavily T_2-weighted image shows the extraosseous endolymphatic sac *(arrowheads)* extending beyond the confines of the vestibular aqueduct into the dura. There is also enlargement of the vestibular aqueduct on the opposite side. Note the good visibility of the nerves within the internal auditory canal.

ments are achieved, MRI may become the preferred modality. However, sedation, often necessary for the pediatric patient, is more of a problem with MRI than with CT.

Superior Semicircular Canal Syndrome

Recent descriptions of Tullio's phenomenon (vertigo with loud sound or pressure) related to a bony defect over the superior semicircular canal are best demonstrated by thin section CT (16,17). Multidetector CT scanning with oblique reformatted images is done in a plane perpendicular and parallel to that of the canal, allowing visualization of small defects in the bone (Fig. 4.18).

Labyrinthitis Ossificans

Labyrinthitis ossificans is a bony replacement of the normal fluids of the labyrinth. The lower, soft tissue CT density is obliterated by bone density or the high T_2 MRI signal of fluid is replaced by lower signal or even a signal void. Early change with incomplete replacement or fibrous obliteration may show the outline of the osseous labyrinth. Magnetic resonance imaging is probably more sensitive in demonstrating earlier fibrous obliteration. More attention is focusing on this evaluation as cochlear implants become more common.

Internal Auditory Canal

Magnetic resonance imaging is the clear choice for imaging of the internal auditory canal and contained neural elements.

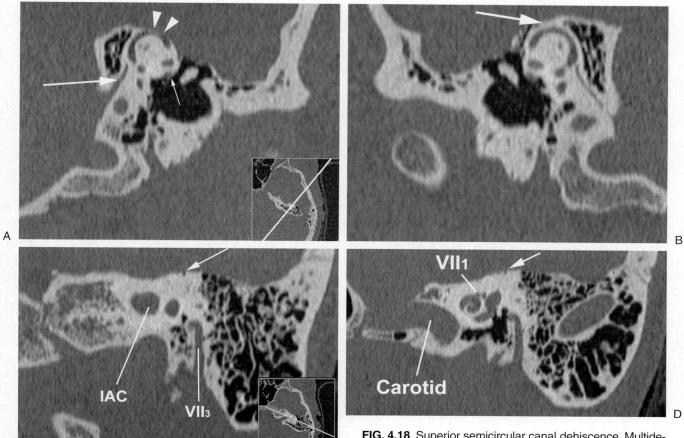

FIG. 4.18 Superior semicircular canal dehiscence. Multidetector CT with oblique reformatted images. The patient had vertigo and abnormal eye movement with loud noise on the left side. **A:** Abnormal side *(left)*. Reformatted image in plane perpendicular to the axis of the petrous apex (see inset). This plane is parallel to the plane of the superior semicircular canal. The bone separating the lumen of the canal from the middle cranial fossa is dehiscent *(arrowheads)*. Compare with the normal left side in **(B)**. Vestibular aqueduct *(large arrow)*. Facial nerve canal *(small arrow)* passing just inferior to the lateral semicircular canal. **B:** Normal side *(right)*. The bone *(arrow)* covering the superior semicircular canal is normal in thickness. **C:** Abnormal side *(left)*. Reformatted image in plane parallel to the axis of the petrous bone (see inset). This plane is perpendicular to that of the superior semicircular canal and shows the canal in cross-section. The image shows the defect in the bone covering the canal *(arrow)*. Compare with the normal side shown in **(E)**. IAC, internal auditory canal **(D)**. VII$_3$, facial nerve canal, third or mastoid segment. **D:** Reformatted image parallel but just anterolateral to **(C)** demonstrates the defect *(arrow)* in the thin bone. VII$_2$, facial nerve canal, tympanic segment. **E:** Oblique reformatted image of the opposite normal side shows the normal bone *(arrow)* covering the canal. This image is taken along the plane of the petrous apex as were **(C)** and **(D)**.

Magnetic resonance imaging can differentiate various soft tissues and fluids and is therefore ideal for this assessment. Gadolinium-enhanced MRI is thought to approach 100% sensitivity (Fig. 4.19). Missing a vestibular schwannoma (acoustic neuroma) is extremely unlikely.

Newer sequences may obviate the need for gadolinium because the nerves themselves are precisely outlined (Figs. 4.17 and 4.19) (18–22). High resolution T$_2$-weighted imaging can follow the nerves from the brainstem to the exit point in the lateral fundus of the internal auditory canal. A

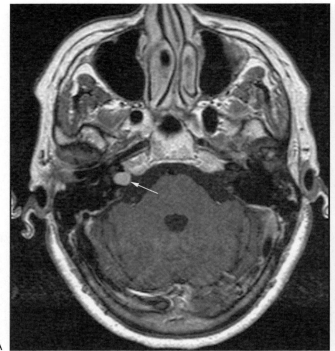

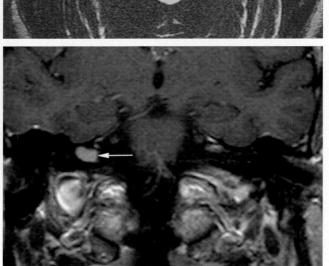

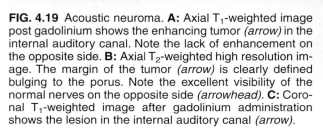

FIG. 4.19 Acoustic neuroma. **A:** Axial T₁-weighted image post gadolinium shows the enhancing tumor *(arrow)* in the internal auditory canal. Note the lack of enhancement on the opposite side. **B:** Axial T₂-weighted high resolution image. The margin of the tumor *(arrow)* is clearly defined bulging to the porus. Note the excellent visibility of the normal nerves on the opposite side *(arrowhead)*. **C:** Coronal T₁-weighted image after gadolinium administration shows the lesion in the internal auditory canal *(arrow)*.

schwannoma produces an enlargement of the nerve. Demonstration of the nerve without an enlargement is an effective method of ruling out a tumor. This method will identify almost all tumors and would represent a cheaper screening method, saving the cost of the gadolinium. However, caution must be exercised, and if all nerves are not clearly seen, gadolinium should be given (Fig. 4.20). Optimal visualization of the nerves may require multiplanar reformatting of the T₂ sequence. The sagittal or sagittal oblique plane is particularly helpful.

The gadolinium-enhanced T₁-weighted sequence remains the gold standard even as the high resolution T₂ sequence continues to improve. The gadolinium-enhanced examination is not perfect, and false positives are possible. Minor inflammation or small vessels can create enhancement mimicking very small schwannomas. In cases where the lesion is not absolutely definite the patient is followed by repeated imaging until the lesion declares itself as a tumor or as inflammation or anatomic variation.

Other lesions can occur in the internal auditory canal. Hemangiomas will enhance. Lipomas are bright prior to contrast. If a lesion is seen as bright after contrast injection, comparison must be made with a nonenhanced scan or a fat-suppressed sequence should be done. Otherwise, a lipoma

cannot be differentiated from a schwannoma. In the cerebellopontine angle, cistern epidermoids follow CSF closely and do not enhance. Diffusion-weighted images may help separate the epidermoid from the contiguous CSF and differentiate the lesion from an arachnoid cyst.

Petrous Apex

The petrous apex can be thought of as a block of bone perforated by air cells (23). The carotid artery passes through the petrous apex. If one can place a lesion in the petrous apex separate from the contiguous structures of the jugular foramen, internal auditory canal, facial nerve, and otic capsule, then the diagnostic possibilities are relatively few. Most disease relates to either the bone or to an air cell.

Cholesterol cyst or granuloma arises in a cell of the petrous apex that is usually well aerated. Usually the other areas of the temporal bone have an extensive air cell system as well. The cholesterol cyst has a very characteristic appearance on MRI (Fig. 4.21). The expanded air cell has high signal (bright or white) on both T₁ and T₂. This reflects blood products found within the lesion. Often there are also small areas of very low signal (dark or black) thought to represent hemosiderin, another breakdown product of blood.

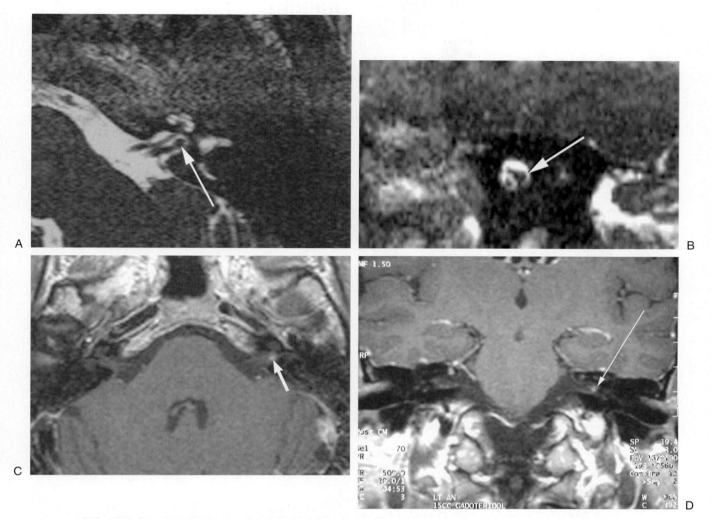

FIG. 4.20 Small acoustic neuroma. **A:** High resolution T$_2$-weighted image shows a very small nodule *(arrow)* on the vestibular nerve. **B:** Sagittal reformatted image through the three-dimensional data set shows the enlargement *(arrow)* of the vestibular nerve. This is posterior to the facial and cochlear nerves. The lesion appears to arise from the superior vestibular nerve. **C:** Post gadolinium T$_1$-weighted image shows the enhancing small tumor *(arrow)*. **D:** Coronal T$_1$-weighted postcontrast image shows the enhancing tumor *(arrow)* in the fundus of the internal auditory canal.

Computed tomography shows an expansile mass with relatively low density (Fig. 4.22). This may be difficult to differentiate from an epidermoid of the petrous apex (see below), giving MRI the advantage.

A mature cholesterol cyst is relatively easy to diagnose because of the very characteristic findings. However, obstruction of the air cells can produce a spectrum of pathology ranging from an opacified but unexpanded air cell through slight expansion to a true mature cholesterol cyst. Indeed, many cases come to the otologist because of a questioned abnormality on the MRI done for headache. Abnormal signal is seen in the petrous apex, and the otologist is asked to evaluate the significance and possible relationship to the patient's symptoms. Here CT can be helpful. If the apex in question shows a pattern of normal air cell development with intact septations and with no internal erosion, then the abnormality is probably a simple effusion or fluid in an air cell. One may elect to follow unless

the patient's symptoms argue strongly for intervention. Computed tomography is then used (at our institution) for follow-up scans to look for subtle remodeling suggesting early expansion (Fig. 4.23). If there is remodeling of bone, the lesion is deemed to possess expansile potential and is approaching the status of mature cholesterol cyst.

When a cholesterol cyst is diagnosed, CT is usually performed, even if the diagnosis is definite by MRI. The radiologist must define the exact position and integrity of the carotid canal to exclude an aneurysm and to warn the surgeon of possible erosion of the carotid canal by expansion (Fig. 4.22). Computed tomography also identifies the most likely air cell tract responsible for the cyst. This often defines the best surgical approach.

An epidermoid or congenital cholesteatoma has an appearance quite similar to that of a cholesterol cyst. On CT an epidermoid may be slightly more lobulated than a cholesterol cyst, appearing to have small podlike extensions,

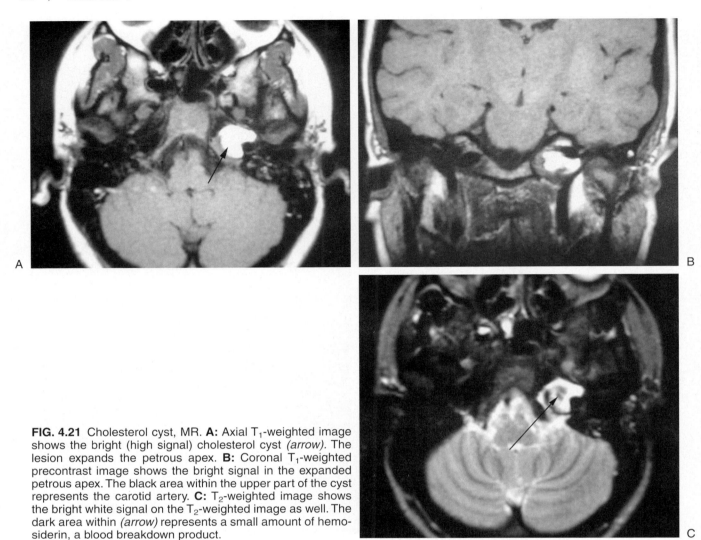

FIG. 4.21 Cholesterol cyst, MR. **A:** Axial T_1-weighted image shows the bright (high signal) cholesterol cyst *(arrow)*. The lesion expands the petrous apex. **B:** Coronal T_1-weighted precontrast image shows the bright signal in the expanded petrous apex. The black area within the upper part of the cyst represents the carotid artery. **C:** T_2-weighted image shows the bright white signal on the T_2-weighted image as well. The dark area within *(arrow)* represents a small amount of hemosiderin, a blood breakdown product.

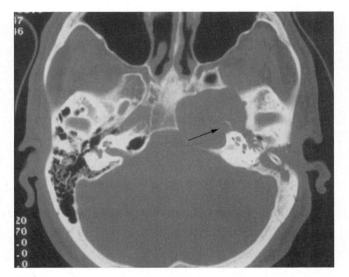

FIG. 4.22 Cholesterol cyst, CT. The expansile abnormality of the petrous apex skeletonizes and partially erodes the carotid canal *(arrow)*. The patient has undergone several attempts to drain this cholesterol cyst.

perhaps along lines of least resistance (Fig. 4.24). The differentiation of a cholesterol cyst from an epidermoid is best made on MRI. On MRI T_1-weighted images the epidermoid is dark (Fig. 4.25), and the cholesterol cyst is bright. This is considered to be a reliable differentiating point. There is slight overlap. Rare epidermoids have been reported as bright on T_1, and an obstructed air cell may simply fill with fluid, giving a dark signal on T_1. The variability in signal of obstructed petrous air cells is analogous to obstruction and mucocele formation in the paranasal sinuses. The contents can have virtually any signal combination on T_1 and T_2 images, depending on the amount of protein or hemorrhage present. Indeed, obstructed and slightly expanded air cells with low T_1 signal have been reported as mucoceles. Though some ambiguity remains, the diagnosis can usually be made.

A petrous carotid aneurysm, though rare, must be excluded whenever there is an expansile abnormality of the petrous apex (Fig. 4.26). An aneurysm can have an appearance similar to that of a cholesterol cyst. T_2 images usually show more blood products with lower signal on T_2.

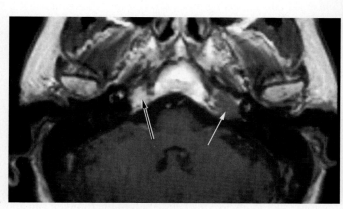

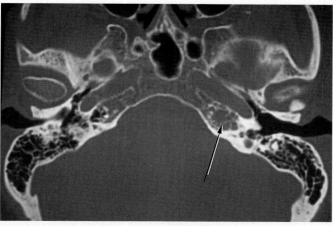

A   B

FIG. 4.23 Fluid in petrous apex air cells. **A:** Axial MR postcontrast. The area of abnormality *(white arrow)* is visualized in the left petrous apex. There is no definite expansion. The area of high signal on the opposite side *(black-on-white arrow)* represents normal fat. **B:** Axial CT shows the opacification of the petrous apex air cells *(arrow)*. There is slight sclerosis of the septations but no obvious destruction and no expansion. This represented a simple effusion in the petrous apex air cells.

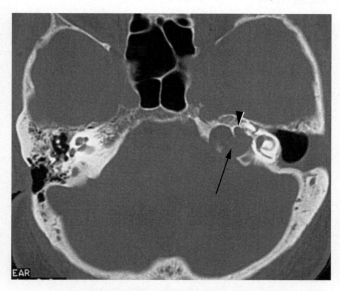

FIG. 4.24 Epidermoid (cholesteatoma) of the petrous apex. There is an expansile lesion of the petrous apex *(arrow)*. Note the slightly lobulated *(arrowhead)* appearance of the margin. The patient has had a mastoidectomy on the left and a mastoidotomy on the right.

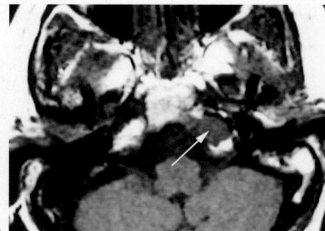

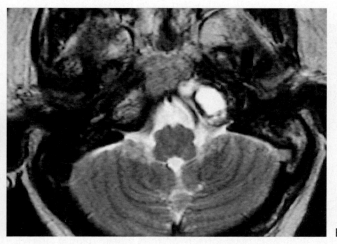

A   B

FIG. 4.25 Epidermoid of the petrous apex, MR. **A:** Axial T$_1$-weighted image shows an intermediate to low signal abnormality *(arrow)* expanding the petrous apex. **B:** The abnormality has high signal on T$_2$-weighted image.

A thrombus may have a laminated appearance, and a flow void of the residual lumen may be visualized. Unless the aneurysm is completely thrombosed, there will be a change in appearance after contrast where part of the aneurysm will usually become brighter. This does not happen in epidermoid nor in a cholesterol cyst. These latter two lesions represent avascular spaces, and the internal portions do not change with contrast.

A meningocele or arachnoid cyst can also form in the petrous apex. These CSF-filled cavities usually fill from the region of the middle cranial fossa, often from the region of Meckel's cave. Small bone defects or free communications through a sizable gap are detected on CT scan.

The previously described lesions, with the exception of the carotid aneurysm, are avascular spaces and do not enhance. If the bulk of a lesion does enhance, a tumor is suspected. A metastasis is considered. Primary bone tumors are rare in this area.

In other areas of the petrous bone, location is a strong determinant in predicting a likely histology. In the petroclival synchondrosis a chondroid lesion such as a low-grade chondrosarcoma is the most likely diagnosis. It may or may not have chondroid matrix identifiable on CT and is usually bright (high signal) on T_2 MRI. A lesion appearing to arise from the surface of the bone is likely a meningioma, though various granulomatous diseases as well as metastasis must be considered. With meningioma, there is usually a "dural tail" with bright enhancement extending away from the obvious mass for a variable distance. This lesion is suspected particularly when there is hyperostosis of the contiguous bone. An adenomatous tumor arising from the endolymphatic sac is considered in lesions arising just medial to the posterior semicircular canal. This lesion is destructive and usually contains hemorrhage.

The jugular fossa is seldom investigated as an isolated entity. Most glomus tumors present because of symptoms related to the middle ear. Occasionally a lesion may be seen incidentally in the area of the jugular fossa or may be detected in an evaluation for vocal cord paralysis. In such an evalua-

tion, one is more commonly trying to exclude a tumor rather than actually expecting to see one. Demonstration of a small protrusion of CSF density on CT or signal intensity on MRI is good evidence that there is no tumor in the neural compartment of the foramen. The vascular segment of the foramen is often difficult to evaluate on MRI because of flow artifacts. The integrity of the lateral bony wall or jugular plate is very reassuring, because tumors do not actually arise from the vascular portion of foramen itself but rather from the margin.

If a lesion is detected, then schwannoma must be differentiated from a paraganglioma. Tumors arising from the nerves in the jugular foramen (Fig. 4.27) enlarge the medial aspect of the foramen and have a smooth expanded margin. The cortex of the bone is usually preserved. The paraganglioma should involve the lateral part of the foramen and appears to smudge the bone rather than smoothly expand it. Occasionally a glomus vagale can extend superiorly and will pass through the medial foramen.

Facial Nerve

In classic Bell's palsy with rapid onset of paralysis, imaging is often considered unnecessary. Imaging may be done if there is anything atypical about the presentation or if a more central lesion is suspected.

In cases of facial paralysis the principal goal is to exclude tumor either in the temporal bone or more centrally. Imaging should include the brain, emphasizing the brainstem and temporal bone, but continue inferiorly to include the stylomastoid foramen and parotid gland. Any distortion of the anatomy must be considered questionable. Enhancement of the nerve is typical in a patient with Bell's palsy. However, the canal should not enlarge. With modern imaging, the resolution is now such that the size of an enhancing nerve can be judged (Fig. 4.28). In questionable cases, CT can be done

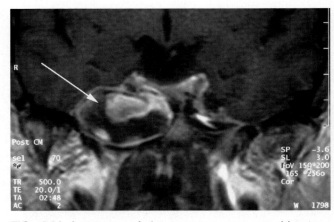

FIG. 4.26 Aneurysm of the petrous apex, carotid artery. Coronal post gadolinium T_1-weighted image shows the expanded abnormality *(arrow)* containing a variable amount of blood product. There is some enhancement seen representing flow in a residual lumen.

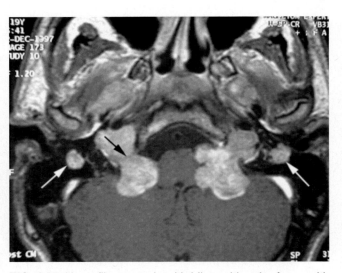

FIG. 4.27 Neurofibromatosis with bilateral jugular fossa with tumors of jugular foramen and facial nerve. Bilateral lesions extend through the medial portion of the jugular foramen. Note the constriction *(black arrow)* as the tumor squeezes through the narrow opening. There is expansion. Note the enlarged facial nerves *(white arrows)* as well.

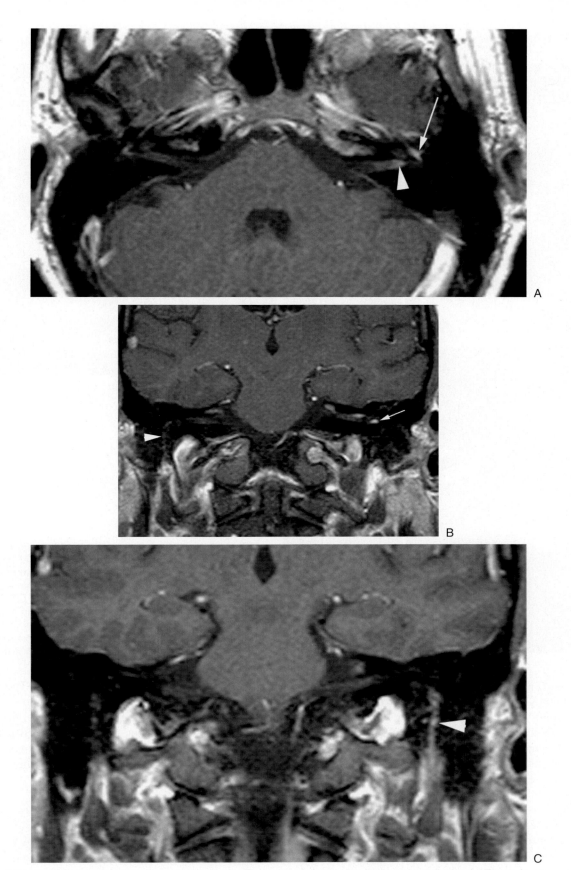

FIG. 4.28 Schwannoma of the facial nerve. The patient has a facial nerve paralysis. **A:** There is enhancement of the anterior tympanic facial nerve *(arrow)* and enhancement in the fundus of the internal auditory canal *(arrowhead)*. **B:** Coronal T1-weighted post gadolinium image. There is enhancement of the tympanic segment of the facial nerve canal *(arrow)*, as well as enhancement within the internal auditory canal. The tympanic segment appears to be slightly enlarged *(arrowhead)*. **C:** There is enhancement of the vertical mastoid segment of the facial nerve canal *(arrowhead)*. It does not appear to be enlarged.

(continued)

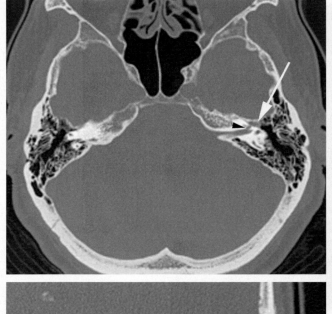

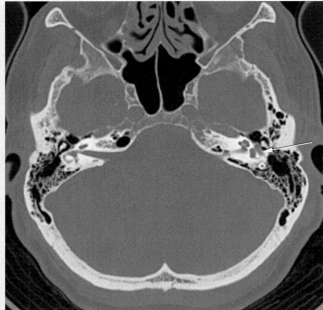

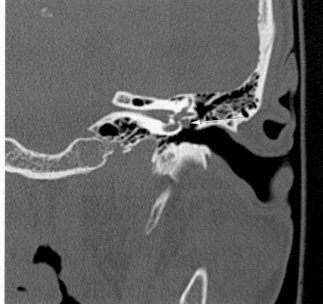

FIG. 4.28, cont'd. Schwannoma of the facial nerve. The patient has a facial nerve paralysis. **D:** Axial bone algorithm CT shows expansion of the anterior tympanic facial nerve canal *(white arrow)*. The labyrinthine segment *(black arrowhead)* is borderline. **E:** Axial CT. There is slight but definite expansion of the tympanic segment of the facial nerve canal *(black-and-white arrow)*. **F:** Coronal image shows the tumor *(black-and-white arrow)* protruding downward from the facial nerve canal into the oval window.

to better assess for any slight enlargement of the canal suggesting tumor. Of note, the segment of the nerve within the internal auditory canal may enlarge in Bell's palsy; this should not be mistaken for a tumor (24). When enlargement is seen in this area, most radiologists recommend a follow-up exam to confirm temporal stability or regression.

If there is a suggestion of enlargement or abnormal enhancement in the region of the facial canal, then high-resolution CT is done to better evaluate the bony architecture. A facial schwannoma will gradually expand the canal (Fig. 4.28), whereas a hemangioma may give a more irregular appearance of the contiguous bone. Perineural spread of malignant tumor can mimic a facial schwannoma with gradual enlargement of the canal. Usually tumor of the parotid is clinically obvious before perineural spread occurs, but this area should be checked.

Finally the facial nerve can be aberrant. The nerve may bulge out of a dehiscent canal, or it may follow an abnormal course. The horizontal segment of the facial nerve may be displaced inferiorly, lying against the superstructure of the stapes, or even pass inferior to the oval window over the promontory. In every case the facial nerve should be identified and its position verified.

SUMMARY

Imaging of the temporal bone is best done by CT and MRI. The first choice of imaging modality or technique of examination may vary among radiologists. The clinical history is extremely important if the examination is to be targeted appropriately. In general, middle ear and mastoid are first imaged with CT; the internal auditory canal is imaged with

MRI. The inner ear may be imaged with either. Magnetic resonance imaging is more specific than CT in the petrous apex. However, few studies are directed specifically at the petrous apex unless a finding is discovered on MRI done for headache or some unrelated reason. In this case, CT can provide important information.

REFERENCES

1. Som PM, Curtin HD. *Head and Neck Imaging,* 3rd ed. St. Louis: Mosby, 1996.
2. Swartz JD, Harnsberger HR. *Imaging of the Temporal Bone,* 3rd ed. New York: Thieme, 1997.
3. Valvassori GE, Mafee MF, Carter BL, et al. *Imaging of the Head and Neck.* Stuttgart, Germany/New York, New York: G. Thieme Verlag, Thieme Medical Publishers, 1995.
4. Fisher NA, Curtin HD. Radiology of congenital hearing loss. *Otolaryngol Clin North Am* 1994;27(3):511–531.
5. Swartz JD, Faerber EN. Congenital malformations of the external and middle ear: high-resolution CT findings of surgical import. *AJR Am J Roentgenol* 1985;144(3):501–506.
6. Yeakley JW, Jahrsdoerfer RA. CT evaluation of congenital aural atresia: what the radiologist and surgeon need to know. *J Comput Assist Tomogr* 1996;20(5):724–731.
7. Curtin HD, Wolfe P, May M. Malignant external otitis: CT evaluation. *Radiology* 1982;145(2):383–388.
8. Grandis JR, Curtin HD, Yu VL. Necrotizing (malignant) external otitis: prospective comparison of CT and MR imaging in diagnosis and follow-up. *Radiology* 1995;196(2):499–504.
9. Curtin HD. Radiologic approach to paragangliomas of the temporal bone. *Radiology* 1984;150(3):837–838.
10. Lo WW, Solti-Bohman LG, McElveen JT Jr. Aberrant carotid artery: radiologic diagnosis with emphasis on high-resolution computed tomography. *Radiographics* 1985;5(6):985–993.
11. Lo WML, Solti-Bohman LG. Vascular Tinnitus. In: Som PM, Curtin HD, eds. *Head and Neck Imaging,* 3rd ed, vol 2. St. Louis: Mosby, 1996:1535.
12. Lemmerling MM, Mancuso AA, Antonelli PJ, et al. Normal modiolus: CT appearance in patients with a large vestibular aqueduct. *Radiology* 1997;204(1):213–219.
13. Antonelli PJ, Nall AV, Lemmerling MM, et al. Hearing loss with cochlear modiolar defects and large vestibular aqueducts. *Am J Otol* 1998;19(3):306–312.
14. Davidson HC, Harnsberger HR, Lemmerling MM, et al. MR evaluation of vestibulocochlear anomalies associated with large endolymphatic duct and sac. *AJNR Am J Neuroradiol* 1999;20(8):1435–1441.
15. Casselman JW, Kuhweide R, Ampe W, et al. Pathology of the membranous labyrinth: comparison of T1- and T2-weighted and gadolinium-enhanced spin-echo and 3DFT-CISS imaging. *AJNR Am J Neuroradiol* 1993;14(1):59–69.
16. Minor LB, Solomon D, Zinreich JS, et al: Sound- and/or pressure-induced vertigo due to bone dehiscence of the superior semicircular canal. *Arch Otolaryngol Head Neck Surg* 1998;124(3):249–258.
17. Mong A, Loevner LA, Solomon D, et al: Sound- and pressure-induced vertigo associated with dehiscence of the roof of the superior semicircular canal. *AJNR Am J Neuroradiol* 1999;20(10):1973–1975.
18. Allen RW, Harnsberger HR, Shelton C, et al. Low-cost high-resolution fast spin-echo MR of acoustic schwannoma: an alternative to enhanced conventional spin-echo MR? *AJNR Am J Neuroradiol* 1996;17(7):1205–1210.
19. Daniels RL, Shelton C, Harnsberger HR. Ultra high resolution nonenhanced fast spin echo magnetic resonance imaging: cost-effective screening for acoustic neuroma in patients with sudden sensorineural hearing loss. *Otolaryngol Head Neck Surg* 1998;119(4):364–369.
20. Fukui MB, Weissman JL, Curtin HD, et al. T2-weighted MR characteristics of internal auditory canal masses. *AJNR Am J Neuroradiol* 1996;17(7):1211–1218.
21. Schmalbrock P, Chakeres DW, Monroe JW, et al. Assessment of internal auditory canal tumors: a comparison of contrast-enhanced T1-weighted and steady-state T2-weighted gradient-echo MR imaging. *AJNR Am J Neuroradiol* 1999;20(7):1207–1213.
22. Stuckey SL, Harris AJ, Mannolini SM. Detection of acoustic schwannoma: use of constructive interference in the steady state three-dimensional MR. *AJNR Am J Neuroradiol* 1996;17(7):1219–1225.
23. Curtin HD, Som PM. The petrous apex. *Otolaryngol Clin North Am* 1995;28(3):473–496.
24. Brandle P, Satoretti-Schefer S, Bohmer A, et al: Correlation of MRI, clinical, and electroneuronographic findings in acute facial nerve palsy. *Am J Otol* 1996;17(1):154–161.

CHAPTER 5

Evaluation of the Vestibular System

Conrad Wall III, Richard F. Lewis, and Steven D. Rauch

A basic understanding of the vestibular system is essential to the otologist, who is often called upon to evaluate symptoms of dizziness. Such symptoms may or may not be manifestations of ear disease. The otologist's first task is to determine if the patient's symptoms are otologic. Symptoms that involve a prominent illusory feeling of motion of oneself or the environment are particularly suggestive of a vestibular abnormality and can include a sense of rotation (most commonly), linear motion, or tilting. Symptoms of imbalance and dysequilibrium can be vestibular in origin, particularly if they are associated with illusory movement of the visual world (oscillopsia), but can also result from many types of neurologic disorders such as Parkinson's disease or cerebellar degeneration. Presyncopal symptoms, typically described as lightheadedness, are rarely due to vestibular dysfunction and usually result from insufficient cerebral perfusion. Finally, symptoms that are primarily cognitive, often described as a "foggy" or "remote" sensation, are unlikely to be vestibular and often result from anxiety, hyperventilation, or related disorders.

Only a limited number of vestibulopathies are managed surgically, and these surgical approaches can be divided into two categories: procedures that correct a specific pathologic abnormality and ablative procedures that eliminate fluctuations in vestibular function. The former category includes perilymph fistula surgery, canal plugging for superior canal dehiscence or intractable benign positional vertigo, endolymphatic shunting for Meniere's disease, acoustic neuroma resection, and, possibly, microvascular decompression of the eighth cranial nerve. The latter category includes labyrinthectomy, vestibular (or ampullary) nerve section, and gentamicin labyrinthectomy. The indications for these different procedures are discussed elsewhere in this volume. It should be stressed that ablative procedures should only be considered when there is clear evidence of spontaneous fluctuations in vestibular function, because their purpose is to eliminate these fluctuations and thereby promote central compensation. Symptoms of vestibular insufficiency, such as transient dizziness and imbalance provoked by rapid head motion or visual stimulation, reflect physiologic activation of a static vestibular deficit and hence are not an indication for an ablative procedure.

This chapter is divided into three sections. First, we present an overview of the organization and function of the vestibular system, relating these features to common vestibular symptoms. We then summarize the methods used during the physical examination to assess the patient with vestibular symptomatology. Finally, we describe the different types of quantitative vestibular testing and indicate how vestibular testing can aid in diagnosis and surgical decision making.

ORGANIZATION AND FUNCTION OF THE VESTIBULAR SYSTEM

The vestibular system senses head motion and orientation (with respect to gravity) and provides information to the brain that is used to stabilize images on the retina and to maintain balance and spatial orientation. Because humans make complex motions in a three-dimensional world, five sensors in each inner ear are required to accurately measure these movements. The three semicircular canals (superior, posterior, and lateral) detect angular acceleration, whereas the two otolith organs (saccule and utricle) detect linear acceleration and gravity. Each sensor has its own bundle of nerve fibers that join to form one nerve before reaching the brain. Figure 5.1 shows the motion-detecting portion of a human left inner ear. Not shown are nerve fibers that attach to each of the five detectors and join together in a region near Scarpa's ganglion (SG) to form the vestibular portion of the eighth nerve. Each semicircular canal responds maxi-

Portions of this chapter were adapted from Wall III C. The sinusoidal harmonic acceleration rotary chair test: theoretical and clinical basis. In: Arenberg IK, ed. *Dizziness and Balance Disorders: An Interdisciplinary Approach to Diagnosis Treatment and Rehabilitation.* Amsterdam/New York: Kugler Publications, 1993:299–313; and Wall III C. Vestibular function and anatomy. In: Bailey BJ, Pillsbury HC, eds. *Head & Neck Surgery—Otolaryngology,* vol. 2. Philadelphia: J.B. Lippincott, 1993:1462–1472.

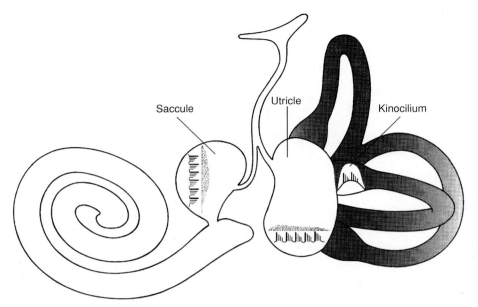

FIG. 5.1 Schematic drawing of the left inner ear. The kinocilium of the lateral semicircular canals adjacent to the utricle. Deflection of the kinocilium toward the utricle is called a utriculopetal deflection. When the kinocilium is bent away from the utricle, the deflection is utriculofugal. Note that the plane of the utricular macula is horizontal, whereas that of the saccular macula is vertical.

mally to head rotations that are in the plane of the canal. The three canals are aligned so that they are approximately perpendicular to each other. The two otolith organs are approximately planar and are mutually perpendicular. Each otolith organ has a multitude of sensors that are maximally sensitive to linear accelerations in the plane of the organ. The right and left inner ear structures are arranged as mirror images of each other.

The geometrical layout of the six semicircular canals is shown in Figure 5.2A and B. Both lateral semicircular canals lie in the same plane, which is tilted approximately 30 degrees from the horizontal and runs parallel to a line drawn between the external auditory canal and the outer canthus of the eye. The four vertical canals lie in planes that are roughly at right angles to the plane of the horizontal canal pair. The superior vertical canal on one side is nearly in the same plane as the posterior vertical canal on the other side. Thus the functional canal pairs are the right and left lateral canals, the right superior and the left posterior canals, and the right posterior and left superior semicircular canals. The neural signals from these pairs of canals converge in a synergistic way in the nervous system, which allows the system to function even in the case of a complete unilateral lesion. The otolith organs are paired in a similar way (Fig. 5.2C). The right and left utricles are in approximately the same plane as the right and left lateral semicircular canals. The right and left saccules are in a plane that is approximately perpendicular to the plane of the utricle.

For both the canals and otolith organs, head acceleration causes a microscopic deflection of one or more microscopic masses in the inner ear. The deflection of the mass relative to its support structure is detected by sensory hair cells, which

have their cell bodies attached to the support structure and their sensory hair bundles (stereocilia) connected to the mass. Motion of the head therefore causes deflection of these hair bundles, which in turn convert their microscopic displacements into electrical signals that are carried by nerve fibers to the brain. Inner ear disease or injury can break the chain of information transfer involving the masses, the hair cells, and the nerves. A malfunction of any element in this process will block the signal. Because there are many parallel transmission links, a significant fraction must be disabled for a true loss of useful sensory information to occur. Persons with this condition have severe vestibular hypofunction.

Semicircular Canals

In the semicircular canals the hair cells attach to the cupula, a gelatinous flap that completely seals one side of the widened region of the canal (the ampulla). The interior of the canal is filled by endolymph, a liquid with the density and viscosity of water. The membranous portion of the canal is attached to the temporal bone. When the head is turned, the membranous labyrinth moves with it, but the inertia of the endolymph tends to oppose the turning motion. This results in a pressure buildup across the cupula, which deflects it from its equilibrium position and bends the stereocilia of the hair cells, thereby transducing the head motion into a modulation of the firing rate of the vestibular nerve. For brief head movements, cupula distortion is proportional to head velocity, and the modulation of afferent activity in the vestibular nerve modulates with cupula distortion. Changes in the spontaneous firing rate of the vestibular nerve are

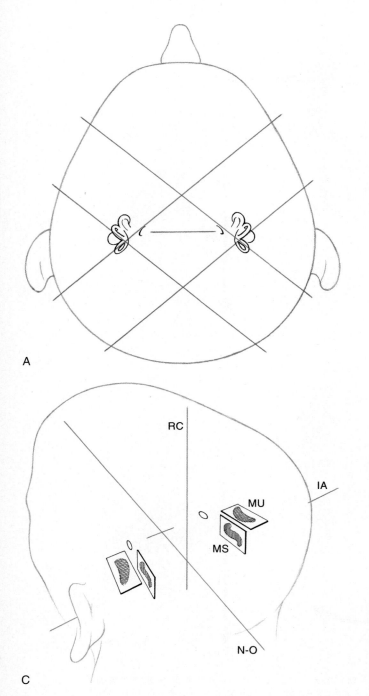

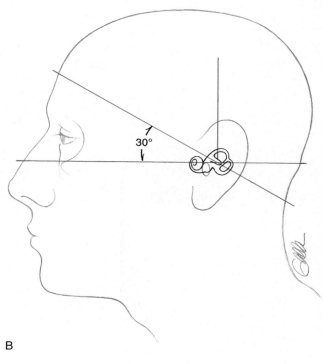

FIG. 5.2 A: Approximate layout of the anterior and posterior vertical semicircular canals. **B:** Approximate layout of the lateral semicircular canals. **C:** Approximate planar layout of the otolith organs. MS, macula sacculi; MU, macula utriculi; IA, interaural axis; N-O, nasal-occipital axis; RC, rostral-caudal axis.

therefore proportional to head velocity. Hence it is not surprising that changes in afferent activity appear closely related to subjective sensations of angular velocity (rotation), and to the velocity of the reflexive eye movements (nystagmus). For long-duration stimuli, such as those experienced while flying, dancing, or in clinical testing, the dynamics introduced by cupula distortion and by the transduction and encoding process become significant and often limit human performance.

Pairs of canals in opposite ears combine into one functional "canal plane." The six semicircular canals therefore combine into three functional canal planes, which are formed by the right and left lateral canals, the right superior and left posterior canals, and the left superior and right posterior canals. Angular rotation in any of these planes produces a maximum response from the two canals that are in that plane. The two canals in each plane operate in a push-pull manner such that a movement that maximally excites one member of a pair produces maximum inhibition in the other member of the pair (Fig. 5.3A and B).

Most vestibular afferents synapse on cells in the vestibular nucleus in the brainstem. The vestibular nucleus is in-

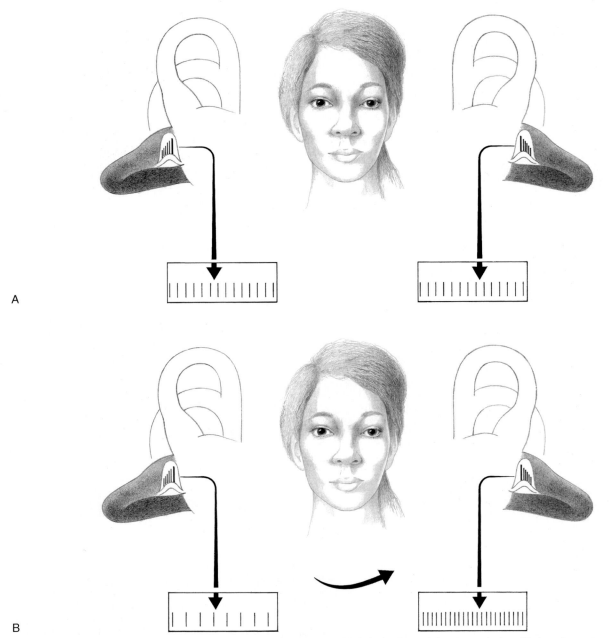

FIG. 5.3 A: Schematic representation of right and left lateral semicircular canals with head erect and stationary. The action potential discharge from each side is equal (90 spikes per second in mammals). **B:** Schematic representation during head rotation to the left. The action potential discharges are increased above the stationary baseline rate on the left side and decreased on the right side.

volved in the processing of both visual and vestibular information, and activity recorded from cells located there can differ markedly from afferent information received from the labyrinth. From the vestibular nucleus, multiple pathways have been identified that project to the cerebral cortex, the cerebellum, and the motor nuclei for the eye and skeletal muscles. The relationship among the vestibular system and the oculomotor and skeletal postural control systems is of particular interest in clinical evaluation.

The vestibuloocular reflex (VOR) stabilizes the images of visual objects on the retina by producing eye movements that are compensatory to the head movement. Thus a motion of the head at l0 degrees per second to the right would produce an eye movement of l0 degrees per second to the left (Fig. 5.4). Measurement of reflexive eye movements resulting from rotation and caloric (thermal) stimulation of the semicircular canals is the primary clinical means of evaluating the status of the human vestibular system, because nerve record-

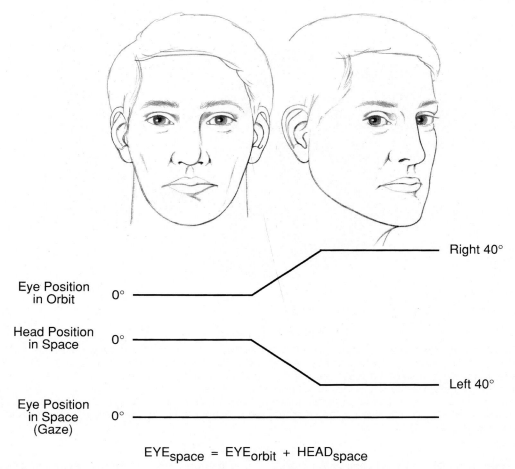

Eye Position in Orbit   0°

Right 40°

Head Position in Space   0°

Left 40°

Eye Position in Space (Gaze)   0°

$$EYE_{space} = EYE_{orbit} + HEAD_{space}$$

FIG. 5.4 The function of the vestibuloocular reflex. As the head is rapidly turned to the left, the eyes execute an arc of rotation equal and opposite to the head movements. Above, head position and eye position in orbit are plotted against time. Because the movements of the head and eye in orbit are equal and opposite the sum, eye position in space (gaze) remains zero *(bottom equation)*. Gaze is held steady; then images and the seen world do not slip on the retina and vision remains clear. (Redrawn from Andres RO, Anderson DJ. Design of a better postural measurement system. *Am J Otolaryngol* 1980;1: 197–206, with permission.)

ing is not feasible. During rotation, vestibular information reaches the motor nuclei of the eye muscles to produce compensatory eye movements, which aid in retinal image stabilization. When angular motions are large, the oculomotor system generates quick movements that recenter the eyes, resulting in the slow-quick, slow-quick motions of the eye that are called nystagmus (Greek *nystagmos,* "head nodding while drowsy"). By convention, nystagmus is said to "beat" in the direction of the fast phase. Nystagmic eye movements can also be elicited by visual stimulation, such as by watching a field of moving stripes (optokinetic nystagmus).

Otolith Organs

In the otolith organs (utricle and saccule), calcium carbonate crystals known as otoconia are embedded in a gelatinous supporting substrate called the otolithic membrane. Both linear acceleration and changes in the orientation of the head, with respect to gravity, shift the otolith membrane and distort the stereocilia of the hair cells that connect to the membrane. The arrangement of sensory hair cells in one otolith organ tends to be laid out in a roughly planar organization. These basic features are illustrated in a simplified diagram of an otolith organ, shown in Figure 5.5. In the diagram each of the sensory hair cells has a polarization vector with a small arrow indicating its direction of maximal excitation in the plane. The large arrow at the top of the otolithic mass represents a linear acceleration that deflects the otolith mass in the direction of the arrow. Thus the hair cells that have polarization vectors aligned with that arrow and in the same direction are excited maximally, whereas hair cells having polarization vectors that are at right angles to the acceleration are not stimulated at all. It is from an array of these hair cells that the brain is able to estimate the magnitude and direction of a linear acceleration. The right and left otolith organs, like semicircular canals, exhibit a mirror symmetry around the sagittal plane.

Utricular and saccular afferents project primarily to the inferior and medial vestibular nuclei. Secondary fibers then

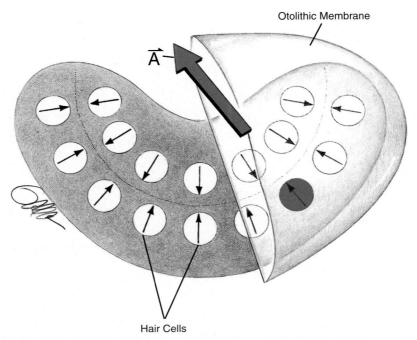

Otolithic Membrane

$\vec{A}$

Hair Cells

FIG. 5.5 A simplified otolith organ. The otolithic membrane is shown suspended above the sensory hair cells in an exploded view. Each hair cell is innervated by one afferent nerve fiber. These join together to form a branch of the vestibular nerve. Each hair cell is shown with a small arrow above it corresponding to the direction of its functional polarization vector. This arrow is always pointing in the direction of the kinocilium. The large arrow above the otolithic mass is a linear acceleration vector. The response of hair cells depends on the cosine of the direction between its polarization vector and the linear acceleration $(\vec{A})$.

carry the otolith information rostrally to ocular motor nuclei, cerebral cortex, and cerebellum and caudally to the spinal levels. Stimulation of the otoliths is known to produce compensatory eye movements. In the absence of rotational cues from the canals, lateral or vertical acceleration causes the eyes to deviate in a direction opposite to the acceleration (referred to as the linear VOR). In addition, head tilts around the nasooccipital axis produce a static torsional motion of the eyes in the opposite direction. These movements, called ocular counterrolling, have been used as an index of otolithic response.

Vestibular Compensation

How well the central vestibular and ocular motor systems readjust following a partial or total unilateral peripheral insult is an important factor of the recovery to several otologic medical and surgical treatments. Under normal conditions, with two intact ears, there is a near balance of tonic activity from the right and left vestibular nerves. This tonic activity bombards the vestibular nuclei, and the total activity available to drive the ocular motor system can be thought of as the difference in activity between the two sides. Under normal conditions, this difference is close to zero. A unilateral insult or lesion on one side tends to reduce the amount of tonic activity from that side and causes an imbalance that can result in spontaneous nystagmus and a subjective sense

of motion. This central nervous system has the potential of correcting the imbalance over time, but the degree of correction varies among individuals. Thus one criterion for "successful" treatment will depend upon the individual patient's ability to make the desired compensation. One approach to accelerate the compensation process is to use a rehabilitation protocol in which patients make voluntary movements of the body, head, and eyes as soon as it is practical after a treatment has been given. Although the vestibular end organs operate using the principle of mirror symmetry, explained previously, there is some evidence that suggests that even in cases of complete vestibular compensation the input from just one ear does not perfectly replace the function of two ears (1).

CLINICAL EXAMINATION

There are four principal components to the clinical examination of patients with vestibular disorders: (i) vestibular tone; (ii) vestibular gain; (iii) positional nystagmus; and (iv) nonvestibular oculomotor function. Vestibular tone is assessed by noting the presence of spontaneous nystagmus (i.e., nystagmus with the head upright and stationary and the eyes centered in the orbits). This should be evaluated in a lit room in the presence of visual fixation and with fixation removed (i.e., with Frenzel glasses). In general, unilateral peripheral vestibular deficits produce a mixed horizontal-torsional nystagmus, with slow phases directed toward the involved ear that are suppressed by visual fixation. In contrast, central vestibular disorders can produce a variety of nystagmoid eye movements (such as vertical or torsional) that are not suppressed by fixation. Central disorders only rarely result in a horizontal-torsional nystagmus that can mimic a peripheral lesion. If any spontaneous nystagmus is present, it typically will vary with orbital eye position, increasing in magnitude with gaze in the direction of the quick phases (Alexander's law). Vestibular tone asymmetry can be amplified by repetitively shaking the head side to side, which produces a horizontal nystagmus with slow phases directed toward the side of the lesion. With several vestibular disorders, a tone imbalance (and associated nystagmus) can be provoked by specific stimuli, such as Valsalva maneuvers (with perilymph fistula, canal dehiscence, or Chiari malformations); modification of pressure in the middle ear (Hennebert's sign, with perilymph fistula, canal dehiscence, or Meniere's disease); or hyperventilation (with central or peripheral demyelinative lesions such as multiple sclerosis or microvascular compression of the vestibular nerve).

Vestibular gain, defined as eye velocity divided by head velocity, is normally close to one, so the eyes remain stationary in space when the head moves. This gain can be assessed by three methods, all of which look at eye position during side-to-side head movement.

1. *Dynamic E test.* Visual acuity is measured with the head stationary and also with the head passively oscillated. Normally, visual acuity is minimally affected by head motion. If vestibular gain is reduced, however, the eyes move in space when the head is oscillated (abnormal gain). Visual acuity during head motion is degraded by two or more lines on the Snellen chart.

2. *Head thrust test.* The patient is instructed to fix his/her gaze on the examiner's nose. The patient's head is then rapidly thrust approximately 20 degrees to one side or the other. If the VOR is normal, the eyes remain stationary on the nose during the head thrust. If the gain is abnormal, the eyes move during the head motion toward the affected side and then make a readily observable "reflection saccade" to bring gaze back to the nose.

3. *Use of ophthalmoscope.* The optic disk is visualized with an ophthalmoscope while the head is turned side to side. If the vestibular gain is normal, the eye (and optic disk) remains stationary during head motion. If the gain is reduced, the disk moves in the opposite direction of the head, because the disk is behind the center of rotation of the eye. Vestibular gain tends to be markedly reduced when the vestibular system is damaged bilaterally. Such bilateral damage is usually peripheral (e.g., with aminoglycoside toxicity) but can be central (e.g., with Wernicke's disease). Asymmetries in gain occur with unilateral lesions and can be deduced with the head thrust test, because the gain is lower when the head is

rotated toward the bad ear (Ewald's second law). Increases in gain are rare; their occurrence usually reflects disease in the vestibulocerebellum, particularly the flocculus and paraflocculus.

Positional nystagmus is elicited with the Dix-Hallpike maneuver, whereby the patient's head is turned 45 degrees to the right or left and is then rapidly moved backward so that the head is tilted 30 degrees below the horizontal. This maneuver provokes vertigo and nystagmus if the subject's disorder is activated by head motion with respect to gravity. The most common positional disorder is benign positional vertigo (BPV) involving the posterior canal, which produces an upbeat, torsional nystagmus when the affected ear is placed undermost. Less common variants of BPV are in the superior canal (producing a downbeat, torsional nystagmus) or lateral canal (producing a direction-changing geotropic horizontal nystagmus). Positional nystagmus can occur with other peripheral disorders, such as perilymph fistula and Meniere's disease, and can also occur with central disorders, such as the static downbeat nystagmus associated with lesions of the cerebellar nodulus.

In addition to the specific tests described earlier, clinical examination of a patient with vestibular symptoms should also include a careful assessment of nonvestibular oculomotor function. A complete discussion is beyond the scope of this textbook but generally includes examination of fixation, gaze holding, saccades, pursuit, and optokinetic and vergence eye movements (2). A thorough neurologic and otologic examination also contributes to the clinical assessment of vestibular disorders.

FUNCTIONAL VESTIBULAR TESTING

Vestibular testing is used to identify the peripheral and central abnormalities of vestibular function that can occur with diseases that affect the labyrinth, the eighth nerve, or the brain. Vestibular tests in isolation are not typically diagnostic, but rather are used in conjunction with other clinical information such as the patient history and the physical examination to reach a meaningful diagnosis. Three options will be described: (i) the basic electronystagmography (ENG) test battery, (ii) postural stability tests, and (iii) rotation about the earth vertical. Each of these tests can be affected by nonvestibular sensory or motor systems in potentially complex ways, and therefore each individual test has somewhat limited value. When several tests are analyzed in concert, however, the results may provide convergent data that allow a specific diagnosis to be reached. An American National Standard for the ENG test battery (ANSI S-3.45) (3) has recently been approved by members of the consortium of users, including the American Academy of Otolaryngology—Head & Neck Surgery (AAO-HNS). Having wider access to results from standardized procedures will become increasingly more important as the medical world becomes more linked—for example, by the computer internet. Accordingly, the ENG test battery will be presented as described in ANSI S-3.45.

ENG Test Battery

The ENG test battery, currently considered to be the standard of practice, consists of the calibration of the electrooculogram (EOG); a test of the saccadic eye movement system; a search for spontaneous or gaze-evoked nystagmus; a test of pursuit eye movements; a search for nystagmus that occurs during or after the patient is positioned in a manner that is apt to provoke nystagmus; and the bithermal, binaural caloric test.

EOG Calibration

This test is used to relate the amplitude of the eye movements in the orbit to the voltage measurements recorded by the electrooculogram. The patient is seated upright with the head level and instructed to stare straight ahead to establish a zero deflection of the recording device. The patient is next instructed to make voluntary saccadic eye movements back and forth between left target and a right target. Eccentric targets are usually placed 10 to 15 degrees from the zero position.

Saccade Test

The saccade test assesses the capacity of the visual and ocular motor systems to make fast and accurate voluntary eye movements. Seated in the upright position with the head level, the patient is asked to make rapid voluntary saccades in the horizontal and vertical planes. These saccades should start from the zero position and go from the center to the left, then return, center to right with return, center to upper position then return, and center to the lower position and return. Deficits in saccadic eye movements can have an effect upon the interpretation of the nystagmus responses to vestibular stimulation and therefore must be assessed separately. In the normal patient, fixation upon the target is steady and the saccadic movements are conjugate, symmetric, and of appropriate latency, amplitude, and velocity.

Spontaneous and Gaze-evoked Nystagmus

A seated patient holding the head level is asked to make repeated eye deviations to real and imaginary visual targets and then to bring the gaze back to the zero position. With the room lights on and the eyes open, the subject looks all the way to the right and to the left in order to record any nystagmus under these conditions. Next the eyes are closed and the patient is told to gaze straight ahead, then to the left, then to the right, then up, then down. Each of these positions is held for 30 seconds in order to determine whether any nystagmus appears. As described earlier, spontaneous nystagmus is nystagmus that occurs with the eyes looking straight ahead, and gaze-evoked nystagmus is nystagmus that is elicited with eccentric gaze and typically beats in the direction of gaze. These forms of nystagmus can be indicative of either central or peripheral vestibular anomalies. A normal response consists of a stable gaze position with no nystagmus.

Pursuit Tracking

This test determines whether a subject can follow a visual target moving in a continuous, predictable path by the use of smooth voluntary eye movements. The patient is seated upright with the head erect and is asked to track a target moving in the horizontal plane. In normal patients the tracking eye movements during pursuit are smooth, symmetric, and conjugate. The pursuit gain (eye velocity divided by target velocity) depends upon the age of the subject and typically decreases with advancing age.

Positioning and Positional Test

This test introduces dynamic vestibular stimulation into the basic test battery and is a search for nystagmus that occurs with either static or dynamic changes in subject orientation with respect to gravity. The patient is placed in a number of head and body positions that are known to produce nystagmus with certain vestibular abnormalities. Frenzel lenses are often used because they eliminate visual fixation cues while allowing for visual observation of nystagmus eye movements. There are three "dynamic" positioning (Hallpike) maneuvers. Each starts in the sitting position and ends up in one of three supine positions: head right, left, and straight. There are five "static" positional maneuvers, of which three are supine (head right, head left, or head straight) and two are done in the lateral position (head and body right or head and body left). Normal responses include eye movements in the compensatory direction of short duration, which are associated with the head movement from one station to another. It is also sometimes normal to observe a weak nystagmus while the eyes are open in the dark after the position has been reached (4). Nystagmus that occurs when visual fixation is allowed is not considered a normal variant.

Caloric Tests

Four sequential irrigations of the external ear canal, using water that is warmer than and cooler than body core temperature, are employed to excite and to inhibit the horizontal semicircular canals of the right and of the left ears; the patient lies supine with the head tilted upward at approximately 30 degrees in order to align the lateral canal with the gravity vertical. The irrigation procedure yields a sequence of four responses to right ear excitation, right ear inhibition, left ear excitation, and left ear inhibition. From this sequence of stimulation, it is possible to make inferences concerning peripheral and central vestibular function.

The response of nystagmus slow-component velocities is quite broad in normal subjects. To decrease the effect of variability in a subject, ratios of response magnitudes are often used, giving a valuable "self-calibrating" aspect (5). These ratios are known as the percent reduced vestibular response (or canal paresis) (%RVR) and the percent directional preponderance (%DP) and are defined as follows:

Percent reduced vestibular response:

$$\%RVR = \frac{(V_{rw} + V_{rc}) - (V_{lw} + V_{lc})}{V_{rw} + V_{rc} + V_{lw} + V_{lc}} \; 100$$

Percent directional preponderance:

$$\%DP = \frac{(V_{rw} + V_{lc}) - (V_{lw} + V_{rc})}{V_{rw} + V_{rc} + V_{lw} + V_{lc}} \; 100$$

where portions of the responses from the right warm, right cool, left warm, and left cool caloric irrigations, respectively. Although individual laboratories usually develop their own normative data, typical normal ranges for %RVR and %DP are 20% to 30%.

Fixation Suppression

Fixation suppression is a way of estimating how well patients can voluntarily suppress their vestibular responses during caloric stimulation by fixating a visual target when their vestibular response is near its maximum intensity.

The index of fixation suppression is computed from the slow-component velocities from one right beating test (rb), rw or lc, and one left beating (lb), lw or rc, test.

$$\%FI_{rb} = [V_{rb}(\text{eyes open fixed upon lit target})/V_{rb}(EOD)] \cdot 100$$

and:

$$\%FI_{lb} = [V_{lb}(\text{eyes open fixed upon lit target})/V_{lb}(EOD)] \cdot 100,$$

where EOD is "eyes open in dark."

Normal patients are able to suppress their responses almost completely and have fixation suppression indices of 5% or less.

Ice Water Caloric Test

Because ice water is such a strong stimulus, this test is usually given only when there is little or no nystagmus response from both the warm and the cold irrigations of one ear. A small amount of ice water, typically 2 ml, is placed into the external canal of the nonresponsive ear while the patient lies with the other ear down. The water is allowed to stand for a short time, typically 20 seconds, and the patient is returned to the normal nose-up recording position, where the eye movements are recorded for at least 1 minute. The slow component is calculated by the same method used for the bithermal stimulation. Many interpret the ab-

sence of any nystagmus in response to ice water testing as being a strong indicator that there is no useful function left in the ear.

Postural Stability Testing

Postural stability testing measures and records estimates of body sway under a variety of conditions. These conditions depend upon the apparatus that is used. The premise for these devices is that three sensory information channels (the visual system, the somatosensory system, and the vestibular system) are normally used to maintain stability. When sensory information to the first or second of these channels is denied or distorted, vestibular information becomes primary. Under these conditions, persons with vestibular anomalies will tend to sway excessively or to fall. Besides varying the sensory input conditions, the sway of the body can be measured during quiet stance and during mechanical disturbances produced by angular or linear motion of the supporting platform. Typical force plate measuring devices measure two or four vertical forces, and some can resolve forces that occur parallel to the support plane (6). Displacement of selective parts of the body can also be simultaneously measured. In addition, muscle activity, primarily in the leg muscles, can be measured using electromyography (EMG).

Currently the prevalent test in North America is a computerized test known as Equitest, which has sensory organization and motor control portions. The sensory portion of the protocol is designed to distort some of the visual and somatosensory information used for maintaining postural stability. This forces the patient to rely heavily upon vestibular cues. In North America the prevalence of Equitest, with its largely preset protocol, has resulted in a de facto standard test that tends to make the results from all test sites comparable. The manufacturer provides users with a normative database that can be used in the clinical evaluations of persons suspected of having vestibular or neurologic deficits.

Postural stability testing is important because it can evaluate the postural reflexes, which are known to be modulated by the vestibular system. Different parts of the vestibular system are thought to modulate this reflex compared with the more commonly tested horizontal canal ocular reflex, which is evaluated during the caloric and rotational tests. Tests of postural stability are often used as evaluations of the efficacy for the rehabilitation of patients having vestibular deficits.

Rotational Testing

The purpose of this test is to evaluate the horizontal vestibuloocular reflex by measuring eye movements in response to a rotary motion about an earth-vertical axis. This test is performed while the patient sits in a chair that is connected to a computer-controlled torque motor. Eye movements are recorded while the chair rotates, and subjects are given simple questions to keep them alert. The test is done in the dark with the eyes open.

The sinusoidal harmonic acceleration (SHA) stimulus is a sequence of sinusoidal angular velocity signals given at several test frequencies. The SHA is intended to evaluate the horizontal semicircular canal reflexive eye movements that can be evoked by rotating a subject about the rostral caudal (yaw) body axis while it is aligned to the gravity vertical (7,8). Usually the head of the subject is tilted forward in order to bring the plane of the horizontal semicircular canals to an orientation that is perpendicular to the axis of rotation, thus ensuring maximum stimulus delivery. Eye movements are usually recorded with bitemporal electrooculography (EOG) or by video. The eye movement signals are usually stored and analyzed with a small computer. Although SHA is not the only stimulus used to evaluate the VOR (9,10), it is probably the most commonly used clinical method. Three other stimuli are (i) a sum of sines, which can combine two or more stimuli; (ii) pseudorandom, which uses a long but finite set of random numbers as its basis; and (iii) velocity trapezoids (steps), which are commonly used in cupulometry.

The SHA stimulus, $\theta(t)$, has the form $\theta(t) = A \sin (2\pi ft)$. The peak amplitude, A, is kept constant, typically at 50 or 60 degrees per second, and the test frequency, f, is varied for a set of sequential runs over a frequency range from approximately 0.0l Hz to l.0 Hz. Perhaps the most compelling clinical reason to use the SHA is that all the energy during each test run is concentrated at only one frequency. This can be important for eliciting responses in patients whose vestibular sensitivity is reduced due to disease.

The response to the SHA stimulus is the slow component velocity (SCV) of horizontal nystagmus. The SCV is customarily extracted from the nystagmus by a computer algorithm. Three parameters used to describe the SCV response to SHA at a single stimulus frequency are gain, phase, and asymmetry. A sinusoidal rotational input, $A \sin (2\pi ft)$, yields an SCV response that is fit with a sinusoid that estimates a response, $B \sin (2\pi ft + \phi)$. Gain is the ratio of the amplitude of the sinusoidal eye movement response sine, B, divided by the amplitude of the sinusoidal chair movement stimulus sine, A. Thus gain is B/A. These amplitudes are both in degrees per second (°/s), so gain is dimensionless. Phase, ϕ, relates the timing between response and stimulus sinusoids based upon the time for one cycle or period of the sinusoid. A common way of measuring asymmetry for each test frequency is to calculate the average value of the SCV response for a data length corresponding to an integral number of whole cycles of the stimulus. This data length is chosen because the value of the stimulus itself when averaged over this length is zero. Thus a completely symmetric response would also average out to zero, but an asymmetric one would not. This estimate of asymmetry is called bias. Sometimes the bias measure is normalized by dividing it by the peak amplitude, A, of the stimulus sinusoid. Pooled data from normal subjects (8,11,12) form the basis of normal/abnormal comparisons. The minimum information for each frequency point is gain, phase, and one or more measures of

asymmetry, such as bias. This information is usually plotted in a frequency response representation known as a Bode plot (Fig. 5.6). Normative data are typically presented using values of gain, phase, and asymmetry for each frequency averaged over the pool of normal subjects.

Simplifying the Interpretation of Rotational Tests Results

Although interpreting the results of SHA rotation can sometimes be straightforward, this is not always the case. The person doing the interpretation has to deal with a large number of data points, some of which may not agree with others. In a test that uses seven test frequencies, 21 separate data points will be generated. Figure 5.7 shows the results for three patients. If all test variables lie clearly within the normal range (Fig. 5.7A), the interpreter has an easy task and, given no other information, would classify the patient's test as normal. Likewise, if most of the data points lie outside their two standard deviation zones (Fig. 5.7B), the test would easily be classified as abnormal. The situation becomes more difficult when some of the data points lie within and some lie outside these normal zones (Fig. 5.7C). In this case the interpreter is forced to deal with conflicting data, thus requiring a subjective decision. To remedy the situation, we have developed an objective method that simplifies test interpretation by using a physiologically based model to capture the trends in the data using just three parameters. The rationale for this approach is explained next.

The results of rotational tests reflect the dynamic responses of the end organs (the horizontal semicircular canals) as "filtered" by the central nervous system (vestibular and ocular motor nuclei and cerebellum). The filtering process is affected by changes in peripheral inputs, by central lesions, and by aging. Figure 5.8 shows a simplified diagram of this filtering process. It illustrates the activity of the semicircular canals (changes in average nerve firing rate) and of the movement of the eyes (slow component velocity of horizontal nystagmus) in response to an abrupt rotation of the head toward the left. This response trajectory represents a convenient way to think of the horizontal angular vestibular ocular reflex and can be applied both to sinusoidal and to impulsive rotational test results.

Figure 5.8 illustrates how the central nervous system processes afferent information from the horizontal semicircular canals to produce the ocular motor signal that generates the slow component of nystagmus during a step of angular velocity toward the left. In healthy subjects this counterclockwise velocity step excites the left horizontal semicircular canal and inhibits the right one, as previously illustrated in Figure 5.3B. This results in a rapid increase in the firing rates of the left vestibular nerve fibers that are connected to the left horizontal semicircular canal. This increase is followed by a slow exponential decay to baseline activity having a time constant of about 5 seconds, which reflects the mechanical properties of the horizontal semicircular canal. This canal response is depicted in the upper left-

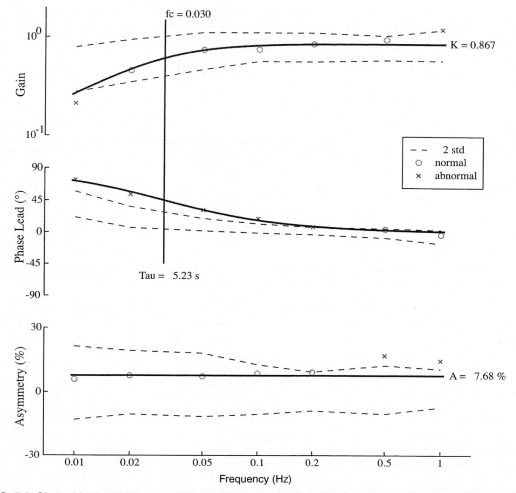

FIG. 5.6 Sinusoidal harmonic acceleration (SHA) test results for a single subject, presented in the form of a modified Bode plot, which plots the response parameters of gain, phase, and asymmetry as a function of the log of the test frequency. *Circles* represent data within normal limits; *x*'s show abnormal data; *dashed lines* mark the ± 2 standard deviation limits of normal responses. The *solid lines* are parametric fits to the actual data, which are used to determine the VOR time constant, the mid-frequency gain, and the asymmetry. The solid vertical line at 0.056 Hz through the gain and phase data marks the calculated corner frequency, f_c.

hand side of the figure next to the left canal as the change in the average firing rate of the afferent nerve fibers versus time with subsequent exponential decay, labeled "T_c" (Fig. 5.8A). The response of the right horizontal semicircular canal resembles a mirror image with an initial abrupt decrease in firing rate, which is followed by an exponential return to baseline. For simplicity, only the response in the left canal is shown.

The central nervous system synergistically combines the signals from left and right canals but contributes another feature that tends to prolong, or perserverate, the slow component response for a longer time than that of the canal responses. This feature, called velocity storage, is highly dependant upon the tone of the peripheral signal and can thus be altered by peripheral lesions of the horizontal semicircular canal and the afferent nerves that connect them to the central nervous system. The essential feature of velocity

storage is to increase the decay time constant of the response compared with the decay time constant of the canal afferent signals. The VOR response, using just the slow component velocity to the right, is depicted versus time on the upper right side of the figure as a rapid increase in slow component velocity that is followed by an exponential decay, labeled T_{VOR}. Thus the VOR response reflects the underlying mechanical dynamics of the canals but with an additional "filtering" by the central nervous system that enhances low-frequency performance. It is this enhancement that can be affected by lesions of the peripheral vestibular system.

Like the canals, the VOR response to a step of velocity is an abrupt increase in compensatory eye velocity followed by a slow exponential decay, but with a much longer decay time constant than that of the canals. The normal VOR time constant averages about 22 seconds (Fig. 5.8B). In the case of

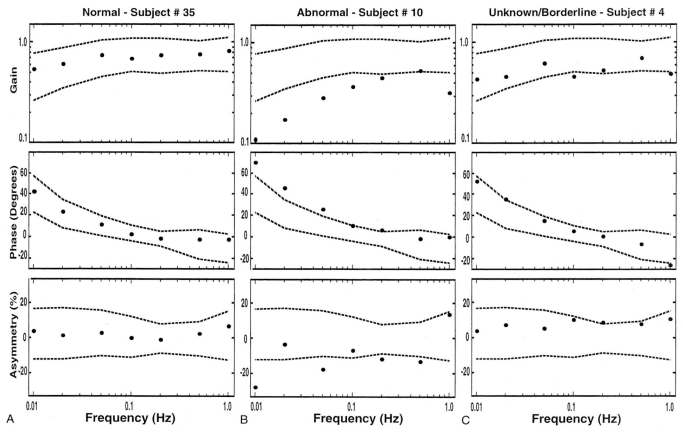

FIG. 5.7 Sinusoidal harmonic acceleration (SHA) test results for the patients who, under the present subjective interpretation methodology, would be classified as **(A)** normal: All points lie clearly within two standard deviation boundaries. **B:** Abnormal: Many points lie outside boundaries. **C:** Unknown/borderline: Points close to edge of boundaries. *Filled circles* mark the patient's test results. *Dashed lines* represent 2 standard deviation boundaries generated from a large group of normals.

unilateral vestibular hypofunction, shown in Figure 5.8C as an X through the left horizontal semicircular canal, the decay time constant of the canal remains essentially unchanged, but the tone and the overall strength of the canal response are reduced. This decreases the action of the velocity storage element. The VOR time constant, while remaining longer than that of the canals, is reduced in comparison to the normal response and averages about 10 seconds (range: 8 to 12 seconds). In the case of bilateral vestibular hypofunction (Fig. 5.8D) the tone and overall strengths of both canal responses are reduced. This further decreases the action of the velocity storage element, yielding a VOR time constant that averages about 5 seconds (range: 3 to 7 seconds).

Several studies have shown that the VOR time constant depends upon the age of the subject. This may be because aging results in a known decrease of hair cell count in the sensory maculae of the canals and otolith organs (13). Thus the age of the subject becomes an important factor in rotational test interpretation. It is possible to correct for the aging effect on the VOR time constant in a way that is independent of the lesion status of the individual (normal, partial unilateral lesion, full unilateral lesion, partial bilateral le-

sion) (14). This age-corrected time constant is a more sensitive measure for classifying a patient's VOR time constant than an uncorrected measure.

We have published an exact method of using a model to fit SHA data in order to get the best estimate of mid-frequency gain and T_{VOR} (14). Here, we present a simplified method that can be easily applied by the reader to most SHA data. The mid-frequency gain may be calculated by taking an average of the three highest frequency gain points unless one point looks significantly lower than the other two. In this case, average just the other two points. To get T_{VOR}, draw a smooth line fit through the three lowest frequency phase lead points and estimate the frequency at which the line has a phase lead of 45 degrees. This is called the corner frequency. In Figure 5.6 the corner frequency is about 0.03 Hz. Look up the value of T_{VOR} for that frequency in Table 5.1. This table gives the age-corrected time constant, τ as a function of corner frequency, and subject age. Calculate the asymmetry estimate by averaging the separate measures, neglecting any single point that looks significantly different from its neighbors.

The amplitude (gain) of the VOR response is also affected by unilateral and bilateral hypofunction. Unilateral lesions

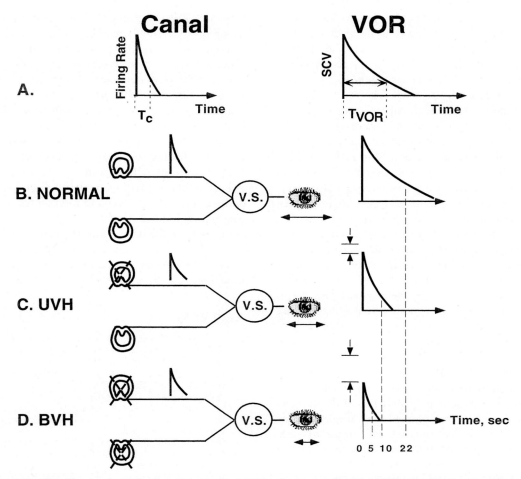

FIG. 5.8 Simplified schematic to compare the VORs of a normal subject **(A),** a subject with unilateral vestibular hypofunction (UVH) **(B),** and a bilateral vestibular hypofunction (BVH) **(C).** For further explanation, see text **(D).**

TABLE 5.1. *Age-adjusted time VOR time constant, τ*, as a function of corner frequency, f_c, and age*

f_c (Hz)	τ^*(sec)												
0.004	74.2	58.5	49.5	44.3	41.5	40.1	**39.8**	40.3	43.1	47.8	53.9	61.3	70.0	79.7
0.005	59.3	46.8	39.6	35.4	33.2	32.1	**31.8**	32.2	34.5	38.2	43.1	49.1	56.0	63.8
0.006	49.4	39.0	33.0	5.0	27.6	26.7	**26.5**	26.9	28.7	31.8	35.9	40.9	46.7	53.1
0.007	42.4	33.4	28.3	25.3	23.7	22.9	**22.7**	23.0	24.6	27.3	30.8	35.1	40.0	45.6
0.007	37.1	29.2	24.7	22.1	20.7	20.0	**19.9**	20.1	21.5	23.9	26.9	30.7	35.0	39.9
0.009	32.9	26.0	22.0	19.7	18.4	17.8	**17.7**	17.9	19.2	21.2	24.0	27.3	31.1	35.4
0.010	29.6	23.4	19.8	17.7	16.6	16.0	**15.9**	16.1	17.2	19.1	21.6	24.5	28.0	31.9
0.0125	23.7	18.7	15.8	14.1	13.3	12.8	**12.7**	12.9	13.8	15.3	17.2	19.6	22.4	25.5
0.0150	19.7	15.6	13.2	11.8	11.1	10.7	**10.6**	10.7	11.5	12.7	14.4	16.4	18.7	21.3
0.0175	16.9	13.3	11.3	10.1	9.5	9.2	**9.1**	9.2	9.9	10.9	12.3	14.0	16.0	18.2
0.020	14.8	11.7	9.9	8.8	8.3	8.0	**8.0**	8.1	8.6	9.6	10.8	12.3	14.0	15.9
0.025	11.8	9.3	7.9	7.0	6.6	6.4	**6.4**	6.4	6.9	7.6	8.6	9.8	11.2	12.8
0.030	9.8	7.8	6.6	5.9	5.5	5.3	**5.3**	5.4	5.7	6.4	7.2	8.2	9.3	10.6
0.040	7.4	5.8	4.9	4.4	4.1	4.0	**4.0**	4.0	4.3	4.8	5.4	6.1	7.0	8.0
0.050	5.9	4.6	3.9	3.5	3.3	3.2	**3.2**	3.2	3.4	3.8	4.3	4.9	5.6	6.4
0.060	4.9	3.9	3.3	2.9	2.8	2.7	**2.7**	2.7	2.9	3.2	3.6	4.1	4.7	5.3
0.080	3.7	2.9	2.4	2.2	2.1	2.0	**2.0**	2.0	2.2	2.4	2.7	3.1	3.5	4.0
0.120	2.4	1.9	1.6	1.4	1.4	1.3	**1.3**	1.3	1.4	1.6	1.8	2.0	2.3	2.7
0.160	1.8	1.4	1.2	1.1	1.0	1.0	**1.0**	1.0	1.1	1.2	1.3	1.5	1.7	2.0
	5	10	15	20	25	30	**35**	40	50	60	70	80	90	100
Subject age in years													

typically reduce the gain for the lowest stimulus frequencies only and may produce an asymmetry in the gain such that the response is greater when the head rotates toward the normal ear compared with the abnormal side (a manifestation of Ewald's second law). Bilateral lesions typically reduce the gain for all stimulus frequencies. The mechanisms of central compensation, however, tend to mitigate the response sensitivity over time after a peripheral lesion, whereas the changes in the time constants are largely unaffected by the compensation process. This makes T_{VOR} a more reliable indicator of peripheral pathophysiology than the VOR gain. The velocity storage element can also be affected by other factors such as central pathologies, which must be accounted for during clinical decision making. For example, lesions involving the nodulus of the cerebellum disinhibit the velocity storage mechanism and increase T_{VOR}. Used appropriately, the T_{VOR} can provide the surgeon with useful information to determine the presence of a unilateral lesion and also to indicate whether there may be bilateral involvement. This information can have a significant impact on the decision to perform surgery, because ablative procedures are usually contraindicated if there is bilateral dysfunction of the vestibular system.

In summary the central nervous system "filters" the peripheral response in normal subjects in a way that tends to enhance the response duration relative to that of the semicircular canals. This results in lengthening of the VOR time constant, which is equivalent to a decrease in the low-frequency phase lead. A peripheral lesion creates an imbalance in sensory input to the central nervous system, which tends to decrease this enhancement, resulting in a shorter-than-normal VOR time constant (strongest effect) and somewhat decreased sensitivity. The time constant can be corrected for aging effects to provide a more accurate basis of normal/abnormal comparisons.

Combining Results from Several Tests

Traditionally, the ENG alone has been the standard for testing dizzy patients. Work by many investigators has shown that ENG alone is inadequate. These findings indicate that (i) ENG alone lacks sufficient sensitivity to detect abnormalities in patients with known lesions or disease states that imply vestibular pathophysiology; (ii) using several tests together (e.g., ENG and rotation) can significantly increase sensitivity and specificity; and (iii) in certain applications the rotation test turns out to be more sensitive than ENG. In 52 patients with Meniere's disease, one study showed that 62% had abnormal ENG tests, whereas the combination of ENG with posturography tests had a sensitivity of 72%, and the combination of rotation with posturography had a sensi-

tivity of 83% (15). Another study was designed to classify a group of 100 patients who had either Meniere's disease or migraine-associated dizziness as defined by strict diagnostic criteria. Classification was based upon test result data from one or more vestibular tests. Using ENG alone, 74% of the patients were classified correctly. This increased to 91% using rotation test data alone. Combining information from both tests yielded a classification rate of 92% (16). Combined vestibular test results can also be used to aid surgical decision making because detection of occult bilateral vestibular hypofunction, a strong contraindication to ablative vestibular surgery, is achieved with greater sensitivity and accuracy using ENG and rotation test results together. The current limitations of the vestibular test battery lie in the complexity of the dataset and subjectivity of the interpretation. Application of multivariate statistical techniques holds promise for developing simplified and more objective interpretations.

REFERENCES

1. Curthoys IS, Halmagyi GM. Vestibular compensation: a review of the oculomotor, neural, and clinical consequences of unilateral vestibular loss. *J Vestib Res* 1995;5:67–107.
2. Leigh RJ, Zee DS. *Neurology of Eye Movements,* 3rd ed. New York: Oxford University Press, 1999.
3. Wall C III, Parker DE, Von Gierke HE. Procedures for testing basic vestibular function. *American National Standard ANSI* S3.45, 1999.
4. Barber HO, Wright G. Positional nystagmus in normals. *Adv Otorhinolaryngol* 1973;19:276–283.
5. Jongkees LBW, Philipszoon AJ. Electronystagmography. *Acta Otolaryngol (Stockh)* 1964;[Suppl 189].
6. Andres RO, Anderson DJ. Design of a better postural measurement system. *Am J Otolaryngol* 1980;1:197–206.
7. Hirsch BE. Computed sinusoidal harmonic acceleration. *Ear Hear* 1986;7(3):198–203.
8. Wolfe JW, Engelken EJ, Olson JW, et al. Vestibular responses to bithermal caloric and harmonic acceleration. *Ann Otol Rhinol Laryngol* 1978;87:861–867.
9. Honrubia V, Brazier MA. *Nystagmus and Vertigo: Clinical Approaches to the Patient with Dizziness.* New York: Academic Press, 1982.
10. Wall C III, Black FO, O'Leary DP. Clinical use of pseudorandom binary sequence white noise in assessment of the human vestibulo-ocular system. *Ann Otol Rhinol Laryngol* 1978;87:845–852.
11. Hixson WC. Frequency response of the oculo-vestibular system during yaw oscillation. *Report AO.NAMRL-1212,* Naval Aerospace Medical Research Lab, Pensacola, FL, 1974.
12. Wall III C, Black FO, Hunt AE. Effects of age, sex and stimulus parameters upon vestibulo-ocular responses to sinusoidal rotation. *Acta Otolaryngol (Stockh)* 1984;98:270–278.
13. Merchant SN, Velazquez-Villasenor L, Tsuji K, et al. Temporal bone studies of the human peripheral vestibular system. Normative vestibular hair cell data. *Ann Otol Rhinol Laryngol* 2000;[Suppl 181]:3–13.
14. Dimitri PS, Wall C III, Oas JG. Classification of human rotation test results using parametric modeling and multivariate statistics. *Acta Otolaryngol (Stockh)* 1996;116(4):497–506.
15. Black FO, Wall C III. Comparison of vestibulo-ocular and vestibulo-spinal screening tests. *Otolaryngol Head Neck Surg* 1981;89:811–817.
16. Dimitri PS, Wall C III, Oas JG, et al. Application of multivariate statistics to vestibular testing: discriminating between Meniere's disease and migraine associated dizziness. *J Vestib Res* 2001;11(1):53–65.

CHAPTER 6

Evaluation of Facial Paralysis

Arvind Kumar, Arlene Barr, and Aftab Patni

A variety of lesions have been reported to cause facial paralysis; these can be broadly classified as traumatic, idiopathic, toxic, metabolic, infective, neoplastic, and degenerative (1). When confronted with a patient suffering from facial paralysis, the immediate task of the clinician is to uncover the probable cause. According to Sir Terrance Cawthorne (2), "all that palsies is not Bells," and it is for this reason that a detailed history with respect to the mode of onset, progression of paralysis, and history of head trauma and associated otologic and neurologic symptoms is important. Facial paralysis can be supranuclear or infranuclear. The latter can be unilateral and acute in onset or chronic, progressive in nature. The acute form could also be bilateral (simultaneous or sequential) or ipsilaterally recurrent. The purpose of this chapter is to discuss the evaluation of facial paralysis as it presents to the clinician in any of the forms just described.

ACUTE PALSIES

Bell's Palsy and Herpes Zoster Oticus

The most common type of acute onset unilateral facial paralysis is Bell's palsy. The cause of Bell's palsy has long been held to be idiopathic, and the diagnosis is made by the characteristic clinical features and by a process of exclusion (3). Today, Bell's palsy is regarded as a neuritis of the nerve within the fallopian canal. Recent studies have demonstrated ample clinical, histopathologic, experimental, imaging, and therapeutic evidence to support a viral infection of the nerve with the herpes simplex type 1 virus (4–8). The infection produces inflammation and edema of the nerve. Fisch (9) proposed that the neural compression and conduction block occurs at the meatal foramen secondary to nerve edema (Fig. 6.1). He defined the meatal foramen as the medial opening of the fallopian canal into the internal auditory meatus (9). His measurements of the fallopian canal showed that the meatal foramen is its narrowest segment (0.68 mm); he termed it the "bottle-neck."(9)

Herpes zoster oticus (Ramsay Hunt syndrome), on the other hand, is caused by the varicella zoster virus. The clinical presentation is characterized by vesicles on and around the pinna (3). The clinical evaluation and diagnostic workup are similar to those for Bell's palsy.

Clinically, two patients may present with an equally dense House-Brackman grade 6 paralysis. One may improve to grade 2, and the other may recover to only grade 5. How can the physician prognosticate the final outcome? Today it is generally accepted that the best method for accurately predicting the final outcome is from the results of serial electrophysiologic tests. The selection of the test most appropriate for a given situation and interpretation of the results will be facilitated by an understanding of the underlying pathologic changes that occur in the facial nerve secondary to injury.

In the facial nerve there are about 10,000 axons, of which 7,000 are branchial motor axons. The rest are afferent taste fibers from the anterior two-thirds of the tongue, as well as efferent parasympathetic secretomotor fibers from the lacrimal, nasal, submandibular, and sublingual glands (10). The structure of each branchial motor axon is similar to that of any peripheral nerve except that the size is different. The axoplasm is surrounded by a *myelin sheath,* and these myelinated fibers are encased in a connective tissue tubule, the *endoneurium* (Fig. 6.2). In peripheral nerves, groups of axons are surrounded by concentric sleeves of flattened polygonal cells called *perineurium.* Each such collection of axons enclosed by perineurium is a *fascicle.* Peripheral nerves are made up of groups of fascicles, which in turn are held together by a condensation of loose areolar connective tissue, the *epineurium.* The structure of the facial nerve, however, has been shown to be different from that of peripheral nerves in that the facial nerve has just a single fascicle in its intratemporal course (11,12).

According to the Sunderland (12) classification (Table 6.1), the least severe nerve injury is designated as first degree and in this there is only a physiologic block to propagation of the nerve impulse. The axon, its myelin sheath, and

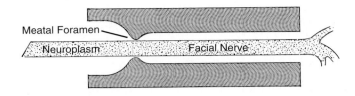

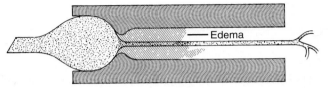

FIG. 6.1 *Top* figure illustrates normal cross-sectional dimensions of the whole length of the fallopian canal. *Bottom* figure illustrates the bottle-neck created by the meatal foramen. The nerve is injured at this site because the edematous nerve is constricted within the fallopian canal.

the endoneural tube distal to the labyrinthine segment are intact. This degree of injury had been described earlier by Seddon (13) as *neuropraxia.* In Bell's palsy, such an injury results from increased intraneural pressure at the meatal foramen (9). Normal nerve impulses are therefore not conducted across the site of compression and hence the face is paralyzed (Fig. 6.3). However, electrical stimulation of the nerve distally elicits a response because the axoplasm and myelin sheath are intact. If the compression is not relieved, venous drainage is obstructed and intraneural pressure continues to increase. This leads to Sunderland's second degree injury (12). Seddon (13) called this degree of injury *axonotmesis.* In this type of injury the axons are destroyed but the endoneural tubules remain intact (Fig. 6.4). Consequently, recovery is prolonged but nerve regeneration is not faulty because the intact endoneural tubes guide the re-

growth of the axons. If the majority of axons suffer this degree of injury, synkinesis is an unlikely sequela of recovery.

The pathologic process in Bell's palsy and herpes zoster oticus usually does not progress past Sunderland's second-degree injury (axonotmesis). The majority of patients with Bell's palsy must suffer this degree of injury because Peitersen observed that 71% of patients with untreated Bell's palsy recovered without any sequelae in a cohort of 1,011 patients (14). With continued increase in intraneural pressure, Sunderland's third and fourth degree injuries may occur. With these degrees of nerve damage, there is axolysis, disruption of the myelin sheath, and loss of endoneurial tubes. The percentage of responding fibers progressively reduced with time, and the graph shown in Figure 6.5 represents these surviving axons. If by the sixth day there are no stimulatable axons (i.e., neuropraxic and surviving fibers), the prognosis for good recovery is poor. In addition, with loss of endoneurial continuity, there is a potential for mismatching of branchial motor and secretomotor fibers during regrowth, resulting in the clinical observation of synkinesis and crocodile tears in grade 3 and 4 injuries. Furthermore, with time, considerable intraneural fibrosis ensues, blocking axonal regrowth. Though both these grades of injury may occur in a case of Bell's palsy, a relatively small number of patients are so affected. Peitersen's (14) study is illustrative because only 16% of untreated Bell's palsy patients showed a poor recovery of function. It is important to note that the various degrees of injury can overlap in any patient with Bell's palsy. Complete or partial nerve transection was described by Sunderland (12) as fifth degree injury (Seddon's *neurotmesis* [13]), but such an injury does not occur in Bell's palsy. Transection is more likely with blunt head trauma, penetrating ear trauma, or trauma during the course of surgery.

Interruption of the axon leads to early retrograde changes in the nerve cell body and the nerve proximal to the site of injury. Anterograde changes in the nerve distal to the site of injury begin within 12 hours of the insult. These anterograde changes are called *Wallerian degeneration*. The axoplasm is destroyed and the myelin sheath disintegrates and is

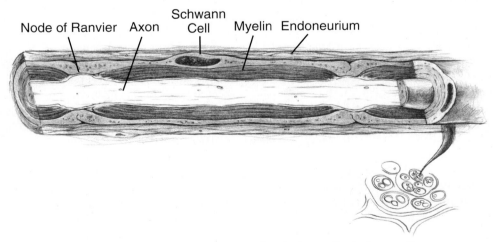

FIG. 6.2 Illustration of the structure of a single myelinated nerve fiber.

TABLE 6.1. *Classification of nerve injuries*

Sunderland (12)	Seddon (13)
First degree	Neuropraxia
• Physiologic block to propogation of nerve impulse	
• Nerve structure intact at site of injury (Fig. 6.3)	
Second degree	Axonotmesis
• Axon degenerate distal to site of injury	
• Myelin sheath disintegrates	
• Schwann cells proliferate	
• Endoneural tubes intact; recovery without synkinesis	
Third degree	
• Axon degenerates	
• Myelin sheath disintegrates	
• Endoneural tubes disrupted	
• Intrafunicular fibrosis	
• Recovery may occur with synkinesis	
Fourth degree	
• Nerve continuity preserved	
• Injured segment converted into a tangled mass of connective tissue, Schwann cells, and regenerating axons, which may enlarge to form a neuroma	
Fifth degree	Neurotmesis
• Complete loss of continuity of nerve	
• Scar tissue may form between cut ends of nerve	
• Bulb formation may occur on both proximal and distal stumps	

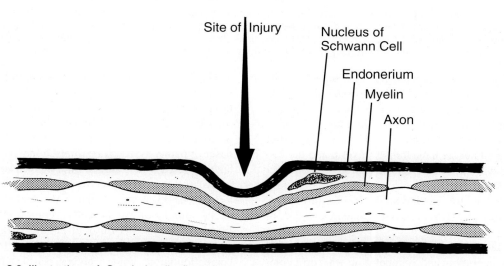

FIG. 6.3 Illustration of Sunderland's first degree injury. Note that the myelin sheath and the endoneurium are intact.

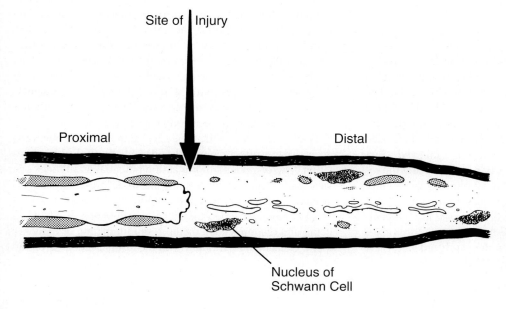

FIG. 6.4 Illustration of Sunderland's second degree injury. The nerve distal to the arrow has undergone Wallerian degeneration. Note that the endoneurium *(outermost thick black lines)* is intact.

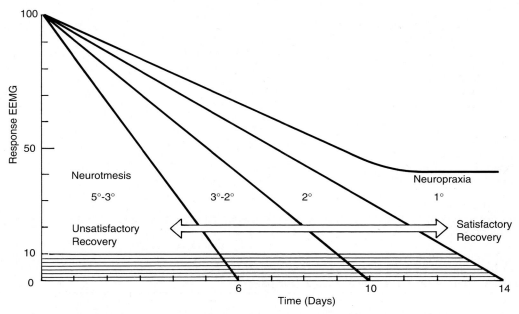

FIG. 6.5 Graphic representation of the percentage of surviving nerve fibers after proximal nerve injury. The x axis represents time in days from onset of paralysis. The y axis represents the percentage of surviving fibers noted on ENoG. On day 1, 100% of nerve fibers on paralyzed side are intact because Wallerian degeneration has not yet begun. $1°-5°$ represents Sunderland's degrees of nerve injury.

phagocytized by activated macrophages. The Schwann cells proliferate and form the bands of Bunger, which fill the endoneural tubes if these are intact. The bands of Bunger strongly support axonal regeneration. In most instances, Wallerian degeneration is complete by 12 to 14 days after injury. Regenerated nerves have thinner myelin and the distance between the nodes of Ranvier are altered (11). As a result, nerve conduction velocity is slowed and there is an increase in the threshold for depolarization. It is for this reason that electroneurography (ENoG) has no value in a regenerating nerve.

With this background information about the events during facial nerve degeneration and regeneration, the principles and scope of electrophysiologic tests can be understood.

Electroneurography

Electroneurography was first popularized by Esslen (15) and Fisch (16). It consists of stimulating the facial nerve percutaneously after its exit from the stylomastoid foramen (Fig. 6.6). The resultant compound motor unit action potential is recorded by surface electrodes at the nasolabial fold. The details of stimulus parameters have been described by Gantz et al (17). Stimulus and recording are first done on the nonparalyzed side. The current strength is gradually increased until the maximum biphasic response is achieved (Fig. 6.7A). The paralyzed side is similarly stimulated and the response recorded (Fig. 6.7B). The amplitudes of the responses from peak to peak on both sides are measured, and the response of the paralyzed side is expressed as a percentage of the normal side. This percentage is a measure of the neuropraxic and surviving fibers on the paralyzed side.

The fibers that have undergone Wallerian degeneration do not respond to electrical stimulation. In principle therefore the test differentiates a Sunderland first degree injury from second to fifth degrees of injury. In any given situation, if the percentage of surviving fibers is still 60% on day 21 after onset of paralysis, it can be inferred that a majority of axons have suffered a first degree injury. Because the majority of axons are neuropraxic, recovery can be expected to be excellent. At the other extreme the responses to maximal percutaneous stimulation can be almost completely lost within the first 5 to 7 days after onset of paralysis. By serially testing patients whose facial nerves have been transected during cerebellopontine angle surgery, Fisch (16) showed that ENoG responses were completely lost by the sixth day. When such a transection pattern is seen in Bell's palsy (even though there is no nerve transection in this condition), the prognosis for satisfactory return of function is poor. The most likely reason is that the nerve has suffered a Sunderland's third or fourth degree injury. In such severe injuries, intraneural fibrosis is more common and regenerating axons are blocked. Electronystagmography can be repeated every other day for 2 weeks after onset of paralysis. Documentation of both the time course and the degree of degeneration is helpful for management and prognostication.

With every electrodiagnostic test there are inherent variables that can affect the results and skew the clinical interpretation. The compound motor action potential amplitudes can vary with electrode placement, electrode pressure, skin resistance, and the strength of the stimulating current. Gantz et al. (17) have discussed the technical problems of ENoG in detail and recommended methods of eliminating or reducing them. Considerable training with the test is needed before an individual can begin to obtain consistent and meaningful results. Even with good training, significant test-retest variability has been reported with studies on normal subjects (18).

Electromyography

Needle electromyography (EMG) is used to demonstrate (i) motor unit action potentials obtained by voluntary facial muscle contraction, (ii) fibrillation potentials seen in denervated facial muscles at rest, and (iii) large polyphasic potentials seen in facial muscle fibers during the process of reinnervation with attempted voluntary motion.

In the early stages of even a complete facial paralysis, some fibers may remain undamaged. They are obviously in a minority because there is no visible facial movement even with forced voluntary contraction. The presence of these voluntary motor unit action potentials can, however, be detected with a needle EMG. The continued presence of these potentials up to day 14 indicates that the degree of injury to the nerve is mild and good recovery can be expected. Axonal loss results in denervation of muscle. If a recording electrode is placed in a field of denervated muscles 3 weeks after onset of paralysis, waveforms called *fibrillation potentials* and *sharp waves* are recorded (Fig. 6.8). Both these waveforms indicate denervation hypersensitivity. It should be noted that the above potentials are recorded with the face at complete rest. *Recruitment* is a term used to describe the activation of a motor unit (axon plus muscle fiber). Figure 6.9 shows recruitment noted in normal muscles. Because the number of motor units that can be activated in a paralyzed face are few, correspondingly fewer motor unit action potentials can be recorded. This phenomenon is called *decreased recruitment* (compare Figs. 6.8 and 6.9).

When nerve regeneration begins weeks or months after the facial nerve injury, regenerating axons branch out to supply a greater number of muscle fibers than would normally be the case. The resultant large *polyphasic potentials* are

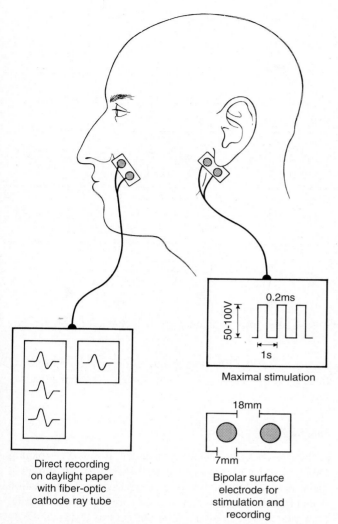

FIG. 6.6 Illustrates the technique of ENoG. The stimulating and recording electrodes are not placed in a fixed position but can be moved around until a maximum response is obtained.

Direct recording on daylight paper with fiber-optic cathode ray tube

Maximal stimulation

Bipolar surface electrode for stimulation and recording

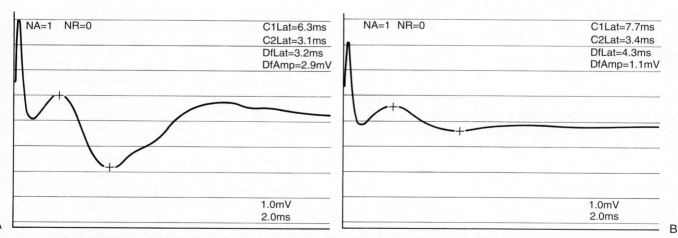

FIG. 6.7 A: Illustrates the biphasic compound action potential induced by stimulation of facial nerve on the nonparalyzed side. The peak-to-peak amplitude is marked with a +. **B:** Illustrates the biphasic compound action potential induced by stimulation of the paralyzed facial nerve. Note the reduced peak-to-peak amplitude compared with the normal side.

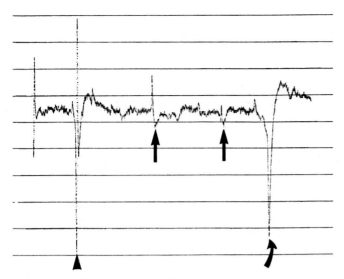

FIG. 6.8 EMG record from a patient with complete facial paralysis 4 weeks after onset. Fibrillation potentials are indicated by *straight arrows.* The *curved arrow* points to a positive sharp wave and the *arrowhead* points to a motor unit. One division is equal to 50 uV.

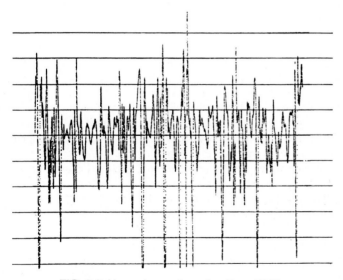

FIG. 6.9 Normal recruitment pattern EMG.

complex in configuration and their presence is a sign that reinnervation is in progress (Fig. 6.10). In summary, EMG is an excellent tool for prognostication of recovery in both the early and later phases of facial paralysis.

Audiogram and Vestibular Evaluation

Though an audiogram is not helpful for prognostication, the presence of the stapes reflex is a positive prognostic finding (19,20). It indicates that even though the face is completely paralyzed, some axons innervating the stapes muscle have escaped injury at the "bottle-neck" (meatal foramen). Thus it can be inferred that the pathologic lesion at the meatal

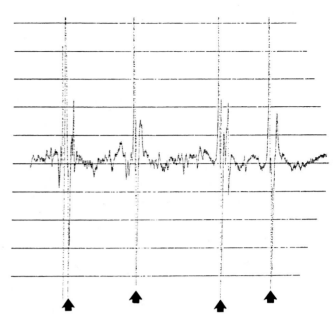

FIG. 6.10 *Arrows* indicate giant polyphasic neurogenic potentials.

foramen is of the first degree and recovery can be expected to be good. In most cases of Bell's palsy a vestibular evaluation is not helpful.

Imaging

Although contrast-enhanced magnetic resonance imaging (MRI) will demonstrate an enhanced signal of the proximal facial nerve (21) in a case of Bell's palsy, such information does not help the physician to either treat or prognosticate. However, if at 6 to 9 months after onset of paralysis the EMG shows no evidence of reinnervation (large polyphasic potentials), other causes for the paralysis must be sought with imaging. In this setting, both computed tomography (CT) of the temporal bones and an MRI with contrast are helpful in evaluating the entire course of the facial nerve (21).

In summary, the conclusions that can be drawn from this discussion on Bell's palsy and herpes zoster oticus are:

1. Facial paresis usually recovers without sequelae because the injury is for the most part neuropraxic.
2. If the ENoG shows the presence of at least 50% surviving fibers up to day 21 after onset of paralysis, an excellent recovery can be expected (Fig. 6.5). In such cases, clinical signs of recovery usually begin early. Such cases usually show some voluntary motor unit action potentials on EMG when facial movement is attempted. By the same token, if the stapes reflex is present, prognosis is good. Needle EMG signs of reinnervation (large polyphasic potentials) often precede signs of clinical recovery.
3. If ENoG shows responses up to day 14, even though the percentage of surviving fibers progressively reduces with time, the prognosis for recovery is good. Recovery, though delayed, occurs without synkinesis because the

underlying pathology in these cases is most likely no more than Sunderland's second degree injury (Figs. 6.4 and 6.5).

4. The prognosis for good recovery in patients showing a "transection pattern" (pathology is most likely Sunderland third and fourth degrees) is only 14% according to Fisch (9). It is highly unlikely that even at an early stage such patients will have voluntary motor action potentials on EMG. A middle fossa decompression of the nerve has been shown to result in a better outcome in 91% of patients in this group, as opposed to 42% of similar patients who were not decompressed (22).

5. Patients who come in for an evaluation 21 days after onset of paralysis need serial EMGs over the next 4 to 5 months with the purpose of seeking evidence of progressive reinnervation (large polyphasic potentials). At this late stage an ENoG neither provides prognostic information for recovery nor guides the surgeon in the decision to decompress the nerve. Patients who have undergone partial recovery also do not benefit from ENoG because regenerating fibers respond poorly to stimulation, as discussed earlier.

6. Finally, if there is no recovery either clinically or on EMG 6 to 8 months after onset of paralysis, a different cause for the paralysis needs to be investigated by imaging the entire course of the facial nerve.

Facial Paralysis Secondary to Trauma

Facial paralysis can result from blunt trauma to the head, from intratemporal and extratemporal penetrating injuries, and from surgical procedures along the entire course of the facial nerve.

Blunt Trauma

Blunt trauma to the head can fracture the base of the skull with resultant unilateral or bilateral facial paralysis. The diagnostic study of choice is a CT scan of the temporal bones. The fracture can either spare the otic capsule or it can traverse it. With the latter, facial paralysis is more common and the auditory and vestibular function is lost. In such injuries, brain concussion is usually severe and therefore electrophysiologic tests are usually deferred until the patient is stabilized. In this delayed presentation the prognostic value of ENoG is lost, but results of EMG studies would guide the surgeon, as shown earlier. Facial paralysis in patients with otic capsule sparing fractures may be profitably studied with serial ENoGs if the patient is available for the study before day 21. However, if serial ENoGs show a transection pattern within 6 days of onset of paralysis (not date of injury), surgical decompression of the perigeniculate area is indicated. If decompression is deferred, extensive proximal intraneural fibrosis has been reported to occur (23). Felix et al. (23) have provided histologic evidence of proximal fibrosis. If no polyphasic potentials are seen on EMG months after onset

of paralysis, decompression or grafting of the facial nerve is indicated. As a general rule, if onset of paralysis occurs hours or days after the trauma, the prognosis for spontaneous recovery is good.

Penetrating Trauma

Bullet wounds and stab wounds can injure the facial nerve in its intratemporal and extratemporal courses. The site of intratemporal injury to the facial nerve is best determined with a CT scan. However, because penetrating injuries can involve the brain and major vessels in this region, the evaluation should include a contrast-enhanced MRI scan with MR angiography and, if necessary, a formal four-vessel angiogram.

Iatrogenic Injury

The facial nerve is susceptible to injury during posterior fossa, intratemporal or extratemporal surgery.

1. If the injury to the nerve is recognized at surgery, neither electrophysiologic nor imaging studies are indicated because the extent of injury and its site are already known.

2. If the nerve was being monitored during posterior fossa surgery and was stimulatable directly before closure, and the patient wakes up with facial paralysis, needle EMG for voluntary motor unit action potentials and serial ENoGs may be obtained. If there is no recovery after 4 weeks, serial EMGs may be obtained to help with prognostication and management.

3. If the patient wakes up with facial nerve paralysis after transtemporal surgery and the surgeon is uncertain about having injured the nerve, reexploration of the facial nerve rather than electrophysiologic tests or imaging studies is probably the more prudent immediate management algorithm. If the nerve is grafted, regeneration can be followed with periodic EMG studies 4 to 6 months after repair.

4. If the paralysis is delayed in onset, good recovery should be expected. However, electrophysiologic test results will reassure the surgeon and patient of a full recovery. Imaging studies are not indicated.

Bilateral Acute Facial Paralysis

Acute onset bilateral facial paralysis is rare. The causes include Guillain-Barre syndrome, head trauma, infectious mononucleosis, sarcoidosis, and Lyme disease, among others. The investigation of such a case will be guided by the suspected underlying condition.

Recurrent Facial Paralysis

Acute facial paralysis may be ipsilaterally recurrent or contralaterally recurrent. In the past, both were regarded as forms of Bell's palsy, chiefly because modern imaging was not available. Even so, in ipsilaterally recurrent paralysis, May and Hardin (24) were able to find tumors as the cause of paralysis in 6 out of 20 patients in 1977 when modern imaging was not available. Figure 6.11 shows a tumor in a patient who had a "Bell's palsy" 16 years prior to presenting with a recurrent acute ipsilateral facial paralysis. The tumor extended from the geniculate ganglion to the second genu. The final histopathologic diagnosis was glomus tumor. Our recommendation for the investigation of recurrent ipsilateral paralysis is therefore to image the entire course of the facial nerve with contrast-enhanced MRI and also obtain a bone window CT scan of the temporal bone. Recurrent contralateral paralysis has not been shown to be caused by mass lesions and in general is considered to be a Bell's palsy. The investigation of such a palsy will be the same as for Bell's palsy.

CHRONIC PALSIES

A slowly progressive facial paralysis is almost always due to a primary tumor of the nerve or its secondary involvement by benign or malignant lesions of the skull base, cerebellopontine angle, or the parotid. Tumors, however, can also present as acute facial paralysis, and May and Schaitkin (25) reported such a presentation in 22 of 104 (21%) patients with benign tumors and in 25 of 93 (27%) patients with malignant tumors. If they present before 21 days, the acute forms should be investigated with electrophysiologic tests, as described earlier. According to May and Schaitkin (25), in such patients the ENoG test shows a transection pattern. The EMG could show both fibrillation and large polyphasic potentials if the tumor growth is slow.

If a tumor is suspected, imaging with both high resolution CT scan of the temporal bone and a contrast-enhanced MRI

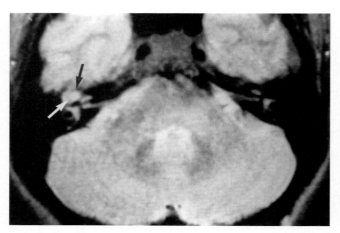

FIG. 6.11 MRI scan of a patient showing a tumor at the geniculate ganglion *(arrows)*. She suffered from ipsilateral recurrent facial paralysis. Recovery from the first paralysis was complete.

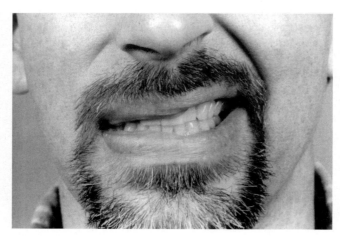

FIG. 6.13 The patient shown in Figure 6.12, seen 42 years later. Recently the patient had noted worsening of paralysis on the right.

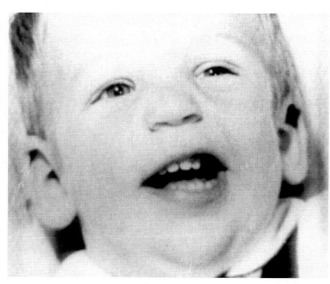

FIG. 6.12 Childhood picture of patient shown in Figure 6.13. The right-sided weakness was diagnosed as Bell's palsy.

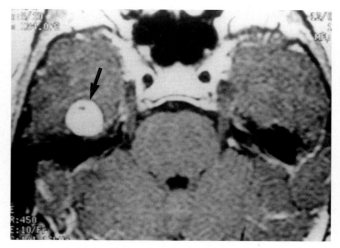

FIG. 6.14 MRI scan of patient seen in Figures 6.11 and 6.12. The facial nerve schwannoma *(arrow)* was removed via a transmastoid–middle fossa exposure.

scan should be performed. The latter is targeted to image the entire length of the facial nerve (21).

A tumor should be suspected in any patient, regardless of age, who has a persistent facial paralysis or paresis or if there is involvement of a particular branch of the nerve. Figures 6.12, 6.13, and 6.14 are illustrative. This patient had a facial weakness since childhood and had been told that he had a Bell's palsy.

REFERENCES

1. Schaitkin BM, May M, Klein SR. Office evaluation of the patient with facial palsy: differential diagnosis and prognosis. In: May M, Schaitkin BM, eds. *The Facial Nerve,* 2nd ed. New York: Thieme Medical Publishers, 2000:179–212.
2. Cawthorne T. Bell's palsies. *Ann Otol Rhinol Laryngol* 1963;72: 774–779.
3. Schaitkin BM, May M, Podvinec M, et al. Idiopathic (Bell's) palsy, herpes zoster cephalicus, and other facial nerve disorders of viral origin. In: May M, Schaitkin BM, eds. *The Facial Nerve,* 2nd ed. New York: Thieme Medical Publishers, 2000:319–338.
4. Murakami S, Mizobuchi M, Nakashiro Y, et al. Bell palsy and herpes simplex virus: identification of viral DNA in endoneurial fluid and muscle. *Ann Intern Med* 1996;124:27–30.
5. Burgess RC, Michaels L, Bale JF Jr, et al. Polymerase chain reaction amplification of herpes simplex viral DNA from the geniculate ganglion of a patient with Bell's palsy. *Ann Otol Rhinol Laryngol* 1994;103:775–779.
6. Proctor B, Corgill DA, Proud G. The pathology of Bell's palsy. *Trans Am Acad Ophthalmol Otolaryngol* 1976;82:70–80.
7. Sugita T, Murakami S, Yanagihara N, et al. Facial nerve paralysis induced by herpes simplex virus in mice: an animal model of acute and transient facial paralysis. *Ann Otol Rhinol Laryngol* 1995;104: 574–581.
8. Adour KK, Ruboyianes JM, Von Doersten PG, et al. Bell's palsy treatment with acyclovir and prednisone compared with prednisone alone: a double-blind, randomized, controlled trial. *Ann Otol Rhinol Laryngol* 1996;105:371–378.
9. Fisch U. Surgery for Bell's palsy. *Arch Otolaryngol* 1981;107:1–11.
10. Van Buskirk C. Seventh nerve complex. *J Comp Neurol* 1945;82: 303–333.
11. Sando I, Takahashi H, Yasumura S, et al. Histopathology of the facial nerve in the temporal bone. In: May M, Schaitkin BM, eds. *The Facial Nerve,* 2nd ed. New York: Thieme Medical Publishers, 2000:127–152.
12. Sunderland S. *Nerve and Nerve Injuries,* 2nd ed. Edinburgh/New York: Churchill Livingstone, 1978:133–141.
13. Seddon HJ. Three types of nerve injury. *Brain* 1943;66:237–288.
14. Peitersen E. The natural history of Bell's palsy. *Am J Otol* 1982;4: 107–111.
15. Esslen E. The acute facial palsies: investigations on the localization and pathogenesis of meato-labyrinthine facial palsies. *Schriftenr Neurol* 1977;18:1–164.
16. Fisch U. Prognostic value of electrical tests in acute facial paralysis. *Am J Otol* 1984;5:494–498.
17. Gantz BJ, Gmuer AA, Holliday M, et al. Electroneurographic evaluation of the facial nerve: Method and technical problems. *Ann Otol Rhinol Laryngol* 1984;93:394–398.
18. Sittel C, Guntinas-Lichius O, Streppel M, et al. Variability of repeated facial nerve electroneurography in healthy subjects. *Laryngoscope* 1998;108:1177–1180.
19. Ide M, Morimitsu T, Ushisako Y, et al. The significance of stapedial reflex test in facial nerve paralysis. *Acta Otolaryngol (Stockh)* 1988; Suppl 446:57–63.
20. Ralli G, Magliulo G, Gagliardi M. Bell's palsy and stapedial reflex. *Clin Otolaryngol* 1986;11:261–265.
21. Kumar A, Mafee MF, Mason T. Value of imaging in disorders of the facial nerve. *Top Magn Reson Imaging* 2000;11:38–51.
22. Gantz BJ, Rubinstein JT, Gidley P, et al. Surgical management of Bell's palsy. *Laryngoscope* 1999;109:1177–1188.
23. Felix H, Eby TL, Fisch U. New aspects of facial nerve pathology in temporal bone fractures. *Acta Otolaryngol (Stockh)* 1991;111: 332–336.
24. May M, Hardin WB Jr. Facial palsy: interpretation of neurologic findings. *Trans Am Acad Ophthalmol Otolaryngol* 1977;84:ORL 710–722.
25. May M, Schaitkin BM. Tumors involving the facial nerve. In: May M, Schaitkin BM, eds. *The Facial Nerve,* 2nd ed. New York: Thieme Medical Publishers, 2000:393–408.

CHAPTER 7

Intraoperative Monitoring of the Facial Nerve and Hearing

Robert A. Levine, Steven F. Ronner, and Aaron R. Thornton

The ideal in any medical intervention is to achieve its purpose with no or minimal adverse effects. For temporal bone surgery, that includes no postoperative cranial nerve deficits. Facial nerve monitoring can minimize the likelihood of injuring the facial nerve intraoperatively for two reasons. First, the nerve can be localized by electrical stimulation when its location may not be visually apparent. Second, electrophysiologic monitoring can detect facial nerve irritation in the absence of any overt facial movement (1–6). Immediate postoperative facial function can also be predicted by stimulation of the most proximal segment of the facial nerve (7–10). However, at present delayed facial weakness cannot be predicted.

For historical reasons, each of the authors' two hospitals has independently developed its own facial nerve monitoring program. Middle ear and mastoid surgery is done at the Massachusetts Eye and Ear Infirmary and suboccipital cerebellopontine angle surgery at Massachusetts General Hospital. As will be apparent from this presentation, the methods are very similar, but by the nature of the different surgical techniques some differences in monitoring have evolved. For example, because rigid head fixation is used in suboccipital cerebellopontine angle surgery, facial movements can be monitored with a motion sensor, but such monitoring is impractical for middle ear surgery because the unrestrained head is relatively free to move.

MIDDLE EAR AND MASTOID SURGERY: FACIAL NERVE MONITORING

Instrumentation and Technique

The facial nerve passes through the internal auditory meatus of the temporal bone and traverses the mastoid through the fallopian canal, passing near several surgical landmarks in the middle ear, including the facial ridge, hypotympanum, and oval window. Although normally protected by bone, the nerve can be exposed due to atypical anatomy, erosion of the bone by disease, or removal of bone from prior surgery. Facial nerve irritation is detected by increased electrical activity of muscles innervated by the facial nerve (*passive* monitoring), and the facial nerve is located by detecting facial muscle contractions from direct electrical stimulation of the nerve from various points in the operative field (*active* monitoring). This electrical stimulation uses 4-per-second, 0.2-msec duration pulses, whose amplitude usually ranges between 0.1 to 0.6 mA. As with any nerve conduction study, a compound muscle action potential (CMAP) is produced (with about a 3-msec latency), and it can be readily detected with an oscilloscope triggered by the stimulus pulse (Fig. 7.1).

Aside from the stapedial nerve, the motor portion of the facial nerve has no other branches before it emerges at the stylomastoid foramen. Consequently, stimulation of the nerve trunk within the mastoid or middle ear may excite any or all of the muscles of the head and neck that are innervated by the facial nerve. Stimulation during surgery, intentional or inadvertent, can be expected to activate muscles over a large portion of the face. Differential recording electrodes placed at the outer canthus of the eye and near the nares and upper lip are sensitive to myogenic activity from all muscle groups in the central portion of the face. The myoelectric signals are relatively strong in this region, providing good sensitivity and signal-to-noise ratio of the recordings. The differential ground is typically placed on the cheek. Surface and needle electrodes perform equally well for this type of broadly spaced, nonspecific array. The monitoring device presently being used by us for mastoid and middle ear surgery, the Xomed Neural Integrity Monitor (NIM), can record two channels simultaneously, typically with one pair of electrodes near the eye and the other near the upper lip. However, this somewhat increased specificity for site of activity provides no greater sensitivity for active or passive

The authors thank B. Kiang for preparing many of the figures and M. Skrip and J. Wilkins for their valuable assistance with the middle ear and mastoid section.

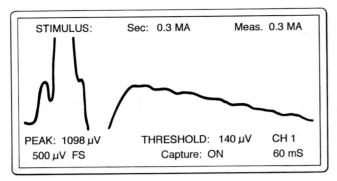

FIG. 7.1 Facial muscle compound action potential (CMAP) elicited by direct electrical stimulation of the facial nerve. Differential recording between surface electrodes at the outer canthus of the eye and near the upper lip. The CMAP is depicted as seen on the display of the Xomed Neural Integrity Monitor. Because of the CMAP's large amplitude (1098 μv) as compared with the screen maximum display of 500 μv, the major upward and downward deflections are clipped. Sweep duration: 60 msec; pulse amplitude: 0.3 mA.

monitoring; furthermore, two channels have the disadvantage of dividing the monitor's attention and thereby increasing the likelihood of missing a fleeting event. For these reasons, we routinely monitor with a single channel.

Surface electrodes are easily applied with the patient just prior to anesthesia. The recording instrument can be then be used to evaluate the amplitude of the EMG (electromyography), which is particularly helpful for patients with a preexisting facial paresis. If necessary, electrodes can be placed satisfactorily even after the start of surgery. Instruments such as the NIM display the ongoing EMG on a small screen and can provide alarms when the waveform exceeds specified criteria. However, electrical artifacts generated by instruments, irrigation, drilling, and manipulation of the patient are mixed with the EMG and are often large enough to set off the alarms, causing unnecessary confusion and irritation. Consequently, the alarms are generally silenced when (i) there is no risk to the nerve or (ii) a monitor operator is present who can observe the waveform to discriminate between artifacts and EMG, so that the surgeon is alerted only when there is evidence of facial nerve stimulation.

Unfortunately, the nerve cannot be monitored reliably under all conditions. Poorly grounded equipment such as electric drills, electrocautery, and anesthesia instruments may increase background electrical noise to such an extent that the facial EMG is obscured, particularly if the EMG is abnormally small. Electrocautery generates signals so large that electrical monitoring is not possible during cautery, even though cautery can damage the nerve. Under these conditions, partial or complete loss of facial function can occur without being detected. At these times, facial muscle contractions are detected by the anesthesiologist placing a hand on the patient's face or by the use of mechanical tranducers to detect facial movement. It is important to note that persistent heating of the nerve by drilling without irrigation and rest will make the nerve less likely to respond if damaged.

The condition of the patient also affects the quality of the monitoring. Preexisting nerve dysfunction may not be readily discerned during a clinical evaluation, but it can reduce EMG amplitudes. Although it may be possible to monitor patients with paresis as low as House grade IV, the procedure will be much more susceptible to artifacts; consequently, reliability will be greatly diminished. These conditions can be anticipated by preoperative electroneurography. Care must be exercised in the use of muscle relaxants, because their very action is to reduce the responsiveness of the muscles being monitored. When excessive, they may prevent monitoring altogether.

During passive monitoring, the role of the operator is to detect any signs of facial nerve irritation. When the nerve is encountered, a sudden burst response, bipolar in morphology, is seen. The underlying timing of nerve firing is slow enough so that when amplified and presented through a loudspeaker a characteristic low-frequency sound can be heard. Such sounds can occur from touching or transecting the facial nerve. The differences in response between a brief touch and complete division of the facial nerve are slight. A continuous "growling" sound has been associated with irritation of the nerve (e.g., stretching of the nerve or sudden change in temperature).

Active monitoring with a stimulating probe may be used by the surgeon whenever there is a need to locate the nerve and differentiate it from surrounding tissue. The monitor assists by adjusting current levels of the stimulator, discriminating CMAPs from artifacts, and reporting on the relative sizes of CMAPs. By varying the probe location and the current, the amplitude of the CMAP can often reveal the precise location of the facial nerve. In the case of a nerve enveloped in cholesteatoma or other soft tissue, for example, the monitor operator will reduce the stimulus current to a very low level (0.1 to 0.4 mA) so that the probe will only stimulate if it is directly on the nerve. In this way the surgeon can systematically probe each piece of tissue before excising it. Because bone is a poor electrical conductor, the nerve within the intact bony canal cannot be reliably stimulated or localized with this method. Very high current levels are nonlocalizing because they can produce a maximum CMAP over a wide area. However, as the bone overlying the nerve is thinned, the stimulator becomes more effective, so that current level can sometimes be used to assess the relative thickness of the remaining bone.

CEREBELLOPONTINE ANGLE SURGERY: FACIAL AND HEARING MONITORING

Facial Nerve Monitoring

Cerebellopontine angle tumor resection is done by our surgeons, employing either the posterior or middle fossa approaches. In the past the posterior fossa approach had been used almost exclusively (11); more recently the middle fossa operation is being used for small intracanalicular tumors when hearing preservation is paramount. However, there may be a small increased risk of facial nerve injury with the middle fossa approach (12).

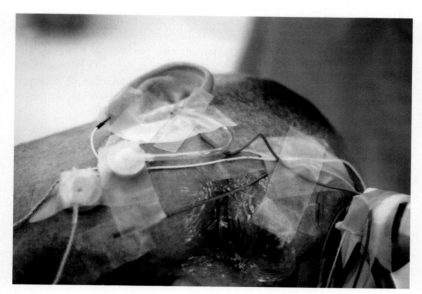

FIG. 7.2 Layout of electrodes and ear phone for facial nerve and hearing monitoring during cerebellopontine angle surgery (1999). After the patient is anesthetized and intubated and the head fixed in the Mayfield frame, needle electrodes are inserted in the ipsilateral orbicularis oculus *(light green wire)*, orbicularis oris *(brown wire)* for facial nerve EMG monitoring. An ipsilateral forehead electrode *(purple wire)* serves as an isolated ground lead. The transtympanic electrode is a 75-mm insulated needle electrode *(red lead)* with a 90-degree crimp so the needle can be securely taped to the face. An electrode *(white)* inserted into the earlobe serves as the reference for the transtympanic electrode and for an electrode *(tan wire)* located in the contralateral forehead (for the far-field auditory evoked responses). Sound is delivered by an earphone *(round white disk)* connected to the ear via clear plastic tubing attached to an ear insert (AstroMed/Grass canal ear tip no. 3). A piezoelectric motion sensor is taped to the cheek halfway between the corner of the mouth and the ear.

Anesthetic Considerations

Although the facial nerve can be stimulated and facial movements detected while patients receive low-dose muscle relaxants (13), to optimize monitoring sensitivity, no muscle relaxant should be used after intubation. Anesthesia is maintained with intravenous anesthetics such as propofol and remifentynl. Once tumor removal is complete and dural closure has begun, muscle relaxants may be used freely.

Localization of the Facial Nerve

Unlike mastoid and middle ear monitoring, direct electrical stimulation of the facial nerve is detected with facial movements rather than the CMAP. The facial nerve is electrically stimulated in the operative field with a Prass flush-tip monopolar handheld probe (Xomed-Treace, Inc.). The probe is connected to a Montgomery nerve-stimulating unit that delivers a continuous 60-Hz constant-voltage sinusoid whose peak-to-peak amplitude can be varied between 0.1 and 1 volt (14). The patient's Bovie pad completes the circuit. This mode of stimulation results in a tetanic facial nerve discharge pattern, which induces a facial movement that can be detected. To locate the facial nerve, stimulation of the tumor capsule is typically initiated with one volt, whereas stimulation within the tumor capsule begins with 0.3 or 0.5 volts. Once facial movements are detected, the nerve is located by remapping the region using progressively lower voltages until only a very restricted region evokes facial movements.

Detection of Facial Nerve Activation

Three complementary techniques are used to detect facial nerve activity.

Electromyography

Electrical myogenic activity from 13-mm intramuscular needle electrodes is recorded routinely from two muscles innervated by the ipsilateral facial nerve, namely, the orbicularis oculi and orbicularis oris (15,16). A contralateral forehead electrode serves as the reference (Fig. 7.2). For larger acoustic neuromas, the trigeminal nerve is monitored with an additional EMG channel recording from an electrode in the trigeminally innervated ipsilateral masseter muscle. An ipsilateral forehead electrode provides the isolated ground for the amplifiers. All electrodes are secured to the face with tape and connected to a biopotential-isolated electrode board. EMG signals are then amplified, filtered (30 to 1,000 Hz), and displayed on both an oscilloscope and a chart recorder. The multichannel oscilloscope sweeps at 5 msec/cm and is triggered by line voltage. An eight-channel pen recorder set to paper speeds of either 5, 50, or 500 mm/min continuously records each EMG channel, as well as electrocardiograph (ECG) and arterial blood pressure. EMG activity is audible from the sound of the chart recorder pen movements. A special circuit shuts off all pens whenever electrocautery is in use.

Mechanical Detection of Face Movements

Because the EMG is swamped by the electrical signal from electrocautery and irreversible facial nerve damage can occur if cautery is too close to facial nerve fibers, alternative methods of detecting facial nerve activation are necessary during cautery. We use a motion detector (accelerometer housed in a button-shaped plastic casing) taped to the ipsilateral cheek (Fig 7.2). It generates a voltage with any movement (17,18); in this way, facial muscle contractions are readily detected. In fact, facial motion due to the cardiac cycle can be detected as well and is useful as an indicator that the motion sensor is operating properly. Other techniques, such as the use of air-inflated rubber sensors (19) or strain-gauge clips attached to the cheek, can serve the same purpose (20).

In our arrangement the output from the motion sensor triggers a strobe light whenever the face moves, thereby immediately alerting the surgeon. The accelerometer output is also recorded on the chart recorder as a permanent record of facial movements.

Video Monitoring of Facial Movements

A closed-circuit video system is routinely used as a third technique for monitoring facial movements (Fig. 7.3). The patient lies supine with the head turned to the side so that the ipsilateral ear is superior and almost horizontal. The head is secured by a Mayfield frame to which all lead wires are taped. The endotracheal tube exits from the contralateral side to avoid distortion of the ipsilateral face. The surgical drapes are kept off the face with a metal frame, so that the face can be observed at all times. A fiber-optic light illuminates the face, and a closed-circuit video system records the image of the face, which is displayed along with the video output from the operating microscope.

When EMG is not available, this technique is most useful as a complement to the motion detector because it can clarify the source of movement. During direct electrical stimulation of the nerve with electrocautery, simultaneous activation of both the facial nerve and the motor division of the trigeminal nerve can occur if a large acoustic neuroma displaces the facial nerve toward the trigeminal. In such a case, viewing the video monitor can indicate whether the motion sensor output is signaling face or jaw movements. Movement of the upper and lower lips indicate facial nerve stimulation, whereas jaw movements point toward trigeminal nerve stimulation. Other occasional uses of directly viewing the face include observing horizontal eye movements (through the closed eyelid), indicating abducens

nerve stimulation. Shoulder and neck movements from spinal accessory nerve activation or tongue movements due to hypoglossal nerve activation can also be observed by closed-circuit monitoring. Fasciculations of facial muscles occurring while tumor is dissected off the facial nerve can be observed synchronous with EMG activity, and signs of facial movements due to light anesthesia can also be detected.

Case Study

Figures 7.4 to 7.9 illustrate for one patient (no. 1123) the use of facial nerve monitoring during the total removal of a 2-cm acoustic neuroma via the posterior fossa approach; the postoperative facial function was normal. The first step prior to any tumor removal is to map the surface of the tumor capsule with the nerve stimulator. When 1 volt was applied to the superior portion of the tumor capsule, facial movement was detected by the motion sensor and could be seen on the video monitor. This area of the capsule was then restimulated using 0.3 volts (Fig. 7.4); facial movements occurred again but in a more restricted region. This result indicated that the facial nerve was displaced over the superior-posterior portion of the tumor—an infrequent finding that can be associated with a poor prognosis. On closer inspection of the region of stimulation, the nerve could be seen as a thin band. By electrically mapping the surface of the capsule prior to dissection, injury to the facial nerve was avoided.

The dissection then proceeded, with special care taken to avoid the region where the facial nerve could be stimulated. While dissecting the tumor in another location using bipolar cautery, movement of the face was detected by the motion

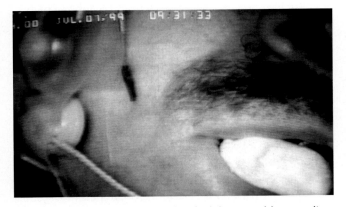

FIG. 7.3 The face as seen during facial nerve video monitoring of cerebellopontine angle surgery. A cotton wad is used as a bite-block and avoids distortion of the ipsilateral lip. The needle hub *(black)* of the orbicularis oris muscle electrode is seen, as well as the motion sensor (with twisted wire leads) and *(above)* the earphone used for generating clicks for auditory monitoring.

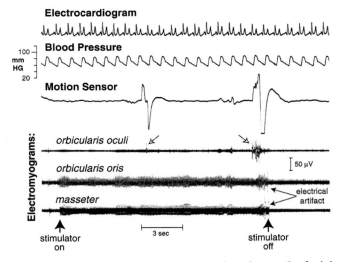

FIG. 7.4 Stimulation of the tumor capsule to locate the facial nerve. Shown are the chart recorder traces while the nerve stimulator is being moved over the tumor surface. The bursts of activity from orbicularis oculi *(open arrows)* that coincide with large changes in the motion sensor signal indicate that facial nerve fibers are near the stimulator tip. Continuous electrical activity on orbicularis oris and masseter channels is electrical artifact from the stimulator.

sensor and the strobe light flashed. The dissection was then halted, and the stimulator was used to locate the course of the nerve in this region (Fig. 7.5).

When the operative field was irrigated with body temperature saline, EMG activity from the facial muscles but not the masseter muscle occurred (Fig. 7.6). However, the EMG activity was not sufficient to cause visible facial movement. No deleterious effect upon postoperative facial nerve function has been noted to occur as a result of saline irrigation. Depth of anesthesia may affect the degree of spontaneous

activity evoked by irrigation. Cold irrigation can cause vagal stimulation with slowing of the pulse. For this reason, only body temperature irrigation fluids are used during cerebellopontine angle surgery.

EMG-like artifacts may sometimes occur (Fig. 7.7A). When scissors touch the retractors, motor-unit–like electrical activity appears. However, it is never associated with motion sensor activity or visible facial movements. Inspection of the waveform of this electrical activity (Fig. 7.7B) confirms that it is artifactual.

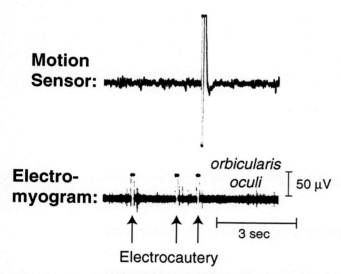

FIG. 7.5 Electrocautery can sometimes discharge facial nerve fibers. Each time cautery occurs, the EMG is shorted out by our system, as shown by the square wave on the orbicularis oculi channel *(arrows)*. With the third electrocautery, the face was activated, as detected by the motion sensor. The surgeon was alerted to this fact by a flash of a strobe light. Surgery was then redirected to avoid any further irritation of the facial nerve.

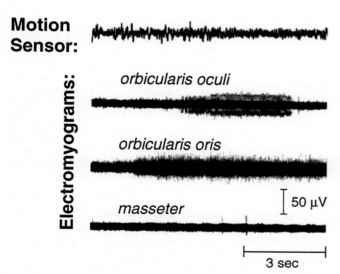

FIG. 7.6 Irrigation can elicit facial nerve activity. Irrigation of the operative field with body temperature saline elicited EMG activity in orbicularis oculi and oris but not in masseter. No motion sensor activity was apparent.

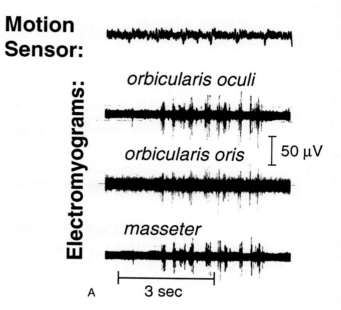

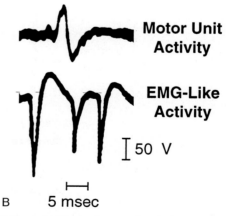

FIG. 7.7 A: EMG-like activity can occur when scissors touch cerebellar retractors. No associated movements of the face occurred. B: Oscilloscope traces of the true EMG activity *(top trace)* and the activity associated with the scissors touching the retractors *(bottom trace)*. Distinct differences in the two types of waveforms confirm that the activity associated with the scissors touching the retractors is artifactual.

At other times, facial movements occur that are not signs of impending facial nerve damage. For example, a facial twitch can occur if the electrically activated bipolar cautery forceps touch the tip of the metal suction tube in contact with cerebrospinal fluid (CSF). This occurs presumably because current passes from the cautery forceps to the CSF and then to the facial nerve.

Drilling open the internal auditory canal can cause facial twitches (Fig. 7.8A), presumably due to mechanical activation of the facial nerve. Proximity of the nerve to the drill can be confirmed by directly stimulating the thinned area of bone and noting if facial movement occurs.

Once the internal auditory canal is opened, tumor dissection usually proceeds in a medial to lateral direction. Depending upon how adherent the tumor is to the facial nerve, facial nerve activity and twitches may occur with the dissec-

tion (Fig. 7.8B). Often the spiking activity seen on the motion sensor channel output can be visually correlated to tiny twitches and fasciculations, especially near the corner of the ipsilateral mouth.

After the tumor is completely removed, the fact that low-voltage (0.2 volts) facial nerve stimulation evokes facial movement confirms that the facial nerve is physiologically intact and predicts good immediate postoperative facial function (Fig. 7.9A). When mastoid air cells within the internal auditory canal are waxed (to prevent a postoperative CSF leak), facial twitching and motor unit activity can occur from touching the facial nerve (Fig. 7.9B). Placement of abdominal fat into the bony defect of the internal auditory canal prior to dural closure can also cause facial EMG activity (Fig. 7.9C) if pressure is applied to the facial nerve. Facial nerve monitoring is discontinued with dural closure.

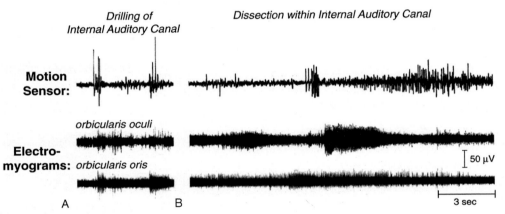

FIG. 7.8 EMG and motion sensor activity occur during **(A)** drilling of the internal auditory canal and then **(B)** dissection of tumor from internal auditory canal.

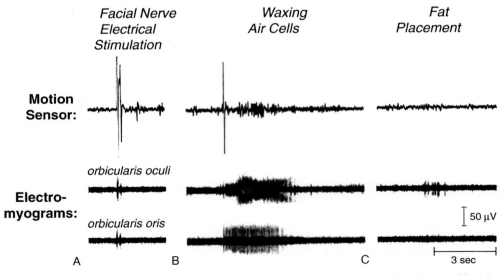

FIG. 7.9 Motion sensor and EMG recordings following total tumor removal. **A:** Stimulation of facial nerve near brainstem. The evoked motion sensor and EMG activity indicates the nerve is physiologically intact and predicts good immediate postoperative facial function. **B** and **C:** EMG activity occurs with both waxing of mastoid air cells and placement of abdominal fat over the internal auditory canal, but motion sensor activity only occurs with the former.

Monitoring of Hearing

Whereas facial nerve monitoring is performed in all cases of cerebellopontine angle surgery, hearing monitoring is only performed in select cases; however, the indications for hearing preservation are beyond the scope of this chapter. Multiple factors appear to be important in hearing preservation for cerebellopontine angle surgery (principally, vestibular schwannoma surgery). Tumor size is one factor; the likelihood for saving hearing is correlated with tumor size for tumors resected via the posterior fossa approach (21–23). Other factors also affect the chances for hearing preservation, most notably whether the internal auditory artery or the cochlear nerve is intimately involved with the tumor (24). In one of our cases, despite the tumor being 3 mm in its entire extent, hearing could not be preserved because the schwannoma arose from the auditory nerve; total tumor resection required sacrifice of the auditory nerve. Like facial nerve function, delayed hearing loss may occur despite hearing preservation in the immediate postoperative period (25,26).

Permanent loss of blood supply to the cochlea will result in hearing loss (27); a delay of about 1 minute occurs between interruption of the cochlear blood supply and change in any of the auditory evoked potentials (Fig. 7.10) (24,28). Other techniques, such as laser Doppler monitoring of cochlear blood flow (24,29) or measurement of otoacoustic emissions, may provide more rapid feedback regarding cochlear blood flow (30). Transient compromise of cochlear blood supply is compatible with preservation of hearing (Fig. 7.11). Vasospasm of the internal auditory artery at the

site of dissection with the tumor sometimes can be reversed by prompt direct application of a vasodilator, such as papaverine (Fig. 7.11) (24,28). Once the compound action potential of the auditory nerve, N-1 of the electrocochleogram (EcochG), has been totally lost for more than 15 minutes, the patient has always been deaf in the operative ear in our experience (Fig. 7.10) (24).

The surgical approach may also influence outcome. Some reports suggest that hearing preservation is more likely with the middle fossa approach (31). The direction of tumor dissection may affect hearing outcome with the posterior fossa approach (32); lateral to medial traction of the tumor sometimes appears to lead to hearing loss (33,34). For patients with neurofibromatosis type II and bilateral acoustic neuromas, tumor resection is usually subtotal because hearing preservation is paramount. The most conservative approach in this setting is decompression of the internal auditory canal only with no tumor removal. Another approach is to proceed with tumor resection until the auditory evoked potentials indicate the first hint of a signal loss (Fig. 7.12). Successful preservation of hearing in patients with neurofibromatosis type II can be achieved by such a protocol (33).

Hearing outcome can be predicted in some but not all cases from the status of the auditory evoked potentials (Table 7.1). Little or no change in the auditory evoked potentials proximal to the tumor (e.g., wave V of the brainstem auditory evoked potentials [BAEPs]) implies that hearing is unchanged (Fig. 7.13). In general, major improvements in hearing have not occurred with cerebellopontine angle

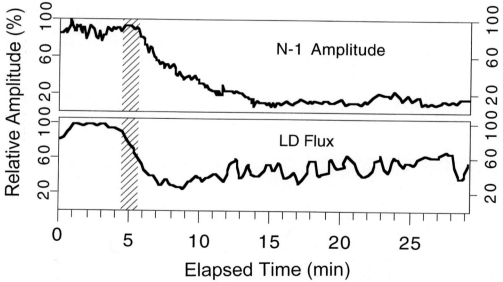

FIG. 7.10 Sudden loss of N-1: laser Doppler evidence for cochlear ischemia. Plotted vertically in the two panels are relative amplitudes of N-1 and the laser Doppler signal over a 29-minute interval, during which the acoustic neuroma was being dissected out of the internal auditory canal. The laser Doppler probe was on the promontory of the middle ear. The 1-minute interval *(crosshatched)* between the drop in the laser Doppler signal and the decrease in N-1 amplitude supports the contention that a minute elapses from the time of cochlea ischemia to any change in N-1. The patient was deaf postoperatively. In general, hearing does not recover if N-1 is lost for more than 15 minutes. Rarefaction clicks, 29/sec, 80-dB hearing loss.

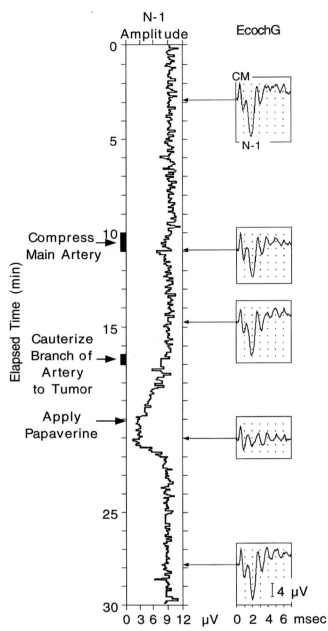

FIG. 7.11 Blood vessel compression identifies internal auditory artery and papaverine (a vasodilator) restores hearing. Plot of N-1 amplitudes obtained during 30 minutes of dissection of tumor from internal auditory canal. To the right of this plot are EcochG waveforms. The main trunk of a small blood vessel passing into the internal auditory canal with a branch going into the tumor was identified as the internal auditory artery, because when occluded for a minute (as indicated by *uppermost solid rectangle*), a small (approximately 20%) reversible decrease in N-1 amplitude occurred. When the branch entering the tumor was cauterized, the main artery went into spasm and a major loss of N-1 amplitude resulted. Applying the vasodilator, papaverine, to the blood vessel, resulted in full restoration of N-1. Postoperatively, pure-tone thresholds were minimally changed and speech discrimination remained good. Rarefaction clicks, 29/sec, 80-dB hearing loss.

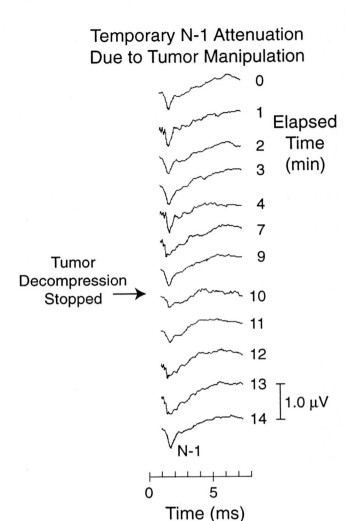

FIG. 7.12 Transient N-1 attenuation during internal debulking of tumor. Patient with neurofibromatosis type II. Successive EcochG waveforms are shown from the 14-minute interval during which the change in N-1 occurred. Because of these changes, further dissection of patient's 2.5-cm left acoustic neuroma was stopped. Postoperatively the patient's audiogram remained normal. Stimulus artifact has been suppressed at the beginning of all traces.

TABLE 7.1. *Hearing outcome as related to the evoked potentials*

N-1	Wave V	Hearing Outcome
Detected	Detected	Hearing
Detected	Not detected	Indeterminate
Not detected	Not detected	No hearing

surgery (35). Changes in but still presence of wave V implies that hearing will be present postoperatively. However, the quality of hearing cannot be predicted; it may be unchanged or may have worsened. Loss of wave V but preservation of the auditory nerve potential (N-1) is indeterminate. Hearing may be absent (Fig. 7.14), unchanged (Fig. 7.15),

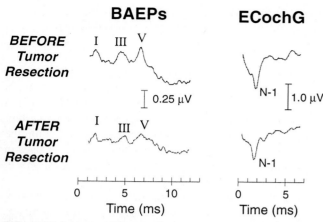

BAEPs   **ECochG**

BEFORE Tumor Resection

AFTER Tumor Resection

0.25 μV   1.0 μV   N-1   N-1

Time (ms)   Time (ms)

FIG. 7.13 Intraoperative auditory evoked potentials before and after tumor resection. The vestibular schwannoma extended 1.5 cm into the cerebellopontine angle. Preoperative and postoperative audiograms and speech discrimination scores were normal. Following tumor removal, N-1 was unchanged, but minor changes in amplitudes and latencies of waves III and V did occur. Stimulus artifact has been suppressed at beginning of all traces.

or something in between these two outcomes (25,36). N-1 may persist for 15 minutes or even days following auditory nerve transaction (24,28). Permanent loss of N-1 (more than 15 minutes) has always been associated with a total hearing loss.

Technique of Hearing Monitoring

Compared with the facial muscle potentials, the auditory evoked potentials are very small, so that optimal detection becomes a major issue. In fact, it was only with advancements in miniaturization of noise reduction instruments that hearing monitoring became possible (37). What must be optimized is *signal-to-noise ratio per unit time*. The technical aspects of optimizing detection of the auditory evoked potentials have been described in detail previously (24), so they will only be summarized here.

Ideally signals from two locations should be monitored: the auditory nerve distal to the tumor and the auditory nerve (or auditory pathway) proximal to the tumor. A major factor is the signal size. Use of a transtympanic electrode whose uninsulated tip is placed on the promontory of the round window is ideal for recording from the distal auditory nerve. As a near-field recording, the EcochG is often large and always present if the patient has some preoperative hearing. Typically with signal averaging, adequate noise reduction can be obtained in a few seconds because the N-1 amplitude is on the order of a few microvolts. In addition, it can record cochlear microphonic and summating potential, which provide additional information regarding the physiologic state of the cochlea.

Recordings of neural activity proximal to the tumor are routinely done using the far-field BAEPs, which are present

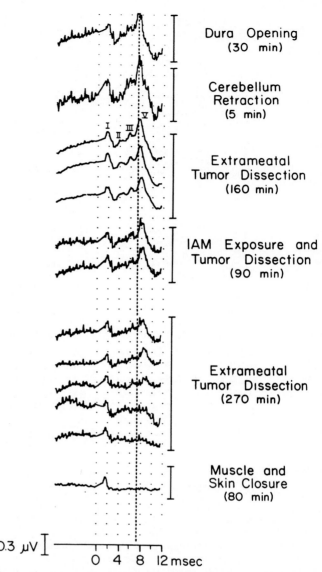

Dura Opening (30 min)

Cerebellum Retraction (5 min)

Extrameatal Tumor Dissection (160 min)

IAM Exposure and Tumor Dissection (90 min)

Extrameatal Tumor Dissection (270 min)

Muscle and Skin Closure (80 min)

0.3 μV   0   4   8   12 msec

FIG. 7.14 Hearing outcome indeterminate: loss of waves II, III, and V and preservation of wave I. No hearing postoperatively. BAEPs obtained successively throughout the six stages of complete tumor removal utilizing the posterior fossa approach. Condensation clicks, 33/sec, 78-dB hearing loss.

in a little more than half the patients we have monitored. Usually wave V, which is generated by the upper pons, is the most robust component. However, because of its submicrovolt amplitude, several hundred responses must be averaged to reliably detect wave V. At a stimulation rate of about 30 per second, a minute or more may be required for each new BAEP. For posterior fossa approaches, but not middle fossa surgical approaches, an alternative to the BAEPs are cerebellopontine angle near-field recordings. Various configurations of electrodes can be used to record from within the

AVERAGED WAVEFORMS

ELAPSED TIME (min)

L Promontory (+)
L Ear Lobe (−)

Vertex (+)
L Ear Lobe (−)

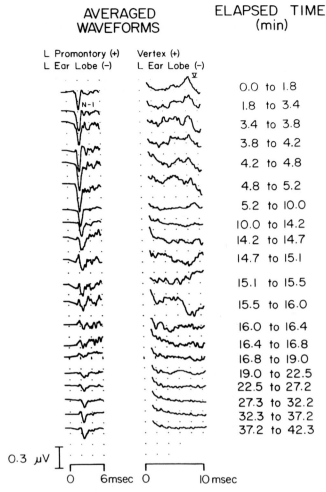

0.0 to 1.8

1.8 to 3.4

3.4 to 3.8

3.8 to 4.2

4.2 to 4.8

4.8 to 5.2

5.2 to 10.0

10.0 to 14.2

14.2 to 14.7

14.7 to 15.1

15.1 to 15.5

15.5 to 16.0

16.0 to 16.4

16.4 to 16.8

16.8 to 19.0

19.0 to 22.5

22.5 to 27.2

27.3 to 32.2

32.3 to 37.2

37.2 to 42.3

0.3 μV

0   6msec   0   10 msec

FIG. 7.15 Hearing outcome indeterminate: loss of waves III, and V and preservation of N-1 and wave I. Speech discrimination scores: 56% preoperatively, 44% postoperatively. Puretone thresholds: unchanged postoperatively except that 4- and 8-kHz thresholds were undetectable postoperatively (had been 70-dB HL preoperatively). EcochG *(left column)* and BAEPs *(right column)* obtained successively over the 42 minutes when the tumor was being separated from the seventh and eighth cranial nerves. Condensation clicks, 44/sec, 78-dB hearing.

operative field (36,38). Although these recording sites improve signal size by a factor of 10 or more, the noise level may increase as well, so that the overall gain in signal-to-noise ratio is less than would be predicted from the larger signal. Furthermore, they do not improve the likelihood of detecting a signal representing neural activity proximal to the tumor; wave V of the BAEPs and the cerebellopontine angle recordings have the same capability in detecting neural activity proximal to the tumor (39). Like the BAEPs, cerebellopontine angle near-field recordings will not detect activity proximal to the tumor in many cases.

Besides the recording site, other factors that can optimize the rapid detection of these auditory evoked potentials are as follows:

1. *Acoustic system.* Adding an acoustic delay of about a millisecond separates the electrical stimulus artifact from the earliest biologic responses so that the two can be distinguished. Use of a stimulus-monitoring system that continuously records the sound pressure within the ear canal is very helpful in deciding whether changes in recordings are due to middle ear problems or failures in the stimulus-generating system.
2. *Choice of stimulus.* Subjects differ in the size of their responses to rarefaction, condensation, or alternating polarity clicks. Therefore each subject's stimulus used for monitoring should be chosen on an individual basis. Signal size also varies with click rate, click intensity, and pulse duration, so these also require optimization. Typical settings are 29-per-second, 100-msec pulses generating 80-dB hearing loss (nHL) clicks; however, the optimal settings will vary from patient to patient. The contralateral ear is always masked with continuous noise at 40 dB below the click level.
3. *Artifact rejection.* Brief, large, extraneous electrical signals are not uncommon in the operating room setting. Every effort should be made to minimize them, but when they do occur they should not be included as part of the averaging; that trial should be rejected.
4. *Bandpass of recordings.* The choice of analog and digital filtering that should be used to facilitate detection of the response will also vary depending upon each patient's recording. Typically, a bandwidth of 30 to 3,000 Hz is used for the BAEPs and 100 to 3,000 Hz for the EcochG.
5. *Exponential averaging.* Computational techniques can be employed so that a completed average is always displayed. Even though in the traditional method it may require minutes to obtain the completed BAEPs, with exponential averaging there is no longer any period of waiting for the buildup of a completed average. Completed BAEPs are always displayed that include only the most recent trials.
6. *Response template.* A template of the expected response waveform can be continuously displayed along with the newly acquired waveforms to facilitate recognition of the subtlest changes in the recordings.
7. *Trending of peaks.* Alongside the waveforms being monitored can be plotted the amplitudes and latencies of the most prominent peaks (or troughs) that have been acquired from the most recent 100 or so completed averages. This complements the response template because at a glance it provides an assessment of the variability of the recordings (40).
8. *Automatic warning.* From applying statistical criteria to the data used for trending, the computer can provide a

warning signal (such as a beep) that indicates when the most recently acquired peak is significantly different from the preceding 100 recordings.

Intraoperative Factors That Affect the Auditory Evoked Potentials

Changes in the evoked potentials are common during tumor dissection, and often no dissection-related event can be pinpointed that is responsible for the change (Figs. 7.10 and 7.14). Nonetheless, whenever a change occurs, the dissection is stopped to allow time for recovery and to reassess the mode of dissection (Fig. 7.12). Others have suggested that retraction of the cerebellum to expose the cerebellopontine angle with posterior fossa surgery can degrade wave V with no change in wave I or N-1 (41); however, this has not been our experience. When the tumor is being separated from the auditory nerve, at times wave V alone is affected with no change in N-1 (Fig. 7.14). Because the auditory nerve can sometimes be incorporated into the tumor, occasionally transection of the auditory nerve is necessary to effect a complete removal of the tumor. When this occurs, wave V is always lost, whereas N-1 can sometimes persist 15 minutes or much longer (24,28). Such observations suggest that N-1 is generated by the portion of the auditory nerve within the cochlea. Because N-1 is the compound action potential of the auditory nerve, its loss will also result in loss of the brainstem potentials and waves III and V.

Drilling of the internal auditory canal often affects the evoked potentials. N-1 may be lost either permanently or, more common, with some later recovery, such as with bone waxing the region of drilling, which had opened the posterior semicircular canal (Fig. 7.16). High-intensity background noise from drilling of the skull or temporal bone acts as a masker and results in either the loss or attenuation of the evoked potentials (Fig. 7.16). Moreover, due to the phenomenon know as temporary threshold shift, even after drilling has stopped, recordings may continue to be suppressed for several seconds in some patients. Because monitoring of hearing is impossible during drilling, in the past we have routinely interrupted the drilling about every 30 seconds to check whether the evoked potentials are stable. The introduction of quieter drills may make this precaution unnecessary.

Often an abrupt loss of N-1 occurs that is complete within about 5 minutes (Figs. 7.10 and 7.11). When cochlear microphonic (CM) is clearly distinguishable from N-1, its loss usually can be seen to begin at the same time as the loss of N-1, to have a longer time course, and to be subtotal. On several occasions this pattern has begun after about a minute of a blood vessel being sacrificed. However, many other times no specific event in the dissection can be identified that might account for the sudden loss of potentials (Fig. 7.10). In one such instance, measurement of laser Doppler flowmetry from the promontory of the middle ear (24) sug-

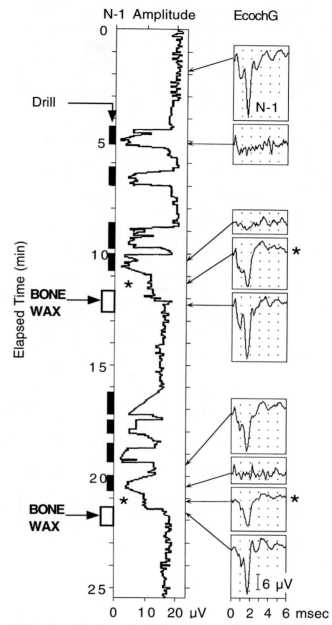

FIG. 7.16 Sealing labyrinth with bone wax restores hearing. Recovery of N-1 with waxing region of drilling during opening of posterior wall of the internal auditory canal. Plot of N-1 amplitudes *(left column)* obtained during 26 minutes of intermittent drilling of internal auditory canal from posterior fossa approach. To the right of this plot are representative EcochG waveforms. The *dark, filled rectangles* along the time (vertical) axis denote when drilling occurred. N-1 amplitude decreases during drilling due to acoustic masking. On two occasions *(asterisks)*, N-1 amplitude recovered only about 50% of its amplitude when drilling was halted. With application of bone wax to the lateral region that had been drilled *(open rectangles)*, N-1 recovered quickly. No changes occurred in the waveforms obtained from the stimulus monitoring system (not shown). Rarefaction clicks, 29/sec, 80-dB HL.

gested that ischemia of the cochlea was the cause of the sudden loss of these potentials, even though no blood vessel was observed to be sacrificed at the time. Before any blood vessel is sacrificed, our practice is to clamp the blood vessel for a full minute to assess whether there is any change in N-1 (Fig. 7.11). Only if N-1 remains perfectly stable will the blood vessel be cauterized. Moreover, when this pattern of an abrupt loss of N-1 does occur, a vasodilator such as papaverine is applied to the blood vessel or, if none is apparent, to the suspicious region of the surgical field on the assumption that vasospasm of the internal auditory artery might be reversed.

Besides insults to the inner ear or nerve, which may cause deafness, middle ear changes can affect the evoked potentials by interfering with sound conduction to the cochlea, yet with no long-term effects on hearing. When a microphone is used to record the sound pressure within the external ear canal, usually a change in the sound conduction properties of the middle ear will also change the waveform of the click as recorded by this microphone. Hence any change in evoked potentials that are accompanied by changes in the external ear canal microphone recordings must be considered to be caused by changes in the sound-conduction prop-

erties of the middle ear and not to a perturbation of the inner ear or auditory nerve (Fig. 7.17).

In summary, monitoring of auditory evoked potentials provides a rapid feedback of the status of the cochlea and distal auditory nerve. Conditions such as vasospasm and entry into the labyrinth can be recognized and corrected to preserve hearing. Feedback regarding the proximal auditory nerve is not as rapid and its implications for hearing less certain. The presence of distal auditory nerve potentials (N-1 or wave I) are necessary but not sufficient for preservation of hearing, whereas the presence of proximal auditory nerve potentials (waves III and V) are sufficient but not necessary for preservation of hearing.

REFERENCES

1. Harner SG, Daube JR, Ebersold MJ, et al. Improved preservation of facial nerve function with use of electrical monitoring during removal of acoustic neuromas. *Mayo Clin Proc* 1987;62(2):92–102.
2. Harner SG, Daube JR, Beatty CW, et al. Intraoperative monitoring of the facial nerve. *Laryngoscope* 1988;98(2):209–212.
3. Leonetti JP, Brackmann DE, Prass RL. Improved preservation of facial nerve function in the infratemporal approach to the skull base. *Otolaryngol Head Neck Surg* 1989;101(1):74–78.

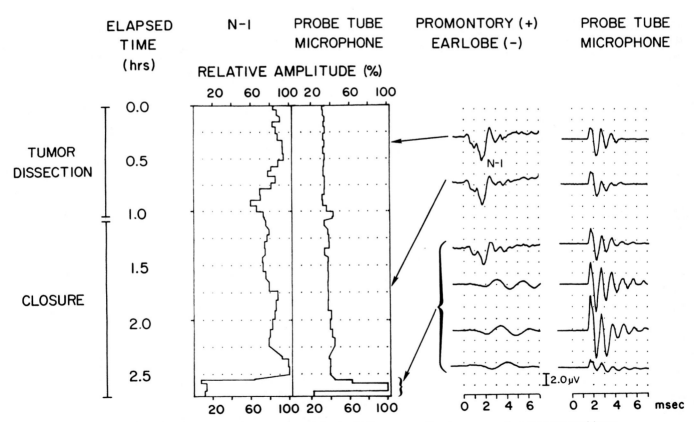

FIG. 7.17 Stimulus monitoring system can detect middle ear or stimulus generating system problems. Plot of peak amplitudes of N-1 and probe tube microphone recordings (stimulus monitoring system) over the last 2.5 hours of surgery. During the last 15 minutes of closure, N-1 became very small; concurrent major alterations in the probe tube microphone recordings indicated that N-1 changes were due to middle ear changes. After surgery, a cerebrospinal fluid leak into the middle ear was identified. Rarefaction clicks, 33/sec, 70-dB HL.

4. Niparko JK, Kileny PR, Kemink JL, et al. Neurophysiologic intraoperative monitoring. II. Facial nerve function. *Am J Otol* 1989; 10(1):55–61.
5. Jellinek DA, Tan LC, Symon L. The impact of continuous electrophysiological monitoring on preservation of the facial nerve during acoustic tumour surgery. *Br J Neurosurg* 1991;5(1):19–24.
6. Dickins JR, Graham SS. A comparison of facial nerve monitoring systems in cerebellopontine angle surgery. *Am J Otol* 1991;12(1):1–6.
7. Silverstein H, Willcox TO Jr, Rosenberg SI, Seidman MD. Prediction of facial nerve function following acoustic neuroma resection using intraoperative facial nerve stimulation. *Laryngoscope* 1994;104(5 Pt 1):539–544.
8. Taha JM, Tew JM Jr, Keith RW. Proximal-to-distal facial amplitude ratios as predictors of facial nerve function after acoustic neuroma excision. *J Neurosurg* 1995;83(6):994–998.
9. Sobottka SB, Schackert G, May SA, et al. Intraoperative facial nerve monitoring (IFNM) predicts facial nerve outcome after resection of vestibular schwannoma. *Acta Neurochir (Wien)* 1998;140(3):235–242.
10. Selesnick SH, Carew JF, Victor JD, et al. Predictive value of facial nerve electrophysiologic stimulation thresholds in cerebellopontine-angle surgery. *Laryngoscope* 1996;106(5 Pt 1):633–638.
11. Ojemann RG. Suboccipital approach to acoustic neuromas. In: Wilson CB, ed. *Neurosurgical Procedures: Personal Approaches to Classic Operations.* Baltimore: Williams & Wilkins, 1992:77–86.
12. Weber PC, Gantz BJ. Results and complications from acoustic neuroma excision via middle cranial fossa approach. *Am J Otol* 1996; 17(4):669–675.
13. Ho LC, Crosby G, Sundaram P, et al. Ulnar train-of-four stimulation in predicting face movement during intracranial facial nerve stimulation. *Anesth Analg* 1989;69(2):242–244.
14. Prass RL, Luders H. Constant-current versus constant-voltage stimulation [Letter]. *J Neurosurg* 1985;62(4):622–623.
15. Miller AR, Jannetta PJ. Preservation of facial function during removal of acoustic neuromas. Use of monopolar constant-voltage stimulation and EMG. *J Neurosurg* 1984;61(4):757–760.
16. Møller AR. Intraoperative monitoring of cranial motor nerves. In: Møller AR, ed. *Evoked Potentials in Intraoperative Monitoring.* Baltimore: Williams & Wilkins, 1988:100–119.
17. Sugita K, Kobayashi S. Technical and instrumental improvements in the surgical treatment of acoustic neurinomas. *J Neurosurg* 1982; 57(6):747–752.
18. Johnson JO, Kern SE. In response to Kopman AF. A piezoelectric neuromuscular monitor. *Anesth Analg* 1994;79(6):1210–1211.
19. Zini C, Gandolfi A. Facial-nerve and vocal-cord monitoring during otoneurosurgical operations. *Arch Otolaryngol Head Neck Surg* 1987; 113(12):1291–1293.
20. Silverstein H, Smouha E, Jones R. Routine identification of the facial nerve using electrical stimulation during otological and neurotological surgery. *Laryngoscope* 1988;98(7):726–730.
21. Frerebeau P, Benezech J, Uziel A, et al. Hearing preservation after acoustic neurinoma operation. *Neurosurgery* 1987;21(2):197–200.
22. Umezu H, Aiba T. Preservation of hearing after surgery for acoustic schwannomas: correlation between cochlear nerve function and operative findings. *J Neurosurg* 1994;80(5):844–848.
23. Nadol JB Jr, Chiong CM, Ojemann RG, et al. Preservation of hearing and facial nerve function in resection of acoustic neuroma. *Laryngoscope* 1992;102(10):1153–1158.
24. Levine RA, Ronner SF, Ojemann RG. Auditory evoked potential and other neurophysiologic monitoring techniques during tumor surgery in the cerebellopontine angle. In: Loftus CM, Traynelis VC, eds. *Intraoperative Monitoring Techniques in Neurosurgery.* New York: McGraw-Hill, 1994:175–191.
25. Levine RA, Ojemann RG, Montgomery WW, et al. Monitoring auditory evoked potentials during acoustic neuroma surgery. Insights into the mechanism of the hearing loss. *Ann Otol Rhinol Laryngol* 1984;93(2 Pt 1):116–123.
26. McKenna MJ, Halpin C, Ojemann RG, et al. Long-term hearing results in patients after surgical removal of acoustic tumors with hearing preservation. *Am J Otol* 1992;13(2):134–136.
27. Sekiya T, Møller AR. Avulsion rupture of the internal auditory artery during operations in the cerebellopontine angle: a study in monkeys. *Neurosurgery* 1987;21(5):631–637.
28. Levine RA. Surgical monitoring applications of the brainstem auditory evoked response and electrocochleography. In: Owen J, Donohoe C, eds. *Clinical Atlas of Auditory Evoked Potentials.* New York: Grune and Stratton, 1988:103–106.
29. Levine RA, Bu-Saba N, Brown MC. Laser-Doppler measurements and electrocochleography during ischemia of the guinea pig cochlea: implications for hearing preservation in acoustic neuroma surgery. *Ann Otol Rhinol Laryngol* 1993;102(2):127–136.
30. Telischi FF, Stagner B, Widick MP, et al. Distortion-product otoacoustic emission monitoring of cochlear blood flow. *Laryngoscope* 1998;108(6):837–842.
31. Irving RM, Jackler RK, Pitts LH. Hearing preservation in patients undergoing vestibular schwannoma surgery: comparison of middle fossa and retrosigmoid approaches. *J Neurosurg* 1998;88(5):840–845.
32. Ojemann RG, Levine RA, Montgomery WM, et al. Use of intraoperative auditory evoked potentials to preserve hearing in unilateral acoustic neuroma removal. *J Neurosurg* 1984;61(5):938–948.
33. Levine RA. Monitoring auditory evoked potentials during acoustic neuroma surgery. In: Silverstein H, Norrell H, eds. *Neurological Surgery of the Ear.* Birmingham: Aesculapius, 1979:287–293.
34. Sekiya T, Møller AR. Cochlear nerve injuries caused by cerebellopontine angle manipulations. An electrophysiological and morphological study in dogs. *J Neurosurg* 1987;67(2):244–249.
35. Nadol JB Jr, Levine R, Ojemann RG, et al. Preservation of hearing in surgical removal of acoustic neuromas of the internal auditory canal and cerebellar pontine angle. *Laryngoscope* 1987;97(11):287–294.
36. Matthies C, Samii M. Direct brainstem recording of auditory evoked potentials during vestibular schwannoma resection: nuclear BAEP recording. Technical note and preliminary results. *J Neurosurg* 1997; 86(6):1057–1062.
37. Levine RA, Montgomery WW, Ojemann RG, et al. Evoked potential detection of hearing loss during acoustic neuroma surgery. *Neurology* 1978;28:339.
38. Colletti V, Fiorino FG, Mocella S, et al. ECochG, CNAP and ABR monitoring during vestibular schwannoma surgery. *Audiology* 1998;37(1):27–37.
39. Levine RA. Monitoring auditory evoked potentials during cerebellopontine angle surgery: relative value of electrocochleography, brainstem auditory evoked potentials and cerebellopontine angle recordings. In: Schramm J, Moller A, eds. *Intraoperative Neurophysiologic Monitoring in Neurosurgery.* Berlin: Springer-Verlag, 1991:193–204.
40. Levine RA. Short-latency auditory evoked potentials: intraoperative applications. *Int Anesthesiol Clin* 1990;28(3):147–153.
41. Grundy BL, Lina A, Procopio PT, et al. Reversible evoked potential changes with retraction of the eighth cranial nerve. *Anesth Analg* 1981;60(11):835–838.

CHAPTER 8

Outcomes Measurements for Ear Surgery

Pa-Chun Wang, Richard E. Gliklich, and Joseph B. Nadol Jr.

QUALITY OF LIFE

Although the evaluation of ear disease has largely relied on the physical and audiologic examination, measurement of treatment success has always included patient-related quality-of-life issues such as the elimination of disease, the achievement of a dry ear, and hearing improvement. Yet other than clinician impression, the rigorous assessment of patient-perceived quality of life has been largely neglected (1,2). Clearly the inclusion of patient-oriented outcomes information will enhance our understanding of the impact of ear disease and the success of treatment (3,4). The development of valid and reliable measures of ear-specific quality of life is the first step in this process. This chapter assesses how far we have come and how far we still must go in measuring the patient's view of ear disease and its treatment.

EFFICACY VS. EFFECTIVENESS

If efficacy is the ability of a specified treatment to achieve a specified result in an experimental setting, then effectiveness is the ability to achieve that result in the real world. The treatment of chronic ear disease is a complex and individualized mix of patient instructions, medications, and procedures. Traditional ways of reporting treatment results for ear disease, meaning audiograms and "objective" ear assessments, are typically inadequate for comparing different treatments (5,6). Patient-perceived quality of life offers another approach to measurement that is useful for a disease that has few fatalities but many sufferers. In this paradigm a standard of ear-specific quality of life is established by developing and testing measurements and applying those measurements to normal and diseased populations. In practice, once such measures are available, quality of life is assessed before and after treatment and the change in quality of life is recorded as the impact of the treatment. Theoretically, different treatment modalities can be assessed by comparing patients on the basis of change in standardized measurements of quality of life. With this ap-

proach, assessment of quality of life becomes a quantitative measurement with known error and confidence intervals (not unlike an audiogram). As our measurements become quantitative and more precise, they can be used for a range of research and practical applications, including identifying the most effective treatments on the basis of absolute results or cost (7).

Patient-based quality-of-life measurements supplement traditional objective measurements and provide a more complete understanding of the effects of a specific ear condition and its intervention.

OUTCOMES MEASURE

Generic vs. Disease-specific

One approach to measuring quality of life is to combine general and disease-specific measurements or surveys. General measures assess the patient's general health status along several lines of functioning and well-being ranging from physical activities to mental health. The Medical Outcomes Study 36-Item Short-Form Health Survey (SF-36) (7), for example, is one of the most widely used general health surveys (8,9). A disease-specific measure focuses more narrowly on the dimensions of disease perceived by the patient with a particular disease (e.g., chronic otitis media). Because of this focus, disease-specific measures tend to be more sensitive to clinical change than general health measures. Combining the two sets of measures provides a broad inventory of health with both the appropriate sensitivity to measure real clinical change and the flexibility to compare across different diseases (10).

Developing general and disease-specific health measures is in itself a rigorous science termed psychometrics (11). Survey content development, item selection, and measurement validation are performed according to standard processes. Each measure has a set of performance characteristics that denote its reliability, validity, and ability to measure clinical change with adequate statistical power (12).

93

Disease-specific Measurements for Ear Disease and Surgery

Chronic Ear Survey

The Chronic Ear Survey (CES) is a patient-based measure for the evaluation of chronic otitis media developed by the Clinical Outcomes Research Unit at the Massachusetts Eye and Ear Infirmary (13). The CES (Table 8.1) is a 13-item Likert scale survey using three subscales. The activity restriction (AR) subscale assesses the impact of chronic otitis media (COM) on the patient's daily life. The symptom subscale (ST) assesses the presence of symptoms such as hearing impairment and drainage. The medical resource utilization subscale (MR) assesses medication usage and office visits.

The CES is a validated chronic ear-specific outcomes measure (13). Test-retest reliability is high, with correlation coefficients ranging from 0.81–0.91 for total scores and subscores. Internal consistency (Cronbach's alpha measurements) is also high at 0.83 for total score and 0.62, 0.8, and 0.75 for AR, ST, and MR subscores, respectively. The CES also correlates with traditional measures such as hearing tests. Survey items on hearing ability are strongly correlated with pure-tone average in the affected ear. The CES correlates well with other measures of hearing-specific and general health. For example, the hearing portion of the CES questionnaire is strongly correlated ($r = 0.54$; $p = 0.0005$) with the Hearing Handicap Inventory for Adults (14,15). The ST and AR sections correlate to the bodily pain and social functioning subscales of the MOS SF-36 general health survey, and the CES total score correlates with the SF-36 general health subscale. The CES also demonstrates sensitivity to clinical change after therapy.

Other Ear-specific Outcomes Surveys

Several other statistically validated outcomes surveys are currently available to evaluate different ear-specific conditions. Stewart et al. (16) have developed a survey to report outcomes on conductive hearing loss. Kuk et al. (17) have developed a tinnitus instrument (Tinnitus Handicap Questionnaire), and Murphy and Gates (18,19) have developed a Patient-Oriented Severity Index (MD POSI) for Meniere's disease. There are also several validated caregiver measures available for acute otitis media in the pediatric population (20,21).

TABLE 8.1. *Chronic Ear Survey (CES)*

Activity Restriction Subscale (AR)

a1. *Because of your ear problem, you don't swim or shower without protecting your ear:* definitely true ___ true ___ don't know ___ false ___ definitely false ___

a2. *At the present time, how severe a limitation is the necessity to keep water out of your ears?* very severe ___ severe ___ moderate ___ mild ___ very mild ___ none ___

a3. *In the past 4 weeks, has your ear problem interfered with your social activities with friends, family or groups?* all of the time ___ most of the time ___ a good bit of time ___ some of the time ___ a little of the time ___ none of the time ___

Symptom Subscale (ST)

s1. *Your hearing loss is:*
very severe ___ severe ___ moderate ___ mild ___ very mild ___ none ___

s2. *Drainage from your ear is:*
very severe ___ severe ___ moderate ___ mild ___ very mild ___ none ___

s3. *Pain from your ear is:*
very severe ___ severe ___ moderate ___ mild ___ very mild ___ none ___

s4. *Odor from your ear is very bothersome to you and/or others:*
definitely true ___ true ___ don't know ___ false ___ definitely false ___

s5. *The hearing loss in your affected ear bothers you:*
all of the time ___ most of the time ___ a good bit of time ___ some of the time ___ a little of the time ___ none of the time ___

s6. *In the past 6 months, please estimate the frequency that your affected ear has drained:*
constantly ___ 5 or more times, but not constantly ___ 3-4 times ___ 1-2 times ___ not at all ___

s7. *The odor from your affected ear bothers you and/or others:*
all of the time ___ most of the time ___ a good bit of time ___ some of the time ___ a little of the time ___ none of the time ___

Medical Resource Utilization Subscale (MR)

m1. *In the past 6 months, how many separate times have you visited your doctor, specially about your ear problem?*
more than 6 times ___ 5–6 times ___ 3–4 times ___ 1–2 times ___ none ___

m2. *In the past 6 months, how many separate times have you used oral antibiotics to treat your ear infection?*
more than 6 times ___ 5–6 times ___ 3–4 times ___ 1–2 times ___ none ___

m3. *In the past 6 months, how many separate times have ear drops been necessary to treat your ear condition?*
more than 6 times ___ 5–6 times ___ 3–4 times ___ 1–2 times ___ none ___

Outcomes Studies for Chronic Otitis Media

Applying these measures to afflicted patient populations provides new insights into the impact of therapy on ear disease. Current literature is limited in COM to recent studies using the CES by the authors.

Study Overview

One hundred and forty-seven patients with unilateral COM were enrolled in a nonrandomized, prospective, longitudinal outcomes study. Patients were administered the CES and SF-36 at enrollment and at 6 months and 1 year after ear surgery. At baseline, COM patients were not significantly different than the U.S. general population in measures of general health. After surgery, the ear-specific CES scores showed significant improvement by 6 months in 73% of patients, which increased to 89% by 12 months. General health measures remained unchanged (Fig. 8.1).

This study illustrates the value of combining a general and ear-specific measure in studies of ear disease. In this case, patients with ear disease do not have significant decrements in general health as compared with patients with other chronic illnesses. However, these patients manifest significant improvement in ear-related quality of life after surgery and no discernible improvements or decrements in general health as a result of their surgery. The use of the SF-36 alone may have led to erroneous conclusions as to the value of therapy in this population.

This study also demonstrated the importance of comorbidity classification and stratification in interpreting the results of ear outcomes studies. It is well described that outcomes data must be properly adjusted for patient and provider characteristics, including comorbidities and other factors, to make fair comparisons (22,23). Which characteristics actually influence outcome? With regard to comorbidi-

ties, none of the major systemic illnesses, ranging from hypertension and diabetes to asthma and depression, were associated with a difference in surgical outcomes in this study. With regard to staging and stratification, using a multivariate regression analysis model, this study also showed that increasing age was associated with better results on total CES scores and MR subscores (although gender, race, smoking, history of sinusitis, etc. had no impact). In other words, older patients appear to have greater economic benefit from ear surgery in that they have a greater reduction in utilization of medical resources following surgery. Although this finding needs to be replicated in other studies, it demonstrates that different subgroups may derive different benefits from the same therapy and that therapeutic decisions in ear disease should be multifactorial.

Appropriate outcomes assessment also requires controlling for stage of illness. This requires a staging system (24,25). Although staging systems exist for cancer and some acute and chronic illnesses, such as heart disease, pneumonia, and sinusitis, there is no universal severity index for COM. In this study, Nadol's classification (26,27) for chronic otitis media was used to stratify patients before and after surgery and found to be useful. The more active the disease process, the greater the impact of surgery in improving quality of life. Surgery for inactive COM had the lowest effect on CES total score, whereas surgery for patients with active COM and granulation or frequent reactivation showed the largest improvements in CES total score.

With regard to predicting success with chronic ear surgery, this study suggests that baseline quality of life was one of the strongest predictors of surgical outcome. Low preoperative CES scores are independently (controlling for other factors) predictive of more significant improvements in quality of life after surgery. Preoperative risk assessment, including quality-of-life scores such as the CES, will become an increasingly important part of surgical decision making.

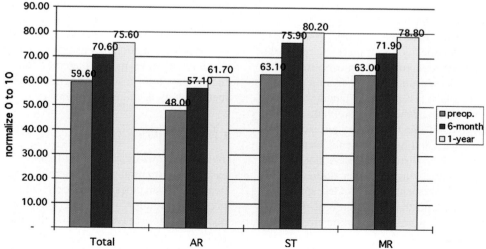

FIG. 8.1 Mean score for CES. Changes between all preoperative and postoperative scores were significant (<0.001). Significant differences were also found between 6 months and 1 year postoperative scores.

Outcomes Studies for Pediatric Acute Otitis Media

Acute otitis media is one of the most common diseases of childhood. Myringotomy with ventilation tube insertion to treat its sequelae, otitis media with effusion, is the most common surgical procedure performed on children. Due to the high prevalence of acute otitis media in children, treatment of acute otitis media in the United States costs $3.2 billion annually. Combined with treating otitis media with effusion, this figure rises to $5.6 billion (28,29).

Evaluating the impact of acute otitis media and otitis media with effusion on patient quality of life is a more difficult undertaking than a pure economic analysis. How does one assess the consequences on a child's daily activities? In recent years the field of psychometrics has developed survey techniques that can be applied to caregivers or parents of patients suffering from illnesses. The Child Health Questionnaire (CHQ) is one example of a general health survey for children that has been applied in otolaryngology patients (30). Using this approach, two surveys have been developed for assessment of otitis media in children (20,21). Rosenfeld et al. (20) used the Otitis Media 6-Item Survey (OM-6) to investigate the impact of tympanostomy tube insertion on the child's quality of life and found tympanostomy tube insertion significantly reduced physical symptoms, caregiver concerns, emotional distress, and hearing loss immediately after surgery. Predictors for poor quality of life were prolonged otorrhea and parents' dissatisfaction with the surgical decision.

Outcomes Studies for Acoustic Neuroma Management

There have been many advances in the diagnosis and treatment of acoustic neuroma during the past several decades. Development of operating microscope, diagnostic imaging technique, and intraoperative cranial nerve monitoring have dramatically reduced mortality rate and significantly improved the chance of facial nerve and hearing preservation. Surgical outcome reporting is now extending beyond survival and complications. Quality of life has become an important consideration for both patients and physicians.

A study of 541 acoustic neuroma patients conducted in late 1980s was the first publicized large survey to report the subjective assessment of symptoms, diagnosis, treatment, and outcomes of acoustic neuroma surgery from a patient's perspective (31). The study revealed that facial weakness, hearing loss, loss of independence, eye problems, altered self-image, difficulty with balance, and fatigue were most difficult aspects of recovery felt by the patients. Depression, anxiety, headache, and sleep disturbance were not uncommon residual complaints after surgery. Other studies (32,33) in acoustic neuroma management have yielded similar results. Rigby et al. (32) found that the degree of disability tends to increase with tumor size, leading some clinicians to favor earlier intervention.

Several quality-of-life studies have gone beyond symptomatology to investigate the socioeconomic impact of acoustic neuroma surgery on patients' financial status, employability, psychologic well-being, daily activity, and social involvement. Chung et al. (34) found that 84% of patients were able to return to normal activity within 6 months after surgery, with ladder climbing and night driving being the most often impaired tasks. Half of patients report reduced quality of life and are involved in fewer social activities after surgery.

Outcomes data have been used to compare different treatment modalities. Several studies (35,36) have compared functional status, patient satisfaction, length of hospital stay, and cost of health care in patients undergoing stereotactic radiosurgery or simple observation to those undergoing surgery. Functioning and well-being, meaning quality-of-life data as an adjunct to survival data, will play an increasingly important role in therapeutic decisions.

Outcomes Studies for Cochlear Implantation

Profound hearing loss has a dramatic impact on a patient's quality of life. Numerous studies have documented the effectiveness of multichannel cochlear implants in improving the auditory and speech function of profoundly deaf individuals who cannot benefit from conventional hearing aids. In this case the issue has not been whether cochlear implants can improve function but whether the improvement justifies the cost. One approach to answering this question is to apply an outcomes methodology known as cost-utility analysis.

Cost-utility analysis is a widely used method of medical technology assessment that permits cost-effectiveness comparisons between medical interventions by determining the cost per quality-adjusted life year (QALY) they provide. The costs, outcomes, and clinical process are incorporated into a decision-analytical model, and the expected cost-utility ratio can be calculated. Health interventions with a cost-utility ratio of less than U.S. $25,000 per QALY are considered to be cost effective (37) in many countries. A meta-analysis (38) investigating the cost-utility data from 14 studies averaged the improvement of 0.26 in health utility, resulting in a cost-utility ratio of $12,787 per QALY. These types of studies provide critical data regarding the cost effectiveness of cochlear implantation that can be used to compare this intervention with other medical interventions. However, translating quality into costs has significant limitations, and the methodology is still in its infancy.

CONCLUSION

To improve quality of care for treatment of various ear diseases, it is important for otolaryngologists to integrate patient-based outcomes information into routine medical practice. The studies presented demonstrate the value of quality-of-life measurement in the therapeutic decision-making process for several ear procedures. Outcomes assessment in ear disease enhances our understanding of the impact of disease on the patient, the likelihood that our therapies will improve the patient's quality of life, and whether one therapy offers substantial benefit over another therapy for a particular population.

REFERENCES

1. Browning GG, Gatehouse S, Swan IR. The Glasgow Benefit Plot: a new method for reporting benefits from middle ear surgery. *Laryngoscope* 1991;101:180–185.
2. Smyth DGL, Patterson CC. Results of middle ear reconstruction: do patients and surgeon agree? *Am J Otol* 1985;6:276–279.
3. Tarlov AR, Ware JE Jr, Greenfield S, et al. The medical outcomes study. An application of methods for monitoring the results of medical care. *JAMA* 1989;262:925–930.
4. Ellwood PM. Shattuck lecture—outcomes management. A technology of patient experience. *N Engl J Med* 1988;318:1549–1556.
5. Piccirillo JF. Outcomes research and otolaryngology. *Otolaryngol Head Neck Surg* 1994;111:764–769.
6. Roper WL, Winkenwerder W, Hackbarth GM, et al. Effectiveness in health care. An initiative to evaluate and improve medical practice. *N Engl J Med* 1988;319:1197–202.
7. Ware JE Jr, Sherbourne CD. The MOS 36-Item Short-Form Health Survey (SF-36): I. Conceptual framework and item selection. *Med Care* 1992;30:473–483.
8. McHorney CA, Ware JE Jr, Raczek AE. The MOS 36-Item Short-Form Health Survey (SF-36): II. Psychometric and clinical tests of validity in measuring physical and mental health constructs. *Med Care* 1993;31:247–263.
9. McHorney CA, Ware JE Jr, Lu JF, et al. The MOS 36-Item Short-Form Health Survey (SF-36): III. Tests of data quality, scaling assumptions, and reliability across diverse patient groups. *Med Care* 1994;32:40–66.
10. Patrick DL, Deyo RA. Generic and disease-specific measures in assessing health status and quality of life. *Med Care* 1989;27[3 Suppl]: S217–32.
11. Nunnally JC. *Psychometric Theory,* 2nd ed. New York: McGraw-Hill, 1978.
12. Cohen J. *Statistical Power Analyses for the Behavioral Science,* 2nd ed. Hillsdale, NJ: Lawrence Erlbaum Associates, 1988.
13. Wang PC, Nadol JB Jr., Merchant SN, et al. Validation of outcomes survey for adults with chronic suppurative otitis media. *Ann Otol Rhinol Laryngol* 2000;109:249–254.
14. Newman CW, Weinstein BE, Jacobsen GP, et al. The Hearing Handicap Inventory for Adults: psychometric adequacy and audiometric correlates. *Ear Hear* 1990;11:430–433.
15. Newman CW, Weinstein BE, Jacobson GP, et al. Test-retest reliability of the Hearing Handicap Inventory for Adults. *Ear Hear* 1991;12: 355–357.
16. Stewart MG, Jenkin HA, Coker NJ, et al. Development of a new outcomes instrument for conductive hearing loss. *Am J Otol* 1997;18: 413–420.
17. Kuk FK, Tyler RS, Russell D, et al. The psychometric properties of a tinnitus handicap questionnaire. *Ear Hear* 1990;11:434–445.
18. Murphy MP, Gates GA. Measuring the effects of Meniere's disease: results of the Patient-oriented Severity Index (MD POSI) version 1. *Ann Otol Rhinol Laryngol* 1999;108:331–337.
19. Gates GA. Clinimetrics of Meniere's disease. *Laryngoscope* 2000;110: 8–11.
20. Rosenfeld RM, Bhaya MH, Bower CM, et al. Impact of tympanostomy tubes on child quality of life. *Arch Otolaryngol Head Neck Surg* 2000; 126:585–592.
21. Alsarraf R, Jung CJ, Perkins J, et al. Otitis media health status evaluation: a pilot study for the investigation of cost-effective outcomes of recurrent acute otitis media treatment. *Ann Otol Rhinol Laryngol* 1998; 107:120–128.
22. Greenfield S, Aronow HU, Elashoff RM, et al. Flaws in mortality data. The hazards of ignoring comorbid disease. *JAMA* 1988;260: 2253–2255.
23. Kaplan MH, Feinstein AR. The importance of classifying initial comorbidity in evaluating the outcome of diabetes mellitus. *J Chronic Dis* 1974;27:387–404.
24. Gonnella JS, Hornbrook MC, Louis DZ. Staging of disease—a case-mix measurement. *JAMA* 1984;251:637–644.
25. Feinstein AR, Landis JR. The role of prognostic stratification in preventing the bias permitted by random allocation of treatment. *J Chronic Dis* 1976;29:277–284.
26. Nadol JB Jr. Causes of failure of mastoidectomy for chronic otitis media. *Laryngoscope* 1985;95:410–413.
27. Nadol JB Jr. Chronic otitis media. In: Nadol JB Jr, Schuknecht HF, eds. *Surgery of the Ear and Temporal Bone.* New York: Raven Press, 1993:155–171.
28. Gates GA. Socioeconomic impact of otitis media. *Pediatrics* 1983;71: 648–649.
29. Gates GA. Cost-effectiveness considerations in otitis media treatment. *Otolaryngol Head Neck Surg* 1996;114:525–530.
30. Cunningham JM, Chiu EJ, Landgraf JM, et al. The health impact of chronic recurrent rhinosinusitis in children. *Arch Otolaryngol Head Neck Surg* 2000;126:1363–1368.
31. Wiegand DA, Fickel V. Acoustic neuroma—the patient's perspective: subjective assessment of symptoms, diagnosis, therapy, and outcome in 541 patients. *Laryngoscope* 1989;99:179–187.
32. Rigby PL, Shah SB, Jackler RK, et al. Acoustic neuroma surgery: outcome analysis of patient-perceived disability. *Am J Otol* 1997;18: 427–435.
33. Van Leeuwen JP, Braspenning JC, Meijer H, et al. Quality of life after acoustic neuroma surgery. *Ann Otol Rhinol Laryngol* 1996;105: 423–430.
34. Chung JH, Rigby PL, Jackler RK, et al. Socioeconomic impact of acoustic neuroma surgery. *Am J Otol* 1997;18:436–443.
35. Pollock BE, Lunsford LD, Kondziolka D, et al. Outcome analysis of acoustic neuroma management: a comparison of microsurgery and stereotactic radiosurgery. *Neurosurgery* 1995;36:215–229.
36. Deen HG, Ebersold MJ, Harner SG, et al. Conservative management of acoustic neuroma: an outcome study. *Neurosurgery* 1996;39:260–266.
37. Kind P, Gudex C. The role of QALYs in assessing priorities between health-care interventions. In: Drummond MF, Maynard A, eds. *Purchasing and Providing Cost-effective Health Care.* Edinburgh, Scotland: Churchill-Livingstone, 1993:94–108.
38. Cheng AK, Niparko JK. Cost-utility of the cochlear implant in adults: a meta-analysis. *Arch Otolaryngol Head Neck Surg* 1999;125: 1214–1218.

PART II

Soft Tissue Approaches and Management

CHAPTER 9

Incisions and Approaches

Joseph B. Nadol, Jr.

GENERAL PRINCIPLES

The selection of an incision is based on the need to obtain adequate exposure and to minimize risk and morbidity for the patient. At times the selection may be obvious. For example, for posterior perforations of the tympanic membrane or stapedectomy or the placement of a ventilating tube, the transcanal canal approach is appropriate. However, for other procedures, the surgeon may well have a choice of incisions and approaches. Thus, for example, in chronic otitis media, an attic cholesteatoma without a history of otorrhea may be accessed via an endaural or postauricular incision. The surgeon should consider the advantages and disadvantages of each. Similarly, a small glomus tympanicum tumor, of which the entire circumference is visible on otoscopy, may be adequately accessed by a transcanal incision. On the other hand, a larger glomus tympanicum tumor that extends into the anterior mesotympanum or hypotympanum may well require a postauricular incision for adequate access. The selection of an appropriate incision will include an assessment of the extent of disease using all modalities available to the surgeon, including inspection and preoperative radiographic assessment. A brief listing of surgical incisions and approaches to the external auditory canal, middle ear, mastoid, and lateral cranial base are presented in Table 9.1 and Figure 9.1. The most common incisions for access to the middle ear and external auditory canal are the transcanal, endaural, and postauricular. The postauricular incision may be modified with superior extensions for cochlear implantation. The most common incisions for access to the lateral cranial base include the extended postauricular, preauricular (lateral facial) variations of the transtemporal incision, and the suboccipital incision.

APPROACHES TO THE EXTERNAL AUDITORY, MIDDLE EAR CANAL, AND MASTOID

Transcanal Incisions and Transcanal Tympanomeatal Flap

The transcanal approach is appropriate for a variety of surgical procedures limited to the tympanic membrane and posterior tympanic compartment. The most anterior aspect of the tympanic membrane may be hidden by an anterior canal bulge and therefore is better approached by an endaural or postauricular incision. One of the most common surgical procedures done using the transcanal incision is stapedectomy (Chapter 22), in which a transcanal, anteriorly based tympanomeatal incision is used (Fig. 9.2).

With either general or monitored intravenous anesthesia, local injections of an anesthetic are helpful. This is done at two levels, at the meatus of the external auditory canal and in the posterior aspect of the osseous canal. The anesthetic used is 1% xylocaine with a 1:100,000 dilution of epinephrine. After cleaning the external auditory canal, meatal injections are accomplished using a 27-gauge needle in four quadrants—that is, superior, anterior, inferior, and posterior. Following these injections, the meatus may be dilated slightly using a nasal speculum to allow the placement of the largest otologic surgical speculum that can be easily inserted. Using a 30-gauge needle, both superior and inferior injections are then made in the osseous canal several millimeters lateral to the tympanic membrane. This provides anesthesia and hemostasis and facilitates dissection of the cutaneous/periosteal flap from the underlying bone. The most commonly used incisions for creation of an anteriorly based tympanomeatal flap are shown in Figure 9.2. The su-

TABLE 9.1 *Surgical incisions and approaches*

Approaches to the External Auditory Canal, Middle Ear, and Mastoid

Incision	Access	Typical surgical procedures
Transcanal tympanomeatal	Tympanic membrane	Tympanoplasty for posterior perforation
		Placement of ventilating tube
	Middle ear	Ossiculoplasty
		Stapedectomy
		Excision of small glomus tumor
Endaural (Fig. 9.1A)	External auditory canal	Canalplasty
	Tympanic membrane	Tympanoplasty for anterior perforation
		Total drum replacement
Postauricular (Fig. 9.1B)	Tympanic membrane	Tympanoplasty
	Tympanomastoid compartment	Tympanomastoidectomy
		Hypotympanotomy
Modified postauricular (Fig. 9.1C)	Tympanomastoid compartment and temporal fossa	Cochlear implantation

Approaches to the Lateral Cranium

Incision	Access	Typical surgical procedures
Extended postauricular (Fig. 9.1D)	Tympanomastoid compartment, upper neck, infratemporal fossa	Temporal bone resection
		Infratemporal fossa lesions (e.g., glomus jugulare)
		Translabyrinthine resection of acoustic neuroma
Preauricular (lateral facial) (Fig. 9.1E)	Upper neck, infratemporal fossa	Excision of lesion of infratemporal fossa
Transtemporal (Fig. 9.1F,G)	Middle fossa surface of temporal bone	Middle fossa approach to acoustic neuroma, facial nerve, or vestibular nerve
Suboccipital (Fig. 9.1H)	Posterior fossa	Suboccipital
		_ Resection of acoustic neuroma
		_ Vestibular nerve section

perior limb should start above the neck of the malleus and extend posteriorly to the mid-tympanic region. This superior limb should always remain several millimeters lateral to the osseous tympanic annulus to provide a sufficient flap width to cover a tympanic ring, which may become enlarged by curettage. The inferior limb should extend anteriorly to a line projected through the axis of the manubrium.

After securing the speculum in a speculum holder, the anteriorly based tympanomeatal flap is elevated using a canal elevator and a 20 F suction tip. Elevation proceeds on a broad front, avoiding "tunneling." The suction tip should always remain posterior to the elevator and not be allowed to traumatize the flap. Elevation is continued until the fibrous annulus of the tympanic membrane is visualized.

Entry into the middle ear should start superiorly at the posteroinferior limit of the notch of Rivinus, where the fibrous annulus extends anterior to the bony annulus. The fibrous annulus is identified and reflected anteriorly, and the mucosa of the middle ear is incised using either a straight pick or a sickle knife. Elevation of the annulus then proceeds inferiorly either using a sickle knife or annulus elevator, keeping the dissection instrument against the osseous canal to avoid perforation of the drum. A properly elevated tympanomeatal flap will allow visualization of the neck of the malleus superiorly, the manubrium of the malleus in the mesotympanum, and the posterior hypotympanum. The flap is folded over the anterior aspect of the tympanic membrane.

The Endaural Incision

The endaural incision provides excellent expanded access to the tympanic membrane, external auditory canal, and epitympanum. Although these structures may also be accessed via a postauricular incision, the endaural incision has several advantages for both the surgeon and the patient. Thus an endaural incision does not interrupt the majority of the cutaneous innervation of the pinna and therefore does not result in a hypesthetic auricle as does the postauricular incision. In general, the endaural incision does not require postoperative drainage or a mastoid dressing, which is of particular benefit to the patient in an age of outpatient surgery. The endaural incision provides direct access to the epitympanum and external auditory canal. In the postoperative period, following a postauricular incision, the auricle has a tendency to migrate anteriorly, potentially creating a collapsing ear canal, whereas this is not the case with the endaural incision. Thus this author prefers the endaural incision for procedures that predictably involve only the external auditory canal and/or epitympanum, such as anterior atticotomy, canalplasty for exostoses, tympanoplasty for anterior perforations, or total

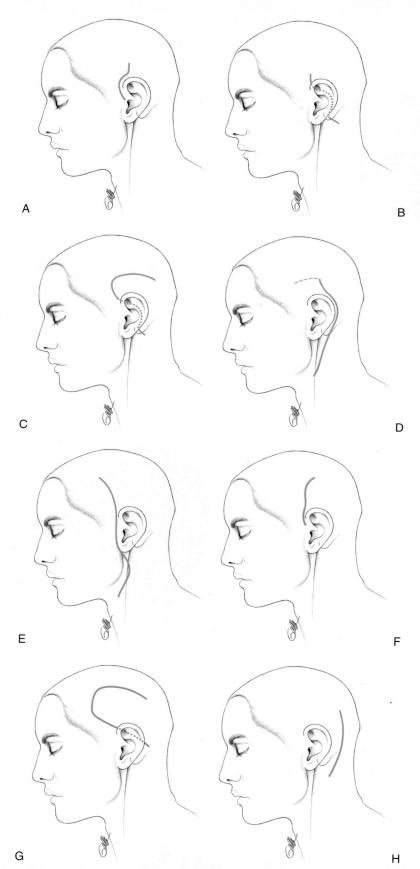

FIG. 9.1 A: The endaural incision for surgery of the external auditory canal and tympanic membrane. **B:** The postauricular incision for surgery of the ear canal and tympanomastoid compartment. **C:** The modified postauricular incision for access to the temporal fossa and for cochlear implantation. **D:** The extended postauricular incision for access to the tympanomastoid compartment, upper neck, and infratemporal fossa. **E:** The preauricular (lateral facial) incision for access to the upper neck and infratemporal fossa. **F:** A preauricular incision for access to the middle fossa surface of the temporal bone. **G:** A postauricular transtemporal incision for access to the middle fossa surface of the temporal bone. **H:** The suboccipital incision for access to the posterior fossa.

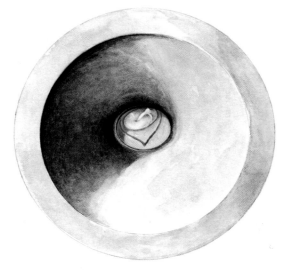

FIG. 9.2 Incisions for the elevation of a tympanomeatal flap via a transcanal approach.

drum replacement. Occasionally an endaural approach may be helpful in middle ear procedures in an abnormally small external canal or meatus. On the other hand, although the endaural approach classically can be used to perform mastoidectomy, particularly with the Heermann extension, if entry into the mastoid compartment is anticipated, the author prefers a postauricular approach.

The endaural incisions were first described by Kessel in 1885 (1) and popularized more recently by Lempert (2,3) and by Heermann (4).

Steps of the Endaural Incision

The endaural approach begins in the distal external auditory canal using an otologic speculum (Fig. 9.3). Two vertical incisions are made with a roller knife and connected by an angled canal knife. The osseous extent of this Koerner flap is then elevated retrograde (Fig. 9.4). Starting the procedure in this way facilitates elevation of the Koerner flap later.

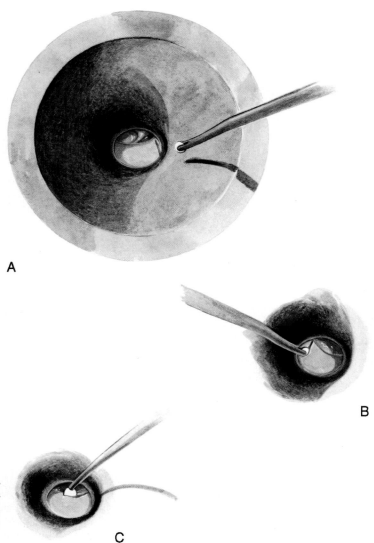

A

B

C

FIG. 9.3 The endaural incisions begin in the bony ear canal through an ear speculum made with a roller knife or similar instrument. After the posterior incisions are made (**A** and **B**), they are connected at the distal ends with an angled canal knife **(C).**

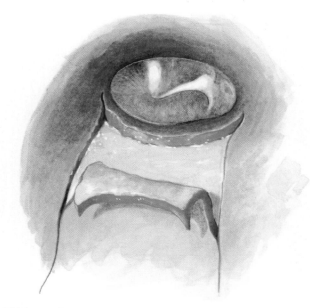

FIG. 9.4 The distal end of the Koerner flap is elevated in the osseous portion of the ear canal.

Using a nasal speculum, the vertical incisions are extended laterally into the conchal bowl with a no. 15 blade (Fig. 9.5). It is important that the incision does not traverse the root of the helix because this will create an unacceptable cosmetic defect. Likewise, as the inferior vertical incision is made, it is important that the knife handle is directed posteriorly, rather than inferiorly. Because the tympanic bone does not extend as far laterally as the mastoid bone, an inferiorly directed knife may pass inferior to the external auditory canal, which results in excessive bleeding and unnecessary risk to the facial nerve. Before attempting to elevate the proximal portion of the Koerner flap, the vertical limb of the endaural incision is created (Fig. 9.6). This should intersect the superior canal incision and extend anterior to the auricular cartilage. It extends superiorly over the temporalis fascia. The skin incision is then deepened to the plane of temporalis fascia (Fig. 9.7), which is done most easily by starting superiorly. The point of union of the vertical limb of the endaural incision and the superior canal incision should be as far anteriorly as anatomically convenient, because any residual skin based anterior to this vertical limb will be difficult to preserve, especially if a subsequent atticotomy is done. Once the level of the temporalis fascia has been exposed, this plane is further developed posteriorly and inferiorly to allow posterior rotation of the auricle. This widens the external auditory canal and tends to straighten the Koerner flap. A no. 15 blade is placed on the plane of the temporalis fascia and is extended deep to the Koerner flap. The knife is then passed posterior to undermine the auricle in the area of the meatus (Fig. 9.8A,B). The knife is then turned, and an incision is made to the level of the lateral mastoid cortex. Using a periosteal elevator, the Koerner flap is separated from the osseous external canal.

The proximal end of the Koerner flap is now freed from the underlying conchal cartilage by elevating the skin from the cartilage using plastic scissors. Care should be taken to use cutting rather than spreading action during this proce-

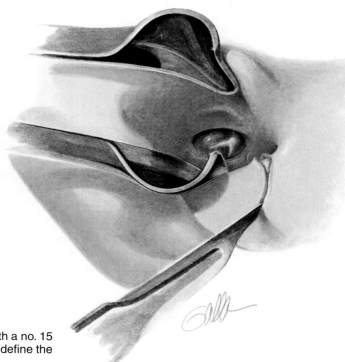

FIG. 9.5 The endaural incisions are extended laterally with a no. 15 Bard-Parker blade through the fibrocartilaginous canal to define the proximal portion of the Koerner flap.

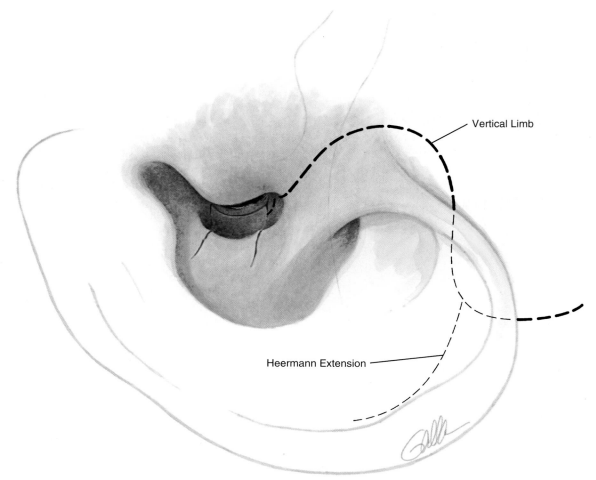

Vertical Limb

Heermann Extension

FIG. 9.6 The vertical limb of the endaural incision is made between the tragus and root of the helix. A Heermann extension can be made in the postauricular area at any time if more exposure to the mastoid is needed.

dure to avoid tearing the Koerner flap (Fig. 9.9). The Koerner flap based on meatal skin is now freed completely from the osseous auditory canal, exposing the conchal cartilage (Fig. 9.10). A meatoplasty is accomplished by removing a crescent of conchal cartilage and underlying soft tissue (see Fig. 9.10). The anatomic rationale for the soft tissue incisions and the rationale for a posterior meatoplasty are depicted in Figure 9.11. The critical planes, in summary, are the plane of the lateral cortex of the mastoid and external auditory canal, the plane of the temporalis fascia, the plane of the conchal cartilage, and finally the overlying skin. Removing a crescent of conchal cartilage posteriorly results in widening of the external meatus of the external auditory canal to match the outlines of the osseous ear canal.

Elevation of Anterior Canal Skin

If an anterior canalplasty or anterior atticotomy is planned, the procedure is facilitated by elevation of the anterior canal skin to expose the tympanic bone around its entire circumference.

This begins superiorly. First the skin of the superolateral external canal wall is separated from the canal wall and tympanic membrane by an anteriorly directed scissor cut. Next, cortical bone is exposed underlying this skin flap using electrocautery. The skin and soft tissue overlying the superior canal wall are then elevated using a large Lempert elevator, freeing them from the underlying tympanosquamous suture line (Fig. 9.12). At this point, using an angled canal knife, an incision is made a few millimeters lateral to the tympanic membrane along the anterior osseous external auditory canal (Fig. 9.13). The skin is then elevated retrograde—that is, from a medial to a lateral direction—to expose the entire circumference of the osseous canal (Fig. 9.14). The elevated skin and soft tissue are retracted using self-retaining retractors. After the completion of surgery, the vertical limb of the endaural incisions is closed in two layers, subcutaneous and cutaneous. No attempt is made to approximate the tissue medial to the helical cartilage. The Koerner flap is then replaced between the canal packing and the posterior osseous canal wall and held in place with antibiotic ointment impregnated Iodoform gauze. It is important that

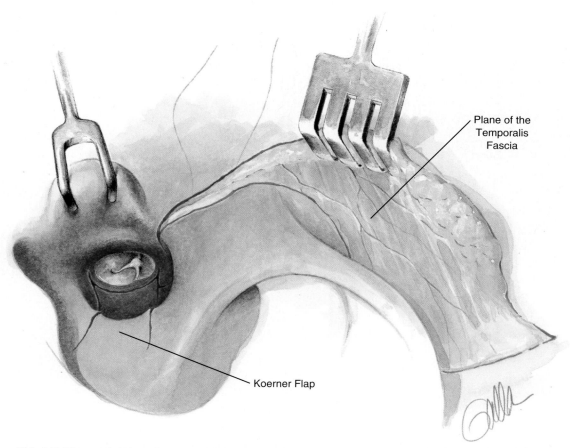

Plane of the
Temporalis
Fascia

Koerner Flap

FIG. 9.7 The vertical incision is deepened to expose the plane of the temporalis fascia and to allow mobilization of the auricle posteriorly.

the skin of the Koerner flap is draped smoothly into the ear canal to avoid a fold at the meatus, which is cosmetically unacceptable. A standard mastoid dressing is applied until the patient is ready for discharge from the hospital. No drain is necessary. Upon discharge, a light dressing over the auricle and superior incision is adequate.

Postauricular Approach

Today the postauricular incision and its modifications are certainly the most widely used in surgery of the temporal bone. The incision was popularized in the nineteenth century by Sir William Wilde (5) and provides a wide exposure of the mastoid portion of the temporal bone. It can be extended anteriorly by transection of the external auditory and elevation in the plane of the parotid fascia for temporal bone resection. Likewise it may be extended posteriorly to allow an extended mastoidectomy for translabyinthine surgery. The postauricular incision may also be extended superiorly for a combined transmastoid/subtemporal approach to the facial nerve. Finally, it may be extended inferiorly into the neck for exposure of the great vessels and to facilitate resection of glomus jugulare tumors and infratemporal fossa sur-

gery. With almost unlimited exposure of the temporal bone possible, there is a temptation to use the postauricular incision for surgery that is anticipated to be limited to the external auditory canal or epitympanum. Although the access for these procedures is certainly adequate, the postauricular incision does have some disadvantages. First, because much of the cutaneous innervation of the auricle approaches it via postauricular skin, the postauricular incision will cause some degree of permanent hypesthesia of the auricle. This is most noticeable to the patient in the first several weeks postoperatively and tends to abate over time. Second the postauricular incision often requires inferior drainage for several hours postoperatively, which may delay hospital discharge or require a postoperative visit for removal of the drain. Third, in general, a postauricular incision requires a bulkier mastoid dressing for approximately 1 week postoperatively. Fourth, over time, despite a two-layer closure, there is a tendency for the auricle to be displaced anteriorly, resulting in collapse of the cartilaginous canal at the meatus if meatoplasty has not been performed. Finally, in the postoperative period, inflammation around the auricular cartilage may produce a protruding ear for several days, which the patient may find cosmetically troublesome.

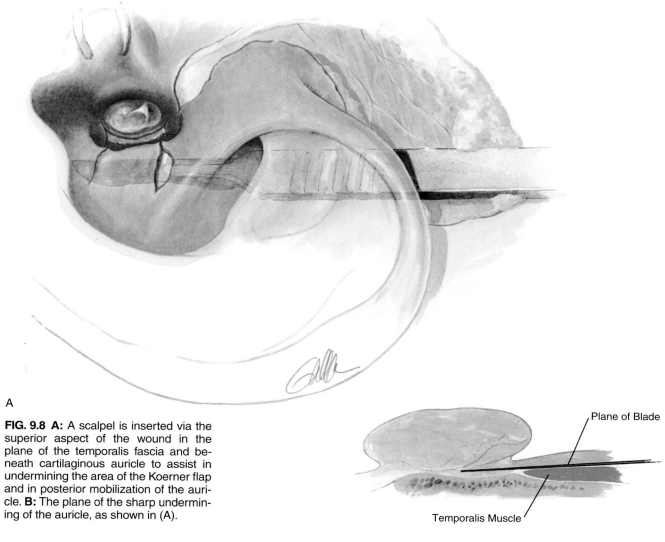

A

FIG. 9.8 A: A scalpel is inserted via the superior aspect of the wound in the plane of the temporalis fascia and beneath cartilaginous auricle to assist in undermining the area of the Koerner flap and in posterior mobilization of the auricle. **B:** The plane of the sharp undermining of the auricle, as shown in (A).

Plane of Blade

Temporalis Muscle

B

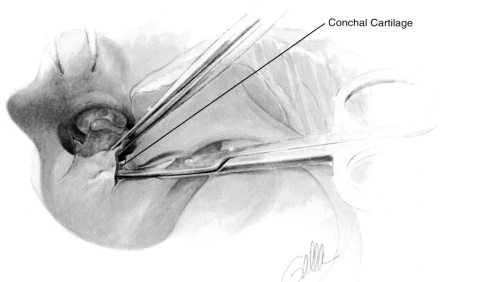

Conchal Cartilage

FIG. 9.9 Using sharp dissection, the proximal end of the Koerner flap is separated from the conchal cartilage.

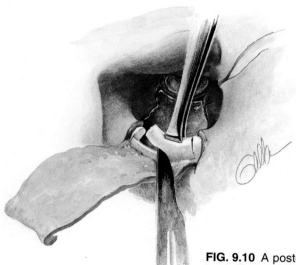

FIG. 9.10 A posterior meatoplasty is created by resecting a crescent of conchal cartilage after elevation of the Koerner flap.

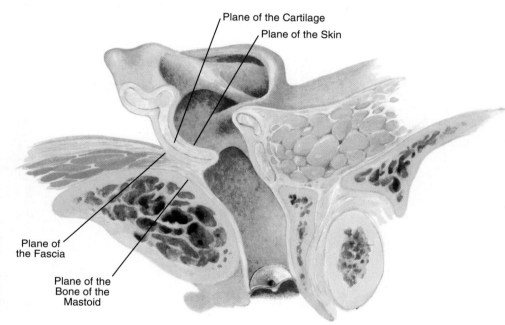

Plane of the Cartilage
Plane of the Skin
Plane of the Fascia
Plane of the Bone of the Mastoid

FIG. 9.11 A coronal view of the external auditory canal, auricle, and tympanic membrane demonstrating the anatomic overhang of the external canal by the conchal cartilage in the area of meatoplasty.

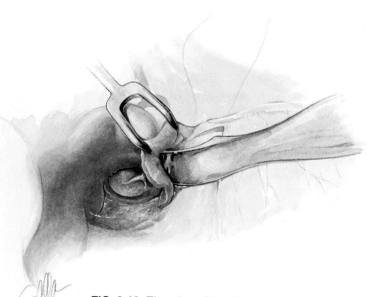

FIG. 9.12 Elevation of the skin of the anterior canal wall begins superiorly, separating skin from the tympanic membrane and from the area of the tympanosquamous suture line.

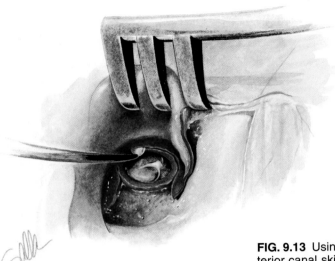

FIG. 9.13 Using an angled canal knife, an incision is made, separating the anterior canal skin from the tympanic membrane to allow elevation of an anteriorly and laterally based flap.

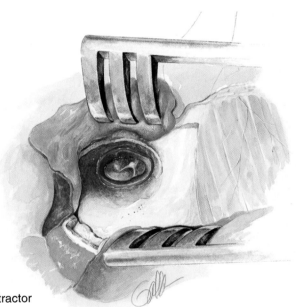

FIG. 9.14 After elevation of an anteriorly based flap, a self-retaining retractor can be used to provide exposure of the entire osseous ear canal.

Details of the Incision and Soft Tissue Management

The standard postauricular incision should be made approximately 2 to 3 mm behind the postauricular crease to facilitate closure at the end of the procedure (Fig. 9.15). Alternatively, the postauricular incision may be placed several millimeters to centimeters behind the postauricular crease to allow wider exposure posteriorly. For mastoidectomy, the postauricular incision should extend to the mastoid tip. A posteriorly directed releasing incision (see Fig. 9.15) allows easier elevation of the posterior flap over the mastoid bone and will provide a convenient location for placement of a drain. The postauricular incision is carried anteriorly to a point superior to the spina helicis. The incision is then car-

ried superiorly to allow easier elevation of flaps and to expose the temporalis fascia and muscle. The incision is then deepened to the plane of the temporalis fascia using electrocautery (Fig. 9.16). The skin edges and subcutaneous tissue are elevated in the plane of the temporalis fascia and its continuation over the musculoperiosteal layer of the lateral mastoid cortex to the level of the mastoid tip. Self-retaining retractors are used to expose the muscle and musculoperiosteal tissues overlying the lateral mastoid cortex (Fig. 9.17). Using electrocautery, soft tissue incisions are made to the level of the lateral mastoid cortex, both anteriorly and posteriorly, to create an inferiorly based musculoperiosteal flap. This flap is extended superiorly to include 3 cm of tem-

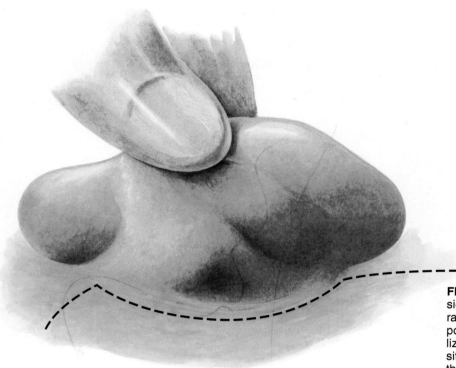

FIG. 9.15 A standard postauricular incision with an extension over the temporalis muscle for exposure of fascia and a posteroinferior extension to allow mobilization of flaps and to provide a suitable site for placement of a drain at the end of the procedure.

poralis fascia superior to the temporal line (see Fig. 9.17). However, in this area, the incision is carried only through temporalis fascia and not through the temporalis muscle, which is preserved. The fascia is then separated from the underlying muscle to the level of the temporal line (Fig. 9.18). From this point inferiorly, the musculoperiosteal flap is elevated in the plane of the lateral mastoid cortex to create an inferiorly based flap that subsequently may be used either to provide a second layer closure over the mastoidectomy in a canal–wall up procedure or to provide obliterative tissue if a canal–wall down procedure is done (Fig. 9.19). The temporalis fascial extension provides adequate length either for reapproximation to the temporalis muscle in the plane of the lateral mastoid cortex or sufficient extension for covering obliterative material such as bone paté.

Modifications for Revision Mastoid Surgery

Although the postauricular incision is appropriate for revision mastoid surgery, as well as primary surgery, certain modifications of the soft tissue technique are advisable. The soft tissue incisions to the level of the lateral mastoid cortex (see Fig. 9.17) are best started posteriorly over an area of previously unoperated lateral mastoid cortex. The musculofascial flap is then elevated posteriorly to anteriorly and the anterior incision made only after underlying tissue has been visualized to avoid laceration of previously exposed lateral venous sinus in the posterior fossa or dura of the temporal lobe in the middle cranial fossa.

Closure of the Postauricular Incision

The postauricular incision is closed in three layers. The inferiorly based musculofascial flap is either reattached to the temporalis muscle or laid into the mastoid bowl. The skin is closed with a subcutaneous interrupted suture and the skin with interrupted nylon sutures. A Penrose drain is placed in the inferior aspect of the wound for 8 to 24 hours.

Modifications of the Postauricular Incision and Other Incisions for Cranial Base Surgery

Extended Postauricular Incisions

The postauricular incision may be extended for cranial base surgery (Fig. 9.1D). It is extended to the neck for exposure of the great vessels and may be extended anteriorly for better exposure of the infratemporal fossa (6–8). A preauricular (lateral fascial) incision may be used to access the infratemporal fossa and upper neck, particularly when the lesion does not involve the tympanomastoid compartment.

Transtemporal Approaches

A transtemporal incision starting at just above the tragus and extending superiorly and vertically over the temporalis muscle may be used to access the middle cranial fossa (see Fig. 9.1F). This incision may be modified to provide opposing flaps of skin and underlying temporalis muscle to allow a wide exposure and a two-layer closure (see Fig. 9.1G).

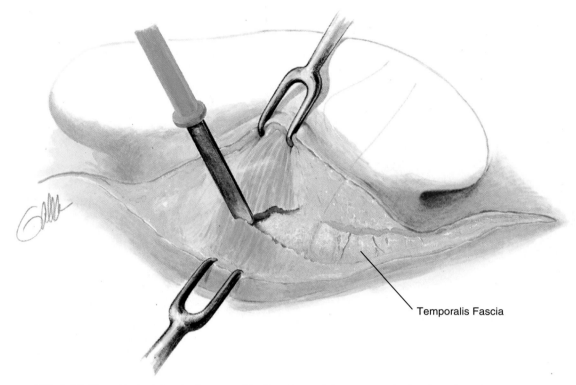

FIG. 9.16 The skin incision is deepened to the plane of the temporalis fascia using electrocautery.

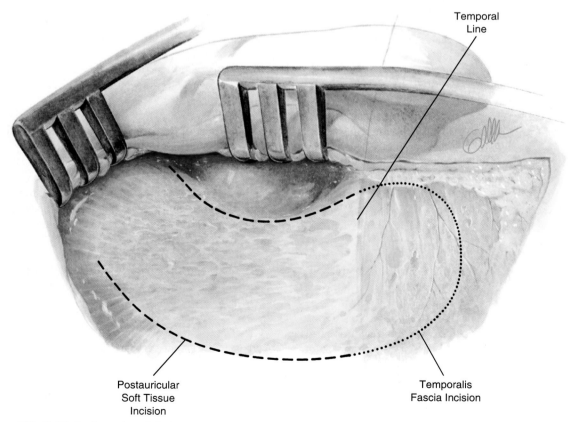

FIG. 9.17 Outline of an inferiorly based musculoperiosteal flap with an extension to include the lower segment of the temporalis fascia.

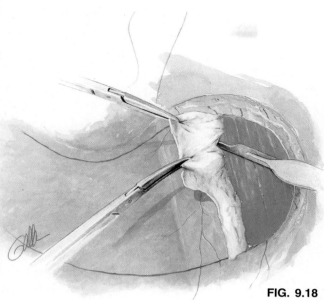

FIG. 9.18 The temporalis fascia extension is sharply dissected from the temporalis muscle to the level of the temporal line.

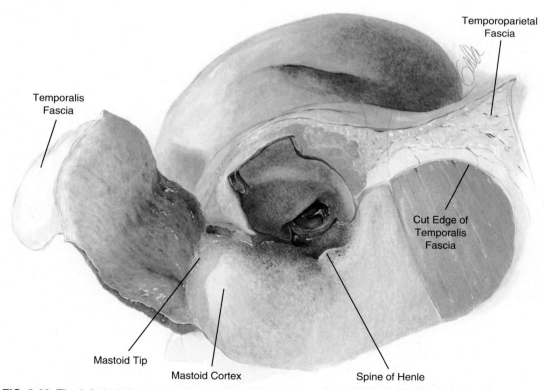

FIG. 9.19 The inferiorly based musculoperiosteal flap with its temporalis fascia extension has been elevated to expose the lateral surface of the mastoid cortex.

REFERENCES

1. Kessel J, 1885, cited by Babbitt JA. The endaural surgery of chronic suppurations. In: Kopetsky SJ. Loose-leaf surgery of the ear. New York: Thomas Nelson & Sons, 1947.
2. Lempert J. Mastoïdectomi sous-corticale. *Ann Mal Oreil Larynx* 1929;48:111.
3. Lempert J. Endaural, antauricular surgical approach to the temporal bone: principles involved in this new approach; summary report of 1,780 cases. *Arch Otolaryngol* 1938;27:555–587.
4. Heermann H. Zur Frage der Plastik bei Gehörgangsradikaloperationen. *Ztsch Laryngol Rhinol Otol* 1930;39:304.
5. Wilde WR. *Practical Observations on Aural Surgery and the Nature and Treatment of Diseases of the Ear.* London: John Churchill, 1853.
6. Glasscock ME III, Jackson CG, Dickins JRE, et al. Panel discussion: glomus jugulare tumors of the temporal bone. The surgical management of glomus tumors. *Laryngoscope* 1979;89:1640–1651.
7. Fisch U. Infratemporal fossa approach for glomus tumors of the temporal bone. *Ann Otol Rhinol Laryngol* 1982;91:474–479.
8. Jackson CG, Glasscock ME III, Harris PF. Glomus tumors: diagnosis, classification, and management of large lesions. *Arch Otolaryngol* 1982; 108:401–406.

CHAPTER 10

Skin Grafting in Otologic Surgery

Joseph B. Nadol, Jr. and Harold F. Schuknecht

Skin grafting performed intraoperatively or postoperatively is essential to the success of some otologic procedures (e.g., atresiaplasty, canalplasty for acquired stenosis) and enhances the success of others (e.g., tympanoplasty or mastoid tympanoplasty).

Before the current method was adopted, skin grafting had passed through two unsuccessful phases: (i) During the 1940s, free grafts of full-thickness or split-thickness skin were used by some surgeons intraoperatively to cover the bony surfaces of mastoid cavities during radical mastoidectomies and fenestration operations. The common donor sites were postauricular for full-thickness skin and the thigh or arm for split-thickness skin. The results were often disastrous because the grafts underwent areas of ulceration and granulation, subcutaneous fibrous thickening, and hyperkeratosis with collection of keratin and caused seropurulent otorrhea. (ii) During the 1940s and 1950s, full-thickness skin grafts from the postauricular area were in common use as tympanic grafts in tympanoplasty procedures. The results were often similar to full-thickness skin used in the mastoid. The subcutaneous fibrous proliferation in itself was destructive to the sound transmission qualities of the newly reconstructed middle ear system.

During the 1960s and 1970s, split-thickness skin grafts from the upper arm came into routine use as a postoperative procedure to cover unepithelialized surfaces. The grafting was performed in the office or, in the case of children, in the ambulatory surgical unit, and was done about 1 month following surgery to allow the healing process to produce a smooth, well-vascularized recipient site.

Since 1980, almost all skin grafting has been done intraoperatively with similar satisfying results. Because these thin split-thickness grafts can be introduced in an overlapping manner, it is technically easy to cover unepithelialized surfaces.

INDICATIONS

The intraoperative split-thickness skin grafting technique is used routinely in the following conditions.

Canalplasty

1. *Chronic stenosing external otitis.* In this case, meatoplasty and canalplasty are followed by skin grafting that includes the bony canal walls and the surface of the pars propria of the tympanic membrane.
2. *Exostoses of the external auditory canal.* Following meatoplasty and canalplasty and removal of exostoses, the unepithelialized surfaces of the bony canal walls are skin grafted.
3. *Traumatic or postoperative stenosis of the external auditory canal.* These cases are often complicated by a canal cholesteatoma distal to the stenotic area. Meatoplasty and canalplasty are often needed to remedy the stenosis, and skin grafting of resulting unepithelialized surfaces is necessary to prevent recurring stenosis.
4. *Congenital aural atresia.* Partial or total atresia of the external auditory canal requires an intraoperative skin grafting technique that completely covers all unepithelialized surfaces. In the case of associated microtia, the grafts must extend to the skin surface to minimize the occurrence of postoperative stenosis at the meatus of the newly created canal.

Tympanoplasty and Mastoid Tympanoplasty

In general, adjunctive split-thickness skin grafting is useful in areas of the canal or mastoid bowl that eventually become epithelialized but are not covered intraoperatively by pedicled flaps or fascial grafts.

115

1. *Anterior perforations and total drum replacement.* Repair of anterior perforations and total perforations nearly always require at least anterior canalplasty to obtain proper exposure of the anterior sulcus between the tympanic membrane and the anterior canal wall. Prompt epithelialization of this area is enhanced by immediate intraoperative skin grafting to prevent fibrosis and blunting of this anterior angle, which in turn may cause fixation of the malleus.
2. *Endaural atticotomy and atticoantrotomy.* This operation is usually performed in association with meatoplasty and canalplasty and is concluded by cartilage reconstruction of the lateral epitympanic wall. It provides adequate access for skin grafting of all unepithelialized surfaces.
3. *Canal wall–up tympanomastoidectomy.* The procedure usually requires canalplasty—for example, in the case of anterior or superior perforations. Prompt healing is enhanced by intraoperative split-thickness skin grafts to exposed bone of the canal.
4. *Canal wall–down tympanomastoidectomy.* Canal wall–down procedures with wide exenteration and saucerization of the mastoid cavity with meatoplasty and canalplasty may be facilitated by intraoperative split-thickness skin grafting to exposed areas of bone in the external auditory canal. In addition, in the type IV tympanoplasty a split-thickness skin graft is invaginated into the oval window directly onto the footplate of the stapes and held in place by a cotton ball to prevent postoperative fibrous obliteration of the oval window niche.

Postoperative skin grafting is used in the following situations.

Postoperative Tympanomastoid Cavity

If the surgeon does not feel comfortable with intraoperative skin grafting, the procedure can be delayed for 4 to 6 weeks. The reasons for delay may be (i) surface undulations or crypts in the walls of the recipient areas, (ii) inability to satisfactorily obliterate the mastoid, (iii) difficulty in controlling bleeding, (iv) inability to completely remove cholesteatoma matrix, or (v) complications of surgery (luxation of footplate of stapes or injury to facial nerve, lateral canal, or sigmoid sinus). Delayed skin grafting is an office procedure for adolescents and adults, whereas children require general anesthesia and therefore are done as outpatients in the ambulatory surgical unit.

In other cases, even when intraoperative split-thickness skin grafting has been done, additional delayed skin grafting may be useful. For example, the temporalis fascia graft placed at the time of surgery does not develop a blood supply and hence will not readily accept a split-thickness skin graft for several weeks. In addition, intraoperative skin grafts that have failed over bony surfaces may survive if done in a delayed fashion once buds of granulation appear on the bony surface. In general, no anesthesia is necessary. The mastoid cavity is prepared by copious irrigation with normal saline, and excessive granulations are debrided with a ring curette prior to skin grafting.

Protracted Granulating Tympanomastoid Cavity

Occasionally a surgically created tympanomastoid cavity that has been healed and dry for years undergoes areas of surface ulceration and granulation characterized by malodorous seropurulent and sometimes blood-tinged otorrhea. Inspection commonly reveals a red vascular granulating area, often in the epitympanic or sinodural areas. If the involved area is small (less than 5 mm), attempts should be made to correct the problem by curettage, chemical cautery, and topical antibiotic eardrops (e.g., gentamicin). If this treatment fails or if the granulating area is larger (more than 5 mm), skin grafting can be done as an office procedure with a high expectation of success.

Even years after the original procedure, the tympanomastoid bowl is hypesthetic or anesthetic; hence local anesthesia is not necessary except for harvest of skin. The mastoid bowl is copiously irrigated with normal saline. Excessive granulation tissue is removed down to a healthy fibrous bed. Bleeding is controlled by the use of cloth wicks wetted by a diluted epinephrine solution before skin grafting is attempted.

If the meatus is narrow, this can be corrected under local anesthesia at the same time skin grafting is done.

TECHNIQUE

The technique of skin grafting is essentially the same for intraoperative, postoperative-delayed, and granulating mastoid bowl conditions. Three surgical principles are the basis for success of this procedure: (i) The split-thickness skin grafts must be very thin, so thin that the lettering on the razor blade can easily be seen through the skin as it slides over the blade during removal. (ii) Because of their thinness the grafts can be expeditiously introduced in an overlapping manner with assurance that overlapping skin will die away. (iii) Firm packing is used to hold the skin tightly against the recipient sites to prevent fluid accumulations and fibrosis underneath the grafts.

HARVESTING THE SKIN GRAFTS

The upper arm from the elbow to the axilla is cleansed with a solution of 70% alcohol, and the arm is draped. When skin grafting is to be done intraoperatively, the arm can be prepared and draped prior to surgery and the skin graft taken when needed. Alternately, the skin grafts may be taken and stored on the operative table until needed at the end of the procedure. A site is selected on the inside of the arm, preferably in a hairless area, nearer the axilla than the elbow (Fig. 10.1).

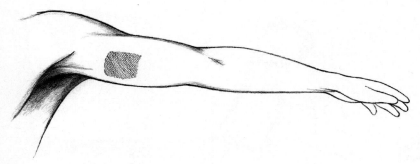

FIG. 10.1 The skin is removed from the inside of the upper arm, preferably nearer the axilla than the elbow and in a hairless area.

It is crucial to the technique to use a very sharp double-edged razor blade that has been broken in half lengthwise and gripped at one end in a small needle holder (Fig. 10.2). The skin is stretched tightly; for thick arms, an assistant may be needed. Do not wet or lubricate the skin. With a gentle to-and-fro movement of the razor blade at a cadence of about one per second, very thin strips of skin are removed that measure about 1 × 3 cm. The strips can be removed side by side so that the donor site appears as a single patch. Two to five such strips are generally adequate. Alternately, a battery-driven or electrical dermatome may be used as long as the technique and instrumentation allow the harvest of very thin split-thickness grafts. A sterile nylon sheathing is supplied as "Owens silk." Alternately, a blue-tinged surgical nylon is available from Boston Medical Products. The blue coloration simplifies removal of the cloth backing during the postoperative period.

The skin strips are placed with epidermis down on nylon cloth that has been lightly coated with an antibiotic ointment of the surgeon's choice. The nylon is cut flush with the edges of the skin grafts to produce cloth-backed patches of skin

that are sufficiently rigid yet pliable enough to make it technically feasible to place them accurately onto the recipient sites (Fig. 10.3).

In the process of sculpting bony surfaces to be eventually covered with split-thickness graft using the otologic power drill, copious suction and irrigation should be used to prevent the creation of a nonviable layer of bone that will interfere with success of skin grafting.

MANAGEMENT OF THE DONOR SITE

There are two methods that can be used to provide rapid healing of the donor site with almost no risk of infection or scarring.

1. The donor site is covered with a transparent dressing (Tegaderm 1620, available from Medical-Surgical Division/3M, St. Paul, MN, 55144–1000), covered by gauze, and the arm encircled by an elastic bandage. Any serum or blood collections that are present under the dressing are aspirated the next morning with a sterile

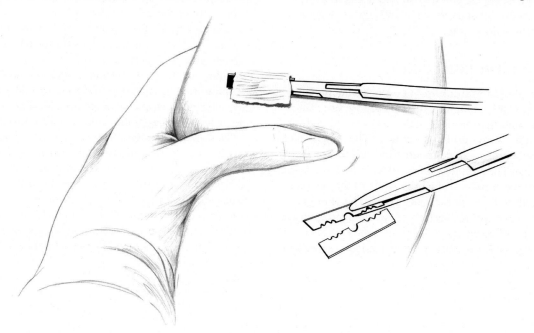

FIG. 10.2 A double-edged razor blade is broken in half lengthwise. Very thin strips are removed that measure about 1 × 3 cm. Alternately, a powered dermatome may be used.

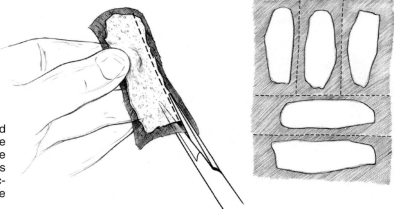

FIG. 10.3 The grafts are placed on ointment-coated nylon cloth, and each strip is then trimmed to remove excess silk. The strips are placed on a moist gauze pad in a covered Petri dish to avoid drying. The strips and attached skin grafts are cut with a scissors to accommodate the dimension of the surfaces to be grafted.

needle, and a bandage is reapplied. The plastic dressing and bandage are removed on the seventh day, by which time the donor site is usually healed. This method of treating the donor site has the advantage of being almost free of pain.

2. The donor site is covered with nylon cloth trimmed to appropriate size to cover the area, covered with gauze, and the arm encircled by an elastic bandage. The following morning the outer bandage is removed and the donor site with nylon attached is exposed to the drying action of mild heat; a 100-watt incandescent light bulb placed 12 to 18 inches from the arm for 1 to 2 hours is usually adequate, but occasionally a second application of drying heat is necessary. Alternately, a hair dryer may be used. The donor site and its attached nylon cloth should now be dry. A dressing should not be reapplied. The silk cloth will separate in 1 to 2 weeks, leaving a dry and healed donor site.

INTRODUCING THE SKIN GRAFTS

The objective of skin grafting is to cover the unepithelialized areas with viable epidermis for the purpose of promoting rapid and controlled healing, reducing fibrosis, and improving the functional result of surgery. The length and width of the skin grafts can be modified to suit the needs of the particular ear. The recipient sites will have been prepared with skin grafting in mind so that the walls of the recipient sites are smooth without pockets or crypts. The skin grafts are laid in place to cover the surface of the enlarged external auditory canal, followed by a layer of nylon strips, and firmly packed in place by large cotton pledgets soaked in

Cortisporin or other antibiotic solution to form a "rosebud" packing. The nylon strips may be cut at the time of surgery from sheets of sterile nylon cloth. Alternately, precut nylon strips (Otosilk, Boston Medical Products) may be used. These have the advantage of a heat-sealed edges preventing fraying of the edges of the cloth strips.

In cases where intraoperative split-thickness skin grafting has been done, the packing is removed in 1 week if no tympanoplasty has been performed and after 2 weeks if tympanoplasty has been performed. In delayed skin grafting the packing may be removed after 7 to 10 days. The nylon strips (rosebud packing) are removed at this time. The nylon cloth backing of the skin grafts are carefully removed. If the underlying skin is not fully adherent, this backing may be left in place for additional 2 to 3 weeks. If epithelial coverage has been completely accomplished, the ear may be left dry. Alternately, if there is evidence of suppuration in some areas, antibiotic otic drops may be used. The patient is generally seen at 2- to 3-week intervals for local hygiene until epithelialization is complete.

Failure of the split-thickness skin graft to survive in the protracted granulating tympanomastoid cavity should raise the clinical suspicion of recurrent disease within residual pneumatized spaces of the tympanomastoid compartment.

The packing should remain in place for 2 weeks, at which time it is carefully removed. Only gentle aspiration of blood or fluid is done at this time. The grafted areas should not be mechanically disturbed because the skin grafts can be easily displaced at this stage. Cortisporin eardrops are prescribed. The surface of the grafted area can be cleaned by aspiration or with cotton swabs 1 month following surgery and then at 2-week intervals until healing is complete.

PART III

Osseous Approaches
to the Temporal Bone

CHAPTER 11

Osseous Approaches to the Temporal Bone

Joseph B. Nadol, Jr.

A variety of osseous approaches are used in surgery of the ear and temporal bone. Presented in this chapter are procedures and their modifications for special surgical problems, the relevant surgical anatomy and landmarks, the factors that must be considered in selecting an appropriate surgical approach, and a uniform method of nomenclature to describe the surgical procedure. Details of the soft tissue incisions are discussed in Chapter 9, and details of each procedure when applied to specific disease processes are described in subsequent chapters.

SURGICAL ANATOMY

Important surgical anatomy of the lateral and basal aspects of the temporal bone is shown in Figure 11.1A,B. The temporal bone is divided into six parts: tympanic, mastoid, squamous, zygomatic, styloid, and petrous. The osseous structures of the lateral aspect of the temporal bone, which are of particular importance as surgical landmarks, are shown in Table 11.1.

PNEUMATIZATION OF THE TEMPORAL BONE

An understanding of the development and variability of pneumatization of the temporal bone is essential for the mastoid surgeon. The pneumatized spaces or potential pneumatized spaces serve as important internal landmarks, guiding the surgeon to the middle and posterior fossa bony plates, facial nerve, jugular vein, carotid artery, and labyrinth. The more medially located tracts may serve as surgical pathways to the petrous apex.

The surgical anatomy of the pneumatized regions of the temporal bone have been described by Allam (1) and Schuknecht (2). Five pneumatized regions of the temporal bone are recognized: middle ear, mastoid, perilabyrinthine cells, petrous apex, and accessory cells (Figs. 11.2 and 11.3; Table 11.2).

Region 1: Middle Ear

The pneumatized middle ear and its extensions are larger than those defined by the bony tympanic ring. Lines drawn tangent to the tympanic ring (Fig. 11.3) help define the approximate limits of the epitympanum, protympanum, hypotympanum, and posterior tympanum.

Clinical Significance

Removal of part of the bony tympanic ring may be necessary for surgical exposure of the middle ear. For example, the transcanal approach to the stapes requires curettage of the posterior tympanic annulus. Similarly, full exposure of the hypotympanum may require drilling of the inferior tympanic annulus in cases of chronic otitis media or glomus tumors. Extension of chronic otitis media to the facial recess and sinus tympani requires surgical access by careful bone removal anterior and anteromedial to the facial nerve (Chapter 17).

In canal wall–up tympanomastoidectomy for chronic otitis media or cochlear implantation, access to the middle ear from the mastoid is achieved through the posterior tympanic (facial recess) cells and the posterior tympanum. For procedures requiring thorough obliteration of the eustachian tube, such as tympanomastoid obliteration for chronic otitis media or for persistent spinal fluid leak, access to the eustachian tube and the peritubal cells, which may enter the eustachian tube several millimeters anterior to the tympanic end of the tube, requires exposure of the protympanum. Symptomatic retraction pockets and early cholesteatoma may be managed by exteriorization of the epitympanum through the ear canal.

Region 2: Mastoid Cells

The growth of the mastoid with age and variations in normal development in the adult have been documented by Eby and Nadol (3). Shortly after birth, only the middle ear and aditus are pneumatized. The central mastoid tract becomes pneumatized in two growth spurts: from 0 to 2 years and again at puberty.

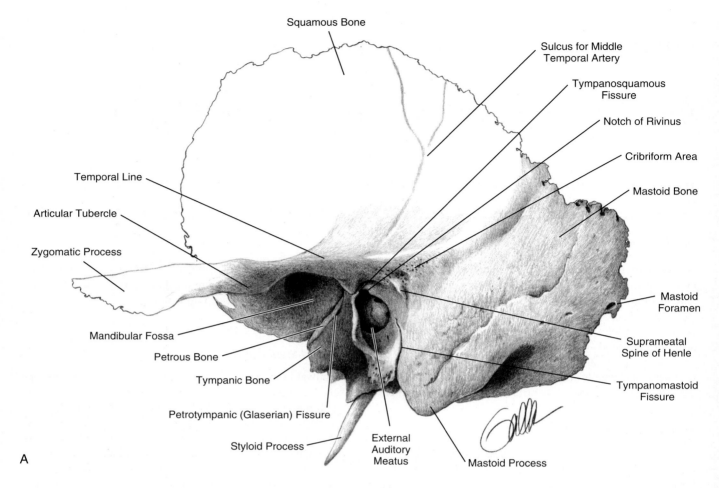

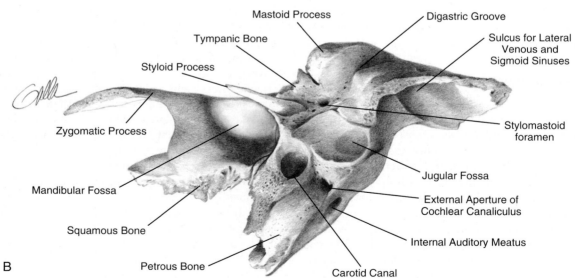

FIG. 11.1 A: Osseous landmarks of the lateral surface of the left temporal bone. **B:** Osseous landmarks of the base view of the left temporal bone.

TABLE 11.1 *Osseous structures of the lateral aspect of the temporal bone that are of particular importance as surgical landmarks*

Structure	Surgical structure
Temporal line	Serves as an approximate guide to the level of the tegmen mastoidea and temporal lobe
Suprameatal spine of Henle	Classically described as a landmark to the location of the antrum
Cribriform area	1. Small foramina that perforate the lateral mastoid cortex in the fossa mastoidea. Particularly in the young, these foramina may provide a pathway for purulence to spread from the pneumatized mastoid to the subperiosteal space. 2. Also used as an approximate guide to the position of the antrum.
Mastoid process	The lateral mastoid aspect of the bone, which serves as an attachment of the sternocleido-mastoid muscle and covers the pneumatized central mastoid tract.
Mastoid foramen	The vascular foramen for the emissary vein to the lateral venous sinus and the mastoid branch of the occipital artery. May be encountered in a wide-field mastoidectomy where vigorous bleeding may be controlled by bone wax or Gelfoam pledgets and pressure.
Tympanomastoid fissure	1. Anatomic division between tympanic and mastoid bone. 2. Serves as a conduit for Arnold's branch of the tenth cranial nerve. 3. May provide a pathway for infection from the external ear canal to the skull base, as in malignant external otitis. 4. Posteriorly based canal skin flaps generally require sharp dissection over this suture.
Digastric groove	1. Origin of digastric muscle. 2. This groove externally and the digastric ridge within the mastoid end anteriorly at the stylo-mastoid foramen and hence serve a useful surgical landmark to the end of the mastoid segment of the facial nerve.
Notch of Rivinus	The tympanic incisure represents a developmental dehiscence in the tympanic ring. On its posterior side the fibrous annulus of the tympanic membrane leaves the bony tympanic annulus and is hence easily identified for elevation of an anteriorly based tympanomeatal flap.
Tympanosquamous fissure	Elevation of a laterally based anterior canal skin flap will commonly be adherent at this suture line between tympanic and squamous bone and require sharp dissection. Troublesome bleeding vessels within the suture can easily be cauterized.

Clinical Significance

The facial nerve exits the stylomastoid foramen on the lateral surface of the mastoid bone and is not covered by the enlarging mastoid process until approximately age $1\frac{1}{2}$ years; hence it is susceptible to injury with a standard postauricular incision.

The tegmental and sinodural areas within the mastoid are common sites of recurrent, chronic, suppurative otitis media. The posterior fossa plate overlying the lateral venous sinus and the middle fossa plate overlying the temporal lobe define the sinodural angle of Citelli (Fig. 11.4A). It is important to remember in the positioning of the patient and in exenterating the mastoid that the tegmental cells may lie medial to the most lateral overhanging extent of the temporal lobe (Fig. 4B,C). In a well-pneumatized mastoid the *sinal cells* may extend both lateral and medial to the sinus. Exenteration of these cells will more fully expose the posterior fossa (cere-

bellar) plate, providing better exposure in the transmastoid approach to the cerebellopontine angle. Exenteration of the lateral and medial *tip cells* will define the digastric ridge between them, which followed anteriorly is an excellent landmark for the stylomastoid foramen. The *retrofacial cells* extend from the central mastoid tract medial to the descending segment of the facial nerve to the infralabyrinthine and hypotympanic cells. In a well-pneumatized mastoid the inexperienced surgeon may follow a well-aerated central mastoid tract into the retrofacial cell tract, not recognizing that the facial nerve is lateral to these cells. Because the retrofacial cells drain into the infralabyrinthine cell tract, complete exenteration of the retrofacial cells in chronic otitis media is not as essential as it is for the central mastoid, sinodural, and tegmental cells. Conversely, exenteration of the retrofacial cell tract provides added exposure to the sinus tympani area for removal of hidden cholesteatoma.

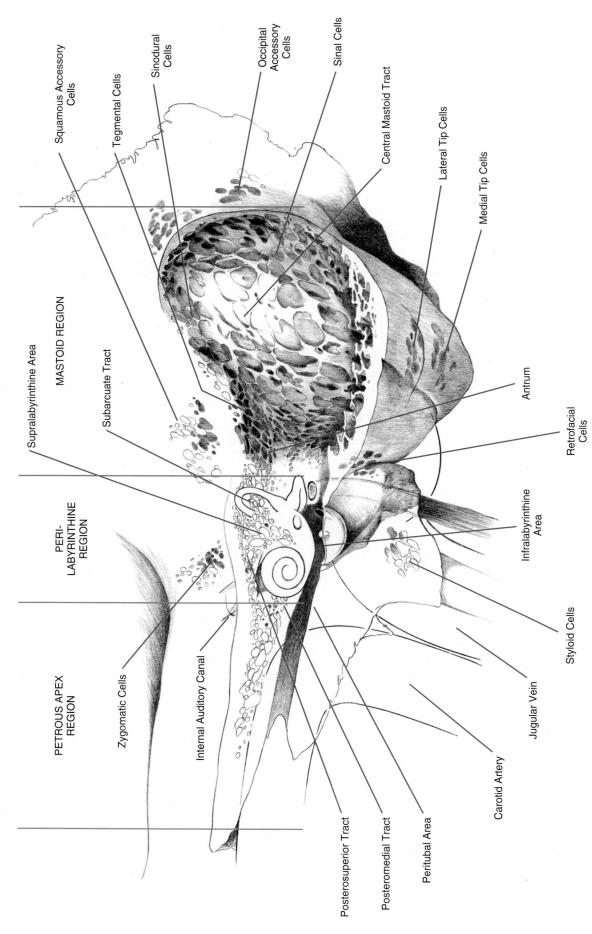

FIG. 11.2 Pneumatization of the temporal bone can be divided into five regions, as presented in Table 11.2. Three of these—the mastoid, peri-labyrinthine, and petrous apex regions—are illustrated here.

Squamous Accessory Cells

Tegmental Cells

Sinodural Cells

Occipital Accessory Cells

Sinal Cells

Central Mastoid Tract

Lateral Tip Cells

Medial Tip Cells

MASTOID REGION

Supralabyrinthine Area

Subarcuate Tract

Antrum

Retrofacial Cells

PERI-LABYRINTHINE REGION

Infralabyrinthine Area

Styloid Cells

PETROUS APEX REGION

Zygomatic Cells

Internal Auditory Canal

Posterosuperior Tract

Posteromedial Tract

Peritubal Area

Carotid Artery

Jugular Vein

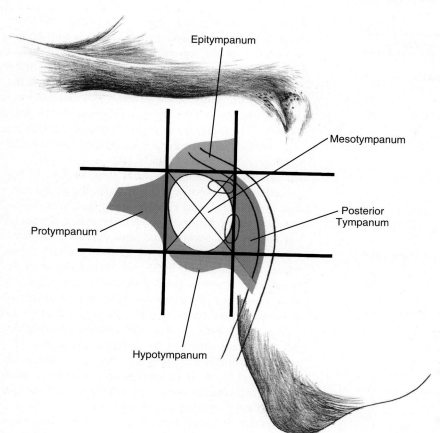

FIG. 11.3 Pneumatization of the middle ear region can be divided into five areas: the epitympanum, hypotympanum, protympanum, posterior tympanum, and mesotympanum. The boundaries of these areas can be roughly delineated by creating horizontal and vertical tangents to the margins of the osseous tympanic ring as indicated.

Regions 3 and 4: Perilabyrinthine Cells and Petrous Apex

The perilabyrinthine region is anatomically divided into supralabyrinthine and infralabyrinthine areas (Table 11.2). The petrous apex may be divided into peritubal and apical areas. Chole (4) has divided the petrous apex into anterior and posterior portions defined by a line drawn through the internal auditory canal in the coronal plane.

Clinical Significance

The clinical relevance of the perilabyrinthine cells relates to their role as a route of communication among the central mastoid tract, middle ear, and petrous apex. Thus suppuration within the mastoid may extend through these pneumatized spaces to the petrous apex, and drainage or access to the petrous apex may be achieved in chronic otitis media and other lesions of the petrous apex without destruction of the membranous labyrinth through the perilabyrinthine cell tracts. Conversely, a spinal fluid leak from the middle or posterior fossae may access the eustachian tube via perilabyrinthine cells. It is important to recognize that the peritubal cells may drain directly into the eustachian tube several millimeters medial to the tympanic orifice (5).

Region 5: Accessory Cells

The accessory cells are extensions of pneumatization from the central mastoid tract and may be divided into zygomatic, squamous, occipital, and styloid areas.

Clinical Significance

Spinal fluid may pass from a suboccipital craniectomy into the occipital and perisinal cells, causing otorhinorrhea even when the mastoid itself has not been entered by the neurosurgeon. Conversely, infection or cholesteatoma may spread beyond the limits of the temporal bone via accessory cells.

OSSEOUS APPROACHES TO THE TYMPANOMASTOID COMPARTMENT

A uniform nomenclature for surgical approaches to the temporal bone is useful for presurgical decision making, record keeping, and communication with colleagues. As shown in Table 11.3, every procedure is comprised of several steps, all requiring a preoperative or intraoperative decision: the incision, the osseous approach, soft tissue and osseous modifications, the pathology found or removed, and reconstructive efforts, if any.

TABLE 11.2

Area	Tract of pneumatization
Region 1: Middle ear	
Mesotympanum	SM (Saccus medius)
	SS (Saccus superior)
Epitympanum	SA (Saccus anticus)
Hypotympanum	SP (Saccus posticus)
Posterior tympanum	SM, SS
Protympanum	SM, SM, SS, SP
Region 2: Mastoid	
Antrum	Aditus
Periantral	CMT (Central mastoid tract)
Central	CMT
Peripheral	
Tegmental	CMT
Sinodural	CMT
Sinal	CMT
Perifacial	CMT, hypotympanic and retro-facial
Tip	
Lateral	CMT
Medial	CMT
Region 3: Perilabyrinthine	
Supralabyrinthine	Posterosuperior
	Subarcuate
	Posteromedial
Infralabyrinthine	Perilabyrinthine
	Hypotympanic
Region 4: Petrous apex	
Peritubal	Peritubal
	Anteroposterior
	Anterolateral
Apical	Subarcuate
	Posterosuperior
	Posteromedial
	Perilabyrinthine
	Peritubal
Region 5: Accessory	
Zygomatic	Epitympanum and CMT (Tegmental)
Squamous	CMT (Tegmental)
Occipital	CMT (Sinal)
Styloid	CMT (Tip)

Commonly used osseous approaches to the temporal bone are illustrated in Figure 11.5.

1. *Anterior atticotomy* (Fig. 11.5A) implies removal of the scutum overlying the epitympanum and wide exposure of the attic and aditus ad antrum. The hypotympanotomy approach also provides excellent exposure for infralabyrinthine approach for drainage of a cholesterol cyst of the petrous apex.

2. *Simple (cortical) mastoidectomy* (see Fig. 11.5B) implies exenteration of the central mastoid tract and preservation of the posterior canal wall without modification of the external ear canal. This approach was common in the preantibiotic era for coalescent mastoiditis and is now used principally as an access to labyrinthine or perilabyrinthine structures such as the endolymphatic sac or the internal auditory canal.

3. *Canal wall–up mastoidectomy* ("intact canal wall technique," "closed technique") (Fig. 11.5C) is a procedure in which a simple mastoidectomy is combined with a transcanal approach, providing both anterior (transcanal) and posterior (transmastoid) approaches to the epitympanum, aditus, mastoid, and middle ear. Such access is facilitated by a posterior tympanotomy (Fig. 11.5B). This technique is commonly used for chronic otitis media and for cochlear implantation via the round window (see Chapters 17 and 27).

4. *Canal wall–down mastoidectomy* (Fig. 11.5D). In this procedure the operative field includes the entire mastoid, middle ear, and epitympanum, and includes removal of the posterior canal wall. The classical "radical mastoidectomy" involves the same approach and bony removal and implies removal of the tympanic membrane, malleus, and incus, without reconstruction, whereas the modern canal wall–down mastoidectomy almost always includes a reconstructive tympanoplasty at the end of the procedure. The Bondy modified mastoidectomy implies a canal wall–down mastoidectomy but with preservation of the ossicular chain and tympanic membrane. This may be effectively used when granulation tissue and cholesteatoma in chronic otitis media are limited to the space lateral to the malleus and incus (lateral epitympanic space) and the aditus and central mastoid tract. The canal wall–down mastoidectomy is commonly used for extensive chronic otitis media and also may be used in the treatment of malignancies of the middle ear and mastoid and glomus jugulare tumors or as a preliminary osseous approach for the transcochlear approach to the petrous apex (Chapters 12, 17–19, 40–41 and 44).

5. *Hypotympanotomy* (Fig. 11. 5E) is a procedure in which the inferior tympanic ring is removed from the tympanomastoid suture line posteriorly and to the anterior canal wall anteriorly. Removal of tympanic bone in this fashion gives wide exposure to the hypotympanum and jugular bulb. It is most commonly used for removal of large glomus tympanicum tumors and may be combined with either canal wall–up or canal wall–down mastoidectomy or performed as a postauricular transcanal procedure, as described by Farrior (6).

SURGICAL ACCESS TO PETROUS APEX

Several surgical approaches most commonly used for drainage of abscesses of the petrous apex common in the preantibiotic era have been described and are listed in Table 11.4 and illustrated in Figures 11.6 and 11.7. These approaches are still useful for relatively uncommon lesions of the petrous apex such as cholesterol granuloma, which is best handled by an extradural technique to avoid contamination of the spinal fluid. The most appropriate approach is dictated by the location of the lesion within the petrous apex, the pneumatization of the mastoid, and the residual

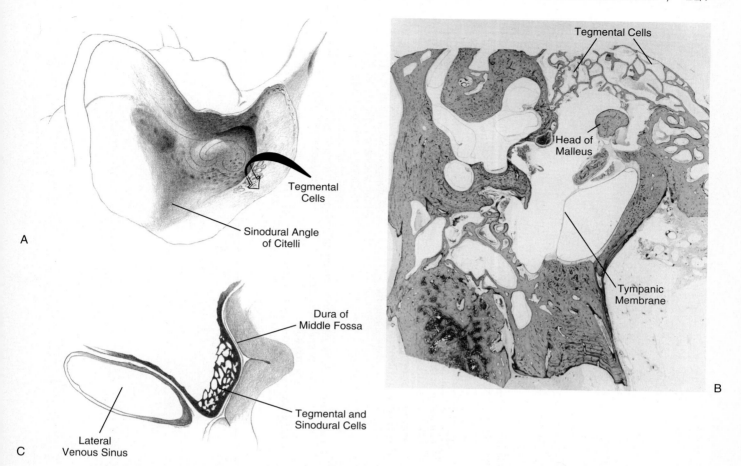

FIG. 11.4 A: The tegmental cells are often hidden from view by the overlying tegmen mastoidea. **B:** Vertical section through human temporal bone demonstrating tegmental cells, superior to the head of the malleus and tympanic membrane (4X). **C:** Diagrammatic representation of tegmental cells near the sinodural angle, which may be partially hidden by overlying temporal lobe.

cochlear function. A canal wall–up approach will allow the creation of a mucosally lined drainage route between apex and mastoid, whereas a skin-lined exteriorization of the apex may be required by the canal wall–down approach.

CRANIOMASTOID PROCEDURES

For certain lesions, a combined cranial and mastoid approach may provide the best exposure. The reader is also referred to Chapter 12 for a more complete discussion of transtemporal and transpetrosal approaches to the cranial base.

Combined Subtemporal Craniotomy with Mastoidectomy

This procedure (Fig. 11.5F) may be used to remove a meningoencephalocele or correct a spinal fluid leakage from the middle cranial fossa into the mastoid. In addition, it provides an excellent exposure of the facial nerve from the meatal to the mastoid segments. A limited subtemporal

craniotomy using an extradural approach may facilitate supralabyrinthine dissection for drainage of a petrous apex lesion.

Combined Posterior Fossa Craniotomy and Mastoidectomy

Excellent exposure for resection of large lesions of the cerebellopontine angle may be obtained by combining a canal wall–up or canal wall–down mastoidectomy, translabyrinthine approach to the cerebellopontine angle, and suboccipital craniotomy (see Fig. 11.5F). When preoperative digital subtraction angiography demonstrates collateral venous drainage, the ipsilateral lateral venous sinus may be sacrificed to improve exposure. This transsigmoid approach is particularly valuable in the removal of large acoustic neurinomas compressing the pontine brainstem or with marked erosion of the internal auditory canal (Chapter 41).

POSTOPERATIVE DOCUMENTATION

TABLE 11.3 *Algorithm and nomenclature for description of surgical procedures of the temporal bone*

Components of every procedure	Incision	Osseous approach	Soft tissue modification	Osseous approach	Pathology addressed	Reconstruction	AS or AD
Examples	Transcanal	Exploratory tympanotomy		Curettage of posterior annulus	Removal of glomus tympanic tumor	Type I tympanoplasty	AS
	Endaural	Anterior atticotomy	Meatoplasty	Canalplasty	Removal of attic cholesteatoma	Type III tympanoplasty (autologous incus graft from stapes to malleus handle) and cartilage graft repair of attic defect	AD
	Postauricular	Canal wall–up mastoidectomy, posterior tympanotomy	Meatoplasty	Canalplasty	Removal of cholesteatoma of epitympanum and mastoid	Type IV tympanoplasty (hydroxyapatite PORP)	AS
	Postauricular	Revision canal wall–down mastoidectomy	Meatoplasty	Canalplasty	Removal of granulation tissue from middle ear and mastoid	Type IV tympanoplasty and obliteration of mastoid with autologous bone paté and musculofascial flap	AD

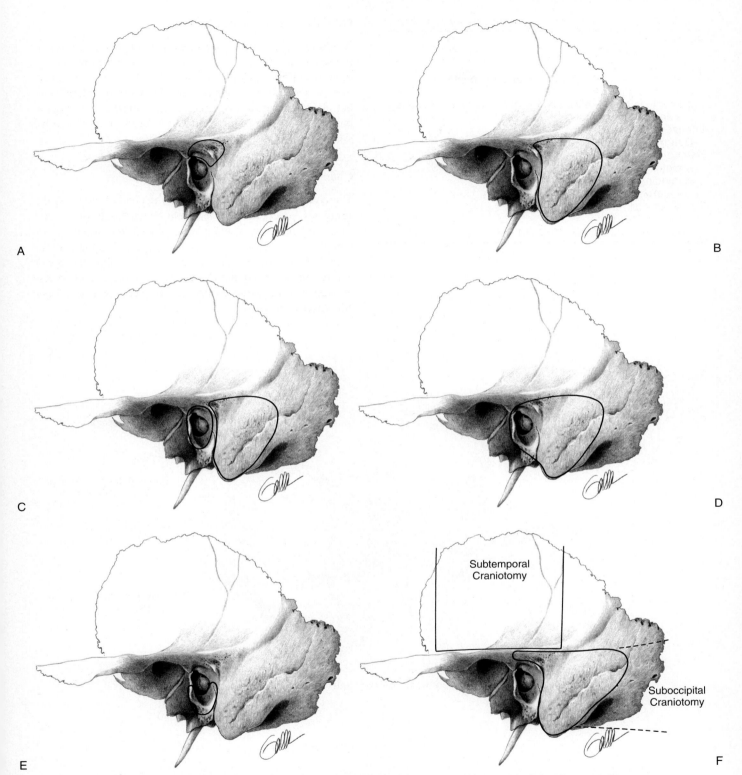

FIG. 11.5 Diagrammatic representation of the limits of osseous removal in a variety of approaches to the mastoid and temporal bone. **A:** Anterior atticotomy. **B:** Simple (cortical) mastoidectomy. **C:** Canal wall–up mastoidectomy. **D:** Canal wall–down mastoidectomy. **E:** Hypotympanotomy. **F:** Craniomastoid osseous approaches. Subtemporal craniotomy and suboccipital craniotomy may be used in conjunction with mastoidectomy for wider exposure of the middle and posterior cranial fossae.

TABLE 11.4 *Transmastoid approaches to petrous apex*

Supralabyrinthine
    Eagleton, 1931 (7)
    Frenckner, 1932 (8)
Anterior to superior semicircular canal and posterior to
    geniculate ganglion
Superior to lateral semicircular canal and posterior to supe-
    rior semicircular canal
Infralabyrinthine
    Dearmin, 1937 (9)
Anterior to cochlea
    Kopetsky and Almour, 1931 (10)
    Ramadier, 1937 (11)
    Lempert, 1937 (12)
Transcochlear
    Gacek, 1975 (13)
    House and De La Cruz, 1977 (14)

OF OPERATIVE PROCEDURE

In addition to a well-written operative note using the format presented in Table 11.3, a drawing of the operative procedure, which includes the operative findings and reconstruction, provides an excellent resource not only for patient care, but also as a means for study and modification of surgical procedures. A preprinted format to be used for the operative sketch (Fig. 11.8) facilitates this process.

Choosing an Osseous Approach

The choice of an osseous approach depends largely on the diagnosis, preoperative assessment of the extent of the disease, and preference and philosophy of the surgeon. Although an encyclopedic guide to the "best" approach for each disease entity is impossible and undesirable, the reader is referred to subsequent chapters for a more complete discussion of surgical approaches in the management of specific disease process.

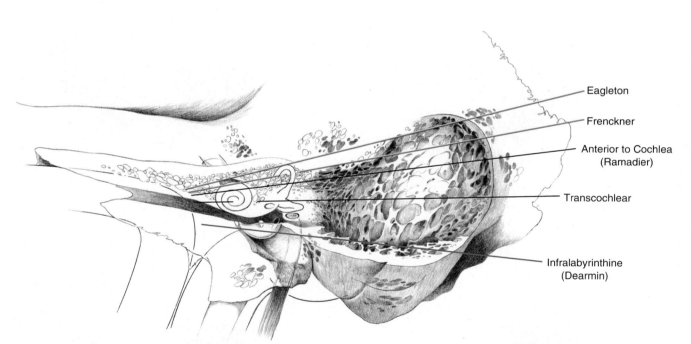

FIG. 11.6 Transmastoid route to the petrous apex shown in the parasagittal plane.

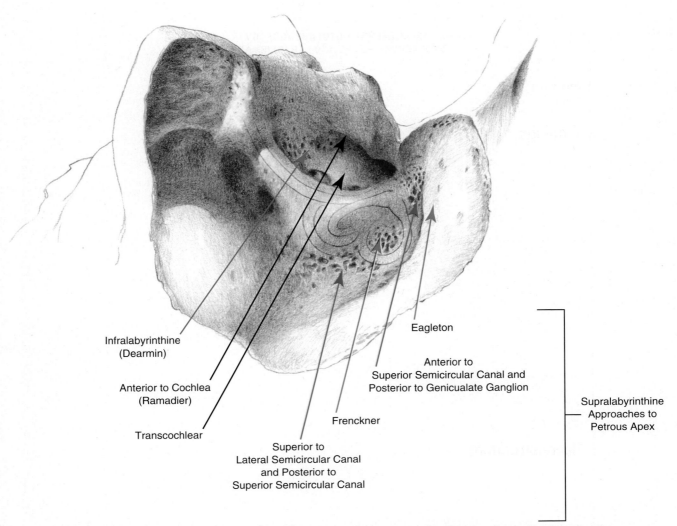

FIG. 11.7 Transmastoid approaches to the petrous apex as demonstrated from the surgical perspective of a canal wall–down mastoidectomy. Some approaches to the petrous apex can be done in conjunction with the canal wall–up mastoidectomy. The infralabyrinthine approach does not require mastoidectomy but can be accomplished via a Farrior hypotympanotomy.

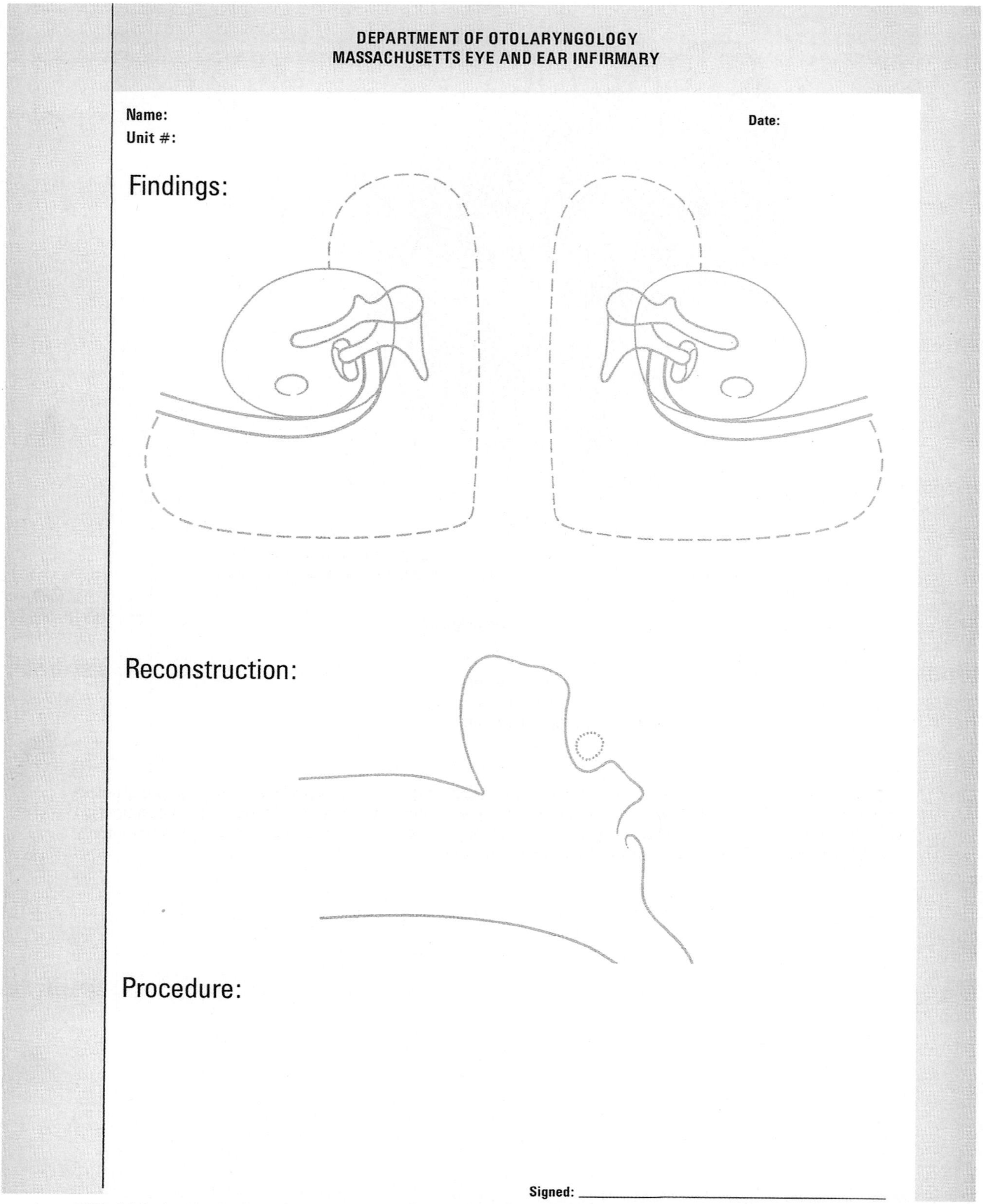

DEPARTMENT OF OTOLARYNGOLOGY
MASSACHUSETTS EYE AND EAR INFIRMARY

Name:
Unit #:
Date:

Findings:

Reconstruction:

Procedure:

Signed: ______________________

FIG. 11.8 A standard form to be used for immediate postoperative drawings of intraoperative findings and reconstruction following middle ear and mastoid surgery.

REFERENCES

1. Allam AF. Pneumatization of the temporal bone. *Ann Otol Rhinol Laryngol* 1969;78:49–64.
2. Schuknecht HF. *Pathology of the ear.* Cambridge, MA: Harvard University Press, 1974;79–92.
3. Eby TL, Nadol JB Jr. Postnatal growth of the human temporal bone: implications for cochlear implants in children. *Ann Otol Rhinol Laryngol* 1986;95:356–364.
4. Chole RA. Petrous apicitis: surgical anatomy. *Ann Otol Rhinol Laryngol* 1985;94:251–257.
5. Saim L, McKenna MJ, Nadol JB Jr. Tubal and tympanic openings of the peritubal cells for cerebrospinal fluid and otorhinorrhea. *Amer J Otol* 1996;17:335-339.
6. Farrior JB. Anterior hypotympanic approach for glomus tumor of the infratemporal fossa. *Laryngoscope* 1984;94:1016–1021.
7. Eagleton WP. Unlocking of petrous pyramid for localized bulbar (pontile) meningitis secondary to suppuration of the petrous apex. *Arch Otolaryngol* 1931;13:386–422.
8. Frenckner P. Some remarks on the treatment of apicitis (petrositis) with and without Gradenigo's syndrome. *Acta Otolaryngol (Stockh)* 1932; 17:97–120.
9. Dearmin RM. A logical surgical approach to the tip cells of the petrous pyramid. *Arch Otolaryngol* 1937;26:314–320.
10. Kopetsky SJ, Almour R. The suppuration of the petrous pyramid: pathology, symptomatology and surgical treatment. *Ann Otol Rhinol Laryngol* Part I:1930;39:996–1016; Parts II,III,IV:1931;40:157–77, 396–414,922–975.
11. Ramadier J. A propos du traitment des petrosites. *Z Hals Nas Ohren-heilk* 1937;40:524.
12. Lempert J. Complete apicectomy (mastoidotympano-apicectomy), a new technic for the complete exenteration of the apical carotid portion of the petrous pyramid. *Arch Otolaryngol* 1937;25:144–177.
13. Gacek RR. Diagnosis and management of primary tumors of the petrous apex. *Ann Otol Rhinol Laryngol* 1975;84[Suppl 18]:1–20.
14. House WF, De La Cruz A. Transcochlear approach to the petrous apex and clivus. *Trans Am Acad Ophthalmol Otolaryngol* 1977;84:927–931.

CHAPTER 12

Transtemporal and Transpetrous Approaches to the Cranial Base

Michael J. McKenna

Advances in surgical technology and technique, intraoperative cranial nerve monitoring, anesthesia, intraoperative stereotactic guidance systems, and stereotactic radiation therapy have made possible the successful management of skull base lesions that were once considered incurable or untreatable without unacceptable morbidity and mortality. During the past 30 years, the limits of resectability have been continuously redefined. These advances have given rise to an evolution of transtemporal approaches to intracranial and skull base lesions and a close collaboration between otologists and neurosurgeons. The acquisition of the necessary skills to successfully perform these procedures requires a thorough knowledge and appreciation of the three-dimensional anatomy of the temporal bone and skull base, hundreds of hours of practice in the dissection laboratory, and an extended period of mentorship and observation. To this end, there are no shortcuts.

Fundamental to the successful management of skull base tumors is the establishment of an accurate preoperative diagnosis, precise determination of the location and extension of the tumor and its proximity to critical anatomic structures, assessment of preoperative deficits, and a realistic estimation of the absolute, likely, and possible deficits associated with each surgical approach being considered. The hallmark of any good surgical approach is the achievement of adequate exposure necessary for safe and complete resection. For most transtemporal approaches, exposure is increased at the cost of function, including hearing and facial function, and the risk of potential neurologic deficits that occur with brain retraction and interruption of central venous flow. An understanding of the advantages and limitations of each approach and a thorough preoperative evaluation provide the basis for surgical planning. Ultimately, the choice of an appropriate surgical approach is determined in large part by the comfort and level of experience and expertise of both the otologic and neurologic surgeons.

PREOPERATIVE EVALUATION

The evaluation of patients who are being considered for surgical treatment of posterior fossa and skull base tumors begins with a thorough physical examination, including a complete neurologic examination, during which the function of each of the cranial nerves must be carefully assessed. Patients who are at risk for developing hearing loss should undergo complete audiometry, including both pure-tone and speech audiometry. Vestibular testing may be helpful in some cases, especially in assessing contralateral vestibular function in patients who are being considered for procedures that result in unilateral vestibular ablation.

Preoperative radiologic evaluation is an essential component of the preoperative assessment (Chapter 4). Both magnetic resonance imaging (MRI) and computed tomography (CT) provide valuable information. Magnetic resonance images are obtained with and without gadolinium contrast in the axial, coronal, and sagittal planes. Magnetic resonance imaging allows for the evaluation of the size, location, and degree of extension for most tumors. In addition, it provides valuable information that is most helpful in establishing an accurate preoperative differential diagnosis, often based on degree of enhancement; enhancement of associated structures, including the dura; signal intensity characteristics; and the location of critical vascular structures, which are seen as flow voids. The sagittal images are especially helpful in gaining an appreciation of the location of prepontine tumors with respect to the brainstem and basilar artery (1). CT scans are valuable in defining the bony anatomy of the temporal bone and skull base, including the degree of pneumatization, location of the venous sinuses, and bony destruction and invasion. These are often critical determinants of the amount of exposure that is achievable. Together, they provide the basis for assessment of the adequacy of exposure to be achieved by the specific approach or approaches under consideration. In

135

addition, preoperative angiography may be helpful in determining the vascularity and blood supply in appropriate cases. It may also be helpful in assessing the venous return and collateral flow through the venous sinuses, as well as the location of the vein of Labbé for procedures in which this structure may be at particular risk. Although some of this information may be obtainable from MRI, in cases where this information is absolutely critical in the decision-making process standard arterial angiography remains the gold standard. In situations where some consideration is given to possible sacrifice of the internal carotid artery, preoperative test occlusion and balloon occlusion may be necessary.

Preoperative review in a multidisciplinary setting with otologists, neurosurgeons, radiologists, and radiotherapists has proven helpful in establishing the most appropriate and advantageous approach. In this setting the geometry of each approach can be reviewed and questions or concerns of each subspecialist discussed. It is particularly helpful in patients who are likely to require postoperative radiation therapy, especially in determining what component of a specific tumor must be removed to provide a critical margin of safety and efficacy for postoperative radiation therapy.

The evolution, development, and modifications of transtemporal surgery were in large part driven by efforts to achieve improved exposure for the removal of posterior fossa tumors, which are not optimally exposed through the suboccipital approach. Although the suboccipital approach is highly versatile, provides a panoramic view of the cerebellopontine angle, and is relatively easy and rapid to perform, it does not allow for complete visualization and exposure of tumors that extend anteriorly into the prepontine space and petroclival junction (Figs. 12.1 and 12.2). Access to these tumors through the suboccipital approach is often blocked by the bridging of cranial nerves V to XI. Also, tumors that extend deep within the cerebellopontine angle and pontomedullary junction are obscured by the cerebellum, which must be either forcefully retracted or partially resected to provide adequate exposure. By approaching the posterior fossa through the temporal bone, a more anterior exposure can be accomplished and the depth of the cerebellopontine angle can be visualized without significant cerebellar retraction. These more lateral and direct approaches result in a shallower surgical field and allow for the use of shorter instruments and improved surgical precision. The degree of required exposure, and hence the size and location of the posterior fossa tumor, and individual variations in pneumatization and location of the venous sinuses determine the approach.

TRANSLABYRINTHINE APPROACH

Indications

The translabyrinthine approach provides exposure to the cerebellopontine angle and internal auditory canal. It has been used extensively for the removal of acoustic neuromas of all sizes when hearing preservation is not a goal. It is a highly versatile approach that has been used for a variety of lesions, including meningiomas and neuromas of the trigeminal and lower cranial nerves, as well as selective gliomas, chondrosarcomas and epidermoid tumors. It offers the distinct advantage over the suboccipital approach in obviating the need for cerebellar retraction (Figs. 12.3 and 12.4). In the past it has been highly criticized for providing inadequate exposure for the removal of large tumors. However, this criticism has been muted over the last two decades as it has gained wide acceptance in numerous centers throughout the world, with excellent results for tumors of all sizes, including even the largest acoustic neuromas. Its successful use for large tumors is absolutely dependent on a complete and thorough removal of bone over the posterior fossa and middle fossa dura and around the internal auditory canal. In cases with poor pneumatization, an extremely anteriorly located sigmoid sinus, or high jugular bulb, exposure may be difficult to accomplish and may be suboptimal for the removal of larger tumors. Under these circumstances, a retrosigmoid approach affords better and safer exposure. The location of the sigmoid sinus and jugular bulb can be assessed with an axial MRI scan. If the MRI scan raises questions regarding the adequacy of the exposure, a CT scan will provide definitive radiographic information. Even under optimal circumstances, the translabyrinthine approach does not provide adequate exposure of the inferior posterior fossa, the view of which is obstructed by the jugular bulb. The jugular bulb also obstructs the view of the neural compartment of the jugular foramen.

Surgical Technique

The translabyrinthine approach is accomplished with the patient in the supine position with the head turned. Some surgeons have advocated the use of a soft headrest so that the head position can be changed intraoperatively to facilitate exposure. Others choose a fixed positioning device, which allows for the use of attached intraoperative retractors. The operation begins with a curved incision approximately 4 cm posterior to the postauricular crease. Inferiorly, the incision is carried down to the bone. Superiorly, the incision is carried down to the level of the temporalis muscle, which is then incised down to bone along the temporal line. The soft tissues overlying the mastoid cortex are elevated with a large periosteal elevator to the posterior aspect of the external auditory canal. Once self-retaining retractors are placed, a large cutting bur and suction irrigation are used to remove the bone of the mastoid cortex. Bone overlying the sigmoid sinus is removed using a combination of both cutting and diamond burs. Some degree of retrosigmoid posterior fossa dural exposure is also necessary, although the degree is dependent on the location of the sinus and the degree of exposure necessary for the task at hand. Mastoid emissary veins are carefully isolated using fine diamond burs and then controlled with bipolar cautery. Avulsion of an emissary vein or inadvertent laceration of the sigmoid sinus is best controlled with

FIG. 12.1 The suboccipital approach is highly versatile and can be used for resection of both large and small tumors. Exposure of the prepontine space is limited by the angle of approach. The pontomedullary junction may be obscured by the cerebellum, requiring cerebellar resection or forceful retraction. Exposure of the entire internal auditory canal cannot be accomplished without transecting the posterior semicircular canal and sacrificing hearing.

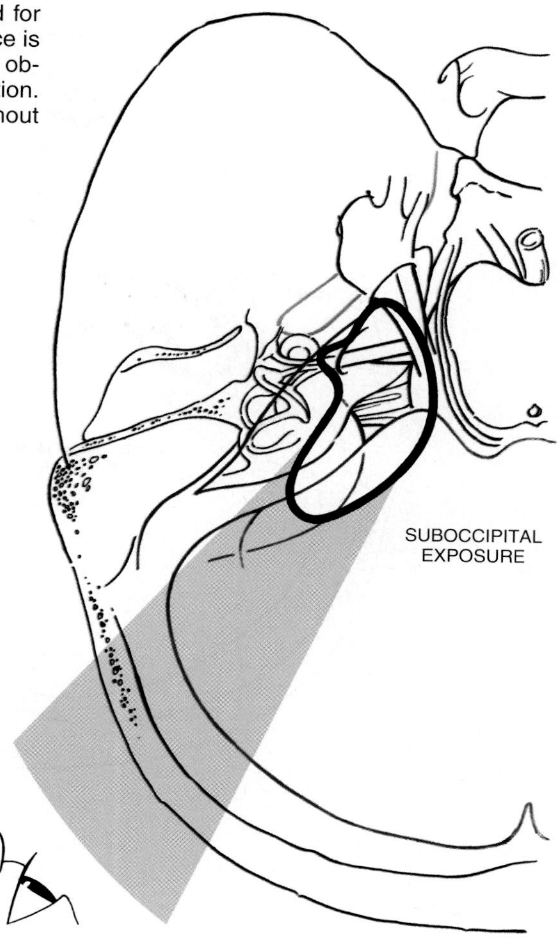

SUBOCCIPITAL EXPOSURE

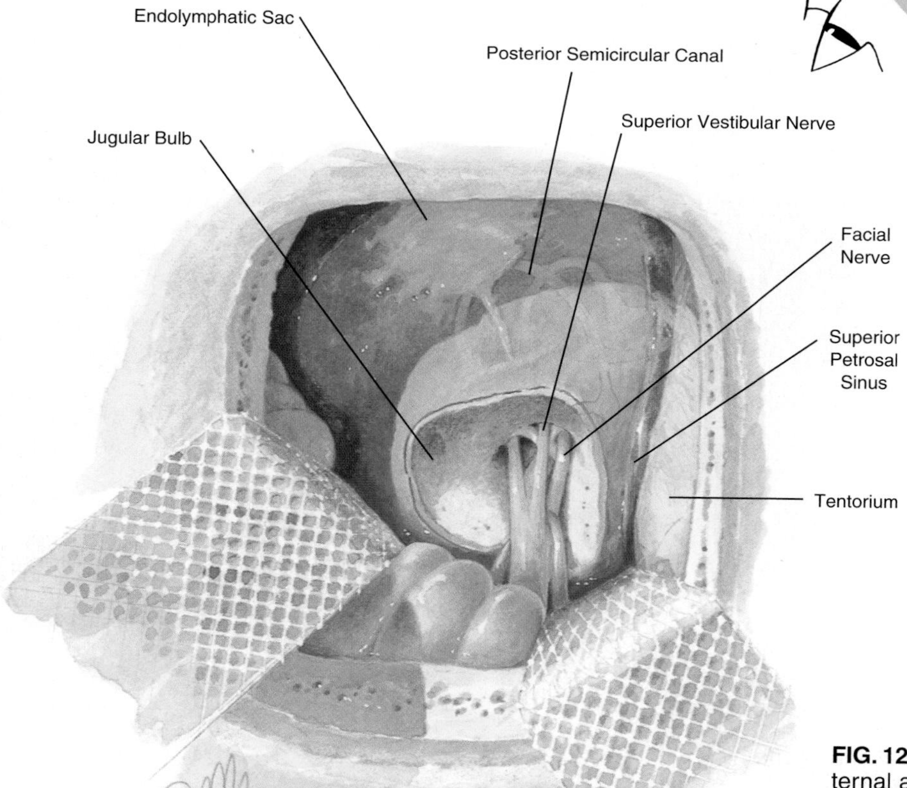

Endolymphatic Sac

Posterior Semicircular Canal

Jugular Bulb

Superior Vestibular Nerve

Facial Nerve

Superior Petrosal Sinus

Tentorium

FIG. 12.2 Exposure of the posterior fossa and internal auditory canal by the retrosigmoid or suboccipital approach. A high jugular bulb may interfere with exposure of the entire internal auditory canal.

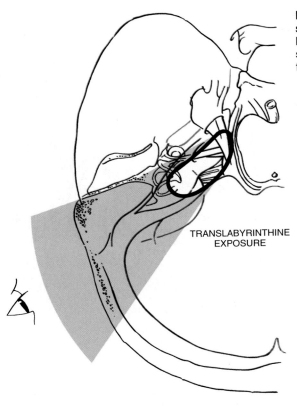

FIG. 12.3 The translabyrinthine approach can be used for tumors of all sizes. It provides excellent exposure of the pontomedullary junction. The lower cranial nerves (IX, X, and XI) may not be well visualized when obscured by a high jugular bulb. A small mastoid cavity may limit its utility for larger tumors.

TRANSLABYRINTHINE EXPOSURE

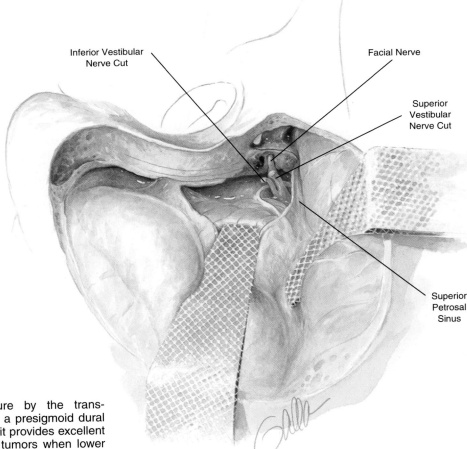

Inferior Vestibular Nerve Cut

Facial Nerve

Superior Vestibular Nerve Cut

Superior Petrosal Sinus

FIG. 12.4 Posterior fossa exposure by the translabyrinthine approach makes use of a presigmoid dural opening. With proper bone removal, it provides excellent exposure for safe removal of large tumors when lower cranial nerve involvement is not a concern.

extra luminal hemostatic packing such as Surgicel. A canal wall–up or canal wall–down (Chapter 11) mastoidectomy is performed with skeletonization without exposure of the descending segment of the facial nerve from the second genu to the stylomastoid foramen. Using diamond burs, bone is removed from the tegmental plate to expose the middle fossa dura, which can later be easily elevated to improve exposure. A labyrinthectomy is then performed and the vestibule entered. The ampulla of the superior semicircular canal is removed last and is an important landmark because it lies in close proximity to the upper tympanic and labyrinthine segments of the facial nerve. Extensive drilling beyond the superior ampulla puts the facial nerve at risk of injury. With completion of the labyrinthectomy, the bone is removed inferiorly to first expose and then skeletonize the jugular bulb. The bony removal is then continued medially to the level of the internal auditory canal. Once the internal auditory canal is identified, bone inferior to the canal and superior to the jugular bulb is removed anteriorly along the posterior fossa bony plate. It is important that bone be removed medial and inferior to the jugular bulb to provide necessary exposure to the anterior inferior aspect of the cerebellopontine angle. Among the most critical aspects of the surgical exposure through the translabyrinthine approach is complete and extensive bone removal around the internal auditory canal. The bone should be removed for approximately 280 degrees around the internal auditory canal and anteriorly along the posterior fossa plate both inferior and superior to the internal auditory canal for several millimeters. Bone is carefully removed from the sinodural angle over the superior petrosal sinus. When completed, there should be no bony restriction to movement of the sigmoid sinus, posterior fossa, and middle fossa dura, all of which should be easily compressible. The last bone to be removed is that which circumferentially surrounds the lateral aspect of the internal auditory canal. This is carefully accomplished until both the transverse and vertical crests are identified and the take-off of the labyrinthine segment of the facial nerve is clearly visualized. Incomplete bone removal at this point in the operation may compromise the early identification of the facial nerve within the fundus of the internal auditory canal. Before the dura is opened, it is essential that the bone removal be complete, because later attempts to remove additional bone with the dura open and the facial nerve exposed significantly increase the risk of neural injury and unnecessarily spills bone dust into the posterior fossa.

The dura over the internal auditory canal is open lengthwise and slightly inferior to the midline to be absolutely certain that the facial nerve is not inadvertently injured. Using a sharp hook or a sharp angled knife, the dura is transected at its bony junction at the fundus of the internal auditory canal. A second curved incision is made in the dura at the level of the porus acousticus and extended anteriorly to the limits of the bone removal. A final T-shaped dural incision is made that extends just anteriorly along the length of the sigmoid sinus with a limb, which extends between the sinus and the opening of the porus. Once reflected, additional exposure can be achieved as needed, depending on the size of the tumor and requirements for exposure.

In cases of large tumors the flow of cerebrospinal fluid (CSF) into the wound may be obstructed and the tumor may begin to protrude into the cavity. At this point, it is essential that CSF decompression be accomplished in order to achieve relaxation of the tumor and cerebellum into the posterior fossa. This can occur by elevating the inferior aspect of the cerebellum and exposing the arachnoid overlying the cisterna magna. The opening the arachnoid in this region with a sharp hook usually results in an immediate flow of CSF and relaxation of both the tumor and cerebellum.

The tumor dissection is begun in the fundus of the internal auditory canal with sharp transection of the superior vestibular nerve and exposure of the facial nerve. With the facial nerve clearly visualized, the tumor and remaining structures of the internal auditory canal are dissected from lateral to medial. The technique for tumor removal is similar to that for other approaches. The capsule of the tumor is incised, an extensive intracapsular debulking is accomplished, and eventually the neural and vascular structures of the posterior fossa are dissected from the capsule using a combination of blunt and sharp dissection with bipolar cautery when necessary. The use of a fenestrated suction irrigator with a constant flow of irrigation is very helpful in dispersing and removing blood and maintaining a clear visual field.

Once the tumor has been completely removed and hemostasis achieved, the craniotomy is obliterated with strips of abdominal fat, which are packed through the craniotomy in layers until eventually a mass of fat is dumbelling through the craniotomy into the posterior fossa. Although it is sometimes possible to narrow the dural defect by partial suture repair, it is rare that a watertight closure can be accomplished. Prevention of egress of spinal fluid is achieved predominantly through fat packing. Additionally, the aditus may be blocked with temporalis fascia or bone wax. Others have advocated opening the facial recess with removal of the incus and packing of the eustachian tube orifice with either fascia or hemostatic packing. Over the past several years, we have nearly eliminated the problem with postoperative CSF otorhinorrhea after translabyrinthine surgery by transection and closure of the external auditory canal with removal of the canal skin and eardrum, removal of the posterior bony canal wall, wide exposure of the eustachian tube orifice, and bone wax packing of eustachian tube as far anteriorly as can be safely accomplished. This maneuver, which requires an additional 30 to 45 minutes of work, has reduced the incidence of CSF leak following this approach from approximately 12% to less than 1%.

Advantages

The translabyrinthine approach offers two distinctive advantages over the retrosigmoid or suboccipital approach. The first advantage is a reduced requirement for cerebellar retraction, especially in cases of larger tumors. However, with a well-performed suboccipital/retrosigmoid craniotomy in which the anterior margin of the craniotomy abuts the posterior aspect of the sigmoid sinus, it is possible to minimize the amount of cerebellar retraction necessary. It is not uncommon for patients to experience some transient postoperative cerebellar dysfunction, especially in the first few weeks following suboccipital surgery. Although this may delay recovery in the immediate postoperative phase, the majority of patients have normal cerebellar function at 1 month following surgery. It is interesting that many of these patients with normal cerebellar function do have evidence of cerebellar encephalomalasia on follow-up MRI scans. It is unclear what effect, if any, this has on long-term cerebellar function as these patients grow older.

The second distinct advantage of the translabyrinthine approach over the suboccipital approach is a significantly reduced incidence of postoperative headache. Although headache can occur following the translabyrinthine approach, the incidence and the occurrence of severe, incapacitating postoperative headache is significantly less than that which occurs with the suboccipital or retrosigmoid approach (2). Several factors have been identified that may contribute to the development of the headache, including injury to the suboccipital musculature and the dispersion of bone dust into the subarachnoid space, which occurs with drilling of the internal auditory canal (3). Over the past several years there have been multiple reports on technical modifications (4,5) to minimize postoperative headache, including modifications of the suboccipital incision, cranioplasty, and packing of the posterior fossa with Gelfoam prior to drilling in an effort to contain bone dust that is liberated from drilling of the internal auditory canal. Although it seems that each of these has resulted in a modest improvement in the postoperative headache problem, it has not been eliminated entirely, and it remains a disabling problem in approximately 5% of patients.

With our modification of the translabyrinthine approach with the canal wall–down obliteration of the eustachian tube and transection and closure of the external auditory canal, the problem of postoperative CSF leak has been nearly eliminated, making this a significant advantage over the retrosigmoid approach, where postoperative spinal fluid leakage still occurs in approximately 10% to 15% of cases. Even in the standard translabyrinthine approach with a canal wall–up technique, the incidence of CSF leakage seems to be less than in the suboccipital approach, which may possibly be attributable to the ability to block the egress of spinal fluid through the attic and at the eustachian tube orifice.

Another potential advantage of the translabyrinthine approach over the retrosigmoid approach is in the event of injury to the facial nerve, which requires repair or grafting. Under these circumstances the labyrinthine and tympanic segments can be mobilized and a proximal stump of the facial nerve made more easily available for anastomosis with a cable graft. It is also possible to mobilize the facial nerve from the stylomastoid foramen to labyrinthine segment, providing 10 to 15 mm of length and thus obviating the need for a cable graft, making possible a primary repair with a single anastomosis (Chapter 36).

Advocates of the translabyrinthine approach have often described an improved ability to identify and dissect the facial nerve beginning at the meatal foramen when it is not possible through the retrosigmoid approach. Our experience with the suboccipital and retrosigmoid approach has proven this not to be a significant issue as long as the internal auditory canal is opened completely, under which circumstances the anatomic relationships of the fundus of the canal are quite similar between the two approaches.

Disadvantages

The primary disadvantage of the translabyrinthine approach over the suboccipital approach is limitation of exposure, especially in the inferior aspects of the posterior fossa. Although this is not a significant problem with acoustic neuromas, which are usually not adherent to the lower cranial nerves and can be delivered from the inferior depths of the posterior fossa, it makes the translabyrinthine approach inadequate or dangerous for other more adherent or invasive tumors, such as meningiomas. Because the inferior aspect of the cerebellopontine angle is not directly visualized, bleeding in this area can be difficult to control and represents a significant potential problem. Occasionally, bleeding can occur from the stump of the petrosal vein, which may be avulsed when it becomes adherent to the superior pole of the tumor capsule and the capsule is delivered from the superior aspect of the cerebellopontine angle. This bleeding, which may be profuse, can be significantly reduced by ligating the superior petrosal sinus.

Another disadvantage of the translabyrinthine approach is the obvious requirement to sacrifice hearing in the operated ear. For large acoustic neuromas, this is not a significant issue, because hearing is not usually preserved with any approach once the size of the tumor exceeds 2.5 cm (6). However, for other lesions, such as meningiomas and epidermoids, this may prove to be a relative disadvantage over the retrosigmoid approach. Unilateral hearing loss is weighted against other potential deficits, which can be avoided by the improved exposure offered by the translabyrinthine approach.

RETROLABYRINTHINE APPROACH

Indications

The retrolabyrinthine approach is a presigmoid approach accomplished by performing a canal wall–up mastoidectomy with skeletonization of the descending segment of the facial nerve, semicircular canals, and jugular bulb. It allows for a relatively small (keyhole) craniotomy, which is well suited for vestibular neurectomy, microvascular decompression, and biopsy procedures (Figs. 12.5 and 12.6). It is generally

FIG. 12.5 The retrolabyrinthine approach provides limited access to the posterior fossa. Although this may be sufficient for selective vestibular neurectomy, some cases of microvascular decompression, and tumor biopsy, it is inadequate for resection of most tumors. Note: the surgeon's view of the eighth nerve complex is proximal to the porus acusticus and the anatomic separation of the vestibular and cochlear nerves.

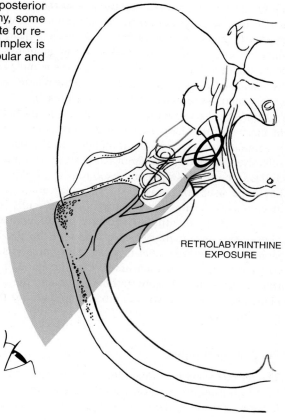

RETROLABYRINTHINE
EXPOSURE

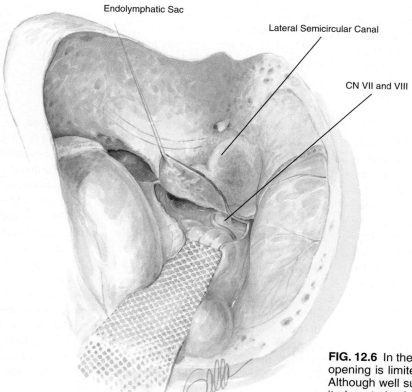

Endolymphatic Sac

Lateral Semicircular Canal

CN VII and VIII

FIG. 12.6 In the retrolabyrinthine approach, the presigmoid dural opening is limited anteriorly by the posterior semicircular canal. Although well suited for selective vestibular neurectomy, the limited posterior fossa exposure makes it inadequate for resection of most tumors. CN, cranial nerves.

inadequate for tumor resection because of the limited exposure achieved. Because the otic capsule is not violated in this approach, the limits of exposure are confined to the region of the root entry zone and proximal course of the fifth, seventh, and eighth cranial nerves. The eighth nerve complex cannot be visualized at the porus acusticus, and the internal auditory canal cannot be accessed through this approach.

Although the retrolabyrinthine approach has been used in the past for microvascular decompression in cases of trigeminal neuralgia, its predominant use at present is for selective vestibular neurectomy in patients with Meniere's disease or other peripheral vestibulopathies. Although it has been used extensively for this indication, we have abandoned it for this use because of the difficulty in being able to clearly identify or separate the vestibular nerve fibers from the auditory nerve fibers in the part of the eighth nerve complex that is proximal to the porus acusticus. Even at the porus acusticus, which cannot be visualized through the retrolabyrinthine approach, the cleavage plane between the vestibular fibers and auditory fibers is not always clear.

Surgical Technique

The retrolabyrinthine craniotomy is performed with the patient in the supine position with the head turned. A curved incision is made in the postauricular area, approximately 3 to 4 cm posterior to the postauricular crease. As with the translabyrinthine approach, the incision inferiorly is carried down to the bone. Superiorly, the incision is carried down to the temporalis muscle, which is incised at the level of the temporal line. Soft tissues over the mastoid cortex are elevated to the level of the posterior aspect of the external canal. Self-retaining retractors are placed, and a canal wall–up mastoidectomy is performed. The sigmoid sinus is skeletonized, as is 1 to 2 cm of posterior fossa dura posterior to the sigmoid sinus. The descending segment of the facial nerve is skeletonized, with the bone left intact. The dome of the jugular bulb is identified, and bone is removed up to the jugular bulb. Superiorly the posterior semicircular canal is skeletonized. Bone is removed from the posterior fossa dura anterior and posterior to the sigmoid sinus from the jugular bulb inferiorly to the superior petrosal sinus superiorly. The sigmoid sinus is retracted posteriorly, and a curved incision is made in the presigmoid dura from the region of the jugular bulb up to the superior petrosal sinus. This dural flap should contain the endolymphatic sac, and efforts should be made not to transect the endolymphatic sac in the incision. Complete exposure of the root entry zones of the seventh and eighth nerves may require gentle retraction of the cerebellum posteriorly.

Upon completion of the intended surgical procedure, the craniotomy defect is packed with fat similar to that which is done for the translabyrinthine approach. In some cases it may be possible to achieve a watertight closure of the durotomy, although this is often technically difficult to accomplish.

Advantages

The retrolabyrinthine approach, which is now used predominantly for selective vestibular neurectomy, offers an advantage over the retrosigmoid or suboccipital approach in that patients have a significantly lower incidence of postoperative headache. When the retrolabyrinthine approach is done for selective vestibular neurectomy in Meniere's disease, a simultaneous endolymphatic sac decompression can be accomplished with some potential for additional benefit.

Disadvantages

The primary disadvantage of the retrolabyrinthine approach is its inadequate exposure of the posterior fossa. In our experience, this even applies to selective vestibular neurectomy. Only the proximal two thirds of the eighth nerve complex can be well visualized through the retrolabyrinthine approach. The most distal segment of the eighth nerve complex that can be visualized through the retrolabyrinthine approach does not have a clearly demarcated separation between auditory and vestibular fibers, making it impossible to be absolutely certain that a complete selective vestibular neurectomy has been accomplished. This problem is evidenced in our own analysis and comparison of patients who underwent selective neurectomy through the retrolabyrinthine approach and a retrosigmoid approach with opening of the internal auditory canal (7). The incidence of recurrent postoperative vertigo and presence of a postoperative ice water caloric response was higher in patients who underwent the retrolabyrinthine approach.

The incidence of postoperative CSF leak is higher with the retrolabyrinthine approach than it is the retrosigmoid approach when the internal auditory canal is not opened.

TRANSCOCHLEAR APPROACH

The transcochlear approach (8) is an extension of the translabyrinthine approach in which the facial nerve is mobilized posteriorly and the craniotomy extended anteriorly through the cochlea and anterior and medial to petrous internal carotid artery (Figs. 12.7 and 12.8). It allows for direct exposure of the most anterior aspects of the cerebellopontine angle, including the petroclival junction and the prepontine space. When complete, the entire lateral aspect of the brainstem, including the pons, and of the medulla can be easily visualized, as well as the midbasilar artery. As is the case with the translabyrinthine approach, the inferior aspect of the cerebellopontine angle is obscured by the jugular bulb. A modification of the transcochlear approach described by Jenkins and Fisch (9) and termed the transotic approach includes an anterior craniotomy, which extends through the cochlea to the level of the petrous internal carotid artery, leaving the tympanic and descending segment of the facial nerve in situ. This approach allows for limited exposure of the anterior cerebellopontine angle be-

FIG. 12.7 The transcochlear approach provides excellent exposure for large tumors with extension anterior to the brainstem. The improved exposure is always at the expense of facial nerve function, which never recovers completely after the required posterior mobilization. The anterior limit of the exposure is the petrous internal carotid artery.

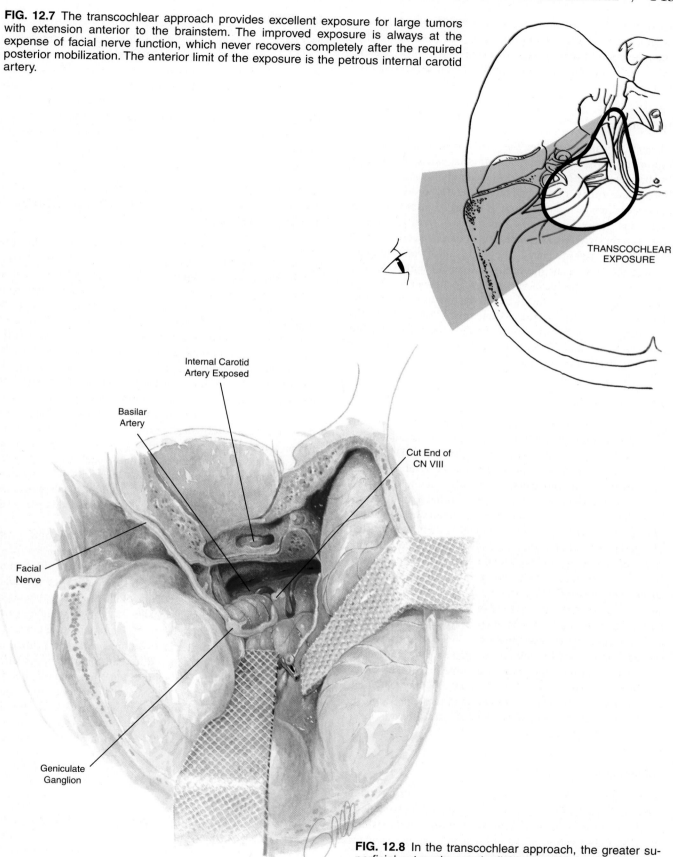

Internal Carotid Artery Exposed

Basilar Artery

Cut End of CN VIII

Facial Nerve

Geniculate Ganglion

FIG. 12.8 In the transcochlear approach, the greater superficial petrosal nerve is divided and the entire temporal facial nerve is posteriorly transposed.

yond that which is achievable by the translabyrinthine approach with anterior extension and has been used for acoustic neuromas with anterior extension. By leaving the facial nerve in situ, the postoperative facial nerve function is improved.

Indications

The primary indication for the transcochlear approach are tumors of the cerebellopontine angle that extend anterior to the brainstem and often medial to the cranial nerves, including meningiomas, chondrosarcomas, and chordomas. It is also occasionally used in cases of large, recurrent acoustic neuromas where facial nerve function has been previously lost. The outstanding exposure, which can be accomplished through the transcochlear approach, must be weighed against the significant morbidity associated with posterior mobilization of the facial nerve. This maneuver always results in postoperative facial nerve dysfunction, with most patients recovering to House-Brackmann grade III or IV. This increased morbidity may be justified for lesions that are adherent to the lateral brainstem and basilar artery, where direct visualization is imperative for safe removal.

Surgical Technique

The transcochlear approach is begun similar to the translabyrinthine approach. In all cases the external auditory canal is transected and a watertight closure achieved. Following the accomplishment of the translabyrinthine exposure, the posterior bony canal wall is taken down to the level of the facial and the facial nerve is mobilized and elevated from the stylomastoid foramen to the geniculate ganglion. The nerve in the labyrinthine segment is then skeletonized. The greater superficial petrosal nerve with its accompanying artery is transected, and the facial nerve is reflected posteriorly from porus acusticus to the stylomastoid foramen. The eustachian tube orifice is opened widely with a diamond bur and tightly packed with bone wax. The petrous carotid artery is skeletonized from just anterior to the jugular bulb to its turn medial to the eustachian tube. The cochlea is then removed, and the craniotomy is extended anteriorly along the face of the petrous bone anterior and medial to the internal carotid artery. The dura is opened, and the eighth nerve complex is divided. Following completion of the tumor removal, the wound is packed with abdominal fat and closed in layers with a watertight closure of the skin.

Advantages

The primary advantage of the transcochlear approach is the panoramic view of the posterior fossa, including the anterior limits, anterior to the brainstem. With closure of the external canal and obliteration of the eustachian tube, the incidence of postoperative CSF leakage is low.

Disadvantages

The primary disadvantage of the transcochlear approach is related to the facial nerve morbidity, which occurs with posterior mobilization. The best expected result following recovery is a House-Brackmann grade 3, with many patients falling into the category of grade 4 (10). This represents a significant deficit and justifies the use of this approach only in cases in which the tumor cannot be approached safely through other routes.

MIDDLE FOSSA APPROACHES TO THE INTERNAL AUDITORY CANAL AND POSTERIOR CRANIAL FOSSA

Lesions of the internal auditory canal, and those with only modest extension into the posterior cranial fossa, can be safely and effectively approached through the floor of the middle cranial fossa. The primary advantage of this approach is the ability to expose the fundus of the internal auditory canal without injury or sacrifice of the inner ear structures, thus making possible the preservation of hearing (Fig. 12.9A,B). This represents a distinct advantage over the suboccipital or retrosigmoid approach, in which only the proximal one half to two thirds of the internal auditory canal can be safely opened without fenestrating the posterior semicircular canal. In recent years the middle cranial fossa approach has been used widely for the removal of small acoustic neuromas when hearing preservation is a goal. Other applications include removal of other tumors, such as facial nerve schwannomas, meningiomas, vascular lesions of the internal auditory canal, and geniculate fossa, and facial nerve decompression of the labyrinthine segment of the facial nerve in selected cases of Bell's or traumatic facial palsy.

Although this approach has been criticized by some for its inadequate exposure of the structures of the posterior fossa, including the blood vessels intimately associated with tumors in this region, when properly performed and when restricted for use in tumors that do not contact the brainstem, the exposure is more than adequate for safe and controlled removal.

The middle fossa or subtemporal approach to the internal auditory canal and posterior fossa has been subclassified by some (11) into the (i) standard middle fossa approach (10); (ii) extended middle fossa approach (12,13); and (iii) middle fossa transpetrous (14) approach. In essence, these approaches are all similar and vary only in the degree of additional exposure achieved by more aggressive bone removal and ligation and division of the superior petrosal sinus and tentorium.

Surgical Technique

The patient is placed in a supine position with his or her head turned. An incision is made in the preauricular area, which extends superiorly into the hairline. The design of the

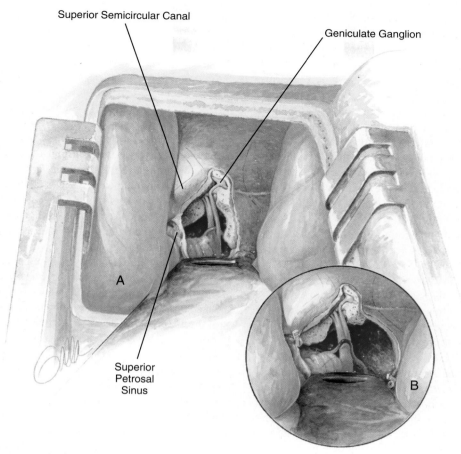

Superior Semicircular Canal

Geniculate Ganglion

A

B

Superior
Petrosal
Sinus

FIG. 12.9 The middle fossa approach is useful for exposure of the entire internal auditory canal when hearing preservation is a goal. **A:** Brainstem exposure is limited, making it unsafe for resection of large tumors with brainstem involvement. The middle fossa exposure can be extended anteriorly with exposure of Meckel's cave. **B:** Exposure of the posterior fossa can be improved by dividing the superior petrosal sinus.

incision may vary depending on the hair pattern of the patient and the preference of the surgeon. The temporalis muscle is incised at its insertion superiorly and is reflected inferiorly. After securing self-retaining retractors, a 5 × 5-cm temporal craniotomy is performed, which is epicentered two-thirds anterior and one-third posterior to the external auditory canal. It is important to ensure that the ascending limbs of the craniotomy be perpendicular to the floor of the middle cranial fossa to allow placement of the self-retaining retractors, which are secured to the craniotomy site for the retraction of the temporal lobe dura. Otherwise, the ultimate placement of the retractor blade may become cumbersome and angulated at its medial perch against the roof of the petrous pyramid. It is also important that the inferior craniotomy margin be lowered to the floor of the middle cranial fossa. This will facilitate elevation of the temporal lobe dura and improve exposure later in the case. We have found that placement of a lumbar drain and siphoning off of spinal fluid following induction of general anesthesia have been helpful in facilitating elevation and retraction of the temporal lobe

dura. Also, by leaving this drain in place for 72 hours and draining spinal fluid for the first few days, the incidence of postoperative CSF leak has been significantly reduced.

The temporal lobe dura is elevated from lateral to medial until the posterior petrous ridge and the groove of the superior petrosal sinus are encountered. It is also important to elevate the temporal lobe dura around the circumference of the craniotomy, so that ultimately when the temporal lobe retractor is placed, bridging dural veins are not torn, which can result in troublesome bleeding. Anteriorly, the dura of the floor of the middle fossa is elevated up to the region of the foramen spinosum. There is tremendous variability among patients in the ease with which the temporal lobe dura may be elevated. Older patients tend to have thinner dura and may be more prone to laceration during elevation. Often the dura is adherent to the greater superficial petrosal nerve as it exits its bony canal just anterior to the geniculate ganglion. In a small percentage of cases the geniculate ganglion itself may be dehiscent and there is a potential risk for injury of the facial nerve from elevation of the dura. It is therefore worthwhile to carefully monitor facial nerve function during this aspect of the case. By elevating the dura from posterior to anterior, the risk of this injury can be minimized. If the dura is densely adherent to the greater superficial petrosal nerve, it is best to separate the two by sharp microdissection under the operating microscope. The elevation of dura in the region of the foramen spinosum may result in troublesome bleeding that can be difficult to control. The bleeding may occur from bridging veins around the foramen, and packing with hemostatic material is difficult because of the trunk of the middle meningeal artery. Occasionally it is necessary to divide the middle meningeal artery and pack the foramen spinosum in order to achieve adequate hemostasis prior to initiating the drilling.

One of the most important and often most difficult aspects of the middle fossa approach is achieving proper placement of the middle fossa retractor. Several retractors have been used for this purpose. For years we have used the House Urban retractor. Recently others (15,16) have described variations or modifications of this retractor system, which may be technically easier to use and result in less obstruction of vision down the length of the retractor blade. Regardless of the retractor system employed, it is important that the retractor blade itself be positioned as superiorly as possible and that the angle between the retractor blade and the floor of the middle fossa be as large as possible. This is accomplished by setting the retractor blades in the superior aspect of the craniotomy and moving the adjustable stage superiorly along the limbs of the retractor. Although this results in a great degree of temporal lobe retraction, failure to do this will place the retractor blade in a cumbersome position, which interferes with the use of surgical instruments, including the drill.

Bone removal for exposure of the internal auditory canal is accomplished using only diamond burs and suction irrigation. Several techniques have been described for identification and exposure of the internal auditory canal (17–19). Some of these rely on early identification of lateral landmarks, including the geniculate ganglion, labyrinthine segment of the facial nerve, and superior semicircular canal. In our experience, the easiest and safest technique is to begin the bony removal as medial as possible and to begin by undercutting in the region of the tip of the retractor blade. Excavation of bone in this area can be safely accomplished without risk of injury to the inner ear or internal carotid artery. Bone is first removed around the internal auditory canal in the region of the porus acusticus, clearly exposing the contour of the canal and its direction. Bone removal around the internal auditory canal is then carried from medial to lateral, initially exposing only the upper half to third of the internal auditory canal up to the takeoff of the labyrinthine segment of the facial nerve. Once the labyrinthine segment of the facial nerve and the region of the geniculate ganglion are identified, the anatomic relationships are well established, making possible safe removal of bone around the remaining portion of the internal auditory canal. It is the most lateral aspect of the bone removal that puts at risk both the

cochlea and the superior semicircular canal. Although some authors have advocated blue lining these structures for their identification, this can be difficult to accomplish and puts them at risk for inadvertent injury. Bone removal in the region of the porus acusticus can be accomplished for 280 degrees around the canal. In the region of the fundus, 180 degrees of bone removal is all that is necessary and it is important not to remove bone deep to the labyrinthine segment of the facial nerve because of its very close proximity to the cochlea. It is essential that the operating surgeon be intimately familiar with the three-dimensional relationships in this region, which can only be accomplished by conducting a series of dissections in the temporal bone laboratory. The failure of this prerequisite will lead to either inadequate exposure of the contents of the internal canal in this critical area or labyrinthine injury.

For tumors that extend beyond the porus acusticus into the posterior fossa, exposure can be improved through the so-called extended middle fossa approach by ligation and division of the superior petrosal sinus, which is relatively easy to control through the middle fossa approach (20) (Fig. 12.9B). Although some have advocated the use of hemoclips, we have used broad bipolar cautery along a significant length of the sinus followed by transection. By dividing the sinus, and in some cases a portion of the tentorium, and removing all the bone around the porus and opening the dura widely, a more than adequate view of the posterior fossa can be achieved with the removal of tumors that extend into the posterior fossa but do not impact or are not adherent to the brainstem. The surgeon's visual field is in direct line with the seventh and eighth nerve complexes from the porus acusticus to the brainstem.

One potential technical disadvantage of the middle fossa approach is that in most cases the facial nerve of acoustic neuromas lies directly atop the tumor. Before tumor removal can be accomplished, the facial nerve is mobilized from the surface of the tumor. This can be accomplished by passing a blunt hook underneath the facial nerve, between the facial nerve and tumor, and gently sliding the hook along the length of the facial nerve and tumor. For it to be adequately freed, this needs to be accomplished on both sides of the facial nerve from the fundus to the porus acusticus. Once this has been done, the facial nerve can be gently rolled over the anterior aspect of the tumor and out of harm's way. As is the case with other approaches and techniques for acoustic tumor removal, the capsule of the tumor is incised and the intracapsular portion of the tumor debulked. Removal of the capsule is accomplished by dissection from medial to lateral in order to avoid traction injury of the cochlear nerve in the fundus of the canal, which can result in the loss of hearing (21). Once the tumor is removed, air cells, which have been exposed during the drilling process, are waxed with bone wax, and a small fat graft is placed in the bony opening and covered by a sheet of Surgicel.

It is also possible through the middle fossa approach to expose a limited portion of the anterior cerebellopontine angle by the removal of bone, which is anterior to the cochlea and medial to the petrous carotid. This so-called middle fossa transpetrous apex approach (22) may be used for removal of trigeminal schwannomas and in some cases for small meningiomas in the region of Meckel's cave. View of the posterior fossa through this approach is partially obstructed by the petrous internal carotid artery, making this a safe approach only for smaller tumors located in this region.

Closure of the wound following the middle fossa approach is accomplished by replacement of the bone flap, which can be either wired or plated in position. Prior to replacing the flap, it is worthwhile to place tenting sutures in the temporal dura around the craniotomy site to avoid potentially catastrophic problems with postoperative epidural hematomas. Following closure of the craniotomy, the temporalis muscle is reapproximated and the wound is closed in layers with a watertight closure of the skin.

Advantages

The primary advantage of the middle fossa approach is in the exposure of the internal auditory canal from the porus to the fundus without injury to the inner ear structures and the potential for hearing preservation. It has been our experience and the experience of others (23,24) that the middle fossa approach results in a higher rate of successful hearing preservation as compared with other methods. Although the reasons for this are not entirely clear, the improved exposure of the fundus of the internal canal and the ability to work under direct vision in this area are a plausible explanation. It has been our experience that even with complete removal of bone over the internal auditory canal up to the fundus, the actual lateral limits of the internal auditory canal are not perfectly visualized. This is in part related to the angle of view that is afforded the surgeon through the middle fossa approach and the fact that the fundus extends for an additional 1 to 2 mm laterally beyond the meatal foramen and takeoff of the labyrinthine segment of the facial nerve (25–27). Despite this, the degree of visualization in this area is significantly superior to that which can be accomplished through the retrosigmoid or suboccipital approach, where only two thirds of the internal auditory canal have been opened to avoid transection of the posterior semicircular canal.

Another advantage of the middle fossa approach is the ability to expose the facial nerve from internal auditory canal to the upper tympanic segment in the same surgical field. This is particularly valuable for tumors involving the facial nerve, including facial nerve schwannomas and geniculate and internal auditory canal hemangiomas. This approach allows for repair and placement of a graft, which could not be accomplished through the retrosigmoid approach.

Disadvantages

One real and potentially significant disadvantage of the middle fossa approach is the requirement for extended forceful temporal lobe retraction, which can result in temporal lobe contusion and memory loss, aphasia, and occasionally, postoperative seizures. Although these problems are relatively uncommon and usually transient, they can be quite worrisome to both the surgeon and patient (28). Another disadvantage of the middle fossa approach is the relatively inadequate exposure for the removal of larger tumors that extend into the cerebellopontine angle. Although some surgeons have advocated the use of the extended middle fossa approach for removal of tumors that extend up to and adhere to the brainstem (20), our experience has been that even with optimized exposure, the view and exposure is inadequate for the removal of larger tumors and the potential need to control bleeding from blood vessels adjacent to the brainstem. For larger tumors, the translabyrinthine and retrosigmoid approaches afford a much better view of the brainstem and are hence safer in this regard.

A relative disadvantage of the middle fossa approach is the location of the facial nerve within the internal auditory canal and the necessity for mobilization of the facial nerve prior to tumor dissection. The facial nerve outcome results in our patients who undergo middle fossa surgery for removal of acoustic neuromas has been similar to that for tumors of similar size removed through the suboccipital and retrosigmoid approaches. However, the incidence of dysfunction in the immediate postoperative period is slightly higher. Also, because of the requirement for dissection of the greater superficial petrosal nerve and often traction of this nerve that occurs with retraction of the middle fossa dura, the incidence of postoperative dry eye is higher in the middle fossa approach than with other approaches. Even patients with normal facial function will sometimes complain of problems with prolonged dryness and sometimes require the use of artificial tears.

TRANSPETROSAL APPROACHES

The terms *petrosal* and *transpetrosal approach* have been used to refer to a variety of combined approaches through both the middle fossa and posterior fossa for exposure and resection of lesions that extend between both the posterior and middle cranial fossae (Fig. 12.10). The two variations that are most commonly used include a combined middle fossa–retrolabyrinthine approach and middle fossa–translabyrinthine approach. Occasionally a transcochlear approach may be combined with a middle fossa approach for wide exposure of lesions that extend from the anterior cerebellopontine angle into the middle cranial fossa. By combining the middle fossa and transmastoid craniotomies with ligation of the superior petrosal sinus and division of the tentorium, a panoramic view of the posterior fossa and middle fossa can be accomplished with a significant reduction in requirement for brainstem retraction than would be necessary for either approach alone. In cases where preservation of hearing is a goal or necessity, the labyrinth and middle ear are left intact and the retrolabyrinthine craniotomy is extended superiorly through the petrosal sinus into the middle cranial fossa. However, preservation of the labyrinth results in a significant compromise of the exposure of the anterior cerebellopontine angle and results in a significant increase in the potential for a postoperative CSF leak. The translabyrinthine petrosal approaches, although they result in loss of hearing, have the distinct advantage of improved exposure in the posterior fossa and the ability to achieve a watertight closure by transection of the external auditory canal and definitive obliteration of the eustachian tube orifice. The petrosal approaches are most commonly used for large meningiomas, which often arise from the tentorium and extend into both the middle and posterior cranial fossa. They may also be used for petroclival meningiomas, under which circumstances either a translabyrinthine or transcochlear petrosectomy is necessary to achieve adequate exposure.

In considering transpetrosal approaches, careful consideration must be given as to whether or not preservation of hearing is outweighed by the additional exposure provided by the translabyrinthine removal of bone and the potential to avoid meningitis in the early postoperative period in patients who are suffering from transient neurologic deficits associated with resection of these large tumors.

A significant potential risk of the petrosal approaches is related to interruption of flow of the vein of Labbé. This vein provides drainage of the posterior temporal lobe and inferior parietal lobe and is at risk with prolonged retraction, especially when the superior petrosal sinus and sigmoid sinus have been divided. It enters the transverse sinus posterior to the takeoff of the superior petrosal sinus and is at risk for occlusion either from retraction of the temporal lobe or propagation of clot along the superior petrosal sinus following ligation (29). Injury to the vein of Labbé or interruption of flow through this structure can result in significant neurologic consequences, including venous infarction of the temporal lobe or significant brain swelling, which can lead to brainstem herniation and death. It is

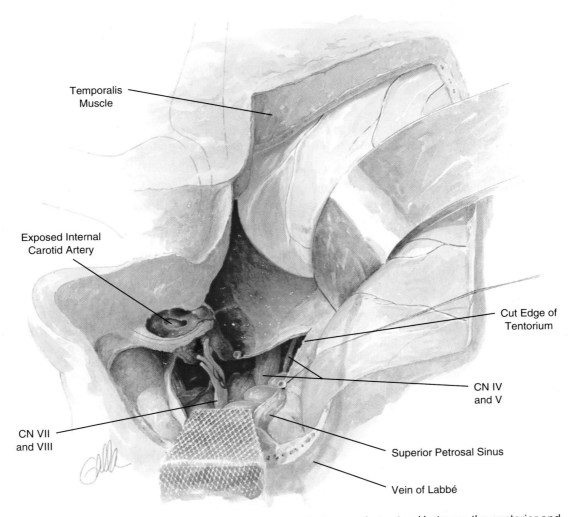

FIG. 12.10 The petrosal approaches provide exposure for tumors that extend between the posterior and middle cranial fossa. Care must be taken not to injure or continuously retract the vein of Labbé and a resultant temporal lobe venous infarct.

therefore prudent to have an accurate preoperative assessment of the venous architecture and collateral venous drainage prior to undertaking such a procedure. It is also worthwhile to minimize retraction of the temporal lobe as much as possible and to release retraction periodically throughout the case to prevent problems with venous stasis and clot formation.

In the petrosal approaches, the superior petrosal sinus is divided with hemoclips followed by division of the tentorium up to the tentorial notch. The trochlear nerve lies in close proximity to the free edge of the tentorium and must be visually identified before the tentorium is completely divided in order to prevent inadvertent injury.

The bone removal that is performed with petrosal approaches is similar to that which has been described for the translabyrinthine, retrolabyrinthine, and middle fossa approaches. Closure of the wound is accomplished by the use of fat grafts, and in the case of the translabyrinthine petrosal approach, canal wall–down mastoidectomy, transection of the external canal with overclosure of the canal, and obliteration of the eustachian tube with bone wax.

Advantages

The primary advantage of the petrosal approach is a wide exposure of the posterior fossa and middle fossa for tumors that extend between the two. By dividing the superior petrosal sinus and tentorium, the amount of brain retraction necessary to achieve adequate exposure is reduced.

Disadvantages

Aside from the unilateral hearing loss, which occurs with the translabyrinthine exposure, the most significant potential morbidity is related to interruption of central venous flow, especially through the vein of Labbé.

INFRATEMPORAL FOSSA APPROACH

The infratemporal fossa approach originally described by Fisch is used primarily for resection of jugular foramen tumors, including paraganglioma, schwannomas, meningiomas, and chondrosarcomas (30). It provides direct visualization of the contents of the jugular foramen, the petrous internal carotid artery, and the lower cranial nerves as they exit the jugular foramen. The exposure is accomplished by mobilization and rerouting of the mastoid and tympanic segments of the facial nerve. Modifications of the infratemporal fossa approach, including varying degrees of facial nerve mobilization and rerouting and preservation of the middle ear structures and auditory function, have been described for use in selected cases, such as glomus jugulare tumors that do not involve the petrous carotid and jugular foramen schwannomas (31–33). The details of the infratemporal fossa approach are described in Chapter 41 on paragangliomas of the temporal bone.

APPROACHES TO THE PETROUS APEX

Transcochlear

Surgical exposure of the petrous apex may be required for removal of cholesteatomas, for drainage of cholesterol cysts, and occasionally for tumor biopsy. Of these lesions, cholesteatomas of the petrous apex are particularly challenging in that successful management involves complete removal of the cholesteatoma, necessitating greater exposure than that which is necessary for either drainage of a cholesterol cyst or biopsy of a tumor. Although the primary goal in the management of cholesteatomas of the petrous apex is complete removal, this may be difficult to accomplish for cholesteatomas, which have eroded the carotid canal. The matrix is often densely adherent to the wall of the internal carotid artery, which may be particularly thin within the petrous bone, especially in elderly patients. Failure to completely remove the cholesteatoma matrix in its entirety results in a risk for recurrence. The risk of recurrence and the potential requirement for future surgery must be weighed against the morbidity associated with the surgical procedure both in terms of hearing loss and injury to the internal carotid artery. The most common site of occurrence for cholesteatomas of the petrous apex is in the anterior petrous apex, anterior and medial to the cochlea and often surrounding the internal carotid artery. As with other benign lesions of the temporal bone, the timing of the surgical procedure and the approach must be carefully considered in the context of the patient's age, general health, hearing in the contralateral ear, and potential for an impending complication based predominantly on the location, size, and radiographic appearance. When surgery is considered, the transcochlear approach affords the best wide-field exposure necessary for potential complete removal.

Surgical Technique

The patient is in a supine position with the head turned. A postauricular incision is made approximately 1 cm posterior to the postauricular crease. The external canal is transected and a blind sac closure accomplished. The remaining skin of the external canal and the tympanic membrane are removed. A canal wall–down mastoidectomy is performed, and the canal wall is taken down to the level of the facial nerve. Using diamond burs, the jugular bulb and petrous carotid artery are identified in the hypotympanum. The carotid artery is skeletonized up to the level of the eustachian tube. The tympanic segment and geniculate portion of the facial nerve are skeletonized. Bone between the dome of the jugular bulb, posterior internal carotid artery, and cochlea is then removed using a diamond bur. Superiorly, care must be taken not to injure the labyrinthine segment of the facial nerve, which lies just superior to the cochlea. Once through the cochlea, bone is removed anterior and medial to the internal carotid artery, providing wide access to the petrous apex. Squamous epithelium adherent to the internal carotid artery may in some cases be difficult to remove. In these cases we feel that it is best to leave a small amount of matrix behind despite the risk for later recurrence. The risk for recurrence and reoperation does not warrant the risk of potential injury to the internal carotid artery for a benign disease. Once the cholesteatoma has been removed, a sheet of temporalis fascia is laid across the length of the internal carotid. The eustachian tube orifice is opened widely with diamond burs and tightly packed with bone wax. The cavity is packed with fat, and the wound is closed. In cases of petrous apex cholesteatomas, it is helpful to obtain a postoperative MRI and CT scan 2 to 3 months following surgery. These studies will serve as a baseline for future studies when recurrence of cholesteatoma is a concern.

Advantages

The transcochlear exposure of the petrous apex provides a field that is potentially wide enough for complete removal of a benign tumor or cholesteatoma. When combined with tympanomastoid obliteration, the potential for postoperative infection is minimized.

Disadvantages

The predominant disadvantage of the transcochlear approach is unilateral hearing loss. Patients may also experience transient vestibular symptoms, although these usually abate over time. There is a potential risk of injury to the labyrinthine segment of the facial nerve, which lies in close proximity to the superior capsule of the cochlea. Preserving the cochlear endosteum in its superior segment can minimize this risk.

TRANSMASTOID INFRALABYRINTHINE APPROACH

The transmastoid infralabyrinthine approach is most often used for drainage of petrous apex cholesterol cysts in cases with advantageous anatomy, such as a low jugular bulb (Chapter 44). The decision to utilize this approach is highly dependent on the CT radiographic anatomy, including location of the bulb and proximity of the petrous apex cyst to the mastoid.

Surgical Technique

A canal wall–up mastoidectomy is performed. The descending segment of the facial nerve from the second genu to the stylomastoid foramen is skeletonized, as is the jugular bulb and posterior semicircular canal. Bone is then removed from the retrofacial cell tract medially between the dome of the jugular bulb and the posterior semicircular canal until the

cyst wall is encountered. The cyst wall is then opened and its contents evacuated. Some have advocated the use of a Silastic stent or tube to maintain patency of the cyst wall fenestra. It has been our experience that these usually become encapsulated in fibrous tissue or granulation tissue. The maintenance of long-term patency of cholesterol cyst fenestras is a potential problem regardless of the technique employed. Reaccumulation is not uncommon, and reoperation may be necessary dependent on radiographic change or the patient's symptoms.

Following fenestration of the cyst wall and evacuation of the contents, the wound is closed in layers as would be done for a routine canal wall–up mastoidectomy.

Advantages

When indicated, the transmastoid infralabyrinthine approach is relatively easy to accomplish with low morbidity. It allows for the preservation of hearing and vestibular function.

Disadvantages

This approach can only be used in a minority of patients with favorable anatomy, which is most often determined by the proximity of the cyst to the mastoid. More typically, these cysts are located more anteriorly and are better accessed through an infracochlear approach.

INFRACOCHLEAR APPROACH

The infracochlear approach may be used for biopsy of petrous apex tumors, as well as drainage of petrous apex cholesterol cysts. It allows for preservation of hearing and the potential for direct drainage of the cyst into the middle ear.

Surgical Technique

The infracochlear approach is accomplished through a postauricular transcanal hypotympantomy described by Farrior for resection of glomus tumors (34). Working through the ear canal and speculum, the skin of the bony canal is incised circumferentially approximately 3 to 4 mm lateral to the tympanic annulus from 3 o'clock to 11 o'clock to facilitate the later development of a superiorly based tympanomeatal flap. A postauricular incision is made approximately 1 cm posterior to the postauricular crease. Soft tissues over the mastoid cortex are elevated with a periosteal elevator, and the skin of the posterior bony canal wall is elevated down to the level of the previous canal incision. The anterior canal wall skin is incised at the bony cartilaginous junction and is removed and placed aside for later use as a free graft. A wide canalplasty is then accomplished with extensive bone removal inferiorly. The tympanic annulus is then elevated from its sulcus and the drum is reflected superiorly. The inferior portion of the bony tympanic annulus is then removed, followed by removal of bone in the hypotympanum to expose the jugular bulb and internal carotid artery. Using diamond burs, bone is then removed between the dome of the bulb and the internal carotid artery inferior to the cochlea. The bony margin of the inferior round window niche is used as a visual landmark for the inferior extent of the cochlea. Bone is removed medially and inferiorly to the cochlea until the cyst capsule is encountered. It is important that this bony opening be made as large as possible to facilitate future drainage. The cyst wall is opened and the cyst contents evacuated. A Silastic tube may be placed within the bony fenestra. Although in our experience it is unlikely that these tubes remain patent, in the event that reoperation is required in the future, removal of the tube may prove useful in reestablishing drainage at a second operation. This is especially helpful when the internal carotid artery has been widely exposed. In subsequent procedures it may be difficult to ascertain the wall of the carotid artery from surrounding soft tissue, which accumulates in this area without the presence of a Silastic tube to mark the path.

Following drainage of the cyst contents, a piece of temporalis fascia is harvested and used to bridge the gap between the inferior aspect of the tympanic membrane and inferior bony canal wall. The anterior canal wall skin is replaced, and split-thickness skin graft is placed over the inferior aspect of the canal and its cover of fascia. A rosebud packing is applied. The postauricular incision is closed, and the vascular strip is tucked posterior to the rosebud; the lateral cartilaginous canal is packed with .25-inch iodoform.

Advantages

The primary advantage of infracochlear approach is that it allows the preservation of hearing and drainage of the cyst contents directly into the middle ear in close proximity to the eustachian tube orifice.

Disadvantages

Disadvantages of the infracochlear approach include potential problems with postoperative infection related to interruption of the tympanic membrane and accumulation of cyst debris within the middle ear. In some cases this may result in a postoperative conductive hearing loss. Another potential disadvantage is related to problems that occur when reoperation is necessary. The internal carotid artery, which may be exposed along its posterior wall, may become covered in dense fibrous tissue over time. The reestablishment of a patent communication between a recurrent and growing cyst and the middle ear may be difficult if the internal carotid artery itself cannot be easily visualized. For this reason, we advocate the placement of a Silastic stent or tube at the time of the initial procedure. Although this may not remain patent, it does provide an important avenue for reexploration when necessary.

INFORMED CONSENT

Preoperative patient education and informed consent vary tremendously depending on the nature of the underlying tumor and the proposed surgical approach. By their nature, these tumors and operations carry with them a very significant potential for serious life-altering complications. Many patients have no idea of the significance of these complications and what to expect even under optimal circumstances for recovery. Failure to accurately review the possible and likely complications, as well as what can be reasonably anticipated for recovery in the postoperative period, will jeopardize the patient's confidence in his physicians, including future recommendations for additional treatment. Informed consent should include the following:

1. Failure to achieve the surgical objective and the possible need for additional therapy. Patients needs to know that in some cases it is not possible to achieve a complete tumor resection without putting them at significant risk for severe neurologic complications, and in some circumstances it may be necessary to leave tumor behind, necessitating the need for additional therapy in the future, including radiation therapy. It is prudent to discuss this with all patients who undergo removal of acoustic neuromas, especially with respect to the facial nerve. In some cases a segment of the tumor may be so adherent to the facial nerve that removal may not be possible without almost certain long-term facial nerve sequelae. A preoperative discussion with the patient will help guide the surgeon in how aggressive to be intraoperatively. Some patients will express a desire for complete tumor removal regardless of the facial nerve consequences, whereas other patients will make it quite clear that all efforts should be made to avoid injury to the facial nerve, even if it necessitates leaving tumor behind and the possibility for additional or future treatment.
2. Potential for neurologic complications both temporary and permanent, including stroke; meningitis; seizures; and cranial nerve injuries such as facial paralysis, aspiration, diplopia, hearing loss, and imbalance. The significance of each of these should be separately discussed.
3. Problems with wound healing, infection, hematoma, and CSF leak. The problem of a potential CSF leak needs to be reviewed in detail with the patient, including the potential requirements for additional treatments if the leak does occur. This should include the possible need for lumbar drainage and reoperation.
4. Pain and headache. Historically, this is one aspect of preoperative education and consent that has been most ignored. Pain and headache are common problems following most of these procedures, especially in patients who undergo suboccipital or retrosigmoid resection of acoustic neuromas (2,3,5,16). A severe, disabling, and persistent headache may occur in up to 5% of these pa-

tients. Although the incidence and severity of headaches following the translabyrinthine and middle fossa approach are less, they may also occur, and patients should be educated accordingly.

POSTOPERATIVE MANAGEMENT

As with other neurologic or neurosurgical procedures, patients who undergo transpetrous approaches to the skull base and posterior fossa require the care of a specialized team of nurses and therapists both intraoperatively and postoperatively. The patients are initially monitored in a neurosurgical intensive care unit. Neurologic monitoring, including motor, sensory, and cognition, is an important component of the early ongoing assessment following surgery. Changes in mental status or neurologic function may be the first sign of an underlying problem. The sooner this is identified and the appropriate diagnostic studies initiated, the better chances for a favorable outcome. There is no substitute for experience in this regard. It is essential that these patients have tight control of blood pressure during the first 48 hours following surgery. Both hypotension and hypertension are potential risks for significant problems. The use of an indwelling arterial catheter with real-time blood pressure monitoring and rapid-acting antihypertensives and pressors may be necessary. Patients should not be discharged from the intensive care unit until all blood pressure problems are under complete control.

Patients who undergo extensive neurosurgical procedures involving the posterior fossa and lower cranial nerves are at increased risk for aspiration both on the basis of lower cranial nerve dysfunction and also from problems related to cerebellar and brainstem dysfunction (35). Patients at increased risk for aspiration should not be allowed to eat or drink until their swallowing function has been adequately assessed.

Patients who undergo transpetrosal surgery are maintained on broad-spectrum antibiotics for the first 72 hours. For cases that are especially long, exceeding 10 to 12 hours, it has been our practice to use intravenous antibiotics that provide antipseudomonas coverage to prevent problems with infection and meningitis in the early postoperative course, which can be of grave consequence.

Patients with facial nerve problems should be seen by an oculoplastic surgeon in the immediate postoperative period for evaluation of their affected eye and recommendations regarding potential management to prevent problems with corneal exposure. Ocular lubricants should be prescribed immediately. In cases where there is incomplete eye closure, a definitive oculoplastic procedure such as the upper lid gold weight implant or lateral canthoplasty should be performed (Chapter 39). Patients with vocal cord paralysis following surgery may benefit from a laryngoplasty prior to discharge, which may or not be done in association with a cricopharyngeal myotomy. Physical therapy, including vestibular physi-

cal therapy, should be initiated as soon as the patient is stable.

REFERENCES

1. Iwata K, Nakagawa H, Hoshino D, et al. Magnetic resonance imaging in the diagnosis of the posterior fossa and the spinal column. *Acta Radiol Suppl* 1986;369:747–749.
2. Pedrosa CA, Ahern DK, McKenna MJ, et al. Determinants and impact of headache after acoustic neuroma surgery. *Am J Otol* 1994;15:793–797.
3. Schessel DA, Nedzelski JM, Rowed DW, et al. Pain after surgery for acoustic neuroma. *Otolaryngol Head Neck Surg* 1992;107:424–429.
4. Schessel DA, Rowed DW, Nedzelski JM, et al: Postoperative pain following excision of acoustic neuroma by the suboccipital approach: observations on possible cause and potential amelioration. *Am J Otol* 1993;14:491–494.
5. Catalano PJ, Jacobowitz O, Post KD. Prevention of headache after retrosigmoid removal of acoustic tumors. *Am J Otol* 1996;17:904–908.
6. Nadol JB Jr, Chiong CM, Ojemann RG, et al. Preservation of hearing and facial nerve function in resection of acoustic neuroma. *Laryngoscope* 1992;102:1153–1158.
7. McKenna MJ, Nadol JB Jr, Ojemann RG, et al. Vestibular neurectomy: retrosigmoid-intracanalicular versus retrolabyrinthine approach. *Am J Otol* 1996;17:253–258.
8. House WF, De la Cruz A, Hitselberger WE. Surgery of the skull base: transcochlear approach to the petrous apex and clivus. *Otolaryngology* 1978;86ORL:770–779.
9. Jenkins HA, Fisch U. The transotic approach to resection of difficult acoustic tumors of the cerebellopontine angle. *Am J Otol* 1980;2:70–76.
10. House WF. Surgical exposure of the internal auditory canal and its contents through the middle, cranial fossa. *Laryngoscope* 1961;71:1363–1385.
11. Kanzaki J, Shiobara R, Toya S. Classification of the extended middle cranial fossa approach. *Acta Otolaryngol Suppl* 1991;487:6–16.
12. Bochenek Z, Kukwa A. An extended approach through the middle cranial fossa to the internal auditory meatus and cerebellopontine angle. *Acta Otolaryngol* 1975;80:410–414.
13. Shiobara R, Ohira T, Kanszki J, et al. A modified extended middle cranial fossa approach for acoustic nerve tumors. Results of 125 operations. *J Neurosurg* 1988;68:358–365.
14. Rosomoff HL. The subtemporal transtentorial approach to the cerebellopontine angle. *Laryngoscope* 1971;81:1448–1454.
15. Driscoll CL, Jackler RK, Pitts LH, et al. Extradural temporal lobe retraction in the middle fossa approach to the internal auditory canal: biomechanical analysis. *Am J Otol* 1999;20:373–380.
16. Garcia-Ibanez E, Garcia-Ibanez JL. Middle fossa vestibular neurectomy: a report of 373 cases. *Otolaryngol Head Neck Surg* 1980;88:486–490.
17. Wigand ME, Aurbach G, Haid CT, et al. Topographical anatomy of the internal auditory canal. Implications for functional surgery in the cerebello-pontine angle. *Acta Otolaryngol* 1991;111:269–272.
18. Jackler RK, Gladstone HB. Locating the internal auditory canal during the middle fossa approach: an alternative technique. *Skull Base Surg* 1995;5:63–67.
19. Matsunaga T, Igarashi M, Kanzaki J. Landmark structures to approach the internal auditory canal: a dimensional study related to the middle cranial fossa approach. *Acta Otolaryngol Suppl* 1991;487:48–53.
20. Wigand ME, Haid T, Berg M. The enlarged middle cranial fossa approach for surgery of the temporal bone and of the cerebellopontine angle. *Arch Otorhinolaryngol* 1989;246:299–302.
21. Sekiya T, Moller AR. Cochlear nerve injuries caused by cerebellopontine angle manipulations. An electrophysiological and morphological study in dogs. *J Neurosurg* 1987;67:244–249.
22. Kawase T, Toya S, Shiobara R, et al. Transpetrosal approach for aneurysms of the lower basilar artery. *J Neurosurg* 1985;63:857–861.
23. Irving RM, Jackler RK, Pitts LH. Hearing preservation in patients undergoing vestibular schwannoma surgery: comparison of middle fossa and retrosigmoid approaches. *J Neurosurg* 1998;88:840–845.
24. Arriaga MA, Chen DA, Fukushima T. Individualizing hearing preservation in acoustic neuroma surgery. *Laryngoscope* 1997;107:1043–1047.

25. Haberkamp TJ, Meyer GA, Fox M. Surgical exposure of the fundus of the internal auditory canal: anatomic limits of the middle fossa versus the retrosigmoid transcanal approach. *Laryngoscope* 1998;108:1190–1194.
26. Silverstein H, Norrell H, Smouha E, et al. The singular canal: a valuable landmark in surgery of the internal auditory canal. *Otolaryngol Head Neck Surg* 1988;98:138–143.
27. Domb GH, Chole RA. Anatomical studies of the posterior petrous apex with regard to hearing preservation in acoustic neuroma removal. *Laryngoscope* 1980;90:1769–1776.
28. Hongo K, Kobayashi S, Yokoh A, et al. Monitoring retraction pressure on the brain: an experimental and clinical study. *J Neurosurg* 1987;66:270–275.
29. Guppy KH, Origitano TC, Reichman OH, et al. Venous drainage of the inferolateral temporal lobe in relationship to transtemporal/transtentorial approaches to the cranial base. *Neurosurgery* 1997;41:615–619; discussion 619–620.
30. Fisch U, Pillsbury HC. Infratemporal fossa approach to lesions in the temporal bone and base of the skull. *Arch Otolaryngol* 1979;105:99–107.
31. Brackmann DE. The facial nerve in the infratemporal approach. *Otolaryngol Head Neck Surg* 1987;97:15–17.
32. Jackson CG. Basic surgical principles of neurotologic skull base surgery. *Laryngoscope* 1993;Suppl 60:29–44.
33. Pensak ML, Jackler RK. Removal of jugular foramen tumors: the fallopian bridge technique. *Otolaryngol Head Neck Surg* 1997;117:586–591.
34. Farrior JB. Anterior hypotympanic approach for glomus tumor of the infratemporal fossa. *Laryngoscope* 1984;94:1016–1021.
35. Poe DS, Jackson G, Glasscock ME, et al. Long-term results after lateral cranial base surgery. *Laryngoscope* 1991;101:372–378.

CHAPTER 13

Management of Soft Tissue and Osseous Stenosis of the Ear Canal and Canalplasty

Steven D. Rauch

The functional characteristics of the ear canal are usually assessed by the practicing otologist on only a subliminal level as part of the general evaluation of a patient with any ear complaint. There are five functional characteristics of a "good" ear canal: (i) admission of sound, (ii) easy inspection, (iii) easy cleaning (or better yet, self-cleaning), (iv) prevention or deterrence or recurrent disease, and (v) admission of a hearing aid.

Admission of sound is permitted as long as there is a patent channel from the meatus to the tympanic membrane. The acoustic characteristics of the sound transmission will necessarily vary with diameter of the canal, as well as the relative bony and soft tissue composition of the walls, but this rarely translates into changes in clinical management. *Easy inspection* refers to the necessity of examining all recesses of the ear canal, particularly in the postsurgical ear, to watch for any sign of disease. A stenotic meatus or canal or a large posterior or superior overhang of soft tissue at the meatus complicates the examination.

The vast majority of normal ears are self-cleaning. Cerumen is produced in the lateral portion of the canal adjacent to the meatus, where it tends to dry and fall out or be washed away. Postsurgical ears, however, often require regular cleaning to manage accumulated cerumen, desquamated skin, and other debris. Most likely this is a result of the loss of normal dermal appendages such as small hairs and cerumen glands, as well as disruption of epithelial migration mechanisms. These dermal appendages are also required to preserve normal skin moisture and integrity as a barrier to infection. Excessive dryness resulting from loss of cerumen glands leads to chronic dermatitis and itching, which in turn leads to scratching, skin breakdown, and infection. A stenotic or misshapen meatus or canal or the presence of chronic dermatitis may preclude the wearing of a hearing aid due to inadequate fit, discomfort, or recurrent infection.

Appropriate management of the ear canal begins with an assessment of these five functional characteristics. Furthermore, they must be kept in mind during treatment of other ear diseases that require alteration of the meatus or canal to gain surgical access to the middle ear or mastoid. Thus every effort can be made to achieve a fully functional ear canal postoperatively. In those cases with a primary ear canal problem, functional assessment provides a clear indication of the site and nature of the disorder and dictates the principles of treatment.

COMMON DISORDERS OF THE EAR CANAL

Senile Meatal Stenosis (the Sagging Auricle)

Progressive soft tissue laxity due to aging often leads to sagging of the pinna relative to the bony external auditory canal. This causes an anteroinferior displacement of the conchal cartilage toward the tragus, with a resultant "fish-mouth" narrowing of the meatus. Simple posterosuperior distraction of the pinna allows examination and cleaning of the ear. Surgical correction is indicated when the deformity results in collapse of the meatus when trying to use the telephone, retention of cerumen, or difficulty in insertion of the ear mold of a hearing aid. A simple meatoplasty under local anesthesia is effective in correcting this condition.

Keratosis Obturans

Current understanding of keratosis obturans is based on the work of Piepergerdes et al. (1), who clearly differentiated this disorder from external auditory canal cholesteatoma. It presents clinically as hearing loss and usually acute, severe pain secondary to accumulation of large plugs of desquamated keratin in the ear canal. Cleaning may require repeated attempts with administration of topical antibiotics and wax softeners or even general anesthesia. Removal of the keratin cast from the ear canal reveals circumferentially erythematous, scaly, canal skin and occasional granulation tissue. In long-standing cases there is diffuse dilation ("ballooning") of the bony canal, presumably from the chronic pressure effect of the keratin plug. The condition typically occurs in children and young adults, is usually bilateral, and has been associated with a high incidence of bronchiectasis and sinusitis (2,3). The underlying pathophysiology is believed to be a desquamative reaction to chronic hyperemia (4–6). The majority of cases will respond to frequent cleaning in conjunction with topical steroids and emollients to reduce desquamation and inflammation. Surgery is indicated for those cases refractory to this conservative approach. Removal of all affected canal skin, a wide canalplasty, and split-thickness skin grafting is curative.

Chronic Stenosing External Otitis

Tos and Balle (7) have reviewed the clinical presentation, pathophysiology, and management of fibrous obliteration of the medial ear canal resulting from chronic inflammation. They believe that recurrent external otitis and granular myringitis lead to fibrous proliferation of the soft tissue of the lateral surface of the tympanic membrane and bony external auditory canal. Patients present with a history of several years of recurrent external otitis and progressive conductive hearing loss. Treatment is surgical and consists of debridement of all abnormal tissue, including the tissue lateral to the lamina propria of the tympanic membrane, a wide bony canalplasty, and split-thickness skin grafting of all denuded areas.

Postsurgical Stenosis

Both postauricular and endaural surgical approaches to the middle ear and mastoid can lead to meatal or canal stenosis. This complication arises from proliferation of scar tissue along surgical planes where skin has been elevated from underlying tissues or where incisions have been made for a Koerner flap or endaural approach. A wide meatoplasty with excision of a crescent of conchal cartilage and adjacent soft tissue and a wide bony canalplasty greatly reduce the incidence of this problem. In the case of endaural incisions, a simple advancement of the pinna side of the incision relative to the facial side at the time of closure complements the meatoplasty/canalplasty to further reduce the likelihood of meatal stenosis. If a developing stenosis is detected in the early postoperative period, it is easily managed by serial dilation with Merocel sponge wicks cut to the largest size the stenotic segment will admit, kept moist with antibiotic drops, and replaced with a larger wick every 7 to 10 days. Very dense or persistent scar tissue will respond better to dilation with the addition of intradermal triamcinolone acetonide injections at the time of each wick change. Complete resolution is expected within 2 to 6 weeks. Surgical correction by meatoplasty is indicated when the problem is detected after meatal healing is complete (more than 3 or 4 months postoperatively) and there is inadequate meatal size for easy inspection, cleaning, or hearing aid insertion.

Exostosis

Exostosis is the most common bony abnormality of the external auditory canal, reported to occur in 6.3 of every 1,000 patients examined for otolaryngologic problems (8). It presents as a gradual narrowing of the bony canal by broad-based mounds of bone arising from both the anterior and posterior bony canal walls. Occasionally a smaller mound may arise posterosuperiorly as well. Histopathologic examination of the bone reveals a dense stratified arrangement of new bone that in time is remodeled, beginning around vascular channels into normal-appearing lamellar bone (Figs. 13.1 and 13.2). The bone deposition is believed to be secondary to a chronic periostitis due to cold temperature. The abnormality is most often seen in cold-water swimmers. It is usually bilateral and asymptomatic. Symptoms may arise, however, if the exostoses become so large as to occlude the ear canal or cause retention of cerumen or desquamated keratin and produce a conductive hearing loss or recurrent external otitis. In such symptomatic cases a wide bony canalplasty with split-thickness skin grafting of all denuded surfaces is indicated.

Because the exostoses extend far medially in the canal, the most common complication of treatment is perforation of the tympanic membrane. This can be avoided by reflecting medially based canal skin flaps down onto the tympanic membrane, covering the tympanic membrane with a shield of Silastic or metal foil, and by using either bone curettes or diamond rather than cutting burs during drilling of the most medial extent of the exotoses.

Osteoma

Osteoma is a discrete pedunculated bony mass arising from the tympanosquamous suture line adjacent to the bony-cartilaginous junction of the external auditory canal (Fig. 13.3). It is a solitary, unilateral, benign, slowly progressive lesion. In contrast to exostoses, the histopathologic appearance is characterized by thick, well-formed lamellae with multiple fibrovascular channels throughout the interlamellar spaces (9). Usually asymptomatic, osteomas require surgical removal only if causing obstructive symptoms of hearing loss, cerumen retention, or recurrent infection. Removal is accomplished simply with a small chisel followed by drilling away the base of the attachment site. Enough overlying skin is easily preserved to resurface the denuded area. Recurrence is unusual but not unknown and requires more aggressive removal of bone at the site of origin during subsequent surgery.

External Auditory Canal Cholesteatoma

Primary cholesteatoma of the external auditory canal presents with chronic dull otalgia, purulent otorrhea, and normal

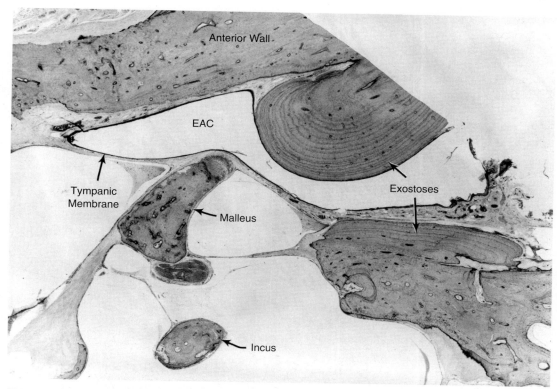

FIG. 13.1 Exostoses of the right external auditory canal. There is a pedunculated lesion located on the anterosuperior wall and a plaque-like lesion on the posterior wall. The laminated appearance is histologically diagnostic for exostoses. EAC, external auditory canal. 13.8X.

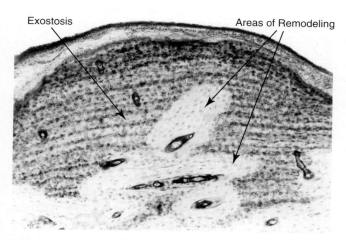

FIG. 13.2 Exostosis in a man who often engaged in water sports in the cold lakes of upper New York state and the Atlantic Ocean. Otoscopy revealed bilateral asymptomatic exostoses. This view shows a flat exostosis on the posterior wall of the right ear that is undergoing remodeling into lamellar bone. This a very slow but normal process that begins around vascular channels. 88X.

hearing. It reportedly occurs in 0.1% to 0.5% of new otologic patients (10). The lesion is a focal area of osteitis with sequestration of bone and surrounding inflammation of canal skin (11) in contradistinction to keratosis obturans, in which the skin is involved circumferentially. Uninvolved ep-

ithelium of the ear canal is normal. The erosive lesion in bone is virtually always in the floor of the bony ear canal (12). In cases of large cholesteatomas the erosion and retained keratin may extend into the mastoid or beneath the tympanic annulus into the middle ear. Anthony and Anthony (12) described the primary lesion as an irregularity of canal bone with local inflammation that causes impairment of normal epithelial migration with subsequent retention of keratin debris and superinfection. Other authors believe the cholesteatoma is a sequel of the periostitis and that the epidermis does not play an active role in this process (13). In small, superficial lesions, conservative management with topical antibiotic/antiinflammatory eardrops and frequent cleaning may improve symptoms. Sequestration of necrotic bone requires surgical debridement by saucerization down to healthy bone, debridement of involved canal skin, and skin grafting of exposed bone. Use of temporalis fascia beneath the split-thickness skin grafts in cases with open mastoid air cells, open tympanic cavity, or large bony defects, as advocated by Anthony and Anthony, improves the reconstruction.

SURGICAL MANAGEMENT

Surgical management of soft tissue and osseous stenosis of the ear canal requires a clear understanding of the anatomic location of the abnormality whether it involves the meatus,

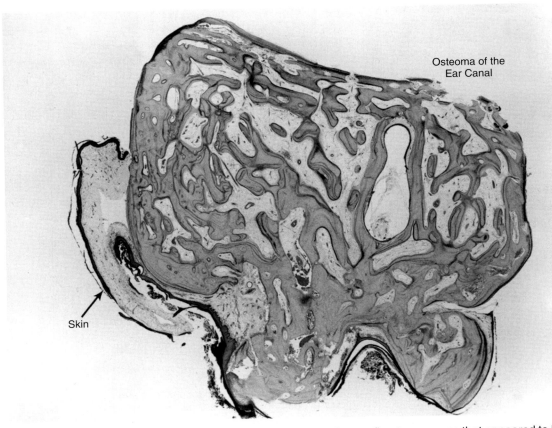

Osteoma of the
Ear Canal

Skin

FIG. 13.3 Osteoma. At age 19 this woman was noted to have a firm tumor mass that appeared to be obstructing 90% of the lumen of the left external auditory canal. On surgical exploration via a transcanal approach, it was found to be pedunculated and easily removed. The denuded area of the canal wall was repaired with a split-thickness skin graft. Histological study reveals a bony mass measuring about 1 cm in diameter. It has a round, slightly nodular configuration and approximately half its surface is covered by normal-appearing squamous epithelium lying on a moderately vascular subcutaneous fibrous layer of varying thickness. The bone is arranged in dense interconnecting trabeculae with a bone/soft tissue ratio of about 60:40. In many areas the trabeculae are lined by osteoid seams and a layer of osteoblasts, indicating active bone growth. The intertrabecular fibrous tissue has a loose stroma infiltrated with scattered round cells and small arteries and veins. 8.3X.

the cartilaginous canal, the bony canal, or some combination of these. In fact, the choice of surgical procedure depends far more on the anatomic distribution of the problem than the particular lesion or disorder. This anatomic consideration coupled with the functional characteristics of a "good" ear canal, as defined earlier, guide the surgeon.

Meatoplasty

Meatoplasty is used primarily as an office procedure for sagging auricles (age related) and minor lateral stenoses, principally postoperative. The meatus should be round to elliptical, with the long axis of the ellipse oriented vertically. It should be located immediately inferior to the root of the helix. If it is positioned too high or posterior, the suspensory support of the pinna is lost and a lop ear deformity results. Excision of a generous crescent of conchal cartilage and an adequate amount of underlying soft tissue is the best means of creating a wide meatoplasty. Access to the cartilage may

be obtained through direct incision of conchal skin in curvilinear fashion along the anterior margin of the anthelix in cases when an isolated meatoplasty is needed (such as for senile meatal stenosis) or via elevation of a Koerner flap in conjunction with an endaural incision or via a postauricular incision when combined with a cartilaginous canalplasty (Fig. 13.4A). Ideally, the meatus should be approximately the same diameter as the bony canal and admit a 6- to 8-mm speculum. The distensibility of meatal soft tissue will allow introduction of a larger speculum than the resting diameter of the meatus, so avoidance of the cosmetic deformity of an excessively large meatal opening is easily accomplished. In cases where a band of scar tissue produces a stenotic web at the meatus, a simple Z-plasty with excision of a wedge of the subcutaneous meatal soft tissue is an effective solution. The central limb of the Z runs in the scar band from superior to inferior along the posterior margin of the meatus. Transposition of the two flaps thus created lengthens the web and relieves the stenosis.

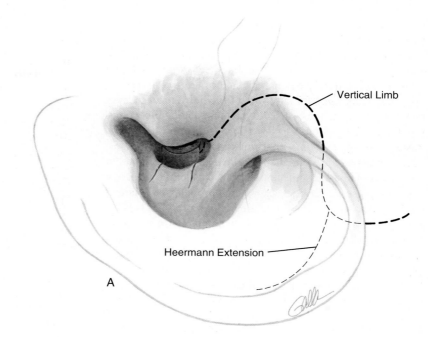

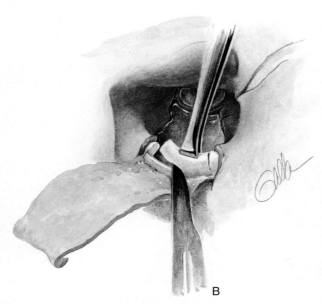

FIG. 13.4 Meatoplasty and cartilaginous canalplasty. **A:** For simple meatoplasty, only the canal and conchal incision are necessary. When a wider exposure is needed, the incision is extended upward, anterior to the helix. **B:** The skin of the posterior cartilaginous canal wall is separated from soft tissue and conchal cartilage by sharp dissection and reflected posteriorly as a laterally based (Koerner) flap. Conchal cartilage and soft tissue are excised sufficiently to provide the desired surgical exposure and to ensure an adequate postoperative meatus.

Cartilaginous Canalplasty

The cartilaginous canal must be large enough to admit a 6- to 8-mm speculum (Fig. 13.4). Preservation of cerumen glands is desirable in order to maintain good canal function with regard to epithelial migration and inhibition of infection. Ideally, the posterior canal wall should drape smoothly from the concha to the isthmus without a posterior or superior overhang. This is best achieved by a wide meatoplasty, including both removal of a crescent of conchal cartilage, as described earlier for the isolated meatoplasty, and resection of a wedge of the underlying fibrous soft tissues deep to the Koerner flap and lateral to the tympanomastoid suture line. The endaural or postauricular incisions provide adequate exposure for canalplasty. When a postauricular incision is used, a slight posterosuperior repositioning of the pinna by excision of a postauricular skin crescent improves the likelihood of avoiding a posterior or superior shelf. Excessive skin excision can produce a "telephone deformity" with the pinna flattened tightly against the side of the head. If a Koerner flap is elevated for exposure of the bony canal, it must be widely based at the concha to maintain a good blood supply. It should be thinned to deep dermis to prevent stenosis postoperatively. It should be trimmed to a length that is just adequate to reach beyond the lateral extent of the rosebud or gelatin packing used in the bony canal. This leaves sufficient length to preserve cerumen glands and provide anterolateral coverage for any mastoid defect or obliteration but is short enough to prevent bunching at the isthmus that can lead to postoperative stenosis. If an anterior canal skin flap has been elevated to expose the bony-cartilaginous junction anteriorly, this flap should be replaced across the isthmus at the time of reconstruction or split-thickness skin graft used to bridge that zone to prevent stenosis. Often after creating a wide meatoplasty and canalplasty, the canal incisions used to create the Koerner flap have several millimeters of gap along the roof and floor of the meatus and cartilaginous canal. Consideration should be given to resurfacing these gaps with split-thickness skin to avoid contracture leading to stenosis. The cartilaginous canal should remain packed with antibiotic-impregnated gauze ribbon for 1 week to stabilize the reconstruction after elevation of Koerner and anterior skin flaps.

Bony Canalplasty

This procedure (Fig. 13.5) is an anatomic continuation of the cartilaginous canalplasty described earlier. The skin of the anterior canal wall is elevated as a laterally based pedicled flap. A Lempert elevator is used to separate the flap from the lateral margin of the bony canal. Thus the entire bony canal down to the tympanic annulus is denuded of skin. To permit wide access to the medial ear canal for inspection and cleaning, a bony canalplasty should expose the entire tympanic annulus to view and extend laterally in a slight conical flare to the bony-cartilaginous junction. The anterior limit of drilling is the temporomandibular joint, and the posterior limit is the air cells of the mastoid. Except for posteriorly located exostosis, little or no drilling is necessary on the posterior bony wall above the tympanomastoid suture line. Superiorly it is rarely indicated to remove bone to approach middle fossa dura, but this is feasible if necessary. Extensive superior bone removal ensures a superior overhang at the meatus, which makes inspection and cleaning more difficult. The inferior extent of tympanic bone removal is dictated by the disease process. Particularly in the case of canal cholesteatoma, in which there is necrosis and sequestration of this portion of the tympanic ring, extensive removal may be necessary. Caution should be exercised because of proximity to the facial nerve as bone is removed inferiorly and posteriorly. The acute angle of the anterior tympanic sulcus where the

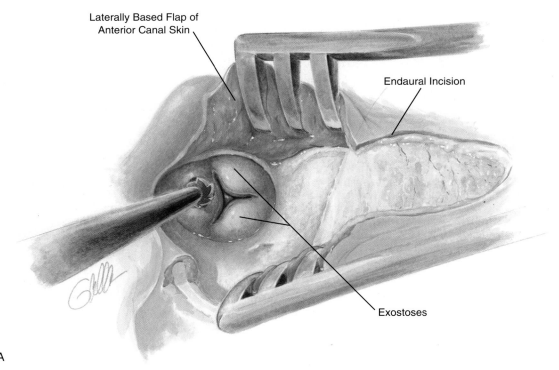

Laterally Based Flap of Anterior Canal Skin

Endaural Incision

Exostoses

A

FIG. 13.5 Bony canalplasty. **A:** Usually the bony canalplasty requires enlarging the entire bony canal.

Continued

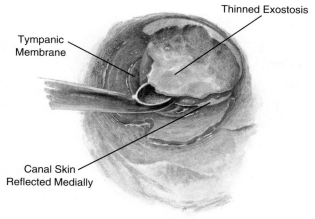

Tympanic
Membrane

Thinned Exostosis

Canal Skin
Reflected Medially

B

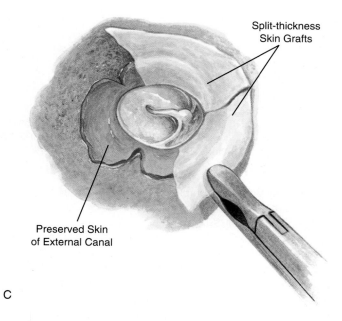

Split-thickness
Skin Grafts

Preserved Skin
of External Canal

C

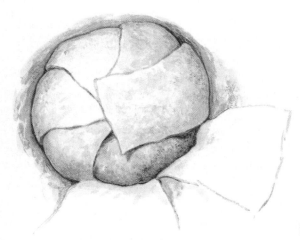

D

FIG. 13.5, cont'd. Bony canalplasty. **B:** When dealing with exostoses, the skin on the medial surface can often be preserved by displacing it toward the tympanic membrane as the operation proceeds, thus protecting the tympanic membrane. Bone curettes are useful when working near the tympanic membrane. **C:** Thin split-thickness skin grafts are arranged to cover all denuded surfaces of the bony canal. **D:** A rosebud packing of silk strips and cotton secures the skin grafts.

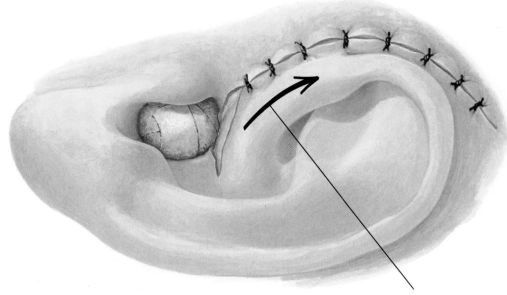

Advancement of Auricular
Side of Incision

FIG. 13.6 In cases utilizing a full endaural incision to gain wide exposure for removal of exostoses, closure includes a 3- to 5-mm rotation advancement of the auricular side of the incision to further widen the meatus and reduce the possibility of postoperative meatal stenosis.

anterior canal wall meets the tympanic membrane exposes the membrane to the risk of perforation by drill burs. A shield made of thin Silastic sheet or metal foil is an effective way to reduce this risk. Bone curettes are also an effective and safe method for removal of bone near the tympanic membrane, particularly for surgeons accustomed to their use. All denuded bony surfaces should be covered with split-thickness skin grafts at the completion of surgery. Healing by secondary intention requires formation of granulation tissue followed by epithelial migration, resulting in thicker scar and slower healing than that obtained by grafting. The incision is closed with a single row of interrupted 4-0 Dermalon sutures (Fig. 13.6). A rosebud pack of surgical silk strips and antibiotic-soaked cotton or a gelatin pack should be left in the bony canal for 2 weeks to stent the reconstruction during preliminary healing. After removal of the pack, antibiotic ear drops are used for an additional 4 to 6 weeks as the overlapping edges of the skin grafts demarcate and slough. Complete epithelialization should be achieved by that time. Any delay of healing will result in granulation tissue, which must be curetted away and the base cauterized lightly with silver nitrate to prevent excessive scar formation and possible stenosis.

REFERENCES

1. Piepergerdes MC, Kramer BM, Behnke EE. Keratosis obturans and external auditory canal cholesteatoma. *Laryngoscope* 1980;90:383–391.
2. Morrison AW. Keratosis obturans. *J Laryngol Otol* 1956;70:317–321.
3. Black JIM, Clayton RG. Wax keratosis in children's ears. *Br Med J* 1958;2:673–675.
4. Green LD. Cholesteatoma-like accumulation in the external auditory meatus. *Arch Otolaryngol* 1933;18:161–167.
5. Costello MJ, Fried S. Keratosis obturans otica; obstructive hollow keratotic cast of external auditory canal. *Arch Dermatol Syph* 1953;67:516–517.
6. McKibben BG. Cholesteatoma-like accumulations in the external auditory meatus. Report of one case. *Arch Otolaryngol* 1958;67:626–628.
7. Tos M, Balle V. Postinflammatory acquired atresia of the external auditory canal: late results of surgery. *Am J Otol* 1986;7:365–370.
8. DiBartolomeo JR. Exostoses of the external auditory canal. *Ann Otol Rhinol Laryngol* 1979;88[Suppl 61]:1–20.
9. Graham MD. Osteomas and exostoses of the external auditory canal. A clinical, histopathologic and scanning electron microscopic study. *Ann Otol Rhinol Laryngol* 1979;88:566–572.
10. Farrior J. Cholesteatoma of the external ear canal. *Am J Otol* 1990;11:113–116.
11. Naiberg J, Berger G, Hawke M. The pathologic features of keratosis obturans and cholesteatoma of the external auditory canal. *Arch Otolaryngol* 1984;110:690–693.
12. Anthony PF, Anthony WP. Surgical treatment of external auditory canal cholesteatoma. *Laryngoscope* 1982;92:70–75.
13. Altmann F, Waltner JG. Cholesteatoma of the external auditory meatus. *Arch Otolaryngol* 1943;38:236–240.

CHAPTER 14

Perforations of the Tympanic Membrane

Dennis S. Poe

Perforations of the tympanic membrane are caused by a number of etiologies, most commonly suppurative otitis media. Perforations cause hearing loss and predispose patients to drainage, pain, and complications from otitis media.

The earliest known evidence of a tympanic membrane perforation was described by Benitez (1) in an Egyptian mummy, Pum II. There was an oval-shaped perforation in which the margins demonstrated histologic evidence of inflammation and repair consistent with otitis media. The process of acute suppurative otitis media leading to perforation of the tympanic membrane was described by Shambaugh (2), who noted that toxins from beta-hemolytic *Streptococcus* were capable of producing rapid necrosis of the tympanic membrane.

Trauma is the second leading cause of tympanic membrane perforations. Injury may be due to direct trauma or to barotrauma. Direct trauma includes self-inflicted injuries with cotton-tipped applicators and other instruments used to clean or scratch the ear canal, iatrogenic injuries from attempts to remove foreign bodies or cerumen, welding slag, waterskiing injuries, temporal bone fractures, and injuries from flying debris. Barotrauma includes aerotitis, waterskiing injuries, slap injuries to the ear, and explosions.

The failure of perforations to heal spontaneously is due to many factors, including size and location of the perforation, severity of tissue injury, approximation of the margins, tendency of epithelial margin to develop squamous ingrowth, presence of infection, and health of the surrounding tympanic membrane. Perforations may persist following the removal or extrusion of tympanostomy tubes and is correlated with the diameter of the tube or duration of the tube in the tympanic membrane (3,4). Spontaneous healing of traumatic perforations occurred in 73% of the cases reported by Kristensen et al. (5).

The severity of the conductive hearing loss due to tympanic membrane perforation appears to be correlated with the size of the defect, with larger perforations generally causing greater hearing loss. The hearing loss is typically worse in the lower frequencies. Perforations overlying the round window are said to have a disproportionately greater hearing loss than a comparably sized perforation located elsewhere on the tympanic membrane due to a lack of phase and amplitude differences between the oval and round windows (6). However, Voss et al. (7) in a cadaveric model have demonstrated that the location of the perforation, at least of those with a diameter of 1 mm or less, had no influence on the size of the conductive hearing loss.

The concept of repairing perforations of the tympanic membrane was revolutionary when it was introduced by Wullstein (8) and Zöllner (9) in 1952 and 1955, respectively. It was realized late in the nineteenth century that manipulation of the ossicles could improve hearing in some cases. The incidence of postoperative deafness and meningitis was sufficiently high that the concept of ear surgery for correction of hearing loss was condemned for decades. The development of fenestration surgery for otosclerosis rejuvenated the concept of hearing restoration by ear surgery, but it remained unthinkable for perforations, because prevention and treatment of infections were the only important goals in chronic otitis media. The very concept of tissue grafting of a tympanic membrane over air seemed to defy the presumed necessity for graft placement on a vascularized base. In 1950 Moritz (10) described the use of pedicle flaps as a staged procedure to close draining perforations and cover the round window before a second-stage fenestration procedure. Zöllner (11) in 1951 adapted the pedicled flap techniques to close simple perforations of the tympanic membrane. Wullstein (8) in 1952 was the first to perform tympanoplasty using a free skin graft placed lateral to the perforation (overlay graft). The success of tympanoplasty gave birth to a new era of reconstructive ear surgery. Skin grafts were complicated by graft eczema, inflammation, perforations, and iatrogenic cholesteatoma. House and Sheehy (12) reported that the skin from the auricular meatus was more suitable than skin from a remote site. Vein graft perichondrium and homograft were employed and offered various benefits (13–15). In 1961 Storrs (16) reported the use of temporalis fascia, which quickly gained widespread acceptance. Techniques to place the graft medial to the tympanic membrane (underlay) using fascia and the loose areolar layer of temporoparietal fascia began to emerge and were popularized by Glasscock (17). Overlay procedures had the technical advantage of being easier to place the graft on the lateral surface of the tympanic membrane, which had been denuded of all epithelium. However, the technique requires a wide canalplasty and precision in packing the tympanic membrane graft in position to minimize scarring and blunting of the anterior canal sulcus or lateralization of the graft. The underlay technique minimizes the possibility of blunting or lateralization because the skin of the anterior ear canal and annulus is left in place. However, placement of the graft medial to the tympanic membrane can be more technically challenging. Given the advantages and disadvantages of both techniques, it is ideal to be well trained in the use of either so that the surgeon may select a technique based on the location, size, and character of perforation. The author prefers the underlay technique for most cases because of the reduced complication rate and reduced time required for performance of the procedure. It is a useful technique even for total tympanic membrane replacement.

OFFICE MANAGEMENT OF TYMPANIC MEMBRANE PERFORATIONS

Tympanic membrane perforations may be symptomatic with hearing loss or otorrhea or present as incidental findings on a routine examination with no symptoms. Pain with infection is unusual because drainage through the perforation will normally prevent the accumulation of pus under pressure. If pain is present with suppurative otitis media, it should be regarded as a potentially ominous symptom of a possible underlying complication (Chapter 18).

Perforations are generally classified as central or marginal. Central perforations occur in the pars tensa and have a rim of tympanic membrane circumferentially. Size is variable, and the shape is typically round, oval, or kidneylike. The edges of long-standing perforations are rounded, with keratinized stratified squamous epithelium of the external surface approximating the middle ear mucosa at the margin of the perforation.

Marginal perforations include defects of the pars tensa that extend to the tympanic annulus and any perforation located in the pars flaccida. Marginal perforations may be preceded by retraction of the tympanic membrane, typically in the posterosuperior portion of the pars tensa or in the pars flaccida.

Chronic perforations may be associated with tympanosclerosis, hyalined plaques embedded in the tympanic membrane (Fig. 14.1). Histologically, there is hyalinization of the subepithelial connective tissue with dystrophic calcification, usually involving the middle fibrous layer of the tympanic membrane and in some cases the middle ear mucosa. Hearing loss usually occurs only when the ossicles become involved and fixed (4,5).

PATIENT SELECTION FOR SURGERY

The principal indications for surgery are hearing loss or infection that may be intermittent or chronic or evidence of early formation of cholesteatoma. Repair of a chronic, sta-

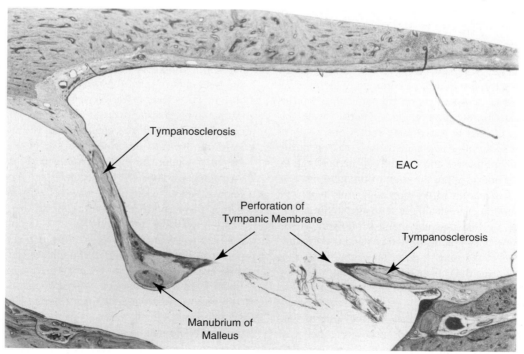

FIG. 14.1 Photomicrograph of chronic perforation of the tympanic membrane with tympanosclerosis. EAC, external auditory canal.

ble, asymptomatic perforation may be done to obviate the need for water precautions. Complicating factors such as allergic rhinitis, sinusitis, other nasal pathology, or immunocompromised state should be managed to the best extent reasonable preoperatively. A comprehensive medical history and physical examination should be completed.

The success of tympanoplasty surgery depends to a large degree on the patient having adequate eustachian tube function. Attempts to objectively evaluate eustachian tube function have not been able to reliably predict which patients will fail tympanoplasty surgery. Many tests use sophisticated means for recording tubal opening pressures in response to varying gradients of applied pressure, but the conditions are actually nonphysiologic and correlate only poorly with clinical success or failure. Bluestone and Cantekin (18) have shown that the simple ability to equalize middle ear pressure by swallowing while the pressure is varied with a tympanometry bridge does correlate well with tympanoplasty success. Failures of equalization tests, however, have not accurately predicted tympanoplasty failures. Other methods of eustachian tube evaluation have shown similar correlations for predicting success when function is good but are poorly correlated with tympanoplasty failures (19–24). Normal tubal function on the contralateral ear does not adequately predict normal tubal function in the perforated ear. Magnuson and Falk (25) observed that variation of tubal function over time is one reason for poor predictive value. It is well known that patients may have successful closure of the perforation for many months, or even years, and suddenly fail after an acute episode of eustachian tube dysfunction.

There is controversy concerning timing of repair of perforations in children. The incidence of otitis media declines sharply after age 6, and the eustachian tube has reached adult length generally by age 7 (26). Symptomatic perforations with infection or hearing loss may be closed at any age. Closure of asymptomatic perforations must be individualized. Generally it is postponed until age 7 when the incidence of upper respiratory infections and dysfunction of the eustachian tube decreases.

The risks and benefits of tympanoplasty should be carefully weighed in all cases. When the perforation involves the better or only hearing ear, repair should be undertaken only when circumstances are compelling, such as with intractable otorrhea, which itself risks inner ear injury.

Examination of the tympanic membrane preoperatively is optimally done with a binocular microscope. Inspection of the perforation edge is done to evaluate the quality of the surrounding tympanic membrane (atrophic or healthy) and to look for additional disease such as migration of skin onto the medial surface of the tympanic membrane, scarring, tympanosclerosis, or myringitis. Examination of the middle ear through the perforation may demonstrate mucosal disease or complications such as cholesteatoma or granulation. The status of the ossicles should be assessed as to their presence, health, and position. Ossicular mobility can be judged by gentle palpation when necessary.

Otorrhea should be treated preoperatively to improve the success rate of tympanoplasty and to reduce postoperative infection. Two weeks of topical antibiotic drops are usually sufficient in those ears that will respond to this treatment. Otic topical drops often contain a corticosteroid to minimize pruritus, inflammation, and edema but are not necessary for successful treatment. A wide range of otic and ophthalmic drops may be used successfully. Drops that contain ototoxic antibiotics are routinely used in inflamed ears, but their use is discouraged in noninflamed ears, in which absorption of the ototoxic medications via the round window may occur more readily. Persistent drainage after adequate topical therapy is an indication for culture. Cultures should include routine and fungal organisms. Tuberculosis should always be considered in endemic areas. If a fungal culture is positive, appropriate treatment may be added to or used to replace the antimicrobial otic drops. When all efforts to dry up the ear fail, mastoidectomy should be considered, but tympanoplasty alone is often successful in cases of uncomplicated chronic otitis media without cholesteatoma (27,28). Ears that persistently drain clear mucoid secretions in the absence of middle ear infection are thought to be of inflammatory or allergic response to airborne allergens and may respond to appropriate allergy therapy (29). Ears that chronically drain clear, watery fluid should always be evaluated for a possible cerebrospinal fluid leak.

Comprehensive audiometry with air-bone and speech evaluations should be done in all patients preoperatively.

The remaining portion of this chapter concerns grafting techniques for the tympanic membrane. Discussion of meatoplasty, canalplasty, canal reconstruction, ossicular reconstruction, and mastoid surgery are presented in Chapters 9–11, 17, 18, and 23.

MYRINGOPLASTY PROCEDURES

Paper Patch Myringoplasty

Paper patches were widely used in the 1940s and 1950s prior to the advent of formal tympanoplasty. The technique usually required multiple treatments in efforts to induce healing. The technique is most successful in traumatic perforations, in which the paper may help to align the injured portions of the tympanic membrane. Chronic perforations require some freshening of the margin of the perforation to deepithelialize it, gently removing the edge of the margin with a sharp pick or by cauterizing the edge by applying a 50% solution of trichloroacetic acid. The acid may be applied using a tiny cotton-tipped applicator or by dipping a 20-gauge suction into the solution, wicking away the excess drops, and applying the residual to the perforation edge. The cauterized edge takes on a white appearance.

Various materials have been used for the actual patch. A small disc just larger than the perforation can be cut out of cigarette paper, an adhesive sterile dressing, or moistened Gelfilm. The procedure is repeated as often as necessary at approximately 2-week intervals. Successful closures often result in a thin, dimeric tympanic membrane consisting of only medial and lateral epithelial layers and lacking the thick fibrous layer.

Fat Graft Myringoplasty

Fat patches are often done to repair small perforations remaining after extrusion of tympanostomy tubes. It is less suitable for larger perforations because the lobular nature of the graft material leads to a thick tympanic membrane repair with higher rates of graft failure. Gross et al. (30) suggested that the technique should be limited to perforations of 4 mm or less. Ringenberg (31) used compressed fat grafts with an overall success rate of 86%.

The procedure may be done either in the office or in the operating room. The patient is placed in the supine position with the head turned approximately 45 degrees, with the operative ear directed upward and the neck extended slightly, which helps position the ear canal away from the patient's shoulder. No shaving of the scalp is done. The ear is prepped with Betadine solution. A 3M no. 1020 adhesive aperture drape is placed around the ear. Sterile drapes are placed around the operative field. The ear is cleaned and carefully inspected under the operating microscope. Lidocaine 1% with epinephrine 1:100,000 is infiltrated through a 27-gauge needle circumferentially into the external meatus and using a 30-gauge needle into the lateral end of the bony canal. A funnel-shaped ear speculum is used to stretch the cartilaginous portion of the canal during infiltration. Injection is also done in the ear lobule. The ear is irrigated with a saline rinse. Lobular fat is first harvested. A no. 15 blade is used to make an incision on the medial surface of the inferior lobule. An incision directly on the free edge may cause a cosmetic deformity. A small portion of fat and fibrous tissue, larger in diameter than the perforation, is harvested. Care is taken to avoid an ear piercing site or including squamous epithelium from the margin of the wound. Hemostasis may be obtained by direct pressure for a few minutes or by use of cautery. The wound is closed with interrupted 6-0 plain catgut or other absorbable suture. The margin of the perforation is visualized under the microscope and freshened using a sharp pick to tease away the marginal epithelium. The margin is carefully inspected to ensure that there is no squamous epithelium remaining on the medial surface of the tympanic membrane. The fat graft is trimmed as needed but should remain wider in diameter than the perforation. The fat is positioned in the perforation such that it takes on the shape of an hourglass pinched in at the waist by the margin of the perforation. The canal is then filled with bacitracin ointment delivered by placing the ointment into a 3-ml syringe fitted with a 14-gauge angiocatheter. A cotton ball is placed in the meatus. Alternatively, a formal rosebud packing may be used. The patient begins using topical antibiotic drops, three drops twice a day, 1 week postoperatively and continues until the postoperative visit at 3 weeks. The patient observes water precautions and is instructed to sneeze with an open mouth and avoid nose blowing for 3 weeks postoperatively. Flying is discouraged for the first 3 weeks postoperatively. Perforations usually heal well but often have a persistent bulky appearance compared with fascia or perichondrial grafts (Fig. 14.2). They are more prone to myringitis than other grafts.

TYMPANOPLASTY PROCEDURES

The choice of approach for tympanic membrane repair depends largely on the size, shape, and location of the perforation, as well as the size and shape of the external auditory canal. In general, the postauricular approach offers wider exposure, particularly of the anterior half of the tympanic membrane and anterior tympanic sulcus. Larger perforations, anterior perforations, or ears with a small external auditory canal are best approached with a postauricular incision. Less experienced surgeons will find the postauricular approach more favorable for successful outcomes. Patients with a wide or inflexible neck and a large shoulder impeding the view into the external canal will be best served with a postauricular approach. The endaural approach is useful for moderately sized perforations and generally favorable anatomy. It eliminates the auricular swelling and hypesthesia that accompany the postauricular approach. The transcanal approach is most useful for small posterior perforations or central perforations with little anterior extension in an ear canal that is relatively straight and will accommodate at least a 6-mm diameter speculum.

The author prefers the loose areolar layer of the temporoparietal fascia as a primary graft material in postauricular cases. The tissue is thin and pliable, making it easy to work with, and it heals as well as true fascia. This layer is usually replaced by scar tissue in revision cases, so true temporalis fascia, periosteum, or a layer of scar tissue (trimmed thinly and compressed with a fascia press) are all excellent alternatives. A tragal perichondrial graft is preferred for repair of smaller defects approached by the transcanal route, because it can be harvested within the immediate surgical field.

Transcanal Approach

The patient is placed in the supine position and prepped and draped in an identical fashion as described for myringoplasty. The posterior tragus is infiltrated with local anesthetic, and a tragal perichondrial graft is harvested. Under the operating microscope, a transverse incision is made on the posterior surface of the tragus, grasping it gently with a small-toothed forceps and displacing it anteriorly to expose the posterior surface. The incision is not made on the lateral edge of the tragus to avoid a cosmetic deformity. The incision is made about 3 mm medial to the lateral edge of the tragus with a no. 15 blade and extended through the posterior surface perichondrium, scoring the cartilage slightly. A McCue knife and Freer elevator are used to develop a subperichondrial plane separating the perichondrium from the cartilage to the root of the tragus medially. The skin on the medial side of the incision is then grasped with the forceps

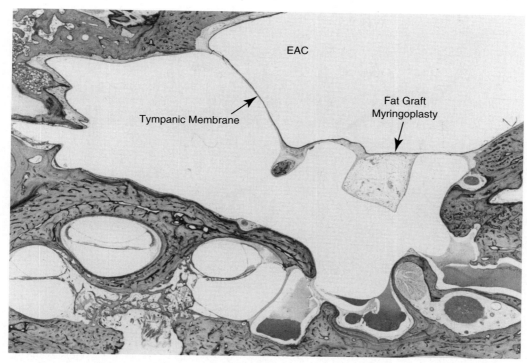

FIG. 14.2 A traumatic perforation of the tympanic membrane in an 18-year-old resulted when an assailant hurled a chunk of ice that struck the auricle. The perforation was repaired 2 days later by a medial onlay adipose graft from the ear lobe. The patient died of unrelated causes 12 years later. Viable adipose tissue is seen as a healthy appearing transplant, and the tympanic membrane is intact. It is not known whether the surviving tissue represents part or all of the originally implanted graft. EAC, external auditory canal. 7.5X.

to put the perichondrium on tension, and a curved sharp scissors is used to sharply and bluntly dissect the perichondrium from the skin. The graft is removed, stretched out on a Teflon cutting block, and kept moist under a wet sponge. The tragus is compressed for hemostasis and the wound closed with interrupted 6-0 plain catgut sutures.

An ear speculum is introduced into the external meatus. If the meatus is too small to accommodate a 7-mm speculum, an incision is made in the 12 o'clock position of the bony canal longitudinally starting from the bony canal meatus and cutting approximately 3 to 5 mm laterally through a soft tissue bulge that normally lies at the tragal-helical incisura. This incision will ordinarily allow the placement of a speculum of 0.5 to 1.0 mm larger in diameter. The speculum is then secured by a holder, and under the operating microscope, a canal skin incision is made using a 45-degree Mc-Cue knife, placing the lateral extent of the incision about 6 mm lateral to the posterior tympanic annulus. The superior limb of the incision continues toward the 12 o'clock position of the tympanic membrane directly superior to the notch of Rivinus and remaining 2 mm lateral to the notch. The inferior limb of the incision is carried toward the 6 o'clock position of the membrane to the tympanic annulus. Elevation of the skin-periosteal flap is done with a Rosen knife and the tympanic cavity is entered either inferiorly or superiorly (within the notch of Rivinus) using a Rosen

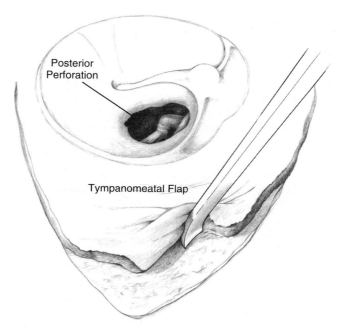

FIG. 14.3 For a posterior perforation, a tympanomeatal flap is elevated in preparation for a medial onlay fascial or perichondrial graft.

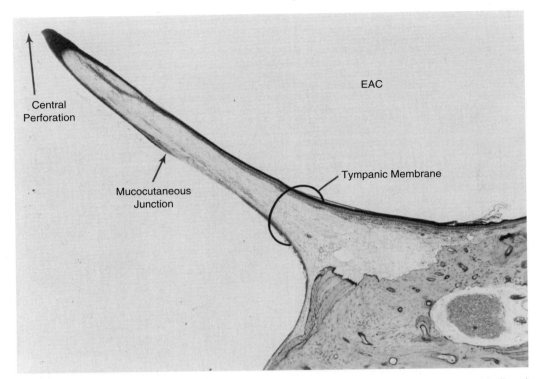

FIG. 14.4 This photomicrograph shows the margin of the inferior perforation. Squamous epithelium has migrated onto the medial surface of the tympanic membrane. EAC, external auditory canal. 39.6X.

needle (Fig. 14.3). The flap is elevated to its attachment with the malleus, and the annulus is elevated inferiorly with a gimmick or drum elevator. Elevation of the inferior annulus is done after inspecting to be sure there is no exposed jugular bulb in the hypotympanum. If hemostasis is required, Gelfoam soaked in 1:10,000 epinephrine solution is packed into the middle ear and external canal for 2 to 5 minutes, removed, and the middle ear irrigated with saline. The medial surface of the perforation is inspected for evidence of squamous epithelial ingrowth into the middle ear (Fig. 14.4). The margin of the perforation is excised using a sharp pick and a cup forceps to tease off the rim of the perforation. Any portion of the tympanic membrane with squamous epithelium fixed to its medial surface is excised to prevent formation of cholesteatoma. The middle ear is carefully inspected for evidence of any pathology such as scarring, inflammatory disease, granulation, tympanosclerosis, or ossicular erosion or fixation (Fig. 14.5). Hemostasis is ensured and the middle ear thoroughly irrigated with saline. Gelfoam moistened with saline or topical antibiotic solution such as sulfacetamide-prednisolone is then placed into the middle ear around the area of the perforation and extending beyond perforation site somewhat to help seal the underlay graft against the tympanic membrane. The perichondral graft is trimmed so that it will extend at least approximately 2 mm circumferentially from the perforation margin. The graft is delivered onto the Gelfoam bed with an alligator forceps and then adjusted into position with a 20-gauge suction and a Rosen needle. The tympanic membrane remnant is laid over the graft and the tympanomeatal flap returned to its normal anatomic position (Fig. 14.6). The graft is carefully inspected to be sure that all margins are smooth and well approximated to the tympanic membrane remnant. A thin layer of Gelfoam moistened with saline or antibiotic drops is placed over the tympanic membrane and the canal filled with bacitracin ointment, as previously described. Alternatively, a formal rosebud packing may be used (Fig. 14.7). A Glasscock dressing is applied and removed the following day. Postoperative care and follow-up is the same as previously described.

Small anterior perforations may be repaired using a "collar-button suture" technique outlined in Figure 14.8.

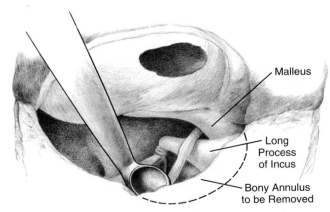

FIG. 14.5 Bony annulus may be removed to improve visualization if there is any suspicion of ingrowth of epithelium from the posterior margin of the perforation.

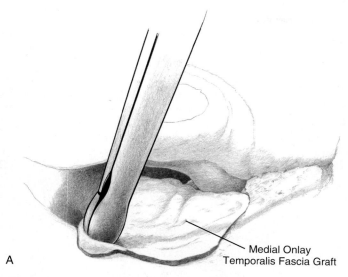

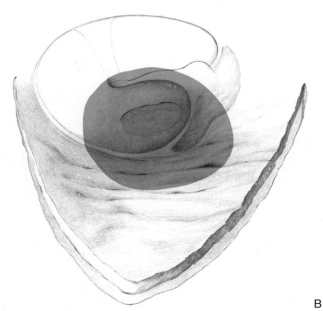

FIG. 14.6 A: A medial onlay fascial or perichondrial graft is introduced. **B:** The tympanomeatal flap is replaced to its original location.

Medial Onlay
Temporalis Fascia Graft

A

B

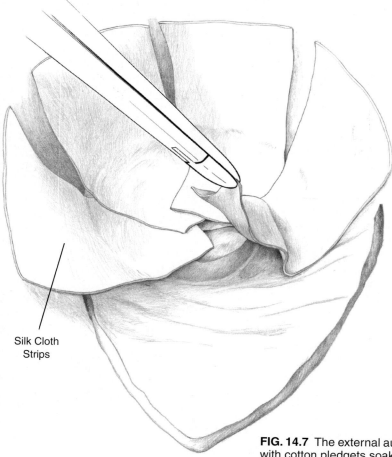

Silk Cloth
Strips

FIG. 14.7 The external auditory canal is lined with silk strips and firmly packed with cotton pledgets soaked in Cortisporin.

Postauricular Approach

The postauricular approach affords optimal exposure and may be used for any tympanoplasty situation. It gives the best exposure of the anterior tympanic membrane, which is often not visible with a transcanal approach. Anterior perfo-

rations can be the most technically challenging simply on the basis of limited exposure. The angle of exposure obtained from posteriorly brings the anterior rim directly into the surgeon's view. Removal of the anterior canal wall bulge is rarely necessary to successfully perform the tym-

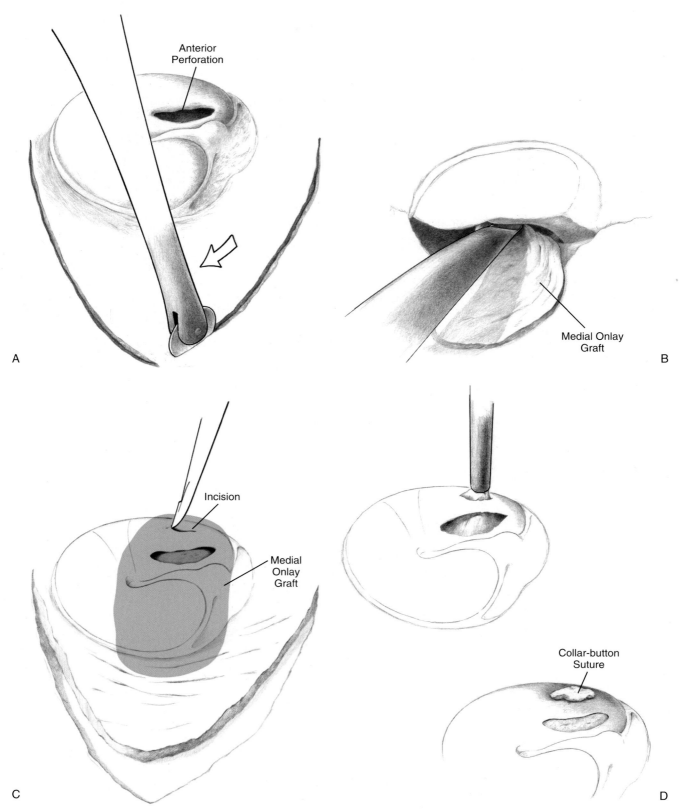

FIG. 14.8 A: For small anterior perforations, the posterior tympanomeatal approach can be used and combined with a collar-button suture. **B:** A medial onlay fascial graft is placed anteriorly. **C:** An incision is made in the anterior drum remnant. **D:** A small segment of the fascial graft is pulled through the perforation to fix it in place anteriorly. This procedure is known as the collar-button suture.

panoplasty, but the surgeon may wish to remove the bulge to facilitate exposure of the entire tympanic membrane for postoperative follow-up.

There are additional advantages to the postauricular approach. Harvest of a fascia graft is facilitated, and canalplasty is easily accomplished. A wider view of the middle ear will facilitate ossiculoplasty. The disadvantages include additional operative time and an incision associated with increased discomfort, hypesthesia of the pinna, postauricular swelling, and a higher risk of wound infection.

The patient is positioned as for a transcanal approach, except that extension of the neck is unnecessary. Shaving of hair behind the postauricular crease is optional but is usually done for hair within 1 to 2 cm of the incision to facilitate placement of adhesive drapes. The ear is prepped and draped, as previously described. Lidocaine with epinephrine is infiltrated into the external meatus and the postauricular area. The ear canal is then irrigated.

Under the operating microscope, the external canal and tympanic membrane are inspected through a handheld ear speculum in the external meatus. A laterally based flap of posterior canal skin is elevated if the ear canal exposure is sufficient. If not, the flap can be created once the postauricular exposure has been obtained. The flap is commonly called a vascular strip because it encompasses many of the vessels running longitudinally with the ear canal in the thicker skin between the tympanosquamous and tympanomastoid suture lines. The first incision is made transversely, immediately lateral to the tympanic annulus, from the 6 o'clock to 12 o'clock positions along the posterior bony canal wall using a 45-degree McCue knife. Longitudinal incisions are made from the tympanic annulus to a few millimeters beyond the lateral extent of the meatus of the bony canal with a no. 57 Beaver blade. This particular blade is curved and is

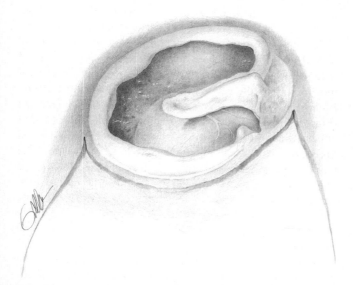

FIG. 14.9 Vascular strip incision outlined in the external auditory canal.

handy for cutting into the often deep canal skin and incising under any overhangs that may be present. Some elevation of the flap is then done using the blade to ensure that the flap is mobilized (Fig. 14.9).

The microscope is set aside to make the postauricular incision. A no. 15 blade is used 0.5 cm posterior and parallel to the postauricular crease. The incision is carried down into the avascular plane just lateral to the temporalis fascia. A skin-subcuticular flap is elevated toward the external canal anteriorly, but it is not necessary to skeletonize the canal cartilage posteriorly. The elevation is carried along the temporal line anteriorly past the anticipated 12 o'clock position of the external auditory canal. The elevation this far anteriorly will be important to allow for adequate elevation of the temporalis muscle and good exposure of the superior external auditory canal and epitympanum if needed. Blunt or sharp dissection is used to elevate the skin flap away from the temporalis fascia superiorly beyond the superior extent of the incision to allow for a large graft if necessary. A small back cut is made along the posterior border of the incision to facilitate closure at the end of the procedure. A Wietlander retractor is placed. Hemostasis is obtained with electrocautery. The loose areolar layer of the temporoparietal fascia or true temporalis fascia is harvested at this time. The author prefers the loose areolar tissue for primary tympanoplasties. The tissue is grasped at the temporal line with forceps and a no. 15 blade used to incise the tissue down to the layer of true temporalis fascia along the temporal line. Elevation of the loose fascia layer is begun with the knife until the true fascia is clearly observed, taking care to remove all the loose fascial tissue from the temporalis fascia. A small blunt-tipped Metzenbaum scissors is used to sharply elevate the loose fascia. The graft is harvested and spread on a Teflon cutting block to dry. It may be placed under an available operating room light for speed drying of the graft if desired. The plane of elevation is avascular so no additional hemostasis is required from the graft harvest, in contrast to the hemostasis required after removal of temporalis fascia.

A no. 15 blade is used to incise a "lazy T" into the periosteum, making a cut along the temporal line and a vertical limb bisecting the mastoid process. Periosteal flaps are elevated in all directions, and the anterior periosteum is elevated into the meatus of the bony external auditory canal. Elevation of the anterior periosteum into the external canal fully mobilizes the vascular strip flap and allows it to be retracted lateral to the surgical field and filled in place by the Weitlander retractor. The operating microscope is repositioned over the field. Anteriorly based skin flaps are developed along the superior and inferior borders of the remaining canal skin. These skin flaps are preserved to help hold the graft in position at the end of the procedure.

A canalplasty may be performed at this time, if desired, because a reasonably straight and wide exposure of the entire circumference of the tympanic membrane is needed. A large tympanosquamous suture may require further anterior elevation of the superior skin flap. Drilling of an anterior canal bulge is done after developing laterally and medially based flaps of the anterior skin. A transverse incision is made directly over the midpoint of the anterior bony bulge. The skin is elevated laterally and medially, making longitudinal relaxing incisions until two rectangular flaps are created, one laterally based and the other medially based on the skin of the anterior sulcus. The entire anterior canal wall can be drilled down as necessary until adequate exposure of the anterior sulcus is obtained. Following completion of the anterior canalplasty, skin flaps are rotated back into normal anatomic position. Small gaps between the skin flaps leaving exposed bone will heal postoperatively without requiring any additional grafting.

Once the exposure of the tympanic membrane down the external canal is considered satisfactory, elevation of the posterior tympanic annulus is done. Elevation of remaining medial skin posteriorly is done with a Rosen knife exposing the tympanic annulus across its entire posterior course and exposing the notch of Rivinus superiorly. Elevation of the tympanic annulus is done with the Rosen needle, teasing the annulus out of its sulcus to carefully look for underlying structures before widely elevating the annulus. While elevating the annulus inferiorly, one should look for a possible dehiscent and high riding jugular bulb. The middle ear may also be entered in the notch of Rivinus, where absence of the annulus facilitates elevation of the tympanic membrane. The neck of the malleus will be immediately visualized. Elevation into the posterior superior quadrant is done carefully because the incus, stapes, and chorda tympani nerve are medial to the tympanic membrane at this level. Once the opening is made to the middle ear, the entire posterior annulus is elevated out of its sulcus using either a needle or Rosen knife. In the inferior half of the middle ear a drum or annulus elevator is most suitable.

The amount of annular elevation anteriorly depends on the location of the perforation. When a perforation involves the anterior half of the middle ear, the inferior annulus is elevated anteriorly up to the junction of the anterior and inferior annulus. This will create a flap of annulus that will help hold the underlay graft. For posterior perforations or perforations with limited anterior extension, the tympanic membrane should be elevated up to the malleus and attachments to the malleus can be left intact (Fig. 14.10). Perforations with significant anterior extension require optimal exposure of the anterior tympanic membrane annulus or bony annulus. The author prefers to maximize the anterior exposure by removing the tympanic membrane from the malleus. Using a sickle knife, the loose adhesions between the malleus neck and the pars flaccida are separated to widely open Prussak's space. The tympanic membrane inserts onto a tiny sesamoid cartilage at the lateral tip of the lateral process. The cartilage is separated from the lateral process, allowing for sharp and blunt dissection of the tympanic membrane off the malleus. The tympanic membrane becomes adherent to the malleus handle at the umbo and can be removed from the umbo with either sharp dissection in the subperiosteal layer or by elevating the skin layer off the umbo and leaving the fibrous layer still attached. The dissection of the tympanic membrane off the malleus is done with great care to minimize movement of the malleus that could cause sensorineural hearing loss. Once the tympanic membrane is separated from the malleus, elevation is continued until visualization of the bony annulus is achieved anterosuperiorly. Diseased portions of the tympanic membrane are excised without regard to the resulting perforation size. The annulus is routinely divided posteriorly to afford an unobstructed view of the entire middle ear. Thickened plaques of tympanosclerosis are excised, but thin plaques not interfering with hearing or healing may be left intact. The middle ear is carefully inspected for any evidence of tympanosclerosis, cholesteatoma, infection, granulation, mucosal edema, or scarring. The course of the facial nerve is identified, and it is noted whether the nerve is bony, covered, or dehiscent and whether it is involved with disease. The chorda tympani nerve is preserved unless it is directly involved in disease. All diseased tympanic membrane is removed without regard to the resulting perforation size. Granulations are debulked, but it is not necessary to remove all granulations, particularly when they involve the ossicular chain or facial nerve. Cholesteatoma in the middle ear is removed, trying to keep the matrix as intact as possible while sharply and bluntly delivering the matrix. An attempt is made to preserve as much mucosa as possible to minimize scarring. The ossicular chain is gently palpated and inspected for any evidence of erosion or fixation. Examination of the round window reflex may be done during ossicular palpation. A severely medialized malleus may be rotated laterally after severing the tendon of the tensor tympani if necessary (Fig. 14.11).

Hemostasis is obtained, when needed, by packing the middle ear with Gelfoam pledgets soaked in 1:10,000 epinephrine solution. A meatoplasty is performed at this time, if appropriate; techniques are presented in Chapter 17. The fascia graft is trimmed into an oval with the smaller axis about 50% larger than the superior to inferior diameter of the tympanic ring. The Gelfoam-epinephrine pledgets are then removed from the middle ear and the ear thoroughly irrigated with saline. If a large amount of middle ear mucosa was removed, the middle ear may be lined with strips of Gelfilm, EpiFilm (Xomed Corp., Jacksonville, FL), or Teflon crescent (Fig. 14.12). The middle ear is filled with Gelfoam soaked in either saline solution or an antibiotic drop that is not known to be ototoxic, such as sulfacetamide-prednisolone. The Gelfoam must be carefully packed to fill the eustachian tube orifice and completely fill the anterior middle ear. Insufficient packing may lead to separation of the graft from the anterior margin. Packing of the ear is done more loosely posteriorly because the graft will be suspended from the posterior bony canal wall.

Grafting of the perforation is now performed. The fascia graft is grasped with an alligator forceps at the anterior leading edge and immersed briefly into saline to moisten it. The graft is placed at the anterior margin of the perforation.

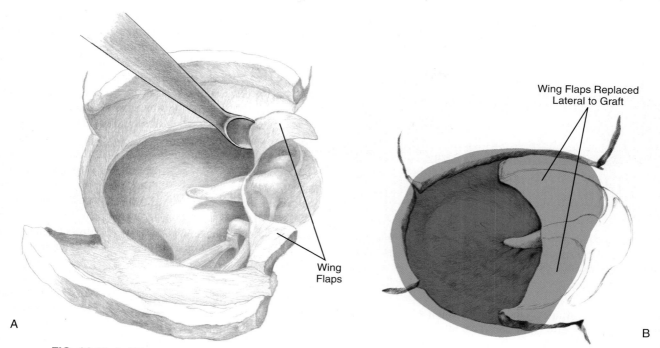

FIG. 14.10 A: When a near-total perforation of the pars tensa exists, it may be possible to perform a winged flap approach. This technique preserves the integrity of a small segment of the pars tensa and the pars flaccida. **B:** The graft is placed medial to the manubrium and wing flaps.

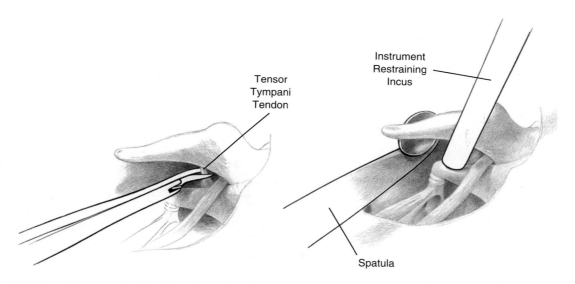

FIG. 14.11 When the manubrium is medially displaced by the unopposed tension of the tensor tympani muscle, the tensor tympani tendon is sectioned and the manubrium is forcibly replaced to its normal position.

Perforations involving the anterior half of the tympanic membrane, including total tympanic membrane perforations, are grafted in a similar fashion. Using a 20-gauge suction in one hand and Rosen needle in the other hand, the graft is inserted medial to the bony tympanic annulus anteriorly at least 2 mm under the annulus. Even in extreme circumstances where there is erosion of the bony annulus, there is always a bony ledge where the tympanic sulcus anteriorly leads to the eustachian tube orifice. This bony

ledge serves equally well for underlay grafting in the absence of a true bony annulus. The graft is smoothed under the bony ledge or annulus using both instruments and spreading in opposite directions as one would flatten a bedsheet. During this spreading motion, the graft is inserted deeper under the bony annulus, which helps it to stay in position. A similar spreading motion is done around the entire anterior half of the tympanic ring. The graft is carefully inserted medial to the annular remnant inferiorly and the

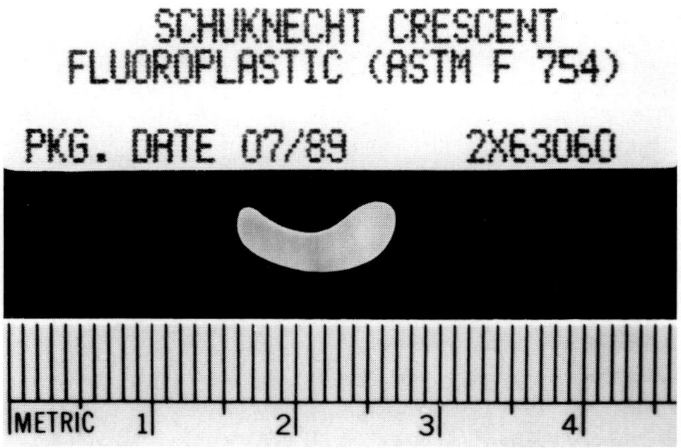

SCHUKNECHT CRESCENT
FLUOROPLASTIC (ASTM F 754)

PKG. DATE 07/89   2X63060

METRIC   1   2   3   4

FIG. 14.12 The Teflon crescent is a thin sheet of Teflon film shaped to fit the space from the eustachian tube to the round window niche (Smith-Nephew Corp., Memphis).

saline or antibiotic drop is packed to fill the entire bony external auditory canal. Alternatively, a rosebud packing may be used.

Wound closure is then performed. The vascular strip flap is stretched and delivered back into normal anatomic position as the pinna is reflected back to normal position. Closure is done with 2-0 vicryl interrupted sutures to approximate the periosteum and 4-0 interrupted subcuticular sutures to approximate the skin. No external sutures are used routinely. Marcaine solution 0.5% with 1:200,000 epinephrine is infiltrated in the skin for postoperative pain control. The canal is reinspected under the microscope to ensure that the vascular strip is in proper position. The canal may be filled with either Gelfoam or bacitracin ointment. When an extensive canalplasty is performed, a rosebud dressing is used instead of Gelfoam. Thin Silastic cut into strips may be used for the rosebud instead of silk to facilitate removal postoperatively.

Grafting of posterior perforations is simpler than for anterior perforations. In these cases the tympanic membrane is left attached to the malleus. The margins are freshened and the leading edge of the fascia graft is simply delivered up to the anterior edge of the perforation. The graft is then inserted medial to the malleus using the same spreading motion as described earlier. The graft is draped up the external auditory canal and skin flaps rotated into normal position to overlay the fascia graft, as described previously.

graft allowed to drape up the external canal wall laterally at the root of the inferior skin flap. The inferior skin flap is rotated back to normal position to overlay the fascia graft. The fascia graft is allowed to overlay the malleus and will drape onto the malleus (Fig. 14.13). The graft is draped up the external auditory canal superiorly at the root of the superior skin flap, which is then rotated into normal position to overlay the fascia graft (Fig 14.14). Gelfoam soaked in

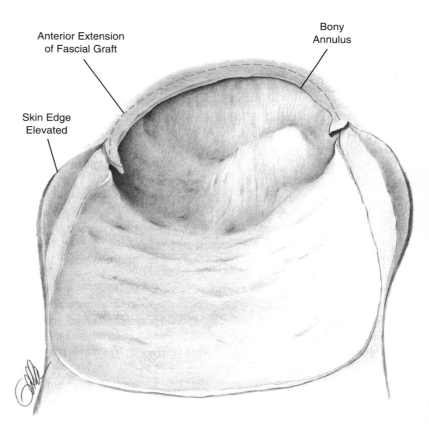

Anterior Extension
of Fascial Graft

Bony
Annulus

Skin Edge
Elevated

FIG. 14.13 Fascial graft being placed medial to the bony tympanic annulus anteriorly and lateral to the malleus to repair a total tympanic membrane perforation.

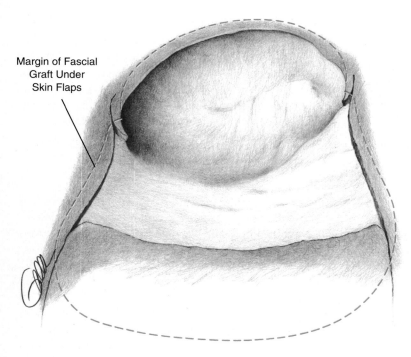

Margin of Fascial
Graft Under
Skin Flaps

FIG. 14.14 Canal skin flaps replaced to overlie the fascial graft.

Tympanic membranes with deep retraction pockets are considered at risk for future recurrence of retraction and may be repaired with cartilage-perichondrium composite grafts. The technique for cartilage grafting is covered in Chapter 15.

Postoperative Care

Patients are usually discharged on an ambulatory basis postoperatively. The mastoid dressing is left in place for the night and removed the following morning. A fresh cotton ball is placed in the conchal bowl to catch drainage and is changed as often as needed. The cotton ball is discontinued when there's no longer drainage from the ear. Showers are permitted on postoperative day 1, observing water precautions by impregnating a cotton ball with petroleum jelly and placing it into the conchal bowl. When there is a postauricular incision, bacitracin ointment is applied to the incision for bathing for the first postoperative week. Topical antibiotic drops are begun 1 week postoperatively on a schedule of three drops twice a day and continued until the first postoperative visit at 3 weeks. Antibiotics intraoperatively and postoperatively are used only in ears that are "wet" at the time of surgery. Patients are instructed to sneeze with their mouth open and avoid nose blowing for 3 weeks. Flights are permitted immediately after surgery, but a 2-week waiting period is preferred.

The first postoperative visit is at 3 weeks. The ear is examined under the operating microscope and cleaned out. Most Gelfoam pledgets are removed with an alligator forceps or suction, some may be left in place if adherent and not obstructing the ear. If a rosebud pack is in place, it is completely removed. The tympanic membrane is inspected for success of the graft and for any evidence of retraction that may indicate the need for a tube. In the unusual case of exuberant granulations, they may be carefully cauterized with a silver nitrate stick and then painted with gentian violet. Patients are allowed to get water in the ear after the entire canal and tympanic membrane are epithelialized. This usually occurs by 4 weeks with a transcanal procedure and 6 weeks for postauricular procedure. The second postoperative visit is normally scheduled for 6 weeks after the first visit, the ninth postoperative week. An audiogram is normally done at both visits, but if the ear is slow to heal at the first visit, testing with a tuning fork and whisper is sufficient.

Complications

Reperforation

A postoperative perforation may be due to a technical failure from an improperly placed graft, infection of the graft or remnant, or poor healing properties such as vascular insufficiency in the remnant. A delayed onset of a new perforation in the tympanic membrane may signify eustachian tube dysfunction with a need for middle ear ventilation through the tympanic membrane. Delayed perforations are generally watched for some time to try to establish whether they will enlarge and whether the patient shows any other evidence for eustachian tube dysfunction.

Canal Stenosis

Narrowing of the external canal from excessive scarring can occur because of hypertrophic or keloid scar formation, ongoing inflammation that causes an excitatory scar response, and circumferential bony exposure. Soft scar in its early stages can be compressed with a blunt instrument to widen the external canal, allowing for placement of a Merocel sponge soaked in antibiotic and steroid otic drops. The patient continues drops three times daily. The compression sponge is changed in the office every 2 weeks for a total of 2 months. If there is a history of hypertrophic or keloid scar formation, triamcinolone 40 mg/ml may also be injected directly into the scar.

Blunting of the Anterior Tympanomeatal Angle

Blunting of the anterior sulcus is also due to excessive scar formation between the denuded anterior canal scan and the tympanic membrane. It is uncommon in underlay grafting techniques because the anterior canal skin is left undisturbed near the annulus. When the skin of the anterior sulcus must be removed for canalplasty, it should be replaced with meatal skin or a thin split-thickness skin graft to prevent this complication. Blunting in the early stages is soft and may be treated the same as for a canal stenosis (Fig. 14.15).

High Frequency Sensorineural Hearing Loss

Injury to the hearing may occur from excessive manipulation of the ossicular chain or by striking the ossicles with a drill.

Conductive Hearing Loss

A conductive hearing loss in the face of a normal ossicular chain at the time of surgery is most likely due to middle ear effusion, middle ear adhesions, retraction of the tympanic membrane, or excessive thickness of the tympanic membrane. If the hearing loss does not improve, a myringotomy may be indicated to rule out a middle ear effusion or excessively thickened tympanic membrane.

Cholesteatoma

Squamous epithelium may present in the middle ear or even within the tympanic membrane as a result of iatrogenic introduction of the squamous epithelium or failure to recognize disease at the time of primary surgery.

Epithelial Pearls

Tiny keratomas may become trapped under otherwise healthy squamous epithelium and will continue to enlarge if left untreated. They may occur on the tympanic membrane or anywhere the external canal skin was elevated. They are due to implantation of tiny bits of squamous epithelium during surgery or epithelialization over a piece of existing skin. They can usually be successfully treated by opening and marsupialization with removal of the contents.

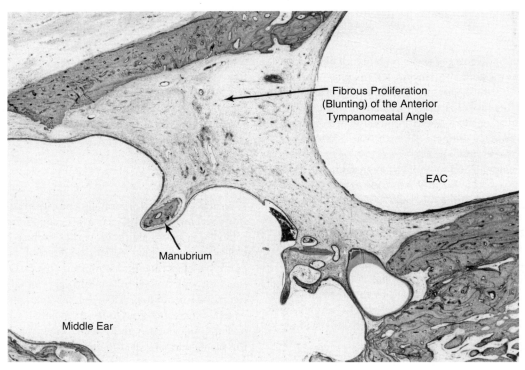

FIG. 14.15 A right myringoplasty was performed for a large central perforation in a 16-year-old patient. A medial onlay technique was used, but the details of the surgical procedure are not known. Hearing was not improved. The patient died at age 19 of unrelated causes. There is severe fibrous blunting of the tympanomeatal angle causing fixation of the manubrium. EAC, external auditory canal. 11.9X.

Lateralization of the Graft

Lateralization of the tympanic membrane is exceedingly rare with underlay techniques. It is possible for a graft to lateralize off of the umbo and may require repair placing the graft medial to the malleus umbo. Occasionally an extreme example of anterior blunting can spread posteriorly, causing blunting of the entire tympanic membrane and medial external auditory canal. When this is recognized early, it can be treated as described for the treatment of blunting.

REFERENCES

1. Benitez JT. Otopathology of Egyptian mummy Pum II: final report. *J Laryngol Otol* 1988;102:485–490.
2. Shambaugh GE Jr. *Surgery of the ear.* Philadelphia: WB Saunders, 1959;164–167.
3. Holt JJ, Harner SG. Effects of large-bore middle ear ventilation tubes. *Otolaryngol Head Neck Surg* 1980;88:581–585.
4. Klingensmith MR, Strauss M, Conner GH. A comparison of retention and complication rates of large-bore (Paparella II) and small-bore middle ear ventilating tubes. *Otolaryngol Head Neck Surg* 1985;93:322–330.
5. Kristensen S, Juul A, Gammelgaard NP, et al. Traumatic tympanic membrane perforations: complications and management. *Ear Nose Throat J* 1989;68:503–516.
6. Yung MW. Myringoplasty: hearing gain in relation to perforation site. *J Laryngol Otol* 1983;97:11–17.
7. Voss SE, Rosowski JJ, Merchant SN, et al. How do tympanic-membrane perforations affect human middle-ear sound transmission? *Acta Otolaryngol (Stockh)* 2001;121:169–173.
8. Wullstein H. Funktionelle Operationen im Mittelohr mit Hilfe des freien Spaltlappen-Transplantates. *Arch Ohr Nas Kehlkopf* 1952;161: 422.
9. Zöllner F. The principles of plastic surgery of the sound-conducting apparatus. *J Laryngol Otol* 1955;69:637–652.
10. Moritz W. Hörverbessernde Operationen bei chronisch-entzundlichen Prozessen beider Mittelohren. *Ztschr Laryngol Rhinol Otol* 1950;29: 578.
11. Zöllner F. Die Radikal-Operation mit besonderem Bezug auf die Hörfunktion. *Ztschr Laryngol Rhinol Otol* 1951;30:104.
12. House WF, Sheehy JL. Myringoplasty. *Arch Otolaryngol* 1961;73: 407–415.
13. Shea JJ Jr. Vein graft closure of eardrum perforations. *J Otol Laryngol* 1960;74:358–362.
14. Goodhill V. Tragal perichondrium and cartilage in tympanoplasty. *Arch Otolaryngol* 1967;85:480–491.
15. Glasscock ME III, House WF. Homograft reconstruction of the middle ear. *Laryngoscope* 1968;78:1219–1225.
16. Storrs LA. Myringoplasty with the use of fascia grafts. *Arch Otolaryngol* 1961;74:45–49.
17. Glasscock ME III. Tympanic membrane grafting with fascia: overlay vs undersurface technique. *Laryngoscope* 1973;83:754–770.
18. Bluestone CD, Cantekin EI. Current clinical methods, indications, and interpretation of eustachian tube function tests. *Ann Otol Rhinol Laryngol* 1981;90:552–562.
19. Virtanen H, Palva T, Jauhiainen T. Comparative preoperative evaluation of eustachian tube function in pathological ears. *Ann Otol Rhinol Laryngol* 1980;89:366–369.
20. Takahashi H, Hayashi M, Honjo I. Direct measurement of middle ear pressure through the eustachian tube. *Arch Otorhinolaryngol* 1987; 243:378–381.
21. Holmquist J, Lindeman P. Eustachian tube function and healing after myringoplasty. *Otolaryngol Head Neck Surg* 1987;96:80–82.
22. Manning SC, Cantekin EI, Kenna MA, et al. Prognostic value of eustachian tube function in pediatric tympanoplasty. *Laryngoscope* 1987;97:1012–1016.
23. Shanks JE. Tympanometry. *Ear Hear* 1984;5:268–280.
24. Honjo I. *Eustachian tube and middle ear diseases.* Tokyo: Springer-Verlag 1988:141–144.
25. Magnuson B, Falk B. Diagnosis and management of eustachian tube malfunction. *Otolaryngol Clin North Am* 1984;17:659–671.
26. Sadler-Kimes D, Siegel MI, Todhunter JS. Age-related morphologic differences in the components of the eustachian tube/middle ear system. *Ann Otol Rhinol Laryngol* 1989;98:854–858.
27. Sheehy JL. Surgery of chronic otitis media. In: English GM, ed. *Otolaryngology.* Philadelphia: Harper and Row, 1984.
28. Glasscock ME III, Jackson CG, Nissen AJ, et al. Postauricular undersurface tympanic membrane grafting: a follow-up report. *Laryngoscope* 1982;92:718–727.
29. Derlacki EL. Aural manifestations of allergy. *Ann Otol Rhinol Laryngol* 1952;61:179–188.
30. Gross CW, Bassila M, Lazar RH, et al. Adipose plug myringoplasty: an alternative to formal myringoplasty techniques in children. *Otolaryngol Head Neck Surg* 1989;101:617–620.
31. Ringenberg JC. Closure of tympanic membrane perforations by the use of fat. *Laryngoscope* 1978;88:982–993.

CHAPTER 15

Granular Myringitis and Tympanic Retraction Pockets

Richard M. Levinson

GRANULAR MYRINGITIS

Granular myringitis is a chronic vascular fibroproliferative and ulcerative dermatitis involving focal or diffuse areas of the tympanic membrane and adjacent canal wall (Fig. 15.1). Synonyms include chronic myringitis, polypoid myringitis, or myringitis granulosa.

Any condition resulting in desquamation and epithelial disruption of the squamous epithelium with exposure of the lamina propria can potentially incite this disorder. This includes local trauma from any source both direct and caustic, dermatologic conditions involving the external auditory canal, such as eczematoid or psoriatic-like skin disorders, or infectious agents. Numerous bacterial agents (*Staphylococcus aureus, Staphylococcus epidermidis, Pseudomonas aeruginosa* and *Proteus mirabilis* being the most common) and fungal agents (predominantly *Candida*) have been implicated. Suppression of reepithelialization with proliferation of inflammatory granulation from the lamina propria of the tympanic membrane ensues and the indolent course then follows (1–3).

Occult chronic suppurative otitis media may sometimes mimic granular myringitis. In this case a small perforation of the tympanic membrane may go unnoticed in the depths of the granulation tissue on the surface of the tympanic membrane only to be discovered after initiation of treatment or upon careful microscopic otoscopy with suction debridement.

The principal symptoms are mild otorrhea, muffled hearing, and occasional itching. The otologic examination typically reveals a cloudy mucoid discharge overlying an area of superficial granulation. There is no predilection for involvement of any particular location on the tympanic membrane. There is no evidence of perforation, and the drum moves well with pneumatic otoscopy.

If left untreated (or unsuccessfully treated), the clinical course may continue for months or years. Initial treatment should include debulking the granulations by either careful debridement with curettage, judicious chemical cautery (e.g., silver nitrate, trichloroacetic acid), or both. Prior to manipu-lation it may be necessary to locally anesthetize the area by injection technique (e.g., infiltrating the skin of the posterior canal wall with a xylocaine-epinephrine or marcaine-epinephrine preparation utilizing a 30-gauge needle) or by applying topical anesthesia (e.g., iontophoresis technique, EMLA cream applied to the area). In many cases the area is strangely insensitive and no anesthetic is required. Water precautions should be instituted, and antibiotic-steroid eardrops should be used a minimum of twice daily. A culture of the area should be obtained to ensure that the chosen pharmacologic therapy is appropriately directed if one or two treatments are not successful in gaining control of the situation.

If three or four courses of therapy are unsuccessful, it is recommended that skin grafting be performed on an ambulatory basis. After anesthetizing the area, granulations are thoroughly removed. Removal of granulations extends down to the pars propria of the tympanic membrane and to the bone of the external canal. Thin skin grafts are harvested from the upper arm or medial surface of the auricle opposite the scapha with a razor blade, as described in Chapter 10, and are applied to the prepared recipient site. It is not necessary to trim the graft to exactly fit the recipient site, because overlapping areas will necrose. The ear canal is then packed firmly with the surgeon's choice of packing (e.g., rosebud type, Merocel). The packing is gently removed in 2 weeks, and cleaning by aspiration is delayed another 2 weeks.

Granular myringitis that leads to stenosis will require more extensive surgery, including meatoplasty, canalplasty, and skin grafting, as described in Chapter 13.

RETRACTION POCKETS

A retraction pocket results from medial displacement of a portion (or all) of the tympanic membrane (Fig. 15.2). Synonyms include atelectatic retraction pocket, atelectatic otitis, adhesive otitis, myringomalacia, middle ear epidermatization, and marginal perforation pocket. If the pocket shows

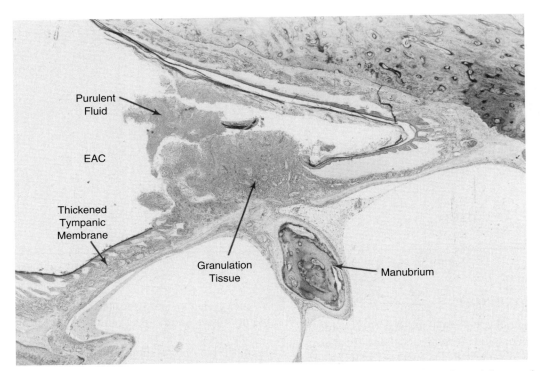

FIG. 15.1 Granular myringitis. A horizontal section through the tympanic membrane of the right ear of a 32-year-old man shows focal granular myringitis. There is a proliferation of highly vascular granulation tissue with ulceration of the skin and seropurulent discharge. The pars propria of the tympanic membrane is intact. There is inflammatory thickening of the subcutaneous layer of the tympanic membrane. EAC, external auditory canal. 19.2X.

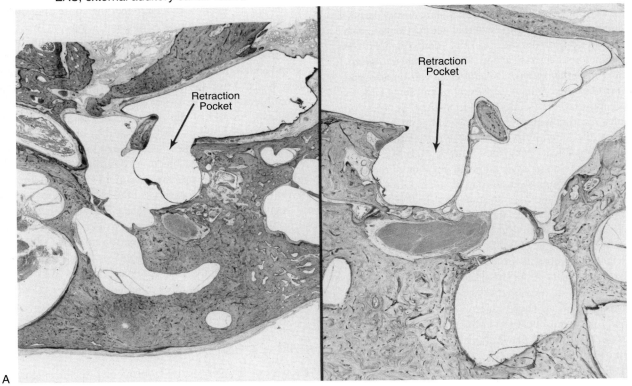

FIG. 15.2 Retraction pockets. **A:** A clean, dry posterior retraction pocket in the right ear of a 67-year-old man. The lining membrane is adherent to the posterior wall of the mesotympanum. 3.4X. **B:** A clean, dry posterior retraction pocket is seen in the left ear of a 47-year-old woman. The lining membrane is adherent to the posterior wall of the mesotympanum and the fallopian canal. 5.5X.

only mild medial displacement and is mobile on pneumatic otoscopy, it is deemed superficial and safe. A deep pocket implies significant extension into the mesotympanum or epitympanum. The epithelium of the retraction pocket may be fixed in position and immobile on pressure otoscopy. Unsafe pockets prone to complications fall into this category. Various grading systems have been proposed for classifying the severity of retraction (4,5). The formation and medial migration of a retraction pocket is a dynamic process and may arrest at any stage (6,7). A seemingly safe and stable retraction pocket, however, may progress and develop complications after years of quiescence.

The pathogenesis of an atelectatic retraction pocket is related to weakening of the structural integrity of the drum from deterioration of the lamina propria associated with negative middle ear pressure from either eustachian tube dysfunction or sniff-induced negative pressure. Middle ear or epitympanic adhesions may also play a role.

Symptomatic retraction pockets include those that are infected and producing otorrhea and granulation tissue and those that retain keratin debris with or without infection (Fig. 15.3). Deep retraction pockets harboring squamous debris and infection often cause osteitis of the ossicles, particularly the long process of the incus. Occasionally a dry, clean pocket will result in ossicular destruction over time.

Conservative management is reserved for those retraction pockets whose limits can be completely visualized, are not fixed to underlying structures, and are causing no complications. Autoinflation techniques for eustachian tube promotion, home politzerization, nasal balloon inflation with an olive-tip adapter, and encouragement for blowing rather than sniffing should be considered. Polyethylene (PE) tube placement can be helpful; however, it is common for the retraction pocket to recur after tube extrusion.

Surgical intervention for a retraction pocket is indicated for one or more of the following reasons: (i) persistent or recurrent otorrhea, (ii) persistent granulation tissue (often associated with otorrhea or bone destruction), (iii) ossicular destruction with significant conductive hearing loss, (iv) noncleansing pocket whose limits cannot be adequately assessed on microscopic otoscopy, and (v) overt cholesteatoma.

Numerous surgical remedies have been proposed for retraction pockets, including simple excision of the retraction pocket with no reconstruction and concurrent PE tube placement in an unaffected part of the drum (8,9), myringoplasty/tympanoplasty with fascia (with and without a PE tube), and canalplasty to prevent accumulation of squamous debris (10). Recurrence, however, is not uncommon, and ongoing treatment is often necessary.

CARTILAGE-PERICHONDRIAL GRAFT TYMPANOPLASTY FOR RETRACTION POCKETS

The concept of the cartilage-perichondrial graft is to create a stiff and structurally secure tympanic membrane that will resist the forces of retraction (11–21; H. Paisner, personal communication) yet allow good hearing (18,22,23). It is applicable to retractions of both the pars tensa and pars flaccida (attic)

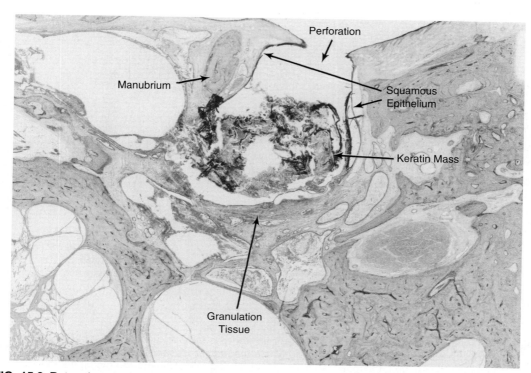

FIG. 15.3 Retraction pocket and cholesteatoma. The right ear of this 67-year-old man shows a deep posterior retraction pocket that is lined partly by squamous epithelium and partly by granulation tissue. A keratin mass (cholesteatoma) occupies the posterior mesotympanum. 10.5X.

areas. The ipsilateral tragus is the preferred cartilage-perichondrial graft donor site, though conchal cartilage can be utilized if the tragus has been previously surgically removed. A horizontal incision is placed approximately 2 to 3 mm medial to the dome of the tragus on the meatal side. This incision goes through the meatal skin, perichondrium, cartilage, perichondrium on the cheek/parotid side, and just into the soft tissue of the preauricular area. A small double-prong skin hook is then used to retract the lateral dome segment of tragus and expose the cut cartilage. The tragal autograft with perichondrium left attached to both sides is then dissected free of attachments by a spreading action with small blunt-tipped scissors. The entire tragus (other than the lateral dome segment) is removed, and one can even "borrow" some additional amounts from the incisura area superiorly and also inferiorly. Sufficient graft tissue can be obtained in this manner to accomplish a total drum replacement if needed. Hemostasis is acquired, the wound is closed, and the graft is placed in saline until it is needed.

For retraction pockets in the posterior aspect of the pars tensa, even those with mild anterior-inferior extension, a transcanal approach can be used provided the canal is of adequate size and the retraction pocket is accessible. Should there be any problem with exposure, a postauricular or endaural approach should be utilized, because inadequate exposure will create difficulty with pocket epithelial elevation and precise graft placement and may lead to failure.

The location and extent of the retraction pocket will dictate the extent of the required dissection (Fig. 15.4). A tympanomeatal flap is elevated, and bony annulus is removed sufficiently to visualize the pocket. At this point a decision may have to be made as to expanding the dissection to include an anterior atticotomy, atticoantrotomy, or intact canal wall tympanomastoidectomy. The retraction pocket is elevated, and granulations and cholesteatoma are removed if encountered. This can be a slow and tedious dissection utilizing various angled instruments because is important to ensure complete removal of all epithelium to prevent it from invaginating itself into the various interstices of the middle ear or attic and draping itself over important structures. All attempts should be made to elevate the retraction pocket intact to ensure there are no vestiges of squamous epithelium left behind. However, it is not uncommon to disrupt the epithelium, particularly where it may be deeply invaginating into the facial recess or sinus tympani. These areas can be assessed with an angled otologic telescope either from the canal side, through a posterior tympanotomy (if performed), or both to ensure that the removal has been complete. After the pocket has been completely elevated, the thin, redundant, flaccid epithelium may be resected with the Bellucci scissors. It is not necessary to preserve and redrape this excess tissue over the graft.

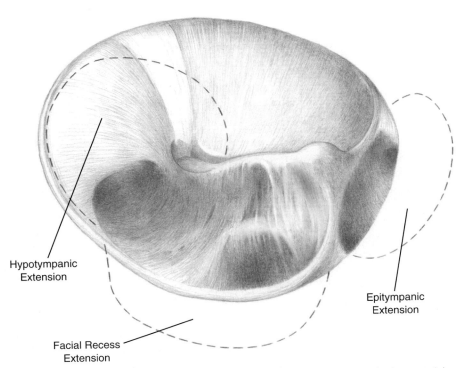

Hypotympanic Extension

Facial Recess Extension

Epitympanic Extension

FIG. 15.4 The most common sites for retractions are the posterior and attic (epitympanic) areas. The squamous epithelial lining may extend posteriorly into the facial recess area and superiorly into the lateral and medial epitympanic compartments, or anteriorly and inferiorly into the hypotympanum as exhibited by the *dotted lines.* The magnitude and location of the retraction will determine the extent and location of the cartilage-perichondrial graft. In all reconstructions the cartilage graft should overlap the bony canal wall and extend just beyond the limits of the original pocket.

The first step in tailoring the graft is to strip the perichondrium off the convex side of the tragal cartilage. This soft tissue can be set aside in case additional grafting material is needed. The cartilage of the composite graft can be thinned if necessary with a no. 10 blade utilizing a shave technique (usually unnecessary, particularly in the pediatric patient). Care must be taken not to thin the cartilage excessively because the graft may curl on itself, making it difficult to position. The graft is trimmed to a size slightly greater than the dimensions of the retraction pocket. Preparing a Silastic template will facilitate this process. In the typical case where the pocket involves the posterosuperior quadrant, the graft is tailored to bridge the area from the manubrium to slightly overlap the posterior canal wall (Fig. 15.5).

If the retracted area extends anteriorly or inferiorly into the hypotympanum, the procedure is simply extended to include these areas (Fig. 15.6). The management of an attic retraction pocket requires the tympanomeatal flap to include an adequate amount of skin that lies superior and anterior to the retraction pocket. This allows the anterosuperior part of the pars tensa adjacent to the malleus to be elevated and also provides the exposure to modify the underlying bone in this area with a drill or currette. The cartilage-perichondrial graft will need a small V-shaped notch (apex superiorly) so that it can be wedged over the neck of the malleus with an anterior extension medial to the elevated anterosuperior portion of the tympanic membrane. The remainder of the graft will then be overlapped onto the superior and posterior canal walls (Fig. 15.7). A drill can be used to sculpture the canal

walls as necessary to accomplish a "best fit." Drilling a slight groove into the medial bony canal wall just lateral, anterior, and posterior to the anterior malleal ligament may facilitate graft placement and positioning.

An alternative method includes using two separate pieces of cartilage-perichondrial graft, one to obliterate the area of pars tensa retraction and a separate piece for the attic blockade.

When the entire tympanic membrane is atelectatic or when a predominantly posterior pocket extends into the anterior quadrants, a total drum or near-total drum replacement may be necessary. To accomplish this the tympanic membrane-periosteal component will have to be incised and elevated off the manubrium of the malleus, skeletonizing the ossicle completely. The graft is also modified by making a small pocket between the perichondrium and the cartilage in the superior central portion (Fig. 15.8). This is usually done with a small duckbill elevator. This allows the surgeon to position the graft by slipping the manubrium into this pocket. A small vertically oriented slit through the cartilage only in the area of the pocket or even a very small V-shaped wedge of cartilage (apex inferiorly) excised from the superior midline area of the pocket may help in placing and positioning the graft around the manubrium. Also, depending on its position, the manubrium may have to be slightly lateralized by sectioning of the tensor tympani tendon.

All grafts are positioned on a bed of moistened Gelfoam in a medial onlay fashion relative to the tympanomeatal flap. A second layer of fascia may be used over the composite

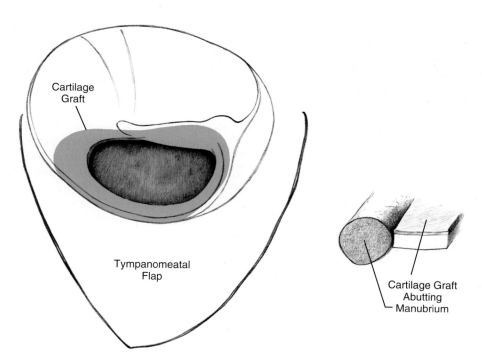

Cartilage Graft

Tympanomeatal Flap

Cartilage Graft Abutting Manubrium

FIG. 15.5 The posterior retraction pocket can be approached via a tympanomeatal flap. Bony tympanic annulus can be removed as necessary to remove ingrowth of squamous epithelium into the posterior mesotympanum.

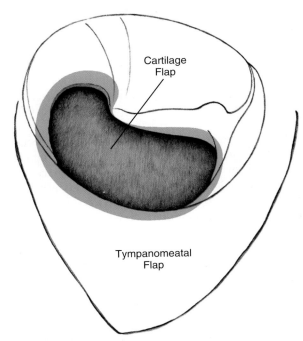

FIG. 15.6 A larger pocket with inferior and anterior extension can be controlled with a larger piece of cartilage that is appropriately modified.

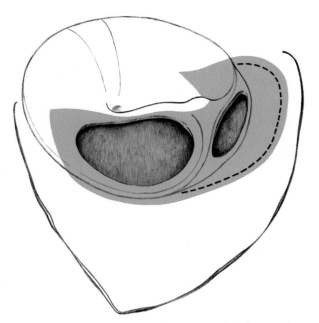

FIG. 15.7 A combined mesotympanic and epitympanic approach can be done by an anterior extension of the superior incision.

graft but is not mandatory for closure of the tympanic membrane defect. There is some experience to suggest that this additional layer may be beneficial in the avoidance of future problems with granular myringitis should there be any squamous epithelial breakdown over the mature graft site. After

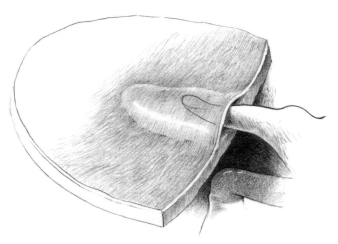

FIG. 15.8 When a large or total retraction is encountered, the cartilage graft can be modified to accommodate the manubrium in a pocket created between the perichondrium and cartilage.

graft positioning is obtained, the edges of the residual perforation are manipulated such that all edges are everted over the graft and the residual epithelium is appropriately redraped. This is technically easy to do because the graft is rigid, providing a firm base over which to roll the edges and manipulate the epithelium. Following graft positioning and replacement of the tympanomeatal flap, standard packing, closure, dressing, and postoperative tympanoplasty care are employed.

Once healing is complete (approximately 6 weeks), the patient should be encouraged to use autoinflation techniques and should be cautioned to avoid chronic sniffing. This will aid in obtaining excellent long-term postoperative results.

Given the opaque nature of the graft, prohibiting visual assessment of the middle ear or attic areas postoperatively, recurrent or residual disease may silently progress until complications occur. Therefore, if a major disruption of the pocket epithelium occurs during elevation or if invasive cholesteatoma is encountered, a second-look procedure is accomplished 9 to 12 months postoperatively. Standard radiologic imaging techniques are, as yet, inadequate to identify early, small, asymptomatic recurrent/residual cholesteatoma. An ossiculoplasty, if necessary, is also usually performed later as a staged procedure. The potential need for these additional surgical manipulations should be discussed with the patient or parents preoperatively.

The most common complication of this procedure is recurrent retraction pocket formation. The area of the graft itself will not retract, but other areas not bolstered by the composite graft are at risk, particularly adjacent to the border of the graft. This may often be due to faulty technique in original graft sizing or placement. One must therefore assure oneself that the composite graft exceeds the dimensions of the original retraction pocket or there will most likely be recurrent retraction between the edge of the cartilage graft and the periphery of the pocket. Also, complete obliteration of the posterosuperior quadrant without leaving a space between the manubrium and the graft is important. Any gap left in this area could allow for a slitlike retraction to occur. Similarly, a retraction can occur between the edge of the graft and the canal wall if the graft does not overlap slightly onto bone. Finally, one must always pay attention to the attic area. A superficial retraction pocket in this area will often deepen and can become unsafe if it is not concurrently blocked with a cartilage-perichondrial composite graft when the original indication included retraction of the pars flaccida.

The ability of the cartilage-perichondrial composite graft to control recurrent retraction dictates that it should be used in tympanoplastic reconstruction of the attic area plus the posterior and superior pars tensa areas of all intact canal wall procedures to avoid future retraction pockets, the most common complication of this procedure and cause of recurrent cholesteatoma.

Technical highlights and pointers:

1. Obtain adequate exposure.
2. There should be a complete and thorough pocket elevation.
3. The cartilage-perichondrial graft should always exceed the dimensions of the original retraction pocket.
4. The composite graft should overlap the bony canal wall posteriorly or superiorly, depending on the location of the pathology being addressed.
5. Ensure complete obliteration of the posterosuperior quadrant, with care being taken to leave no gap between the manubrium and the graft.
6. Pay attention to the pars flaccida. Don't ignore a seemingly safe attic retraction pocket when repairing pars tensa pathology.
7. Perform a second-look procedure (9 to 12 months) if there is significant disruption of epithelium during elevation or if invasive cholesteatoma is encountered.
8. Ossiculoplasty is performed as a staged procedure.

REFERENCES

1. Makino K, Amatsu M, Kinishi M, et al. The clinical features and pathogenesis of myringitis granulosa. *Arch Otorhinolaryngol* 1988;245(4): 224–229.
2. Stoney P, Kwok P, Hawke M. Granular myringitis: a review. *J Otolaryngol* 1992;21(2):129–135.
3. Kunachak S. Intractable granular myringitis: possible etiology and management. *J Otolaryngol* 1992;21(4):297–298.
4. Sadé J. The atelectatic ear. In: *Secretory otitis media and its sequelae.* New York/London: Churchill-Livingstone, 1979:64–88.
5. Charachon R, Barthez M, Lejeune JM. Spontaneous retraction pockets in chronic otitis media: medical and surgical therapy. *Ear Nose Throat J* 1992;71(11):578–583.
6. Avraham S, Sadé J. Surgery of atelectatic ears and retraction pockets. In: *Acute and secretory otitis media.* Proceedings of the International Conference on Acute and Secretory Otitis Media, part 1. Amsterdam: Kugler Publications, 1986:551–554.
7. Sadé J, Avraham S, Brown M. Dynamics of atelectasis and retraction pockets. In: Sadé J, ed. *Cholesteatoma and mastoid surgery.* Amsterdam: Kugler Publications, 1982:267–281.
8. Sharp JF, Robinson JM. Treatment of tympanic membrane retraction pockets by excision. A prospective study. *J Laryngol Otol* 1992; 106(10):882–886.
9. Walsh RM, Pracy JP, Harding MB, et al. Management of retraction pockets of the pars tensa in children by excision and ventilation tube insertion. *J Laryngol Otol* 1995;109(9):817–820.
10. Garside JA, Antonelli PJ, Singleton GT. Canalplasty for chronic tympanic membrane atelectasis. *Am J Otolaryngol* 1999;20(1):2–6.
11. Linde RE. The cartilage-perichondrium graft in the treatment of posterior tympanic membrane retraction pockets. *Laryngoscope* 1973;83: 747–753.
12. Sheehy JL. Surgery of chronic otitis media. In: *Otolaryngology,* vol 1, rev ed. Philadelphia: Harper and Row, 1989.
13. Heerman J. Tympanoplastik mit Vergrosserung der Pauke in den Gehorgang zur Verhinderung von Verwachsungen bei schlechten Schleimhautverhaltnissen oder massiger Tubenfunktion. *Z Laryngol Rhinol Otol* 1962;41:235–241.
14. Martin H. A propos de la chirugie de renforcement du tympan. *J Fr Otorhinolaryngol Audiophonol Chir Maxillofac* 1979;28:195–196.
15. Glasscock ME III, Jackson CG, Nissen AJ, et al. Postauricular undersurface tympanic membrane grafting: a follow-up report. *Laryngoscope* 1982;92:718–727.
16. Adkins WY, Osguthorpe JD. Use of a composite autograft to prevent recurrent cholesteatoma caused by canal wall defects. *Otolaryngol Head Neck Surg* 1984;92:319–321.
17. Schwaber MK. Postauricular undersurface tympanic grafting: some modifications of the "swinging door" technique. *Otolaryngol Head Neck Surg* 1986;95:182–187.
18. Levinson RM. Cartilage-perichondrial composite graft tympanoplasty in the treatment of posterior marginal and attic retraction pockets. *Laryngoscope* 1987;97:1069–1074.
19. Adkins WY. Composite autograft for tympanoplasty and tympanomastoid surgery. *Laryngoscope* 1990;100:244–247.
20. Poe DS, Gadre AK. Cartilage tympanoplasty for management of retraction pockets and cholesteatomas. *Laryngoscope* 1993;103(6): 614–618.
21. Gilain C, Gersdorff M, Decat M, et al. The relevance of using tragal cartilage in tympanoplasty. *Acta Otorhinolaryngol Belg* 1997; 51(3): 195–196.
22. Salen B. Tympanic membrane grafts of full-thickness skin, fascia and cartilage with its perichondrium. An experimental and clinical investigation. *Acta Otolaryngol (Stockh)* 1968;[Suppl 244].
23. Dornhoffer JL. Hearing results with cartilage tympanoplasty. *Laryngoscope* 1997;107(8):1094–1099.

PART IV

Surgery for Disorders of the Ear Canal and Tympanic Membrane

CHAPTER 16

Acute Mastoiditis

Michael J. McKenna and Roland D. Eavey

Acute mastoiditis remains a contemporary disease with significant morbidity and even mortality. The clinical diagnosis of this disorder is so entrenched within the fabric of otolaryngology that it almost symbolizes the specialty. In the preantibiotic era, most patients with acute mastoiditis required surgical drainage. Although most cases can now be managed medically, morbidity and complications of acute mastoiditis continue to be reported.

With the development of newer antibiotics and modern imaging techniques, the diagnosis and treatment of acute mastoiditis and its complications is in constant evolution. Paradoxically, however, because of the comparative diminution in frequency of the disease, studies to test the efficacy of the newer antibiotics are more difficult. Therefore treatment cannot be standardized but must be based on the logical use of an expanding armamentarium.

Acute mastoiditis is defined in variable terms throughout the literature. Although different degrees of mastoid inflammation accompany episodes of acute and chronic otitis media, for purposes of this discussion acute mastoiditis is defined as an acute bacterial infection of the mastoid, often in association with a preceding acute otitis media, that exceeds mere mucosal involvement. Untreated, acute mastoiditis results in osteolytic changes of the mastoid trabeculae and cortex and extension beyond the tympanomastoid space.

As is the case with other bacterial infections, antibiotics have greatly reduced the morbidity and sequelae associated with acute otitis media. Prior to the advent of antibiotics, acute mastoiditis was among the most common admission diagnoses to a hospital. Davison (1) reported that the number of simple mastoid operations for acute mastoiditis at Geisinger Memorial Hospital in Pennsylvania dropped from 119 in 1937 to only 6 from 1951 to 1954, which he attributed to the use of sulfa drugs and, later, penicillin. In 1936, 45.9% of patients admitted to Los Angeles County Hospital with acute otitis media required mastoidectomy as compared with 17.6% of patients in 1946 (2). In 1959 the incidence of acute mastoiditis arising from acute otitis media was as low as 0.4% in a series of 12,000 cases reported by

Palva et al. (3). An excellent analysis of the influence of sulfa drugs and penicillin on acute mastoiditis was provided by Rudberg in 1954 (4). With conservative therapy of acute otitis media, the percentage of patients who required surgery in various series ranged from 9.3% to 69.5%. With the introduction of sulfa drugs, the need for mastoidectomy dropped to a range of 1.5% to 28% for the same institutions.

The incidence of serious complications due to acute mastoiditis, including brain abscess and meningitis, has also declined substantially since the introduction of antibiotics (5). Improved imaging modalities in the form of computed tomography (CT) and magnetic resonance imaging (MRI), along with improved surgical technique, have significantly reduced the fatal and serious neurologic sequelae associated with brain abscesses and meningitis.

Despite the influence of antibiotics on the overall incidence of acute mastoiditis, it is by no means a rare disorder of only historical significance. The emergence of resistant strains of bacteria, an increased incidence of gram-negative infections, and a reduced clinical experience justify the consideration of acute mastoiditis as among the most serious and life-threatening infectious disorders of the head and neck. In addition, present concerns surrounding the overuse of antibiotics and even the need to treat acute otitis media with antibiotics may lead to a resurgence of complications (6,7).

RELEVANT ANATOMY OF THE MIDDLE EAR AND MASTOID

The middle ear and mastoid are contiguous spaces connected by the aditus ad antrum. Pneumatization of the temporal bone begins at birth with aeration of the eustachian tube and tympanic cavity. By 4 weeks of age, a central antral air cell is present. If undisturbed by infection or inflammation, pneumatization will proceed with expansion from the antrum and epitympanum into the zygomatic root, mastoid process, and perilabyrinthine areas. Mastoid pneumatization progresses by resorption of bone adjacent to aerated spaces. Details of the pneumatized spaces of the temporal bone are described in Chapter 11. Pneumatization may be slowed or arrested by infection, which disturbs the physiologic relationship between the mucosa and underlying bone. This arrest of pneumatization may have a partially protective effect in limiting the spread of infection to surrounding structures. In the infant, the lateral mastoid cortex over the mastoid antrum is cribriform in character, and hence infections of the middle ear and antrum readily spread to the postauricular soft tissue.

The stylomastoid foramen in the infant is in a lateral position, unprotected by the mastoid process, which begins to develop during the second year of life. Therefore the standard postauricular incision must be modified to avoid injury to the facial nerve.

PATHOPHYSIOLOGY OF ACUTE MASTOIDITIS

Acute mastoiditis most commonly results as the sequela of acute otitis media or, less commonly, complicates chronic otitis media with cholesteatoma (8), leukemia, mononucleosis, sarcomatous lesions of the temporal bone, and Kawasaki's disease (9–12). With prolonged inflammation, the mucoperiosteum becomes hyperemic and edematous, causing obstruction and sequestration of the infection. Obstruction may occur in the aditus ad antrum or in other smaller periantral tracts. As pus begins to accumulate under pressure, active bone remodeling with osteoclastic bone resorption occurs. As a result, much of the calcified trabecular network and periosteal bone may be replaced by noncalcified woven bone, which is soft and richly vascularized, and may simulate necrotic bone and granulation tissue. At this stage the radiographic appearance of the mastoid begins to change; it is often referred to as the coalescent stage of acute mastoiditis. These bony changes involve the mastoid trabeculae, as well as the thin plates of cortical bone that separate the mastoid air cells from the middle cranial fossa, the sigmoid sinus, the external auditory canal, and the postauricular soft tissues. The clinical diagnosis of acute mastoiditis is usually made when the infection spreads beyond the tympanomastoid space to the soft tissues of the postauricular region. Complications of acute mastoiditis are the result of spread of infection to the intracranial cavity, the sigmoid sinus, the labyrinth, the fallopian canal, or the soft tissues of the neck.

Acute mastoiditis may occur in the absence of an obvious middle ear infection when an aditus block segregates the middle ear and the mastoid air cells. Usually there is an antecedent acute otitis media with apparent resolution of the middle ear process followed by activation of a smoldering mastoid infection. Extension through the postauricular cortex results in a cellulitis of the postauricular soft tissues with protrusion of the auricle (Fig. 16.1). When breakthrough occurs in the zygomatic root, the auricle is deflected inferiorly by cellulitis or abscess formation. Extension through the posterior wall of the external auditory canal results in sagging of the external canal skin. When the tympanic membrane is intact, this presentation may be confused with an acute external otitis. A Bezold abscess occurs deep to the sternocleidomastoid muscle when infection breaks through the mastoid tip.

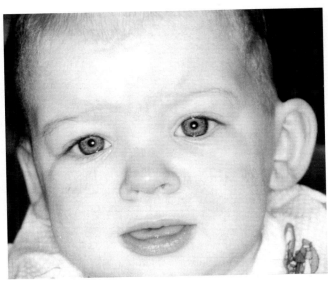

FIG. 16.1 A proptotic left auricle in an infant with acute mastoiditis.

MICROBIOLOGY

The organisms responsible for acute mastoiditis are not identical to those found in acute otitis media.

In one series of 35 consecutive cases of acute mastoiditis reported in 1987 by Maharaj et al. (13), mixed cultures of aerobes and anaerobes were the most common. Occasionally, anaerobes were the sole organism isolated. Most common anaerobes included gram-positive cocci, gram-positive bacilli, and gram-negative bacilli. The most common aerobes were group A beta-hemolytic *Streptococcus, Staphylococcus aureus, Proteus mirabilis, Staphylococcus epidermidis,* and *Pseudomonas aeruginosa. Haemophilus influenzae* and *Streptococcus pneumoniae,* common in acute otitis media, were uncommon in acute mastoiditis.

Other investigators have reported less disparity between cultures in acute otitis media and acute mastoiditis. In a study of 30 children with acute mastoiditis between 1973 and 1984, cultures were positive for *S. pneumoniae* in 7, *S. epidermidis* in 5, *H. influenzae* in 3, group A beta-hemolytic *Streptococcus* in 3, anaerobes in 3, *S. aureus* in 3, and *P. aeruginosa* in 1 (14). Predominance of *S. pneumoniae* was found by Prellner and Rydell (15). However, the remaining organisms were almost evenly divided between *H. influenzae,* beta-hemolytic *Streptococcus, S. aureus, P. mirabilis,* and *Pseudomonas* and *Bacteroides* species. The bacterial spectrum of acute otitis media has changed radically in the last half of the twentieth century. Prior to 1940, almost half the cases of acute mastoiditis were caused by a group A beta-hemolytic *Streptococcus* compared with a 0% to 10% incidence from 1970 to 1983. In addition, there is evidence to suggest the serotypes of pneumococcus isolated from patients with acute otitis media have changed over time (16). Although the incidence of acute mastoiditis caused by *Mycobacterium tuberculosis* has declined, there has been an increase in acute otitis media and mastoiditis caused by *Mycobacterium fortuitum* (17) and *Mycobacteria chelonae* (18). It is also uncertain whether these changes are in part responsible for the decline in the incidence and severity of acute mastoiditis.

DIAGNOSIS AND MANAGEMENT OF UNCOMPLICATED ACUTE MASTOIDITIS

Diagnosis, Signs, and Symptoms

In its most classic presentation, acute mastoiditis is readily diagnosable (19). The clinical diagnosis is based heavily on history and physical examination. It occurs more commonly in children than adults and may occur with or without a history of recurrent infections. Physical findings include pain, swelling, and tenderness over the mastoid process with proptosis of the auricle. Other common findings include fever and sagging of the superior external canal skin. At times this clinical picture may be difficult to distinguish from severe external otitis with retroauricular extension. However, diffuse pain and inflammation of the external canal is usually a more prominent feature in external otitis than in acute mastoiditis. Evaluation of the patient should include a complete physical examination in addition to otolaryngologic evaluation. Neurologic evaluation should include examination of the cranial nerves; relevant motor, sensory, and cerebellar examination; and a search for meningeal signs and nystagmus. Acute mastoiditis occurs without obvious abnormalities of the tympanic membrane or middle ear in 10% to 20% of cases. This unusual finding results from blockage of the aditus ad antrum from edematous mucosa, causing an anatomic partition of the tympanomastoid compartment with resolution of infection within the tympanic cavity.

Laboratory Investigation

Mastoid radiographs are of limited value in confirming the diagnosis, particularly early in the course of the disease. Radiologic evidence of coalescence of the mastoid trabeculae occurs late in the course of the acute illness and days after active remodeling has begun. CT scans usually demonstrate clouding of the mastoid air cells, a nonspecific finding that also occurs in serous, acute, and chronic otitis media (Fig. 16.2). The greatest utility of CT and MRI is in the evaluation of possible complications such as epidural abscesses (Fig. 16.3), brain abscesses, and lateral sinus thrombosis (Fig. 16.4).

Audiometry or auditory evoked response testing should be obtained if the patient's condition permits. Laboratory

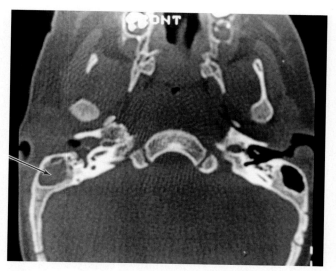

FIG. 16.2 CT scan of an infant with acute mastoiditis demonstrating the single mastoid cell involvement (*arrow*).

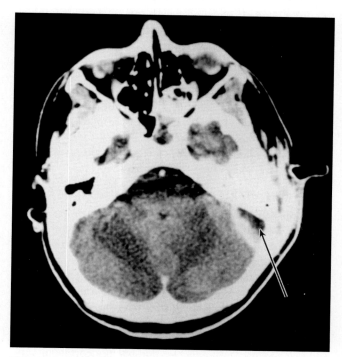

FIG. 16.3 A CT scan demonstrates an epidural abscess in a patient with acute mastoiditis.

examination should include a complete blood cell count (CBC) with a differential white cell count and blood cultures.

Because there is a broad spectrum of organisms and antibiotic sensitivities in acute mastoiditis, an attempt should be made to obtain pus for Gram stain and aerobic and anaerobic culture and sensitivity. In cases with accompanying otorrhea, the ear canal should be cultured after gentle cleansing with sterile saline. In cases with an intact tympanic membrane and evidence of middle ear effusion, a wide

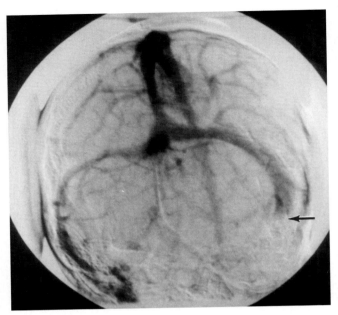

FIG. 16.4 Sigmoid sinus occlusion *(arrow)* demonstrated by digital subtraction angiography.

myringotomy ideally should be performed, followed by culture of the middle ear contents. Insertion of a tube can assist with drainage, as will administration of a topical antibiotic. In the mildest cases, especially if the middle ear is not yet involved, empirical antibiotic selection is appropriate.

Antibiotic Therapy

Acute mastoiditis without evidence of complication or subperiosteal abscess should be treated initially with intravenous antibiotics. The choice of antibiotic should be based on the results of Gram stain and modified according to the results of the culture and sensitivity. Before definitive culture results and sensitivity are obtained, the first choice of antibiotics is a combination of a semisynthetic penicillin and chloramphenicol. This combination provides broad-spectrum coverage for gram-positive organisms such as *Staphylococcus, Streptococcus,* and pneumococcus in addition to organisms such as *H. influenzae* and gram-negative bacteria. These antibiotics also penetrate the blood-brain barrier. The culture results and patient response will determine whether an alteration of the antibiotic regimen is necessary. Treatment for *Pseudomonas* is best achieved by two agents, including an aminoglycoside such as gentamicin or tobramycin and a third-generation cephalosporin such as amikacin or ceftazidime. When the tympanic membrane is open, antibiotic eardrops should also be employed. In uncomplicated cases, significant clinical improvement should occur within 72 hours as indicated by decline or resolution of fever and reduction of the postauricular pain, swelling, and tenderness.

Intravenous antibiotics should be continued until fever and inflammation resolve, usually requiring treatment for approximately 1 week, but ranging from 3 days to 3 weeks. Because acute mastoiditis is an osteitis and not an osteomyelitis, a protracted course of intravenous antibiotics is usually not required. After cessation of intravenous antibiotics, an oral antibiotic is continued for approximately 2 additional weeks. In cases of *Pseudomonas* infections, there is no safe and effective oral antibiotic for children, and hence these young patients may require extended periods of intravenous antibiotics.

One study has reported success with outpatient management of periosteitis. Intramuscular ceftriaxone was utilized to avoid hospitalization. Further experience will be required to evaluate efficacy of this management of less complicated cases (20).

Surgical Intervention

Surgery is indicated in uncomplicated cases of acute mastoiditis that fail to respond to intravenous antibiotics within 72 hours and in cases presenting with subperiosteal abscess or certain other complications. This may represent approximately half of patients admitted with acute mastoiditis. The surgical goals include: (i) drainage of subperiosteal and epidural abscesses; (ii) procurement of representative material for Gram stain, culture, and sensitivity; (iii) debridement of infected material and edematous mucosa from the mastoid to provide drainage through the mastoid antrum into the middle ear; and (iv) ventilation of the middle ear.

When urgent surgery is indicated, antibiotics should be withheld until purulent material has been aspirated or surgically obtained. If a patient's medical condition does not permit early surgical intervention and culture material is not easily available, nafcillin and chloramphenicol may be administered. If gram-negative rods are identified in material obtained for culture, anti-*Pseudomonas* antibiotics should be administered.

Surgery for uncomplicated acute mastoiditis involves three fundamental steps. First the tympanic membrane is inspected, a myringotomy is performed, and a pressure-equalization tube is placed. This should be done even in the presence of a normal tympanic membrane, because removal of the attic obstruction may result in delayed drainage into the middle ear. Second a postauricular incision is made and the swollen soft tissues are explored for collections of pus. The periosteum over the mastoid cortex and zygomatic root is elevated. Third a simple mastoidectomy is performed. Unlike surgery for chronic otitis media, a thorough exenteration of air cells is not necessary. The objective is to safely remove the bulk of osteitic bone and inflamed mucosa and ensure patency of the aditus. The osteitic trabecular bone encountered will be soft and can easily be removed by bone curettes. When the antrum is poorly visualized, this may be preferable to a drill to minimize the risk of dislocating the short process of incus. The cells of the zygomatic root should be explored. Material removed at surgery should be sent for culture and pathologic study. The postauricular incision can be closed in one layer with 3.0 chromic suture material and the wound and mastoid drained with a Penrose drain. The canal should be stented with a wick for 1 to 2 weeks to maintain patency.

Modification of the soft tissue technique of mastoidectomy is necessary for an infant. First, in a child less than 2 years old, the facial nerve exits the stylomastoid foramen on the lateral aspect of the temporal bone, unprotected by an overlying mastoid process. Therefore the incision is more superoposterior in position than in an adult (Fig. 16.5). Second the external auditory canal is often so small in the infant that transcanal instrumentation is difficult. To visualize the middle ear and also to permit adequate postauricular exposure of the mastoid region, the following approach is advocated in children from birth to 2 years of age.

The postauricular incision is made starting superiorly and descending inferiorly behind the postauricular crease to the level of the inferior margin of the external auditory canal. When the incision has been carried to the inferior extent of the external auditory canal, a nerve stimulator is used to evaluate the proximity of the facial nerve in the more caudal soft tissue. Using fine scissors, the incision can be extended by a few millimeters, which provides adequate exposure. Elevation of the soft tissue from the underlying bone of the external canal with a drum elevator and anterior displacement of

the posterior canal skin allows visualization of the tympanic annulus (Fig. 16.6). The annulus is easily elevated in the infant. The view of the middle ear may be more oblique in the infant than in the older child, resulting in visualization of the undersurface of the tympanic membrane and malleus rather than the incus and stapes (Fig. 16.7). The middle ear, like the mastoid, may also be filled with edematous mucosa, making it difficult to insert a ventilating tube. Following exploration of the middle ear, a simple mastoidectomy is performed.

TREATMENT OF COMPLICATIONS OF ACUTE MASTOIDITIS

Complications of acute mastoiditis are due to extension of infection beyond the mastoid air cells to contiguous areas such as the labyrinth, sigmoid sinus, facial nerve, intracranial cavity, and soft tissues of the neck. The infection may spread via the microvasculature of the mucosa or remodeling bone or through preformed spaces such as bony fissures or old fractures.

Subperiosteal Abscess

The most common extracranial complication of acute mastoiditis is a subperiosteal abscess (21). This occurs most commonly in the posterior-superior aspect of the external canal, over the lateral mastoid cortex, or in the region of the

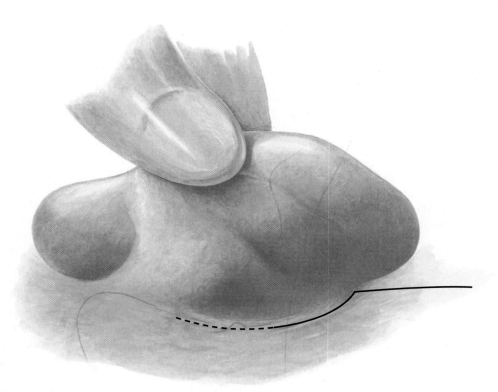

FIG. 16.5 Postauricular incisions for the infant. Compare with that for an adult in Figure 9.15. The incision immediately posterior to the postauricular sulcus is preferred in order to better visualize the middle ear. *Dashed line* indicates that the facial nerve stimulator assists the surgeon during the inferior extension caudad to the level of the external auditory canal.

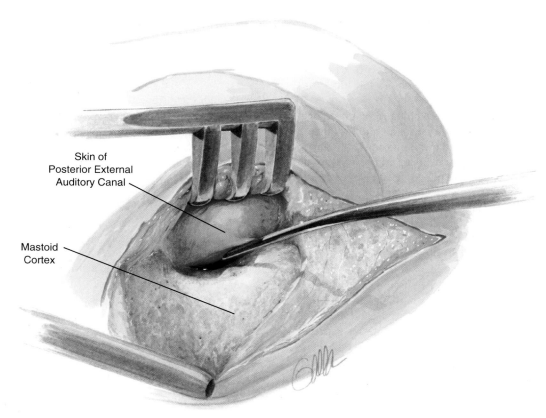

Skin of
Posterior External
Auditory Canal

Mastoid
Cortex

FIG. 16.6 A postauricular transcanal route is used to enter the middle ear.

zygomatic root. Less commonly, a Bezold's abscess will form medial to the mastoid tip, deep to the sternocleidomastoid muscle. In most cases the presence of an abscess is obvious on physical examination. Obvious fluctuance will be noted in the postauricular or supraauricular soft tissues or of the skin of the external canal. However, a patient with a Bezold's abscess usually develops painful rigidity and fullness of the ipsilateral neck without an obvious fluctuant mass. CT is useful in demonstrating a subperiosteal abscess. Needle aspiration is a useful diagnostic maneuver, as well as a means of obtaining material for culture, allowing immediate administration of intravenous antibiotics.

In the presence of an abscess, surgery should be conducted in an expeditious fashion, optimally within hours of diagnosis if the patient's condition permits. Surgery should include postauricular incision and drainage, simple mastoidectomy, and drainage of the wound. If a Bezold's abscess is suspected, the mastoid incision should be continued inferiorly and anteriorly over the anterior border of the sternocleidomastoid muscle. The investing fascia of the sternocleidomastoid muscle is incised along the anterior border and, with blunt dissection, the space deep to the posterior belly of the digastric muscle is explored. If encountered, material from the abscess should be separately cultured, the abscess wall opened widely, and the contents irrigated with copious amounts of antibiotic solution. The abscess may be adjacent to the facial nerve as it exits the stylomastoid foramen. The abscess cavity should be drained through the wound, preferably in the postauricular area to prevent unsightly scarring. The drain is left in place until the drainage diminishes, usually requiring 2 to 3 days.

Facial Paralysis

Intratemporal complications of acute mastoiditis, such as facial nerve paralysis, and suppurative labyrinthitis should raise suspicion of a particularly virulent organism or an immunocompromised patient. A higher incidence of gram-negative organisms, especially *P. aeruginosa,* has been reported in association with these complications (22). Many of these patients have insulin-dependent diabetes mellitus. Although facial paresis complicating acute mastoiditis may be managed initially with wide myringotomy and intravenous antibiotics, progressive paresis and paralysis requires surgical intervention. Surgical exploration of the nerve should be performed within 72 hours of paralysis to allow stimulation of the nerve to determine the extent of neural degeneration. The goal of surgery is to remove any inflammatory nidus from the region of the nerve and to obtain material for culture. The presence of diffuse hyperemic granulation and remodeling bone make complete decompression difficult and often dangerous.

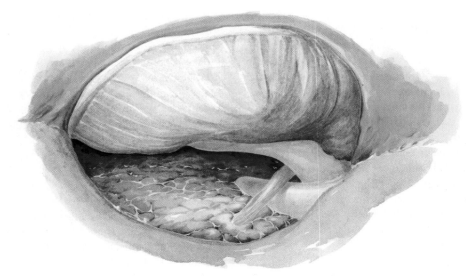

FIG. 16.7 Postauricular transcanal view of the middle ear.

Suppurative Labyrinthitis

The clinical signs of suppurative labyrinthitis include acute vertigo, tinnitus, and profound sensorineural hearing loss. Suppurative labyrinthitis can usually be distinguished from serous (toxic) labyrinthitis, which is often associated with less severe vestibular symptoms and only partial hearing loss. Serous labyrinthitis usually requires only intravenous antibiotics. Patients with suppurative labyrinthitis are at risk for developing meningitis and should be explored surgically to obtain accurate culture material and provide drainage to reduce the chance of intracranial spread of infection. In cases of suppurative labyrinthitis the point of entry of infection into the labyrinth should be explored to be certain that no intralabyrinthine abscess or granulation tissue is overlooked.

Intracranial Complications

Meningitis

The most common intracranial complication of acute mastoiditis is meningitis (23). Physical findings include fever, meningismus, headache, nausea, vomiting, and lethargy. In infants, irritability, fever, a bulging fontanel, and failure to feed may occur. A high index of suspicion for this potentially lethal complication is essential. Older patients should have CT of the brain to rule out other intracranial complications such as an abscess that might lead to brain herniation during lumbar puncture. A lumbar puncture is then performed to obtain cerebrospinal fluid (CSF) for Gram stain and culture. In infants, lumbar puncture usually takes precedence over CT scanning unless focal neurologic deficits are present. Intravenous antibiotics should be administered after CSF is obtained for culture. Surgery may be delayed for 24 to 48 hours while intravenous antibiotics are administered. Surgery should consist of a simple mastoidectomy with

careful inspection of the tegmen. The posterior fossa plate and the lateral sinus are examined for evidence of thrombophlebitis. Separate cultures from the mastoid should be obtained.

Epidural Abscess

Epidural abscess of the middle or posterior fossa as a complication of acute mastoiditis may be diagnosed by preoperative CT scan or may not be suspected until encountered at operation (24). The management of a large epidural abscess is best accomplished as a combined neurosurgical-otologic procedure. Following evacuation of the abscess, a simple or modified radical mastoidectomy may be done to facilitate drainage into the mastoid. Serial CT scanning and prolonged intravenous antibiotics may be necessary to ensure complete resolution of infection. Despite a negative CT scan, a search for a small epidural abscess should be performed in acute mastoiditis complicated by meningitis.

When an epidural abscess is encountered at surgery, the surrounding tegmental bone should be carefully removed to promote drainage. Granulation may be densely adherent to the dura and difficult to remove.

Brain Abscess

The most serious intracranial complication of acute mastoiditis is brain abscess. Even with the administration of antibiotics and surgical intervention, death has been reported to occur in one third of patients (25). The abscess may result from direct extension from the adjacent infected mastoid or occur deep within the brain parenchyma as a result of retrograde septic thrombophlebitis. In 17 temporal bone specimens from patients who died from brain abscesses secondary to mastoid infections, the route of extension to the brain parenchyma appeared to be either blood-borne or directly through the meninges rather than via the labyrinth (26). Abscesses occur most commonly in the temporal lobe and cerebellum (27). Clinical signs and symptoms include headache, fever, and neurologic deficits depending on the site of abscess formation. Once identified by CT scan or on MRI, a brain abscess is best managed by neurosurgical intervention. Abscesses that are located in accessible regions may be surgically drained, usually after a prolonged period of intravenous antibiotic administration. Less accessible abscesses may be aspirated with CT guidance or treated with intravenous antibiotics only. Aspiration may be required several times before complete resolution occurs. Residual neurologic deficits are common. Mastoidectomy should be done after the abscess has been successfully managed and the patient's general condition permits.

Lateral Sinus Thrombophlebitis

Lateral sinus thrombosis or thrombophlebitis is now a relatively uncommon, but serious, complication of acute mastoiditis. From 1928 to 1934, 0.3% of all deaths coming to autopsy were due to lateral sinus thrombosis. Between 1956 and 1960 the incidence was 0.01% (23). In 1935 Meltzer (28) reviewed the experience at the Massachusetts Eye and Ear Infirmary and reported a mortality of 24% in patients with lateral sinus thrombophlebitis. Despite improved diagnostic modalities and antibiotics, the mortality has not significantly changed (29,30). The spectrum of sinus pathology includes intrasinus empyema, thrombophlebitis, and phlebitis without thrombosis. Thrombosis often occurs in association with other intracranial complications, especially epidural abscess. Symptoms include headache, severe otalgia, and neck pain. On examination, neck and mastoid tenderness are usually present. If extension to the mastoid emissary vein occurs, there may be a tender mass over the mastoid cortex, called Griesinger's sign. Spiking fevers demonstrating a "picket fence" pattern on the temperature chart is characteristic. If lateral sinus thrombophlebitis is suspected, CT scan with rapid contrast infusion may help establish the diagnosis (31). Other useful diagnostic tests include digital subtraction angiography (32) (Fig. 16.4) and MRI scanning or MR venography. On MRI scan, the absence of a sigmoid sinus flow void is highly suggestive of sigmoid sinus thrombosis. These imaging modalities may not demonstrate early phlebitis before thrombosis has occurred. Lumbar puncture is necessary to rule out meningitis. A Queckenstedt's or Tobey-Ayer test may provide further clinical evidence of lateral sinus thrombosis.

Patients with suspected lateral sinus thrombosis should undergo surgical exploration as soon as possible. The sinus should be uncovered and inspected from the sinodural angle to the jugular bulb. The sinus should be aspirated. If free flow is encountered, the sinus need not be incised. If no flow is obtained, the sinus should be incised. The clot should be sent for culture to ascertain if the thrombus is septic or sterile. An empyema should be exteriorized into the mastoid. If bleeding is encountered upon evacuation of pus or thrombus, the sinus can be packed extraluminally at the region of the jugular bulb and the superior petrosal sinus with Surgicel. Ligation of the internal jugular vein should be reserved for patients with evidence of jugular empyema determined on aspiration and in patients with septic pulmonary emboli. The use of anticoagulation in lateral sinus thrombosis is controversial and not yet supported by clinical studies (33,34).

Otitic Hydrocephalus

Otitic hydrocephalus is an uncommon intracranial complication associated with acute mastoiditis. Although the cause of otitis hydrocephalus is not known, it occurs as a common sequela of lateral sinus thrombosis. However, most cases of lateral sinus thrombosis do not result in elevated intracranial pressure. Clinically, patients usually present with headache, vomiting, blurred vision, diplopia, and decreased consciousness in association with other signs of acute mastoid infection. Examination reveals papilledema and, occasionally, sixth nerve paralysis. Lumbar puncture demonstrates elevated pressures with normal CSF composition. It is critical that other causes of elevated intracranial pressure be ruled out, especially the presence of a brain abscess. Once the diagnosis of increased intracranial pressure is made, and space-occupying lesions have been ruled out, the patency of the lateral sinuses should be assessed with either rapid contrast infusion CT, venous subtraction angiography, or MRI. Treatment of otitic hydrocephalus involves management of the underlying otologic disease and prevention of complications from increased intracranial pressure. Mastoidectomy with exploration of the lateral sinus from the sinodural angle to the jugular bulb should be accomplished as soon as the patient is medically stable. Treatment of the increased intracranial pressure usually consists of steroids, acetazolamide, hyperosmolar agents, and occasionally a CSF drainage procedure. Patients usually have a prolonged clinical course ranging from weeks to months, even after resolution of the mastoid infection.

ACUTE MASTOIDITIS AND CHOLESTEATOMA

Acute mastoiditis can occur as a complication of chronic otitis media. This was a relatively unusual occurrence in the preantibiotic era, compared with the incidence of acute mastoiditis in patients with acute otitis media. It is unlikely that there is an actual increase in the incidence of acute mastoiditis complicating cholesteatoma, but rather a decrease in the incidence of this process complicating acute otitis media. There is a thicker barrier of sclerotic bone that must be penetrated before postauricular inflammation or other complications can develop. In more recent times, several cases of acute mastoiditis have been reported in patients with chronic otitis media with cholesteatoma (35,36). In most of these cases the cholesteatoma resulted in bone erosion with extension of infection beyond the mastoid. Once identified, surgery should be done as soon as possible. Unlike surgery for acute uncomplicated mastoiditis without cholesteatoma, the surgeon must attempt to eradicate all cholesteatoma and more closely adhere to the principles of surgery for chronic otitis media.

SUBACUTE OR MASKED MASTOIDITIS

The use of antibiotics in the management of otalgia and otitis media has resulted in a subgroup of tympanomastoid infections with a clinical course frequently overlooked or unrecognized until a serious complication occurs (37). In such cases, there is often a history of an antecedent acute otitis media or upper respiratory tract infection that may have been treated with an oral antibiotic resulting in apparent improvement. This clinical entity is referred to as subacute or masked mastoiditis. In this condition, serious complications of meningitis, epidural abscess, brain abscess, and facial paralysis occur without the heralding clinical signs of pain, fever, otorrhea, and postauricular inflammation or abscess formation. Once mastoid infection is identified in these patients, surgery should be performed as soon as the patient's general condition permits. The principles of surgery are unchanged.

ACUTE MASTOIDITIS IN IMMUNE-COMPROMISED PATIENTS

The occurrence of acute otitis media and acute mastoiditis in immune-compromised patients represents a potentially life-threatening process. The incidence of associated complications, including facial paralysis and brain abscess, is significantly higher than that which occurs in individuals with healthy immune systems (38). The increasing incidence of human immunodeficiency virus (HIV) infection and acquired immunodeficiency syndrome (AIDS) throughout the world has led to an increase in identification of unusual pathogens in HIV patients with acute mastoiditis (39). Acute mastoiditis caused by *Aspergillus* is particularly common in HIV-infected individuals (38,40). The identification of *Aspergillus* in patients with acute mastoiditis should raise immediate concerns of HIV or other causes of immune compromise.

Early surgical intervention may be particularly important in determining a successful outcome in immune-compromised patients with signs and symptoms of acute mastoiditis (38). Aside from the therapeutic value afforded by drainage and removal of infected tissue, it provides an opportunity to obtain representative tissue for culture, which may be critical in choosing appropriate antimicrobial therapy. These important advantages far outweigh concerns regarding wound healing and risks of anesthesia in these patients.

REFERENCES

1. Davison FW. Otitis media—then and now. *Laryngoscope* 1955;65: 142–151.
2. House HP. Otitis media. A comparative study of the results obtained in therapy before and after the introduction of the sulfonamide compounds. *Arch Otolaryngol* 1946;43:371–378.
3. Palva T, Pulkkinen K. Mastoiditis. *J Laryngol Otol* 1959;73:573–588.
4. Rudberg RD. Acute otitis media: comparative therapeutic results of sulphonamide and penicillin administered in various forms. *Acta Otolaryngol Suppl (Stockh)* 1954;113:1–79.
5. Proctor CA. Intracranial complications of otitic origin. *Laryngoscope* 1966;76:288–308.
6. Klein JO. Management of acute otitis media in an era of increasing antibiotic resistance. *Int J Pediatr Otorhinolaryngol* 1999;[Suppl 1]: S15–17.
7. Thoroe J, Lous J. Acute otitis media and antibiotics. Evidence-based guidelines for antibiotic therapy? *Ugeskr Laeger* 1999;161:5413–5417.
8. Kacker SK, Sinha A. Role of cholesteatoma in the etiology of acute mastoiditis. *J Otolaryngol Soc Aust* 1968;2:45–48.
9. Wright JL. Acute leukaemia presenting as acute mastoiditis. *J Laryngol Otol* 1971;85:1087–1091.
10. Michel RG, Pope TH Jr, Patterson CN. Infectious mononucleosis, mastoiditis, and facial paralysis. *Arch Otolaryngol* 1975;101:486–489.
11. Agarwal PN, Mishra SD, Pratap VK. Primary liposarcoma of the mastoid. *J Laryngol Otol* 1975;89:1079–1082.
12. Puczynski MS, Stankiewicz JA, Ow PE. Mucocutaneous lymph node syndrome mimicking acute coalescent mastoiditis. *Am J Otol* 1986;7:71–73.
13. Maharaj D, Jadwat A, Fernandes CM, et al. Bacteriology in acute mastoiditis. *Arch Otolaryngol Head Neck Surg* 1987;113:514–515.
14. Ogle JW, Lauer BA. Acute mastoiditis: diagnosis and complications. *Am J Dis Child* 1986;140:1178–1182.
15. Prellner K, Rydell R. Acute mastoiditis. Influence of antibiotic treatment on the bacterial spectrum. *Acta Otolaryngol (Stockh)* 1986;102: 52–56.
16. Hansman D. Serotypes of pneumococci in pneumonia, meningitis and other pneumococcal infections. *Aust N Z J Med* 1977;7:267–270.
17. Neitch SM, Sydnor JB, Schleupner CJ. Mycobacterium fortuitum as a cause of mastoiditis and wound infection. *Arch Otolaryngol* 1982;108: 11–14.
18. Avery RK, Eavey RD, Della Torre T, et al. Bilateral otitis media and mastoiditis caused by a highly resistant strain of *Mycobacterium chelonae. Pediatr Infect Dis J* 1996;15:1037–1040.
19. Gliklich RE, Eavey RD, Iannuzzi RA, et al. A contemporary analysis of acute mastoiditis. *Arch Otolaryngol Head Neck Surg* 1996;122: 135–139.
20. Niv A, Nash M, Peiser J, et al. Outpatient management of acute mastoiditis with periosteitis in children. *Int J Pediatr Otorhinolaryngol* 1998;46:9–13.
21. Hawkins DB, Dru D, House JW, et al. Acute mastoiditis in children: a review of 54 cases. *Laryngoscope* 1983;93:568–572.
22. Ostfeld E, Rubinstein E. Acute gram-negative bacillary infections of the middle ear and mastoid. *Ann Otol Rhinol Laryngol* 1980;89:33–36.
23. Courville CB. Intracranial complications of otitis media and mastoiditis in the antibiotic era. *Laryngoscope* 1955;65:31–46.
24. Rubin JS, Wei WI. Acute mastoiditis: a review of 34 patients. *Laryngoscope* 1985;95:963–965.
25. Samuel J, Fernandes CM, Steinberg JL. Intracranial otogenic complications: a persisting problem. *Laryngoscope* 1986;96:272–278.
26. Quijano M, Schuknecht HF, Otte J. Temporal bone pathology associated with intracranial abscesses. *ORL J Otorhinolaryngol Relat Spec* 1988;50:2–31.
27. Wright JL, Grimaldi PM. Otogenic intracranial complications. *J Laryngol Otol* 1973;87:1085–1096.
28. Meltzer PE. Treatment of thrombosis of the lateral sinus. A summary of the results obtained during twelve years at the Massachusetts Eye and Ear Infirmary. *Arch Otolaryngol* 1935;22:131–142.
29. Jeanes A. Otogenic intracranial suppuration. *J Laryngol Otol* 1962;76:388–402.
30. Seid AB, Sellars SL. The management of otogenic lateral sinus disease at Groote Schuur Hospital. *Laryngoscope* 1973;83:397–403.
31. Rizer FM, Amiri CA, Schroeder WW, et al. Lateral sinus thrombosis: diagnosis and treatment—a case report. *J Otolaryngol* 1987;16: 77–79.
32. Scully RE, Mark EJ, McNeely WF, et al, eds. Case records of the Massachusetts General Hospital. Weekly Clinicopathological Exercises. Case 20-1988. *N Eng J Med* 1988;318:1322–1328.

33. McNeill R. Internal jugular vein thrombosis. *Head Neck Surg* 1981;3: 247–250.

34. James PM Jr, Bevis A, Myers RT. Experiences with central venous and pulmonary artery pressure in a series of 3,500 patients. *South Med J* 1972;65:1299–1307.

35. Shaffer HL, Gates GA, Meyerhoff WL. Acute mastoiditis and cholesteatoma. *Otolaryngology* 1978;86:ORL394–399.

36. Primrose WJ, Cinnamond MJ. Acute mastoid abscess and cholesteatoma. *Int J Ped Otorhinolaryngol* 1987;12:229–235.

37. Holt RG, Gates GA. Masked mastoiditis. *Laryngoscope* 1983;93: 1034–1037.

38. Chen D, Lalwani AK, House JW, et al. Aspergillus mastoiditis in acquired immunodeficiency syndrome. *Am J Otol* 1999;20:561–567.

39. Kim SC, Jorgensen J, Graybill JR, et al. Otomastoiditis caused by *Rhodoccus equi* in a patient with AIDS. *P R Health Sci J* 1999;18: 285–288.

40. Yates PD, Upile T, Axon PR, et al. Aspergillus mastoiditis in a patient with acquired immunodeficiency syndrome. *J Laryngol Otol* 1997; 111:560–561.

CHAPTER 17

Chronic Otitis Media

Joseph B. Nadol, Jr.

The management and selection of an appropriate surgical procedure for a patient with chronic otitis media requires that the clinician identify the proper subclassification of the disease process, to have prioritized the objectives of surgery, and, finally, to be aware of the histopathological limitations imposed on reconstruction by the disease process. Failure of surgery for chronic otitis media, because of either residual or recurrent disease, can be ascribed to improper selection of a surgical procedure as much as to failure of the surgical technique itself. Likewise, much of the current controversy concerning the surgical method of choice and the differences in results is due to comparison of disparate types of chronic otitis media. Assignment of a particular patient in the subclassification presented in Table 17.1 will help guide the otologic surgeon in the selection of surgical procedure and the timing of surgery (1).

Chronic active otitis media implies an active and hence potentially progressive process. Chronic active otitis media includes cases with cholesteatoma, with or without otorrhea, and cases without cholesteatoma but with chronic otorrhea. Except for medically unstable patients, the diagnosis of cholesteatoma almost always implies the need for surgical treatment. On the other hand, the diagnosis of chronic active otitis media without cholesteatoma should engender a trial of medical management in an attempt to arrest the otorrhea and convert the process to chronic inactive otitis media. Medical management includes culture of the suppuration, parenteral and topical antibiotics as indicated by culture and sensitivity tests, and frequent cleaning of the ear canal and removal of exuberant granulation if present. Failure of medical management in chronic active otitis media without cholesteatoma constitutes an indication for surgical treatment.

The presence of a complication of chronic otitis media, such as labyrinthine fistula or facial nerve paralysis, generally implies the need for urgent surgical management, with or without the presence of cholesteatoma (Chapter 18).

Chronic inactive otitis media implies stable, nonprogressive pathology of the tympanic membrane, middle ear, and mastoid cavity caused by previous suppuration and/or eu-

stachian tube dysfunction. In most cases, chronic inactive otitis media represents a relative indication for elective surgery generally directed toward reconstructive procedures for the tympanic membrane and ossicular chain.

Chronic inactive otitis media with frequent reactivation refers to an ear without cholesteatoma, but with a perforated tympanic membrane and a history of episodic mucopurulent drainage. In this condition, although the drainage may cease with oral and/or topical antibiotics, it recurs without an obvious inciting event such as exposure to water. The significance of this diagnosis is that attempts to repair the perforated tympanic membrane without exploration of the mastoid, antrum, and epitympanum to eliminate active infection, granulation, or obstruction of the aditus ad antrum ("attic block") will often result in graft failure and recurrent suppuration. Therefore, before recommending simple tympanoplasty or ossiculoplasty as an elective procedure in a case of chronic otitis media that has only recently been rendered inactive by medical management, a waiting period is advisable to minimize the risk of spontaneous reactivation.

CLASSIFICATION OF RECURRENT CHRONIC OTITIS MEDIA FOLLOWING TYMPANOMASTOIDECTOMY

The classification outlined in Table 17.1 can be used either for primary disease or for recurrent disease following mastoid tympanoplasty. Thus recurrent cholesteatoma with or without otorrhea or recurrent chronic otorrhea can easily be subclassified as chronic active otitis media (recurrent). Occasionally, both with canal wall–up and with canal wall–down procedures, intermittent suppuration may occur and therefore fall under the category of chronic inactive otitis media with frequent reactivation (postoperative). Following canal wall–down procedures, this may take the form of an unstable epithelium. On an intermittent basis, granulation tissue may appear commonly in the sinodural angle or tegmental area but responds to local hygiene and topical antibiotics. On the other hand, a canal wall–down "mastoid bowl" with continuous otorrhea but without cholesteatoma,

TABLE 17.1 *Subclassification of chronic otitis media*

I. *Chronic active otitis media* (primary or recurrent)
   With cholesteatoma
      With otorrhea
      Without otorrhea
   Without cholesteatoma
      With otorrhea
II. *Chronic inactive otitis media*
   With retraction pocket
   With perforation
   With ossicular resorption or fixation
   With adhesive otitis media
      (Nonpneumatized middle ear)
III. *Chronic inactive otitis media with frequent reactivation*
   Primary
   Postoperative

in which the otorrhea does not respond to local hygiene and topical antibiotics, should be classified as chronic active otitis media (recurrent) and usually implies residual or recurrent disease in remaining pneumatized spaces of the temporal bone.

ROLE OF RADIOGRAPHIC STUDIES IN THE SUBCLASSIFICATION OF CHRONIC OTITIS

The classification presented in Table 17.1 is based on clinical observation, either immediate or over time, and generally does not require radiographic studies for classification. However, there are special cases in which computed tomography (CT) of the temporal bone will aid in the subclassification. For example, in a case with an attic retraction pocket, if the superior and posterior limits of the pocket are not visible, CT may indicate an epitympanic soft tissue mass consistent with an attic cholesteatoma, thus allowing subclassification of chronic active otitis media with cholesteatoma. Study of the temporal bone plays a much larger role in the selection of a surgical technique in the evaluation of complications of chronic otitis media and in the evaluation of patients with recurrent chronic active otitis media following mastoid tympanoplasty.

OBJECTIVES AND PRIORITIZATION IN SURGERY FOR CHRONIC OTITIS MEDIA

In addition to appropriate subclassification of the disease process, the selection of an appropriate surgical procedure also requires the surgeon to have adopted specific objectives and priorities in the treatment of chronic ear disease. With few exceptions, the major objectives, in order of priority, are (i) elimination of suppuration and other manifestations of chronic active otitis media, (ii) alteration of the anatomy of the ear and mastoid in an attempt to prevent recurrent disease and to optimize subsequent cleaning and otologic monitoring of the ear, and (iii) reconstruction of the tympanic membrane and ossicular system in order to achieve serviceable and stable postoperative hearing.

It is generally recognized that failure to achieve the first objective will become manifest by residual disease and require revision surgery. However, it should be pointed out that failure to achieve the second objective is also a common cause for revision surgery for recurrent disease. Therefore, paradoxically, a surgical attempt to restore the eardrum and canal to a normal anatomic condition in an inappropriately selected patient may predispose to recurrence of the disease process.

For example, in cases with attic cholesteatoma managed either by anterior atticotomy or by canal wall–up tympanomastoidectomy, substitution of the removed bony scutum by a fascial graft may result in recurrent attic retraction and cholesteatoma formation. However, the placement of free cartilage grafts in the epitympanum following such a procedure is effective in preventing such reretraction.

CLINICAL FACTORS INFLUENCING THE SELECTION OF SURGICAL APPROACH

Several factors, including the clinical history, otologic findings, and hearing, both in the diseased and contralateral ear, are important considerations in surgical decision making. For example, a limited attic cholesteatoma with no suppuration may be adequately treated by anterior atticotomy. Extensive disease, as indicated by the presence of complications, radiographic evidence of significant bone destruction, profuse purulent drainage, and otologic history consistent with progression over many years, usually is best handled by a postauricular mastoidectomy. Table 17.2 presents relative indications for various surgical approaches. Surgery for chronic otitis media should be individualized depending upon the clinical circumstances. It should be emphasized, however, that these indications are relative ones and must be modified by the experience of the particular operating surgeon. Also playing significant roles in the choice of the surgical procedure are such factors as the reliability of the patient in conforming to the otologic follow-up necessitated by a given surgical procedure, age of the patient, presence of usable hearing in the operated on and contralateral ears, evidence for poor eustachian tube function such as the presence of bilateral chronic otitis media, uncontrolled allergic rhinosinusitis, and a history of cranial base anomalies. In general, the surgeon should strive to eliminate the disease process, as well as perform a reconstructive procedure in one surgical procedure unless there is strong indication that staging and multiple procedures will offer a significant benefit to the patient. Although the surgeon should have a specific, planned procedure in mind preoperatively, including the elements of the surgical procedure outlined in Table 17.2, he or she should prepare the patient and allow time for intraoperative revision of the surgical plan.

RECURRENT CHRONIC ACTIVE OTITIS MEDIA: CAUSES, EVALUATION, AND MANAGEMENT

The estimated incidence of recurrent chronic active otitis media when no residual disease was left at the time of the first surgery ranges from 3% to 18% of all surgical proce-

TABLE 17.2 *Relative indications for common surgical approaches to the middle ear and mastoid in chronic otitis media.*

Procedure	Relative Indications	Relative Contraindications
Anterior atticotomy	Limited attic disease Symptomatic retraction pocket	Mucopurulent drainage Radiographic evidence of significant mastoid involvement History of previous ipsilateral otologic surgery
Canal wall–up mastoidectomy	Chronic inactive otitis media with frequent reactivation Limited atticoantral disease Well-pneumatized mastoid Clinical evidence for good eustachian function Ability to preserve tympanic membrane and ossicular chain anticipated	Previous ipsilateral surgery for chronic active otitis media Extensive granulomatous disease or large cholesteatoma Sclerotic, poorly pneumatized mastoid Clinical evidence for poor eustachian tube function
Canal wall–down mastoidectomy	Extensive disease Poorly pneumatized mastoid Presence of complications (e.g., labyrinthine fistula) Clinical evidence of poor tubal function History of previous failure of canal wall–up mastoidectomy for chronic active otitis media	Disease limited to attic or antrum

dures for chronic otitis media (2–5). The causes of failure of mastoidectomy include residual or recurrent cholesteatoma and residual or recurrent suppuration of the middle ear and mastoid compartments.

Residual Disease

Residual cholesteatoma with or without suppuration or residual chronic infection without cholesteatoma may be attributed to inadequate exposure during the previous surgical procedure, failure to recognize the extent of primary disease, or failure to exenterate disease during the previous procedures. Common examples of this include cholesteatoma in the sinus tympani or oval window or round window niches, which are notoriously difficult to access; failure to exenterate obstructed and infected air cells, principally along the tegmen, sinodural angle, facial recess, and mastoid tip (6); and failure to recognize significant disease in the hypotympanum and infralabyrinthine cells (7).

Recurrent Disease

Mastoid tympanoplasty may also fail because of recurrence rather than residual disease. The causes of failure due to recurrent disease are somewhat different following canal wall–up versus canal wall–down tympanomastoidectomy. The most common cause of failure in canal wall–up procedures is failure to alter the anatomy of the ear and mastoid and to make recurrence less likely. Common examples of this include recurrent attic retraction and cholesteatoma due to failure to insert stiff grafts such as free cartilage to prevent reretraction, postoperative sequestration of the mastoid from the middle ear space due to attic block, and failure to maintain an adequate communication between the mastoid and middle ear via the facial recess. In contrast, in canal wall–down tympanomastoidectomy the most common causes of recurrent chronic suppuration are postoperative ob-

struction, sequestration, and reinfection of residual air cells of the tegmen, sinodural angle, facial recess, or mastoid tip; or inadequate meatoplasty or inadequate removal of the bone over the facial ridge, resulting in a mastoid bowl in which it is difficult or impossible to provide local hygiene. It is important to recognize that in this sense the objectives of canal wall–up surgery differ from that of canal wall–down procedures. Thus in a canal wall–up procedure the objective is clearly to remove all disease, both granulation tissue and cholesteatoma, but to allow remucosalization of the pneumatized space of the mastoid in the postoperative period. In contrast, remucosalization of the mastoid not only is not the objective in canal wall–down procedures but in fact commonly results in recurrent disease due to obstruction, sequestration, and reinfection. This principle is best illustrated by the example of the fenestration cavity. The fenestration procedure in which a canal wall–down mastoidectomy was performed for the purpose of hearing improvement in otosclerosis commonly resulted in a chronic draining mastoid bowl (8). Thus in an ear in which there was originally no suppuration whatsoever, the development of a draining mastoid bowl must be attributed to the surgical procedure itself. It is important to remove most or all residual pneumatized cells principally in the sinodural angle tegmen and facial recess, particularly in the canal wall–down technique, because such residual cells may become easily obstructed and then reinfected.

EVALUATION OF RESIDUAL RECURRENT DISEASE FOLLOWING FAILURE OF PREVIOUS MASTOID SURGERY

The evaluation and management of cases in which there is either a residual or recurrent cholesteatoma or persistent or recurrent suppuration requires careful clinical and radiographic evaluation. In failed canal wall–up technique, CT of the temporal bone will help to reveal the extent of recurrent

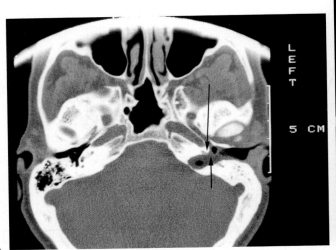

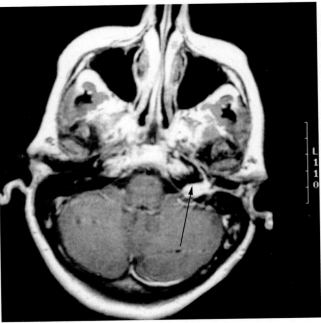

A

B

FIG. 17.1 Chronic otitis media of the left ear with extension to the hypotympanum (*short arrow*). **A:** A CT scan demonstrated expansion of the hypotympanic cell system by chronic otitis media. A cochlear fistula (*long arrow*) resulted in profound sensorineural loss. **B:** An MR scan with gadolinium enhancement also demonstrates granulation tissue in the hypotympanum in the left ear (*arrow*).

cholesteatoma or the location of obstructed and infected residual air cells.

The clinical situation of recurrent suppuration without cholesteatoma following previous canal wall–down technique requires special consideration. Skin grafts placed over bone rather than a thick, subcutaneous soft tissue layer are relatively unstable and are prone to ulceration and suppuration, even in the absence of deep-seated recurrent disease. In such cases, local hygiene, debridement, and delayed split-thickness skin grafts (Chapter 10) may result in a dry mastoid bowl. The bacteriology of chronic suppurative otitis media, particularly following canal wall–down procedures, includes a high prevalence of anaerobic pathogens (9–11). In this regard it is important to recognize that commonly used topical otologic antibiotics have poor anaerobic coverage. Failure of delayed skin grafting and topical or parenteral antibiotics based on culture and sensitivity implies more deep-seated sequestrated disease and should engender a radiographic study. Despite the localization implied by the term *chronic otitis media,* insufficient clinical attention has been paid to the role of the hypotympanum in chronic active otitis media (6,7).

CT and magnetic resonance imaging (MRI) may demonstrate significant disease in the hypotympanum (Fig. 17.1A, B). Imaging may also demonstrate that unsuspected residual or recurrent disease is no longer contiguous with the previous surgical site (Fig. 17.2) or unsuspected contiguous disease in the petrous apex (Fig. 17.3A,B) (12).

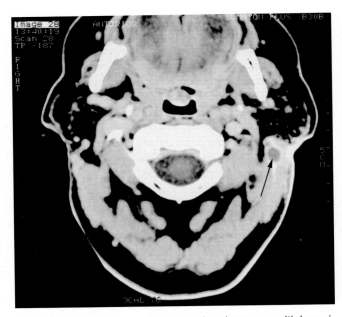

FIG. 17.2 This 65-year-old man had undergone multiple revision surgical procedures for chronic otitis media with cholesteatoma of the left ear complicated by postoperative neck abscesses. Before the final revision, a CT scan with soft tissue windows demonstrated a cholesteatoma (*arrow*) in the soft tissue of the neck below the left mastoid. In retrospect, an extensive cholesteatoma had broken through the mastoid cortex with extension to the neck. This component of the cholesteatoma had been overlooked in multiple revision surgeries.

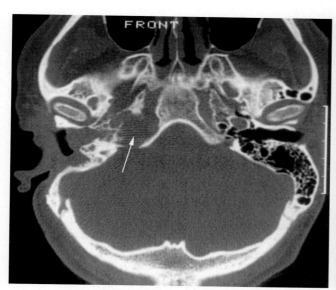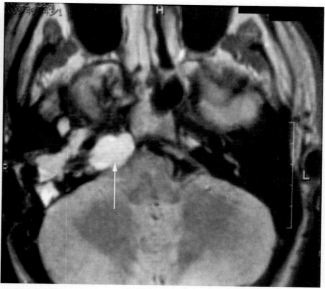

FIG. 17.3 A 35-year-old man had undergone multiple mastoidectomies for chronic otitis media with otorrhea. After multiple failures, a CT scan (**A**) and MRI (**B**) clearly demonstrated a large petrous apex cyst (*arrows*), which was in continuity with the infected tympanomastoid compartment via the hypotympanic cell system and had served as a reservoir for continued otorrhea.

HISTOPATHOLOGY OF MIDDLE EAR AND MASTOID IN CHRONIC OTITIS MEDIA

A knowledge of the histopathology of chronic otitis media as found in the mesotympanum and mastoid is important for the otologic surgeon in the selection of surgical procedures and a realistic appraisal of the possibilities for reconstruction. For a more complete description of the histopathology of chronic active otitis media, the reader is referred to published atlases of ear pathology (13,14).

Tympanosclerosis

Deposition of hyalin may occur in ossicular ligaments and in the submucosal layers of the tympanic membrane, middle ear, epitympanum, and mastoid. When extensive, tympanosclerosis may fix the ossicles and may be accompanied by new bone formation (Figs. 17.4 to 17.6).

Rarefying Osteitis

Osteoclastic resorption of the bone of the mastoid, ossicles, and otic capsule is a common consequence of chronic active otitis media with or without cholesteatoma. It may result in discontinuity of the ossicles, exposure of the dura of the middle and posterior fossae, and dehiscences in the otic capsule, resulting in labyrinthine fistulas, labyrinthitis, and meningitis (Fig. 17.7).

Fibrocystic Sclerosis

As granulation tissue matures, fibrous tissue may be deposited in the submucosal area and cause obliteration of the round window niche and loculation of previously pneumatized spaces of the middle ear and mastoid, exacerbating the obstructive aspects of chronic otitis media (Fig. 17.8).

Fibro-osseous Sclerosis

Deposition of fibrous tissue and new bone is characteristic of the reparative process in chronic active otitis media. This may result in obstruction and sequestration of disease and may seriously limit the potential for reconstruction. Extensive fibro-osseous sclerosis may be recognized as "sclerotic" changes in a poorly pneumatized mastoid (Fig. 17.9).

Cholesteatoma

Although the osteolytic potential of cholesteatoma is well known clinically, there is still disagreement as to the exact pathophysiology of bone resorption. Bone resorption is thought to be secondary to both enzymatic and cell-mediated processes (15,16). Superinfection of a cholesteatoma and increased pressure caused by entrapment in a closed space seem to potentiate the osteolytic potential of cholesteatoma (Fig. 17.10). Although enzymatic processes inherent to a cholesteatoma are at least in part responsible for bone resorption, decompression or exteriorization of the cholesteatoma without total removal may halt bone resorption. This is an important fact to bear in mind when a cholesteatoma intimately involves structures that cannot be sacrificed, such as posterior fossa dura, jugular bulb, or carotid artery, or has caused dehiscences in the vestibular or cochlear bony labyrinth. In such cases cholesteatoma may be decompressed and exteriorized or the residual chole-

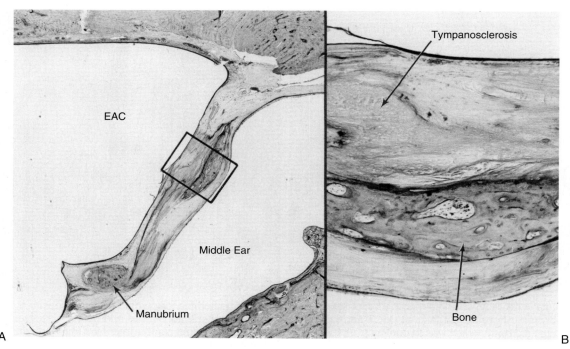

FIG. 17.4 Histologic section through the tympanic membrane of a 73-year-old woman with chronic inactive otitis media of the left ear. There is a subepithelial deposit of tympanosclerosis and new bone formation within the thickened tympanic membrane. EAC, external auditory canal. **A:** 23.5X. **B:** 83.8X.

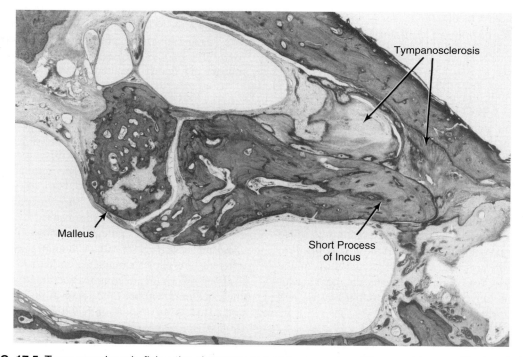

FIG. 17.5 Tympanosclerosis fixing the short process of the incus in a 69-year-old man with chronic inactive otitis media of the right ear. 15.6X.

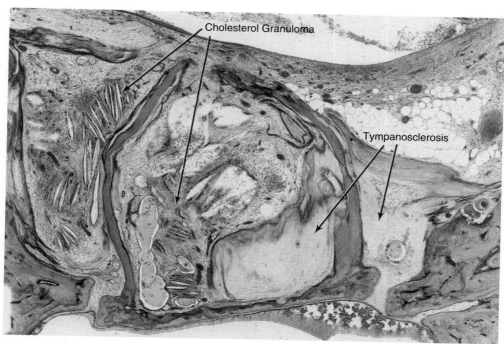

FIG. 17.6 The stapes is embedded in cholesterol granuloma and tympanosclerosis, and the head of the stapes has been reabsorbed in a 67-year-old woman with chronic active otitis media of the left ear who had undergone canal wall–down mastoidectomy 8 years prior to her death. 28.7X.

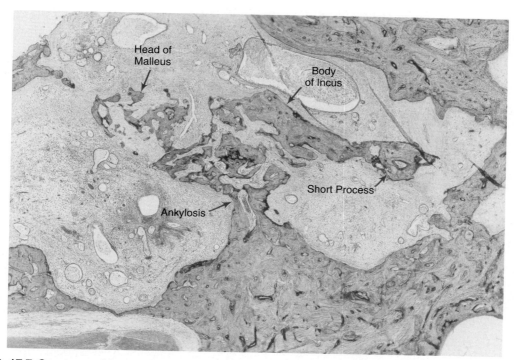

FIG. 17.7 Severe rarefying osteitis of the malleus and incus and surrounding fibrous tissue in the epitympanic space of a 44-year-old man with chronic otitis media of the right ear. 18.2X.

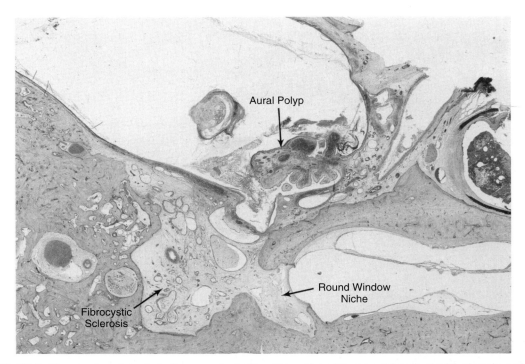

FIG. 17.8 Fibrocystic sclerosis in the round window niche of an 83-year-old patient with chronic active otitis media of the left ear. An aural polyp arises from the mucosa overlying the promontory. 5.9X.

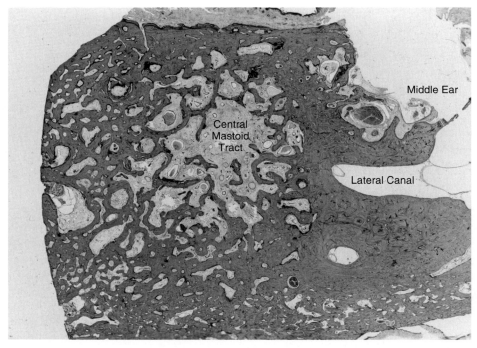

FIG. 17.9 Fibro-osseous sclerosis of the central mastoid tract in a 68-year-old woman with chronic otitis media of the left ear. The pneumatized space has been greatly reduced by subepithelial fibrosis and new bone formation. 3.7X.

steatoma may be removed at a subsequent, staged surgical procedure. Despite the persistence of the cholesteatomatous matrix, bony healing may occur subjacent to it once the pressure and suppurative aspects have been eliminated.

SURGICAL TECHNIQUE

Informed Consent for Mastoidectomy for Chronic Otitis Media

Informed consent for mastoidectomy for chronic otitis media includes delineating the specific surgical procedures that are planned and informing the patient that intraoperative findings may dictate modifications of this plan.

The planned incision, extent of the surgical field, use of split-thickness skin grafting from a separate site, and planned reconstruction should be discussed.

Therapeutic options, if any, should be disclosed. It is important to inform the patient that the healing phase following mastoid tympanoplasty is prolonged and extends far beyond healing of the incision. For example, in canal wall–down tympanomastoidectomy, final healing may take many weeks, and in fact subsequent procedures such as delayed split-thickness skin grafting, may be required before epithelialization is complete and the wound is fully healed. Preoperative discussion of this important aspect will help to ensure that the postoperative visits are kept and to maintain the patient's confidence in the therapy during the weeks following the initial procedure.

Specific risks of tympanomastoid surgery include damage to hearing, balance, or facial nerve function; residual or recurrent disease; postoperative hematoma or infection; and dysgusia secondary to injury or sacrifice of the chorda tympani nerve; these should be discussed. Alteration in the appearance of the auricle and scarring or infection at donor sites should be mentioned.

Specific aspects of surgical techniques applicable to chronic otitis media are presented in Chapter 9 (soft tissue techniques), Chapter 10 (skin grafting), Chapter 11 (osseous approaches), and Chapter 23 (tympanoplasty and ossiculoplasty in conjunction with mastoid surgery). In addition, surgical principles in dealing with complications of chronic active otitis media are presented in Chapter 18. In this section the important details of surgery and modifications of technique for canal wall–up and canal wall–down mastoidectomy as performed for chronic otitis media are presented. In addition, the technique for tympanomastoid obliteration are discussed.

Techniques of Simple Mastoidectomy and Canal Wall–Up Mastoidectomy for Chronic Otitis Media

A postauricular incision provides the best access to the lateral mastoid cortex, although an endaural incision with a Heermann extension may be used. The bony exposure of the

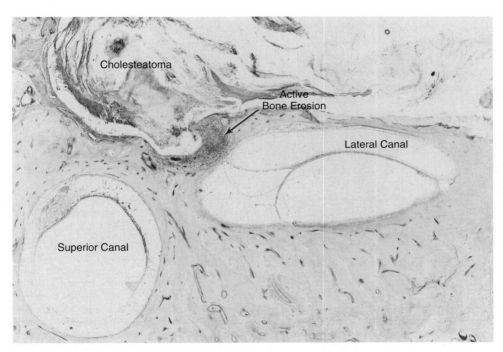

FIG. 17.10 Active rarefying osteitis subjacent to middle ear cholesteatoma in a 65-year-old man with chronic active otitis media of the left ear. The focus of rarefying osteitis is beginning to cause a bony dehiscence of the lateral semicircular canal. 20.3X.

lateral mastoid cortex should include the temporal line superiorly (Chapter 9), at least the posterior half of the circumference of the bony meatus, and should extend inferiorly to the mastoid tip. The field is maintained with self-retaining retractors. Drilling is commenced with a large cutting bur over the mastoid antrum with continuous suction irrigation. The location of the antrum is best determined by the intersection of imaginary lines tangent to the superior and posterior limits of the external bony meatus (Fig. 11A). The middle fossa and posterior fossa plates and the sinodural angle

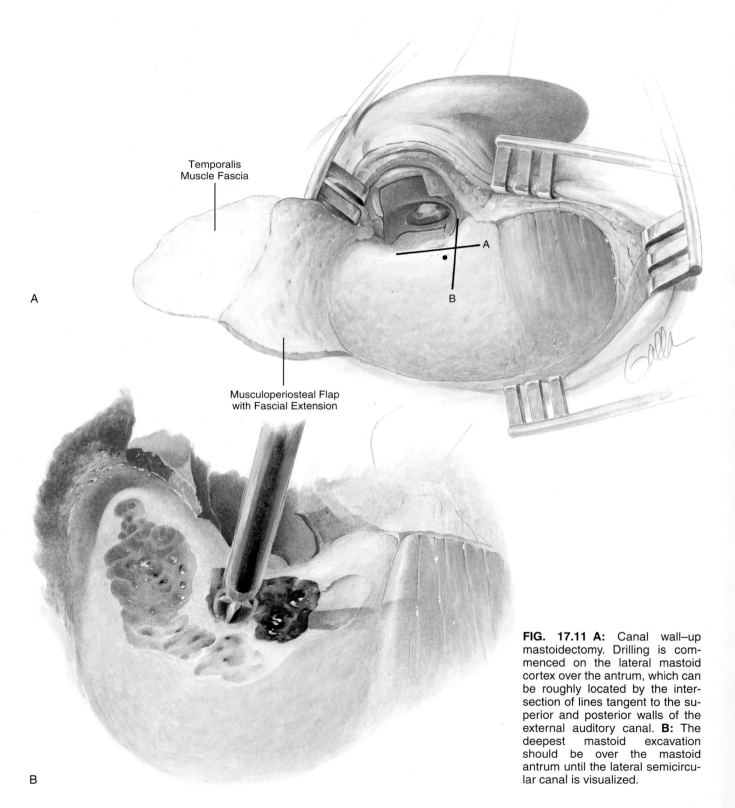

Temporalis
Muscle Fascia

A

B

Musculoperiosteal Flap
with Fascial Extension

A

B

FIG. 17.11 A: Canal wall–up mastoidectomy. Drilling is commenced on the lateral mastoid cortex over the antrum, which can be roughly located by the intersection of lines tangent to the superior and posterior walls of the external auditory canal. **B:** The deepest mastoid excavation should be over the mastoid antrum until the lateral semicircular canal is visualized.

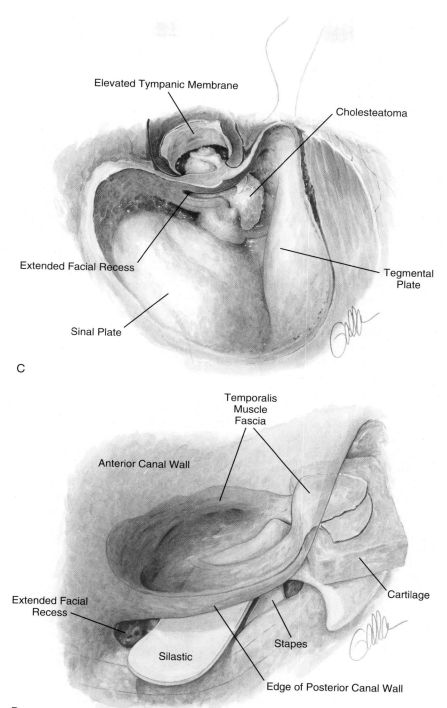

Elevated Tympanic Membrane

Cholesteatoma

Extended Facial Recess

Tegmental Plate

Sinal Plate

C

Temporalis Muscle Fascia

Anterior Canal Wall

Cartilage

Extended Facial Recess

Silastic

Stapes

Edge of Posterior Canal Wall

D

FIG. 17.11, cont'd C: Canal wall–up mastoidectomy completed. The tegmental and sinal plates have been skeletonized and a posterior tympanotomy accomplished. The posterior tympanotomy or "facial recess" is limited by the tympanic annulus laterally, facial nerve medially, chorda tympani nerve inferiorly, and posterior process of the incus superiorly. An extended facial recess approach allows increase in the size of the posterior tympanotomy by sacrifice of the chorda tympani nerve. **D:** During the reconstructive phase of a canal wall–up tympanomastoidectomy, Silastic sheeting is placed through the extended facial recess to ensure aeration of the mastoid compartment.

are then defined. Completion of the exenteration posteriorly will allow better access and instrument angle to the more critical anterior structures. The lateral semicircular canal is identified. This provides a landmark to the facial nerve anteriorly and the incus anterosuperiorly (Fig. 17.11B). Dissection is carried anteriorly, thinning the posterior canal wall using the drill in a superior to inferior direction parallel to the facial nerve. Facial nerve monitoring, either electrophysiologic or visual, is highly desirable during bone removal and subsequent surgery in the vicinity of the facial nerve. The facial canal is delineated using the lateral semicircular canal superiorly and the digastric ridge inferiorly as landmarks. Constant irrigation and use of polishing or diamond burs are necessary as the facial nerve is delineated. Unless facial nerve exploration is contemplated, a thin plate of bone should be left intact over the facial nerve.

The petrosal portions of the central mastoid tract are exenterated, with special attention to the tegmental cells (Fig. 17.11C). If the retrofacial cells are entered, care must be taken to avoid injury to the descending segment of the facial nerve as the drill is withdrawn from the depths of the cavity. The mastoidectomy is extended anteriorly behind the preserved posterior canal wall to perform a posterior atticotomy. A posterior tympanotomy is performed by opening the facial recess. An extended facial recess approach may be accomplished by resection of the chorda tympani nerve and removal of bone lateral to the facial nerve inferior to the chorda (Fig. 17.11C). The remnant of the tympanic membrane is elevated anteriorly, and an anterior atticotomy is performed. Granulation or cholesteatoma is removed from the mastoid, attic, and middle ear, working on both sides of the preserved canal wall and through the posterior tympanotomy. Section of the head of the malleus or removal of the incus may be necessary to eliminate disease from the medial epitympanic compartment.

Once removal of the disease has been accomplished, reconstruction of the tympanic membrane and ossicular chain is performed (Chapter 23). In an effort to prevent postoperative retraction of the tympanic membrane into the attic and antral areas, the tympanoplasty is reinforced by cartilage harvested from the concha or tragus and used to either reinforce the superior aspect of the tympanic graft or to partially obliterate the epitympanic space, particularly when the head of the malleus and incus have been removed. Medium-weight Silastic sheeting is placed in the middle ear and mastoid through the posterior tympanotomy to maintain aeration of the mastoid (Fig. 17.11D). An extensive meatoplasty is avoided to prevent a mastoid cutaneous fistula at the meatus.

The postauricular soft tissue incision is closed by reuniting the superior and inferior musculofascial pedicles, thus reinforcing the conchal area to prevent a mastoid-cutaneous fistula. The postauricular incision is closed in two layers using a 3.0 chromic inverted interrupted subcutaneous suture and 5.0 nylon interrupted cutaneous suture. Working through the enlarged meatus, the Koerner flap is placed between the preserved posterior bony canal wall and the rose-bud packing overlying the tympanic graft. The anterior canal skin is returned to the anterior canal wall, and the unepithelialized surfaces of the superior, inferior, and anterior canal walls are skin grafted, primarily with split-thickness skin grafts. The mastoid incision is drained by placement of a Penrose drain in the inferior aspect of the postauricular wound. A mastoid dressing is applied.

Staging and "Second Look" in Canal Wall–Up Mastoidectomy

Residual or recurrent cholesteatoma, as discovered at a second-stage exploration at 6 to 24 months after canal wall–up mastoidectomy, has been found in up to 30% of procedures (17–19). Because of this high incidence of recurrence, many authors advocate a routine second look procedure in cases of canal wall–up mastoidectomy for cholesteatoma of the central mastoid tract. For cholesteatoma limited to the attic, a second look procedure may not be necessary (20). Austin (21) argues that limiting canal wall–up technique to cases with a large mastoid makes planned second look procedures unnecessary.

Canal Wall–Down Mastoidectomy

The postauricular approach provides the best access. Soft tissue should be retracted to expose the temporal line superiorly, the anterior wall of the external auditory canal anteriorly, the mastoid tip inferiorly, and the mastoid-occipital suture posteriorly. Drilling begins with a large cutting bur using continuous suction irrigation as for a simple or canal wall–up mastoidectomy. A canal wall–up mastoidotomy may be done first to determine whether canal wall–down technique is necessary (Fig. 17.11A–C). Alternately, if a canal wall–down mastoidectomy is planned from the beginning, the drilling over the mastoid antrum is extended anteriorly to include the posterior canal wall. The deepest point of exenteration should be over the antrum until subsequent landmarks are found. The superior, posterior, and inferior limits of exenteration are determined by delineating the tegmental and posterior fossa plates, sinodural angle, lateral venous sinus, and digastric ridge. Thorough exenteration of mastoid cells is particularly important in canal wall–down technique in order to avoid recurrent drainage (6). Cells of particular importance include cells of the tegmen, sinodural angle, and mastoid tip (Fig. 17.12A,B).

In removal of the posterior canal wall, the "bridge" overlying the aditus ad antrum is removed first. This gives wider exposure to the facial nerve, which may be followed inferiorly. Monitoring of the facial nerve visually or electrophysiologically will decrease the incidence of facial nerve injury. For drilling over the fallopian canal, either a polishing or diamond bur with continuous suction irrigation should be used. Using as landmarks the facial nerve identified at the second genu and the digastric ridge inferiorly, the facial canal is thinned using the drills in the superior to inferior di-

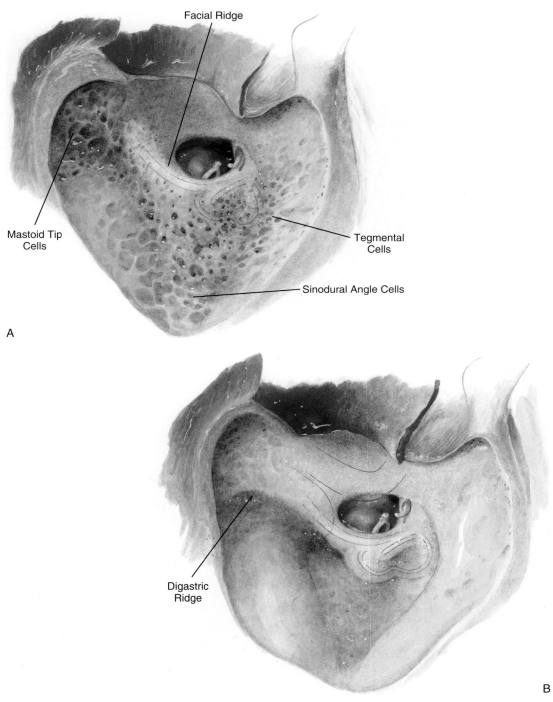

Facial Ridge

Mastoid Tip
Cells

Tegmental
Cells

Sinodural Angle Cells

A

Digastric
Ridge

B

FIG. 17.12 A: Canal wall–down mastoidectomy. The dissection is incomplete in that the cells of the mastoid tip, sinodural angle, and tegmental area remain unexenterated, the facial ridge has not been brought down to the level of the facial nerve, and the canalplasty is inadequate with incomplete exposure of the hypotympanum and mesotympanum. **B:** Canal wall–down mastoidectomy. The dissection is complete. The sinal and tegmental plates have been skeletonized and the cells of the sinodural angle exenterated. The mastoid tip has been developed to demonstrate the digastric ridge. The facial ridge has been taken down to the level of the facial nerve and an anterior and inferior canalplasty have been completed to widely expose the hypotympanum and mesotympanum.

Continued

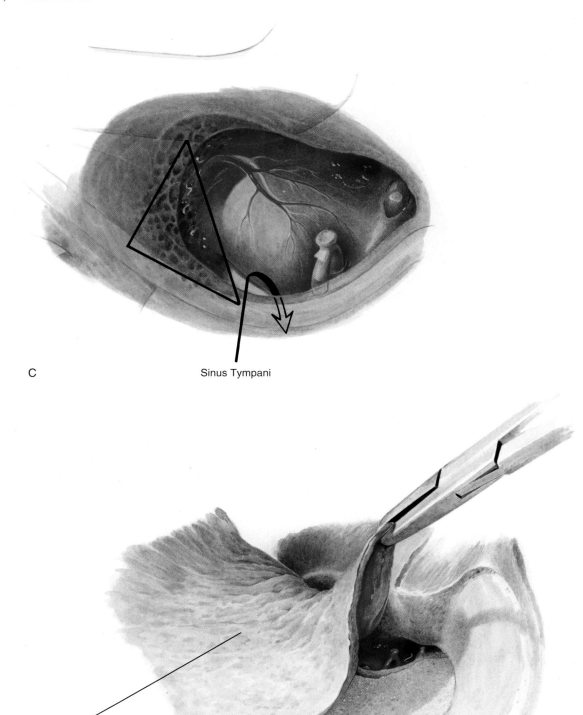

C

Sinus Tympani

Inferiorly Based
Musculoperiosteal Fascial
Pedicled Flap

Bone
Paté

D

FIG. 17.12, cont'd. C: Removal of bone anterior and medial to the facial nerve (*triangle*) will allow exposure of the hypotympanum and increased access to the sinus tympani. **D:** After mastoid exenteration and tympanoplasty, the mastoid may be obliterated using bone paté and an overlying musculofascial pedicle.

rection, avoiding drilling across the nerve. The facial recess cells are exenterated lateral to the facial nerve.

Canalplasty is performed without violation of the temporomandibular joint. The superior aspect of the canal and scutum are removed. The tympanic bone anteriorly and inferiorly is thinned to further expose the middle ear, hypotympanum, and sinus tympani. The bone anterior and medial to the facial nerve is removed (Fig. 17.12C). After the bony exposure has been completed, the residual cholesteatoma is removed first from the mastoid segment and then from the oval window area. Cholesteatoma is easily dissected from underlying bony otic capsule and from the fallopian canal even when the facial nerve is dehiscent. The hypotympanum is carefully inspected for residual chronic otitis media, including granulation tissue. Unexenterated granulation tissue in the hypotympanum and infralabyrinthine cell tract may result in recurrent suppuration without mastoid involvement (6). When all visible disease has been removed, the bony margins of the mastoid and epitympanum are burnished with a diamond bur.

All drilling should be done with continuous suction irrigation. The irrigation should be copious while using diamond burs, because these burs generate more heat than a cutting bur. Thermal injury to the facial nerve can occur when excessive heat is generated by drilling. In addition, a nonviable layer of bone due to excessive heat will delay healing and will interfere with the survival of split-thickness skin grafts that are applied at the termination of the case. The facial nerve may be more vulnerable in revision cases because of distorted anatomy or previous exposure of the facial nerve, with subsequent adhesions to postoperative cicatrix. In general, identification of the nerve in the horizontal segment and second genu is most reliable. The nerve may be then followed proximally toward the geniculate ganglion in the epitympanum, where it may have been exposed by previous surgery or chronic otitis and followed distally toward the stylomastoid foramen.

Details of tympanoplasty are described in Chapter 23. If the middle ear mucosa is in poor condition, Silastic sheeting or a Schuknecht Teflon crescent may be used to maintain aeration of the hypotympanum and patency of the tympanic end of the eustachian tube. The fascial graft should comfortably extend to the superior, anterior, and inferior canal walls but should not reflect more than 1 mm onto those walls to avoid lateralization, blunting of the anterior sulcus, or deep canal stenosis. The fascial graft should extend into the mastoid cavity covering the lateral semicircular canal. The anterior canal skin is returned to the modified anterior canal wall, and previously obtained split-thickness skin grafts backed on silk strips are placed on unepithelialized bone anteriorly, superiorly, and inferiorly. Skin grafts may be placed on the lateral surface of the tympanic graft. The tympanic graft, ossiculoplasty, and split-thickness skin grafts are held in place with a rosebud packing. If all disease has been removed from the mastoid, it may be obliterated using bone paté or musculofascial pedicles. Bone paté is collected from the uninfected lateral mastoid cortex at the outset of the bony dissection using the Sheehy collector. The bone paté is segregated from

the rosebud packing by an inferiorly based musculoperiosteal-fascial pedicled flap (Fig. 17.12D). Alternately, or in conjunction with bone paté, the mastoid bowl may be reduced in size by obliteration with inferiorly or superiorly based muscle pedicles. Removal of bone from the mastoid tip to the level of the digastric muscle will allow easier rotation of the muscle pedicle inferiorly and also will provide some obliteration of the mastoid by decreasing its depth.

The postauricular incision is closed in two layers using a 3.0 chromic inverted interrupted subcutaneous suture and a 4.0 nylon cutaneous suture. The wound is drained with a Penrose drain. The previously elevated Koerner flap is reflected into the mastoid bowl anterior to musculofascial flaps and posterior to the rosebud packing. The lateral meatus is filled with Aureomycin-impregnated iodiform gauze and a standard mastoid dressing applied.

Modifications of Surgical Procedure for Revision Canal Wall–Down Mastoidectomy

Revision mastoid surgery requires modification of the standard primary surgical procedure in order to avoid injury to structures such as the dura, lateral venous sinus, and the facial nerve, which may remain exposed after primary surgery. A longer postauricular incision will allow identification of the plane of the temporalis fascia superiorly above the area of previous surgical exposure. This will also allow wider exposure posteriorly. In revision mastoid surgery, fibrous tissue tends to obliterate and obscure surgical planes. Incisions through the postauricular subcutaneous tissue to the lateral mastoid cortex should be done superior and posterior to the previous mastoid defect in order to find a clean surgical plane and to avoid injury to dura and lateral venous sinus that may have been exposed in the previous procedure.

Elevation of the musculofascial pedicles proceeds from the posterior aspect toward the mastoid bowl. Adhesions between the pedicles and underlying tissue are sharply cut rather than avulsed in order to avoid injury to the underlying dura. Generally, resistance met in elevation of the previous obliterative musculofascial flaps implies adhesion to exposed dura. Identification of dura through the thinned bone superiorly and posteriorly will allow delineation of the surgical field, and extension from these known landmarks into the disturbed previous surgical field will help to avoid injury to dura, semicircular canals, and facial nerve. In revision procedures, particular attention should be paid to exenteration of tegmental, sinodural, and mastoid tip cells, as well as wide canalplasty, maximal lowering of the facial ridge, and removal of bone anterior and inferior to the facial nerve to widely expose the hypotympanum (20).

Tympanomastoid Obliteration

Total tympanomastoid obliteration (22–24) may be performed in cases of chronic otitis media with no useful cochlear function and in which the surgeon is confident of total removal of disease. It may also be used successfully in severe trauma to the temporal bone to repair cerebrospinal fluid otorhinorrhea and may be combined with facial nerve exploration for concomitant injury to the facial nerve. In addition, tympanomastoid obliteration may be performed after extended radical mastoidectomy for neoplastic disease of the middle ear and mastoid. Total tympanomastoid obliteration may also be used in conjunction with cochlear implantation, either as a primary staged procedure in an ear with chronic active otitis media or as part of a primary procedure when osseous obliteration of the cochlear duct requires extensive drilling of the cochlear capsule (Chapter 27).

The obliteration allows rapid healing and provides a thick soft-tissue protection for underlying bone, both in preparation for postoperative radiotherapy (25). In addition to a meticulous canal wall–down mastoidectomy, this procedure includes the following:

1. In removal of malleus and incus and all accessible middle ear mucosa, the mastoid bowl and middle ear are burnished with a diamond bur with suction/irrigation. Visible cell partitions must be meticulously removed.
2. To close the external meatus primarily, the external canal is transected, and the cartilage of the auricular segment of the external canal is removed in conjunction with elevation of the remaining skin at the meatus (Fig. 17.13A,B).

3. The skin of the external ear canal is closed by joining short anterior and posterior laterally based skin flaps and suturing with interrupted nylon or resorbable suture (Fig. 17.13C).
4. The meatal closure is reinforced medially by closure of soft tissue underlying auricular cartilage (Fig. 17.13D).
5. The eustachian tube orifice is cleaned of all mucosa and obstructed with a fascial plug held in place by bone wax, and the tympanomastoid compartment is obliterated with fat harvested from the abdominal wall. Superiorly and inferiorly based muscle pedicles, if available, may be used to help obliterate the mastoid or may be used to reinforce the meatal closure. The temporoparietal fascial flap provides a well-vascularized pedicle, which may be used to supplement other obliterative techniques, particularly in cases in which poor vascularization of bone may be anticipated, such as with preoperative radiotherapy. A postauricular incision is closed in two layers and the wound drained for 1 day.

The *Bondy-modified mastoidectomy* (26–28) involves a canal wall–down approach with preservation of the tympanic membrane and ossicular system. It is a good procedure for the relatively unusual circumstance when chronic otitis media is limited to the lateral epitympanic space and mastoid, but spares the middle ear and medial epitympanic

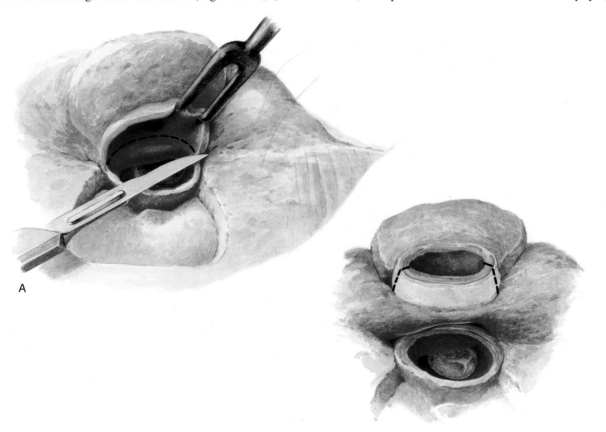

FIG. 17.13 A: Tympanomastoid obliteration. The external auditory canal is identified via a postauricular incision. Retaining a small anteriorly based musculofascial pedicle, the external auditory canal is transected and reflected anteriorly.

Continued

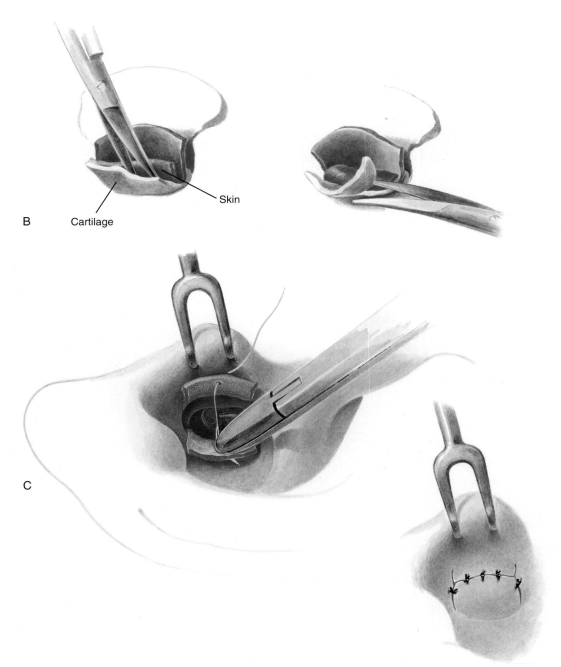

B Cartilage Skin

C

FIG. 17.13, cont'd. B: Cartilage is resected from the auricular segment of the external auditory canal. **C:** Anteriorly and posteriorly based skin flaps are closed in an H pattern after resection of underlying cartilage. The external auditory meatus is closed by suturing the anteriorly and posteriorly based skin flaps.

Continued

space. It is particularly useful in a poorly pneumatized mastoid that makes the canal wall–up approach difficult and in which the creation of a mastoid bowl creates little postoperative problem. It has the advantage of combining preservation of the ossicular chain and tympanic membrane with exteriorization of the mastoid space for otologic follow-up.

The *radical mastoidectomy* is a canal wall–down approach with sacrifice of the tympanic membrane, malleus, and incus and without obliteration of the mastoid or reconstruction of the ossicular system or tympanic membrane. Today this procedure should be done very rarely. The indications are limited to very extensive cholesteatoma or other disorders in which exteriorization of the mastoid and tympanic compartments is desirable.

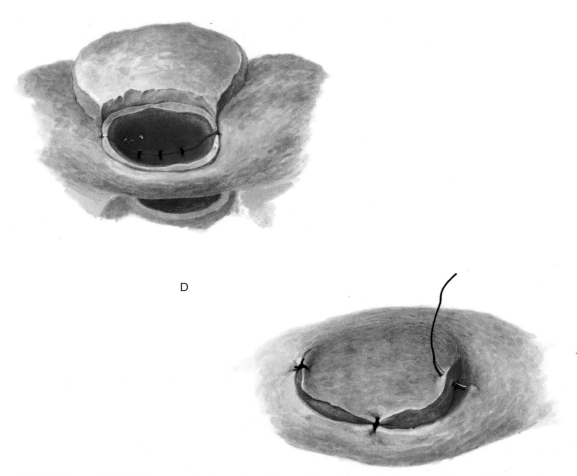

D

FIG. 17.13, cont'd. D: The meatal closure is reinforced from the medial aspect of the auricle by reflecting the anteriorly based musculofascial pedicle over the suture line at the meatus.

Postoperative Care Following Mastoidectomy

After a mastoidectomy (canal wall–up or canal wall–down or tympanomastoid obliteration), the postauricular drain is removed on the first postoperative day and the patient is generally ready for discharge. There is a paucity of information on the utility of perioperative and postoperative antibiotic usage. However, in most cases an oral antibiotic with coverage for *Staphylococcus aureus* is selected for 1 week postoperatively.

The postauricular sutures and outer packing are removed at 1 week, and the inner rosebud packing is removed at the end of 2 weeks. The donor site for split-thickness skin grafts is usually inspected at week 1 and usually is fully healed by week 2. The patient is then followed at 2- or 3-week intervals to monitor the healing process. Use of an antibiotic ointment or antibiotic topical otic drops will help prevent superinfection. It is important that the patient be followed closely until complete epithelialization is accomplished. Prolonged periods of excessive granulations may cause postoperative stenosis or blunting of the anterior sulcus, severely compromising postoperative care and hearing results. Delayed split-thickness skin grafting (Chapter 10) may be required. Granulation tissue in pediatric patients in general is more exuberant than in adults, requiring even more careful postoperative follow-up. It is essential to stress the importance of postoperative care with patients beginning in the preoperative phase.

SURGICAL COMPLICATIONS

Intraoperative Complications

Injury to the Dura, Spinal Fluid Leakage

Exposure of the dura is a common finding during mastoid surgery as a result of bone resorption or surgical exenteration and is therefore subject to injury. If significant injury to the dura or spinal fluid leakage occurs intraoperatively, a culture of mastoid contents should be done and the procedure completed as planned. Injury to the dura is repaired by an overlay graft of temporalis fascia reinforced with musculofascial pedicles. Intravenous antibiotic prophylaxis is continued through the first postoperative day and then converted to oral coverage. If there is no continued leakage, the patient may be discharged at the usual time. Discharge instructions should specifically include the signs and symptoms of meningitis.

Surgical Fistulization of a Semicircular Canal

If fistulization of a semicircular canal occurs during the process of drilling or removal of disease, the fistula should be immediately repaired, preferably with a tissue graft such as temporalis fascia, perichondrium, or fat, and the repair site protected with a neurosurgical patty or Surgicel while the procedure is completed. To prevent chronic postoperative vestibular symptoms, the area of repair should be covered with bone paté or musculofascial flaps.

If the presence of a dehiscence either of the vestibular or cochlear labyrinth is suspected preoperatively based on clinical symptoms and signs and preoperative radiologic evaluation, the dissection in the area of suspect sites of dehiscence should be delayed as long as possible toward the termination of the procedure.

Accidental Removal of Stapes Footplate

If, in the course of removal of granulation of cholesteatoma, the stapediovestibular joint is breached or the footplate fractured, the stapes footplate should be removed in its entirety and replaced immediately with a fat graft to prevent contamination of the inner ear. This area should be protected with a small neurosurgical patty while the mastoid procedure is completed. The fat graft is left in the oval window and temporalis fascia placed lateral to it to create a type V tympanoplasty. Surgical manipulation of granulation tissue and/or cholesteatoma in the oval window niche should be delayed as long as possible toward the end of the procedure so that the potential duration of contamination of the inner ear may be minimized.

Injury to the Facial Nerve

Facial nerve monitoring, either visual or electrophysiologic, should be performed during the course of mastoid surgery to prevent accidental injury. Use of electrical stimulation will aid in the identification of the course of the nerve. It is important to recognize that standard electromyography (EMG) monitoring of the facial nerve may not detect thermal injury or electrocoagulation injury to the facial nerve. Although EMG monitoring is sensitive to compression of the nerve that may occur with surgical instruments, including a drill, it may not detect a transsection of the nerve with a sharp instrument such as a surgical blade. Use of suction irrigation will prevent thermal injury to the facial nerve. If during the course of mastoid surgery an iatrogenic injury to the nerve is suspected, additional bone overlying the fallopian canal on both sides of the site of suspected injury should be removed to thoroughly inspect the facial nerve. A contusion requires only this decompression; however, severance of the nerve is treated primarily by end-to-end anastomosis or nerve grafting (Chapter 36).

The site of injury should be examined at the time of initial surgery in order to avoid unnecessary reexploration if facial paralysis is found postoperatively.

Injury to the Lateral Venous Sinus or Jugular Bulb

If in the course of removal of disease from the central mastoid tract, retrofacial cell tract, or hypotympanum, the lateral venous sinus is entered, a patch of Surgicel and Gelfoam, reinforced by applied pressure for a few minutes, will generally suffice. The patch should be considerably larger than the rent to prevent accidental embolization. Ligation or total occlusion is rarely necessary. The patch site is protected with a neurosurgical patty while the mastoid procedure is completed, and the area of repair is then covered with musculofascial pedicles in the mastoid or reinforced with temporalis fascia in the hypotympanum.

Postoperative Complications

Facial Nerve Paralysis

For a patient who awakes in the recovery room with facial nerve paralysis, when the cause of the injury was unrecognized intraoperatively, reexploration of the ear should be done, generally within 2 days. The operating surgeon should be capable of nerve grafting if necessary. Occasionally, lidocaine (Xylocaine) during the course of a mastoid procedure may produce temporary facial paresis or paralysis, but this effect should resolve within a few hours postoperatively. If iatrogenic injury to the nerve was recognized intraoperatively and the nerve was explored and assessed, reexploration is unnecessary.

If postoperative paresis without total paralysis is present and does not clear within 2 hours postoperatively, removal or loosening of the packing is in order. The use of corticosteroids may reduce postoperative swelling and lessen the pressure on the nerve. If the paresis progresses to a full paralysis with degeneration, as assessed by electroneuronography, identification and examination of the injured segment and decompression of that segment should be performed.

Postoperative Stenosis

Postoperative fibrosis, which is particularly exuberant in children, may result in meatal or canal stenosis. The progress of healing should be carefully followed at 2- to 3-week intervals after the inner packing is removed. Granulation should be removed and cauterized and, if recurrent, a delayed split-thickness skin graft should be performed to avoid blunting and meatal or canal stenosis (Chapter 10).

REFERENCES

1. Nadol JB Jr. The chronic draining ear. In: Gates GA, ed. *Current therapy in otolaryngology—head and neck surgery*, 3rd ed. Philadelphia: BC Decker, 1987;18–22.
2. Ort HH. On recurrence in cavities after radical mastoidectomy with special reference to the complications which may arise. *Acta Otolaryngol (Stockh)* 1957;47:346–352.
3. Jepson O, Swergius E. Cavities after retro-auricular radical ear operations with special reference to significance of primary factors. *Acta Otolaryngol (Stockh)* 1951;39:388–394.

4. Smyth, GD. Postoperative cholesteatoma combined approach tympanoplasty. *J Laryngol Otol* 1976;90:597–621.

5. Sheehy J, Brackmann DE, Graham MD. Cholesteatoma surgery: residual and recurrent disease. A review of 1,024 cases. *Ann Otol Rhinol Laryngol* 1977;86:451–462.

6. Nadol JB Jr. Causes of failure of mastoidectomy for chronic otitis media. *Laryngoscope* 1985;95:410–413.

7. Nadol JB Jr, Krouse JH. The hypotympanum and infralabyrinthine cells in chronic otitis media. *Laryngoscope* 1991;101:137–141.

8. Rambo JHJ. The use of musculoplasty advantages and disadvantages. *Ann Otol Rhinol Laryngol* 1965;74:535–554.

9. Jokipii AM, Karma P, Ojala K, et al. Anaerobic bacteria and chronic otitis media. *Arch Otolaryngol* 1977;103:278–280.

10. Erkan M, Aslan T, Sevuk E, et al. Bacteriology of chronic suppurative otitis media. *Ann Otol Rhinol Laryngol* 1994;103:771–774.

11. Kenna MA, Bluestone CD, Reilly JS, et al. Medical management of chronic suppurative otitis media without cholesteatoma in children. *Laryngoscope* 1986;96:146–151.

12. Merchant SN, Wang P-C, Jang CH, et al Efficacy of tympanomastoid surgery for control of infection in active chronic otitis media. *Laryngoscope* 1997;107:872–877, 1997.

13. Schuknecht HF. *Pathology of the ear.* Cambridge, MA: Harvard University Press, 1974.

14. Nadol JB Jr, Arnold WJ. Ear. In: Arnold WJ, Laissue JA, Friedmann I, et al. *Diseases of the head and neck. An atlas of histopathology.* New York: Georg Thieme Verlag, 1987;22–54.

15. Chole RA. Cellular and subcellular events of bone resorption in human and experimental cholesteatoma: the role of osteoclasts. *Laryngoscope* 1984;94:76–95.

16. Moriyama H, Huang CC, Abramson M, et al. Bone resorption factors in chronic otitis media. *Otolaryngol Head Neck Surg* 1984;92:322–328.

17. Glasscock ME, Miller GW. Intact canal wall tympanoplasty in the management of cholesteatoma. *Laryngoscope* 1976;86:1639–1657.

18. Sheehy JL, Crabtree JA. Tympanoplasty: staging the operation. *Laryngoscope* 1973;83:1594–1621.

19. Smyth GDL. Surgical treatment of cholesteatoma: the role of staging in closed operations. *Ann Otol Rhinol Laryngol* 1988;97:667–669.

20. Tos M, Lau T. Attic cholesteatoma. Recurrence rate related to observation time. *Am J Otol* 1988;9:456–464.

21. Austin DF. Single-stage surgery for cholesteatoma: an actuarial analysis. *Am J Otol* 1989;10:419–425.

22. Bartels LJ, Sheehy JL. Total obliteration of the mastoid, middle ear, and external auditory canal. A review of 27 cases. *Laryngoscope* 1981;91:1100–1108.

23. Gacek RR. Mastoid and middle ear cavity obliteration for control of otitis media. *Ann Otol Rhinol Laryngol* 1976;85:305–309.

24. Rambo JHT. Primary closure of the radical mastoidectomy wound: a technique to eliminate postoperative care. *Laryngoscope* 1958;68:1216–1227.

25. Nadol JB Jr, Schuknecht HF. Obliteration of the mastoid in the treatment of tumors of the temporal bone. *Ann Otol Rhinol Laryngol* 1984;93:6–12.

26. Bondy G. Totalaufmeisselung mit Erhaltung von Trommelfell und Gehorknoch-elchen. *Monatschr Ohrenheilk* 1910;44:15.

27. Baron SH. Modified radical mastoidectomy. Preservation of the cholesteatoma matrix; a method of making a flap in the endaural technic. *Arch Otolaryngol* 1949;49:280–302.

28. Shambaugh GE Jr. Primary skin graft in modified (Bondy) radical mastoidectomy. For preservation of hearing in cases of genuine cholesteatoma. *Arch Otolaryngol* 1936;23:222–228.

CHAPTER 18

Complications of Chronic Otitis Media

Jeffrey P. Harris, David W. Kim, and David H. Darrow

A mastoid abscess was first opened. A sinus persisted; bony sequestra were then removed to expose the dura. After probing, an incision was made into the dura and a finger introduced; this resulting in a release of pus. The cavity was irrigated with barley water containing a little turpentine and balsam. A silver tube was made and this was inserted for drainage. The patient recovered.

—S.F. Morand, 1768 (1)

Complications of chronic otitis media (COM) occur when chronic infection and/or cholesteatoma within the middle ear and mastoid spaces extend to regions beyond their bony confines. They result from the erosion of bone by cholesteatoma or by the spread of infection through intact bone via small venules or preformed pathways. They may involve adjacent sites within the temporal bone, the posterior or middle cranial fossae, or the extratemporal soft tissues or more distal sites reached by hematogenous spread (Fig. 18.1).

Once considered commonplace in the course of otitis media and mastoiditis, otogenic complications have become rare sequelae in these disorders. The advent of modern antibiotic therapy has brought a dramatic decline in the incidence and morbidity of otogenic complications. In 1935 Kafka (2) studied a series of 2,100 patients with acute mastoiditis and 1,125 patients with chronic mastoiditis and reported an intracranial complication rate of 6.4%; mortality was 76.4% among those with complications. In contrast, a series of 100 patients with central nervous system (CNS) complications of active ear disease studied by Gower and McGuirt (3) in 1983 represented less than 0.5% of all admissions coded for intracranial complications or mastoid surgery, and mortality was 10% in this group. Similarly, an autopsy review by Courville (4) found a tenfold reduction in the death rate from acute and chronic ear disease attributable to the development of antibiotics. Prellner and Rydell estimate a reduction of the incidence of intracranial complications from 2% to 0.02% with the advent of antibiotics (5).

An unfortunate consequence of the decline of otogenic complications has been a decreased recognition of the impending complications of otitis media. Fever and inflammation, which once heralded the progression of disease, are now often suppressed by medical therapy. Thus the effectiveness of modern therapy and the low incidence of complications have led to complacency in the treatment of middle ear infections and a lack of familiarity with the manifestations of complications.

The otolaryngologist must bear in mind that complications of COM, especially in the immunocompromised host, may rapidly result in death. Therefore it is imperative that he or she be familiar with the clinical manifestations of these complications.

FACTORS IN THE SPREAD OF INFECTION

Most reports published during the antibiotic era suggest that otogenic complications are more likely to arise from cases of chronic middle ear disease rather than from acute processes, though complications due to acute otitis media may be more common in the pediatric age group (6–8). The pathophysiology and initial management of COM have been enumerated in previous chapters. However, several factors determining the spread of infection beyond the middle ear space bear mention here:

1. Species and virulence of the organism. Aerobic bacteria may be cultured from some 70% of middle ears with COM, and *Proteus* sp. and *Pseudomonas aeruginosa* are the most common offending organisms (9). Anaerobes are present in nearly equal frequency, most notably *Bacteroides* sp., *Peptococcus/Peptostreptococcus* sp., and *Propionibacterium acnes*. Mixed infections are present in more than 50% of these cases. Many organisms cultured from chronic suppurative effusions may represent colonization of the ear, and their preponderance may mask the presence of more virulent organisms.

2. Host conditions. The host tissue responds to the release of toxic substances from the infecting organisms by mounting an inflammatory reaction, and cells involved in the response assist in the removal of the offending bacteria. Several conditions associated with immune

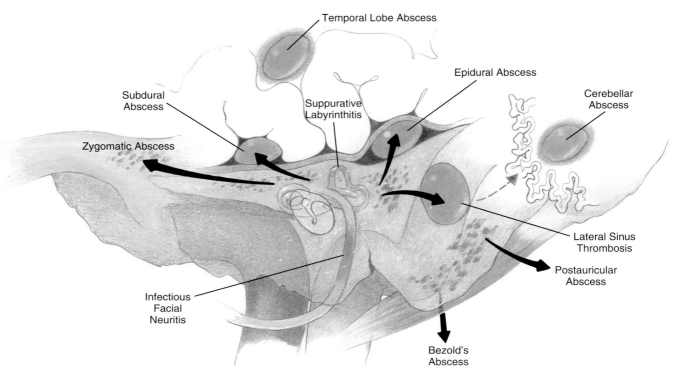

FIG. 18.1 Pathways by which complications result in chronic otitis media.

compromise, such as infancy, old age, diabetes, malnutrition, malignancy, acquired immunodeficiency syndrome (AIDS), and immunodeficiency, are known to diminish the effectiveness of this response and therefore increase the likelihood of spread and the risk of complications. Under these conditions, opportunistic organisms may predominate among the tympanic flora and colonizing organisms may become more virulent. Recent work suggests that patients with complications of COM are more likely to be younger (less than 25 years old) and that younger patients undergoing mastoid surgery for COM were more likely to have complications (10). Disease may be more aggressive in the pediatric population because of increased exposure to respiratory pathogens, chronicity of disease, and immaturity of immune defenses.

3. Prior therapy. Although topical antibiotic combinations are commonly used to treat COM, they are often met by resistant organisms and are unreliably distributed to the affected area. Ciprofloxacin, an antipseudomonal antibiotic, has demonstrated efficacy in the control of chronic ear disease in adults (11,12). However, timely surgical intervention, aimed at debridement of the middle ear and mastoid spaces, establishment of adequate drainage, and reconstruction of defects in the tympanic membrane, remains the cornerstone of therapy in the prevention of otogenic complications. In tympanomastoid surgery, Merchant et al. reported poorer control of infection after surgery for COM with granulation tissue

compared with COM with cholesteatoma. This may be due to an inherent problem of the mucosa. Thus even after disease and unfavorable anatomy are removed, the abnormal mucosa predisposes to the production of more granulations. This variant of COM would therefore be more likely to produce complications (13).

PATHWAYS IN THE SPREAD OF INFECTION

When the mucosal defense system is unable to deter the progression of disease, the integrity of the bone of the middle ear becomes critical. Infection must extend through this bone for complications of middle ear disease to occur. Spread of infection through the osseous barrier may occur in the following several ways:

1. Direct erosion through bone demineralized by cholesteatoma or chronic inflammation.
2. Thrombophlebitic spread through small veins and haversian canals to the dural sinuses.
3. Extension through normal anatomic pathways, including the oval and round windows, the cochlear and vestibular aqueducts, and bony dehiscences and fissures.
4. Extension through iatrogenically or traumatically created bony defects.

Direct extension is the route most commonly implicated in complications due to COM. Extradural abscesses, subperiosteal abscesses, and lateral sinus thrombosis usually occur by this mechanism. Patients will commonly present with a prodrome of partial or intermittent impairment of structures affected by the advancing infection, most notably pain, abducens palsy, facial paralysis, and vertigo. Thrombophlebitic spread is more common in acute infections, in acute exacerbations of chronic infection, and in brain abscess formation. A prodromal period is often absent, and intact bony walls are often found at surgery.

CLASSIFICATION

Complications of COM are generally grouped into two main categories:

1. Complications involving the cranial cavity, including the following:
   Extradural abscess
   Lateral sinus thrombosis
   Brain abscess
   Meningitis
   Subdural infection
   Otitic hydrocephalus
2. Complications involving the temporal bone and extratemporal soft tissues, including the following:
   Subperiosteal and Bezold's abscesses
   Facial paralysis
   Petrous apicitis
   Labyrinthitis
   Sensorineural hearing loss

Among the intracranial complications, meningitis is probably the most commonly encountered (3,7,14), although some authors report more cases of brain abscess (15) and epidural abscess (16) in their series. Brain abscess is generally considered to have the highest rate of mortality (6,14). Similar data regarding the relative incidence of temporal bone complications have not been reported.

In approximately one third of cases, two or more otogenic complications are present concomitantly (17), usually reflecting the path of least resistance chosen by the spreading infection. During an exploration for lateral sinus thrombosis, for example, it is not uncommon to also find a perisinus abscess from which it may have originated or a brain abscess to which it may have progressed. It is therefore incumbent upon the otolaryngologist to thoroughly investigate all potential complications prior to the initiation of therapy.

With the rapid spread of human immunodeficiency virus (HIV) and AIDS in the last quarter century, a growing number of immunosuppressed patients have incurred certain complications of COM that were not commonly seen before. The spread of disease in this patient population tends to be more extensive and follow a more fulminant course. In addition, opportunistic pathogens not usually found in the ear and adjacent structures are more likely to flourish in the immunocompromised host. As more and more severely immunocompromised patients live longer, recognition of these rare complications of COM will become increasingly important.

SYMPTOMS AND SIGNS OF IMPENDING COMPLICATION

The presentation of complicated COM is well described by Neely (8) and Snow (18) and has been reviewed by Schwaber et al. (16). Early signs and symptoms include fetid otorrhea, deep pain, and headache. The development of malodorous, purulent discharge from the ear is highly suggestive of bone destruction. It is postulated that the longer the period of drainage, the greater the amount of bone destruction that has occurred (16). Pain is generally not associated with COM but may arise in exacerbations of the disease or with progressive destruction of bone or obstruction of drainage of purulent material from the mastoid space via the aditus. Uncomplicated exacerbations are associated with transient pain, whereas bone erosion or obstruction to drainage causes deep and constant pain. The latter may suggest a developing complication.

The appearance of the tympanic membrane may provide important information about the condition of the middle ear. Although the presence of chronic perforation with associated otorrhea is classically cited as the tympanic membrane feature in COM, other abnormalities may herald middle ear disease. Pathologic correlates between tympanic membrane and middle ear findings in temporal bones with COM reveal that myringosclerosis even without perforation is significantly associated with middle ear granulation tissue and ossicular pathology. Although both retraction pockets and perforations are associated with middle ear disease, the presence of both together have an additive effect on predicting cholesteatoma, ossicular pathology, and cholesterol granuloma. In addition, a significant fraction of middle ear problems may be hidden behind a normal-appearing tympanic membrane, particularly in infants (19). This underscores the need for tests such as tympanometry or imaging in patients with persistent aural symptoms and normal findings on otoscopic examination.

Fever, nausea, and altered mental status may be present at the time that a complication of COM is diagnosed, but generally these symptoms occur later in the course of the infection. Rarer findings at presentation include dysequilibrium, hearing loss, subperiosteal abscess, cranial neuropathies, nuchal rigidity, and seizures and imply that a complication is imminent or has already occurred.

INITIAL MANAGEMENT

A thorough history and physical examination should be performed on all patients suspected of having a complication of COM. Symptoms of headache, neck pain, and visual changes suggest intracranial involvement, and patients with signs of papilledema, impaired extraocular movement, nuchal rigidity, or hemiparesis warrant immediate neurosurgical evaluation. When intracranial extension is uncertain, lumbar puncture may be helpful in arriving at a diagnosis. All patients suspected of having intracranial disease should undergo a period of observation by qualified neurosurgical personnel.

Computed tomography (CT) scanning with intravenous contrast is the imaging modality of choice in screening for complications of COM. Magnetic resonance imaging (MRI) and MR angiography (MRA) are useful in the definitive diagnosis of certain of these complications. However, CT is almost uniformly positive in cases of intracranial extension and gives the most accurate assessment of bone involvement. CT scanning is therefore an indispensable part of the evaluation of all patients suspected of having otogenic complications.

Intravenous antibiotic therapy should be started as soon as possible. Polymicrobial infection is common in COM and its complications, and broad-spectrum coverage is indicated. Multiple drug therapy may be necessary to accomplish this goal. Traditionally, the penicillins, in combination with stronger anaerobic coverage such as metronidazole, were considered standard primary therapy. However, the high incidence of *Pseudomonas* in these infections, as well as the increasing resistance of gram-positive organisms to penicillins, have prompted the use of alternative agents. Chloramphenicol has often been used and provides exceptional broad-spectrum coverage but has numerous side effects. Its use may be most appropriate in complications of acute otitis media in which *Haemophilus influenzae* is the likely causative organism. Ticarcillin/clavulanic acid provides excellent coverage for the organisms most commonly implicated in these infections (including *Pseudomonas*) and achieves reasonable cerebrospinal fluid (CSF) levels in the presence of meningeal inflammation (20). Ceftazidime, a third-generation cephalosporin with enhanced efficacy against *Pseudomonas,* may be useful in combination with anaerobic coverage. Ciprofloxacin, a fluoroquinolone, is also excellent against *Pseudomonas* and has the added benefit of having similar circulating concentrations in the oral and parenteral routes.

In general, it is desirable to delay surgical treatment of the infected ear until the patient is neurologically and systemically stable. However, judicious surgical intervention at the first signs of clinical deterioration and progression of infection may be lifesaving.

INTRACRANIAL COMPLICATIONS

Extradural Abscess

Cholesteatoma and granulation tissue often complicate chronic suppurative otitis media and have a propensity to erode adjacent bony structures. When these processes reach the periphery of the mastoid space, erosion often proceeds until dura is exposed but is then impeded by this relatively resistant structure. The result is an inflammation of the dura known as pachymeningitis, which is often followed by the production of granulations along the dura. The accumulation of purulent material in this area results in a collection of pus between the dura and the bony wall known as an extradural or epidural abscess (21) (Fig. 18.2).

Commonly, resorption of bone will occur in the region of the tegmen, resulting in an extradural abscess of the middle cranial fossa (Fig. 18.3). The infectious process in such cases begins lateral to the attachment of the dura at the arcuate eminence, which serves to limit the extent of the abscess. An abscess developing medial to the arcuate eminence may abut the petrous apex, involving the fifth and sixth cranial nerves and resulting in facial pain and diplopia (Gradenigo's syndrome). In the middle fossa, lateral to the arcuate eminence, the dura is loosely attached and large abscesses may develop, accompanied by neurologic signs of mass effect. Lateral erosion through the cranium produces the subperiosteal abscess known as Pott's puffy tumor. Posterior fossa extradural abscesses usually result from the erosion of bone in Trautmann's triangle or over the lateral sinus. The latter, known as a perisinus abscess, is often associated with the development of lateral sinus thrombosis. Untreated posterior fossa abscesses may also extend to the neck via the jugular foramen.

Symptoms of extradural abscess may include temporal headache, ear pain, or low-grade fever, but often both physician and patient become aware of its presence only after exposure during elective mastoidectomy. Extradural abscesses of long standing are an exception to this rule and are often accompanied by mild nuchal rigidity and meningismus. Characteristically, when symptoms are present, they are suddenly relieved during periods of spontaneous drainage into the mastoid. Exacerbation of the aural discharge on compression of the ipsilateral jugular vein is also highly suggestive. Lumbar puncture may reveal an increased white cell count, but usually with lymphocyte predominance. Glucose levels are normal, and no organisms are seen. When extradural abscess is suspected prior to surgery, CT scanning is preferred for confirmation of the diagnosis.

Treatment

Surgical intervention is indicated whenever physical examination or CT scan is suggestive of extradural abscess; antimicrobial therapy will not effectively penetrate the walls of the abscess. Mastoidectomy is performed, and the tegmen and sinus plates are removed. Loose granulation tissue is removed, and a border of normal dura is exposed peripherally around the affected site. Cautious manipulation of adherent granulations is necessary to avoid violation of the dura. Cholesteatoma matrix covering a dural exposure may be left behind if well exteriorized. Removal of cholesteatoma is otherwise completed, and a Penrose drain is placed into the mastoid cavity at the end of the procedure. Culture-specific systemic and topical postoperative antibiotics help to prevent the spread of residual organisms throughout the tissues and the incised auricular cartilage and help to prevent postoperative wound breakdown and perichondritis. A 6-week course of antibiotic therapy is generally recommended in cases where a diagnosis or suspicion of osteomyelitis is made.

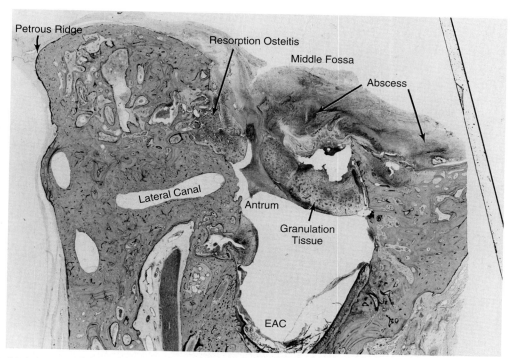

FIG. 18.2 Male, age 58. This man had purulent left otorrhea for many years. At the age of 58 he was hospitalized for left otalgia, vertigo, fever, chills, and vomiting. He became semicomatose and showed left facial weakness. Intensive antibiotic therapy was instituted, and several days later a left radical mastoidectomy revealed chronic granulomatous mastoiditis without cholesteatoma. The tegmen was found to be dehiscent, and granulation tissue extended into the middle cranial fossa. The patient improved temporarily, but 12 days later he became aphasic. Angiography showed an avascular area in the left temporal lobe. A left temporal craniotomy was performed to drain a large abscess of the temporal lobe that appeared to communicate with the mastoid. The patient died the following day. Autopsy revealed a large temporal lobe abscess. Left ear, vertical section: An extensive defect in the tegmen of the mastoid is filled with granulation tissue and a large extradural abscess. EAC, external auditory canal. 5.8X.

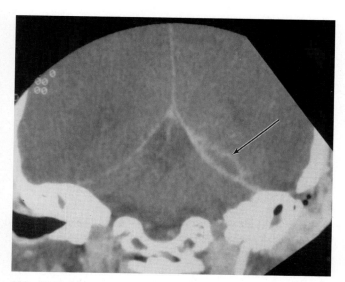

FIG. 18.3 Coronal CT demonstrating extradural abscess extending along tentorium (*arrow*) in a patient with chronic mastoiditis.

Lateral Sinus Thrombosis

Extension of mastoid cavity disease to adjacent venous sinuses may occur through direct extension through the dura or by spread along mastoid or middle emissary veins. The transverse sinus, which begins at the internal occipital protuberance, exits the tentorium as the sigmoid sinus. The sigmoid is joined by the superior and inferior petrosal sinuses before leaving the cranium as the internal jugular vein. The lateral sinus is the segment of the transverse-sigmoid complex immediately beneath the mastoid air cells and is the region most susceptible to thrombosis or thrombophlebitis due to mastoid disease (Fig. 18.4). However, otogenic involvement of other dural sinuses has been reported (22).

Septic lateral sinus thrombosis was first described in the mid-nineteenth century and carried a mortality rate of 100% until the first successful surgical intervention by Lane in 1888 (cited by Tveteras et al. [23]). With improvement in surgical technique, this rate fell to less than 30% to 50% by the early 1900s (14,24). Mortality in the antibiotic era remains in the range of 10% to 36% (14,22,25,26). Thus lateral sinus thrombosis continues to be a significant and lethal complication of COM.

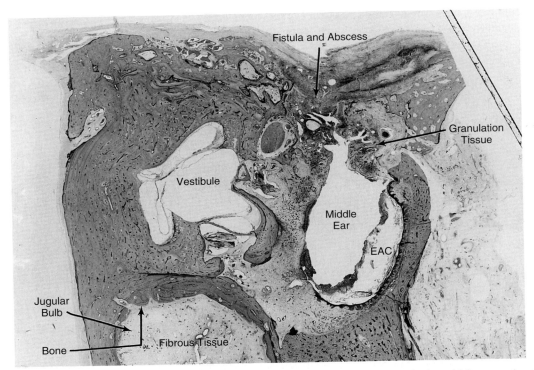

FIG. 18.4 Same case as Fig. 18.2. Left ear, vertical section. Granulation tissue in the middle ear extends superiorly through a large defect in the tegmen into the middle cranial fossa. There is fibrocystic obliteration of the oval and round window niches. Fibro-osseous obliteration of the jugular bulb is evidence of chronic healed phlebitis of the jugular vein. 6.6X.

Thrombosis of the dural sinuses usually begins as a result of damage to the tunica intima by an adjacent inflammatory process, most commonly an extradural perisinus abscess. Damage to the vessel wall initiates fibrin formation and platelet aggregation. This process is enhanced by the thrombogenic capacity of the neighboring bacteria (27). Classically, the thrombus becomes infected by spread of the abscess through the dura and vessel wall. However, it has also been suggested that seeding occurs primarily due to thrombophlebitic spread from the pneumatized spaces and that dural inflammation and fibrosis due to perisinus abscess actually serve to improve resistance to direct spread of infection (18). Thrombus may then propagate along vessel walls, causing local invasion, or it may produce bacteremia, septicemia, or septic embolization. Involvement of the cerebrum, meninges, and cerebellum has been reported in 45% of patients with lateral sinus thrombosis (28).

Recent publications indicate an evolving microbiology in this disorder. Once dominated by beta-hemolytic *Streptococcus* and *Pneumococcus,* cultures now reflect the flora of COM, revealing multiple pathogens, including *Proteus* sp., *Staphylococcus aureus, Bacteroides* sp., and *Escherichia coli,* as well as aerobic and anaerobic streptococci (17,22,23). These results suggest a higher incidence of dural sinus thrombosis in chronic ear disease (17,22,23,25), although in one recent series acute ear disease was the more common etiology (3).

The use of aggressive antibiotic therapy has altered the presentation of this disease to one of a less acute nature. The classical high, spiking "picket fence" fever and rigor are now rarely seen. Cervical or orbital extension of the clot, resulting in paralysis of cranial nerves or proptosis of the eye, is now also an unusual finding.

Typically, patients present after approximately 2 weeks of symptoms with headache that is usually lateral (17,22). The headache is often preceded by ear pain or discharge on the ipsilateral side and may be accompanied by nausea and vomiting. Visual changes, nuchal rigidity, and dysequilibrium are rare complaints.

Physical examination will almost always reveal purulent drainage through a perforated tympanic membrane. Pitting edema and tenderness over the postauricular area due to involvement of the mastoid emissary vein (Griesinger's sign) may be present. Fever remains a prominent feature in most patients, and papilledema due to increased intracranial pressure is present in more than 50% of cases (17,22). Less commonly the clinician may note palsy of the abducens nerve, believed to result from compression of the nerve by a distended inferior petrosal sinus within the closed space of Dorello's canal (Gradenigo's syndrome) (22). Nuchal rigidity and nystagmus are rarer findings.

Routine blood work usually reveals an elevated white cell count with a left shift and an elevated erythrocyte sedimentation rate. Blood cultures are usually negative. Lumbar puncture should be performed unless uncal herniation is likely to result from the procedure. Commonly, an elevated CSF pressure is noted, probably due to impaired CSF reabsorption through the arachnoid granulations. Cerebrospinal fluid chemistry and cell counts are usually unremarkable. A positive Queckenstedt's or Tobey-Ayer test, once considered pathognomonic of the disorder, has been found to be unreliable and to elevate intracranial pressure to dangerous levels (17). The test is considered positive when compression of the internal jugular vein on the side of the thrombosis fails to raise CSF pressure, but compression of the contralateral vein results in a rapid and marked increase in pressure.

Definitive diagnosis of dural venous thrombosis is now based primarily on radiographic studies. Cerebral angiography, the gold standard study, is particularly effective in delineating the cerebral venous anatomy, as well as in demonstrating the presence of vascular occlusion. Traditionally a venous phase arteriogram is performed, and the study may be enhanced by subtraction techniques. More recently, subtraction venography has been employed to avoid the risks associated with arteriography (17).

CT provides a less invasive examination of the dural sinuses and is useful in screening for concomitant otogenic complications. Increased density of the sinus on noncontrast scans suggests the presence of fresh clot, whereas contrast enhancement reveals filling defects and highlights inflamed sinus walls and dura. Soft tissue changes such as cerebral edema, decreased ventricular size, and hemorrhage or abscess may be detected. CT is unquestionably the method of choice for assessment of bony changes.

MRI and MRA have emerged as highly accurate modalities in the diagnosis of venous thrombosis (18,29–32). The defect is determined by the absence of flow-induced signal loss (29). These modalities have the additional advantage of reconstruction from several angles of view.

Treatment

Modern treatment of lateral sinus thrombosis is based on controlling infection with minimal surgical debridement and intensive antibiotic therapy. When thrombosis of the sinus is suspected, intravenous antibiotics should be started to minimize hematogenous spread. Until specific organisms and sensitivities are isolated, empiric therapy should target *Staphylococcus,* aerobic and anaerobic *Streptococcus,* and upper respiratory anaerobes. Historically, a combination of penicillin and chloramphenicol was often used. Given new understanding of relative drug penetration of the blood-brain barrier, it has been recommended to start with a combination of intravenous penicillin or nafcillin, intravenous ceftriaxone, and oral or intravenous metronidazole (25). Surgical intervention is directed by radiographic studies. Mastoidectomy is performed with wide exposure of the sigmoid sinus. Bone is removed until normal dura is exposed peripherally around the region of suspected thrombosis. Dural granulations are carefully removed and the sinus wall is inspected.

A normal-appearing, compressible sinus wall requires no further surgical treatment. If the sinus wall is inflamed or immobile on palpation, however, evaluation of the sinus lumen is indicated. A small-gauge needle may be used to aspirate the sinus, and, if bleeding is encountered, no further surgical treatment is necessary. Failure to obtain blood on aspiration suggests thrombosis, and aspiration of pus indicates infection of the thrombus. The discovery of pus upon aspiration requires drainage of the collection. Under these circumstances, evacuation of the infected clot should be performed. Control is gained distally and proximally within the mastoid cavity by extraluminal compression using absorbable sponges between the sinus wall and the overlying bone. An incision is then made in the lateral sinus wall in the direction of the vessel. If blood is obtained, the incision may be simply covered with absorbable sponge or temporalis muscle. If infected thrombus is noted, it is removed until only healthy clot or bleeding is encountered.

The patient is maintained on intravenous antibiotics. Ligation of the internal jugular vein, once popular in the management of lateral sinus thrombosis, is now reserved only for cases that are unresponsive to initial surgical and antibiotic therapy or those in which septic emboli are developing (14,26). Anticoagulation is still used by many clinicians to prevent extension of the thrombus and to reduce the risk of thrombosis of the cavernous sinus (30). Use of anticoagulant therapy, however, incurs the risks of septic embolization and hemorrhage due to clot breakdown (14). Also controversial is the dry tap of the sinus, which may be managed conservatively by aggressive antibiotic therapy or by opening the sinus and evacuating the clot (Fig. 18.5).

Brain Abscess

Abscess formation within the parenchyma of the brain, once considered the cause of suppurative otorrhea, has been

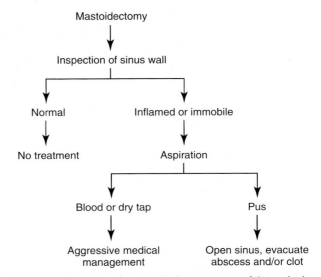

FIG. 18.5 Algorithm for surgical treatment of lateral sinus thrombosis.

recognized as a sequela of otitis media since the time of Morgagni (1682–1771, cited by Glasscock and Shambaugh [7]). Its successful treatment was first described by Morand in 1768 (1) and advanced by numerous nineteenth century surgeons, most notably MacEwen (31), who reported favorable outcomes in 18 of 19 operated cases of brain abscess. Treatment by aspiration through a bur hole was described by Dandy in 1926, and complete excision of an abscess was reported by Vincent in 1936 (cited by Haines et al. [32]).

For many years brain abscess was most commonly associated with otitic infection, and its management lay primarily with the otologist. In 1931 Evans (33) attributed 56% of brain abscesses at autopsy to otitis media, and in 1955 Courville (4) reported an otitic etiology in 46% of these cases. The development of antibiotics during the early part of the twentieth century, combined with improved neurosurgical management of early intracranial complications, has led to a dramatic decline in the incidence of otogenic brain abscess. In 1969 Beekhuis and Taylor (34) reported an asso-

ciation with otitis media in just 12.8% of all cases of brain abscess treated during the years 1956 to 1965. Bradley et al. (35) more recently reviewed cases of otogenic brain abscess at three hospitals between 1950 and 1980 and found an incidence of 25%.

Despite the decreased incidence of otogenic brain abscess, the mortality of the disorder remains high. Death rates in the literature of the last 30 years range from 14% to 47% (14,34,35), making brain abscess the deadliest complication of otitis media. It is therefore essential that the otologist consider the possibility of brain abscess when treating any otogenic complication.

Retrograde venous thrombophlebitis, often in association with extradural abscess, is the mechanism most commonly implicated in the development of a brain abscess. Temporal lobe abscesses, which usually result from spread through the tegmen (19) (Fig. 18.6), occur twice as often as cerebellar abscesses, which are associated with suppurative labyrinthitis or lateral sinus thrombosis (18). Local pachymeningitis

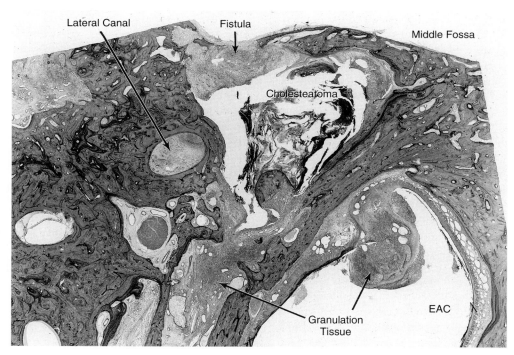

FIG. 18.6 Male, age 23. At the age of 23 this man complained of right otorrhea, otalgia, tinnitus, and dizziness. Examination revealed bilateral aural discharge. A diagnosis was made of bilateral chronic suppurative otitis media, and antibiotic therapy was instituted. Twelve days later he was hospitalized for drowsiness, headache, vertigo, and vomiting. Examiners reported no meningeal signs or nystagmus. Radiologic studies showed probable right attic cholesteatoma. In spite of intense antibiotic therapy, his condition deteriorated and he died on the eighth day of hospitalization. Autopsy showed an abscess of the right temporal lobe in the right ear. Vertical section. A granulation tissue polyp protrudes into the external auditory canal. The mesotympanum contains a combination of thick, inflamed mucosa, cystic spaces filled with acidophilic fluid, granulation tissue, and pools of pus. The mastoid antrum is lined by squamous epithelium on a layer of granulation tissue, and the space is occupied by a large cholesteatoma. There is a 3-mm defect in the tegmen and a fistulous tract containing granulation tissue that leads to the middle cranial fossa. The lateral and superior semicircular canals contain granulation tissue and pus originating from a fistula of the superior semicircular canals. Although the sense organs are intact, the endolymphatic and perilymphatic spaces in the remainder of the inner ear contain acidophilic fluid consistent with diffuse serous labyrinthitis. 8.8X.

induces thrombophlebitic or periarteriolar spread to the cortex of the temporal lobe or the cerebellum. Edema and encephalitis subsequently develop within the white matter, causing softening of this layer. A reactive collagen capsule, formed by fibroblasts, localizes the process over a period of approximately 2 weeks, while liquefaction and infection of entrapped brain tissue progresses. Rarely, a well-encapsulated abscess will become latent, only to be reactivated months or even years later.

Expansion of the abscess generally proceeds in the direction of the ventricle and produces an increase in intracranial pressure with localizing symptoms and signs. Cerebellar abscesses occur within the restricted space of the posterior fossa adjacent to the brainstem and therefore produce earlier symptoms and more lethal sequelae than their temporal counterparts. Respiratory arrest may result from herniation of the cerebellar tonsils through the foramen magnum. Temporal abscess, left untreated, will ultimately rupture into the ventricular or subarachnoid spaces, resulting in a fatal meningitis. Occasionally, rupture onto the surface of the brain may result in the formation of a fistulous tract between the abscess cavity and the ear.

Although numerous pathogens have been implicated in the formation of otogenic brain abscesses, the flora of such an abscess does not necessarily reflect that of the otitic infection from which it arose. Multiple organisms are isolated in one third to one-half of cases (18,36). Recent data suggest that anaerobic gram-positive cocci (*Peptococcus, Peptostreptococcus,* unspecified anaerobic streptococci) are most commonly involved (35,37). However, aerobic gram-positive cocci and gram-negative bacilli are often isolated. *Streptococcus* sp., *Staphylococcus* sp., and *Proteus* sp. are most common among the organisms in this group.

Signs and symptoms of brain abscess progress through four stages, as described by Neely (8) and Mawson (38). The first stage corresponds to the initial encephalitis, which results from the invasion of brain tissue. The symptoms are largely constitutional, consisting of malaise, headache, fever, chills, nausea, and vomiting. They are usually mild and may often mimic an exacerbation of COM or even a viral syndrome. Not uncommonly, they will go unnoticed, especially in the presence of another intracranial complication. During the second or "latent" stage, the abscess localizes and the symptoms abate or disappear.

The third stage (or stage of enlargement) is characterized by signs and symptoms of increased intracranial pressure and irritation and compression of specific locations in the brain. As a rule, the features of mass effect are more constant and present earlier than those of a more focal nature. Severe headache refractory to symptomatic therapy is the most constant symptom and is present in 70% to 90% of patients (32). Nausea and vomiting, often projectile in this stage, occur in 25% to 50% of cases (32), and 30% to 50% of patients present with seizures (32). Visual changes may result from ocular paralysis or from visual field defects due to temporal lobe lesions. Other symptoms associated primarily with temporal lobe abscess include hemiparesis and aphasia. Patients with cerebellar abscess may present with intention tremor or ataxia, with a tendency to fall toward the affected side. Later symptoms may include drowsiness and stupor.

Generalized abnormalities may be apparent on physical examination. Meningismus is present in 20% to 25% of cases and papilledema is present in 23% to 50% (39). Fever is usually low grade to subnormal (7). Pressure on the vagus center may cause a bradycardia, and arrhythmic respirations may result from compression of the respiratory center.

Neurologic examination is helpful in localizing the abscess. Aphasia associated with temporal lobe abscess is usually of the nominal type, in which the patient cannot name an object but can demonstrate its use. Visual field defects in these patients are usually quadrantic homonymous hemianopias, involving the upper quadrants more commonly than the lower. Motor examination confirms weakness of the contralateral side. Patients with cerebellar abscess demonstrate ipsilateral dysmetria and dysdiadochokinesia and spontaneous nystagmus, which increases on ipsilateral gaze. Any of these symptoms should prompt an early MRI scan.

In the final stage, the abscess ruptures into the ventricle or the subarachnoid space. This event usually results in a rapid clinical decline and death.

Routine laboratory testing adds little to the diagnosis of brain abscess. The white cell count may be elevated but is normal or mildly elevated in 40% of cases (39). The results of lumbar puncture are usually abnormal but nonspecific, and transtentorial herniation has been reported in up to one third of cases in which the procedure was performed (32).

CT scanning has revolutionized the diagnosis of these lesions and is now the standard of care in the diagnosis of brain abscess. On contrast-enhanced scans, the pyogenic material appears as an area of decreased density and is surrounded by a high-density ring representing the collagenous wall. The abscess is encircled by an area of low density, representing edema in the surrounding brain tissue. The findings of gas within the lesion and ventricular or meningeal enhancement are also common. MRI appears to be equally diagnostic and may offer certain advantages over CT. First, better contrast between the area of peripheral edema and the surrounding brain is noted on MRI and may suggest the diagnosis of brain abscess at an earlier stage (40). In addition, MRI appears to give more accurate assessment of extraparenchymal spread as demonstrated by intraventricular hyperdensity and periventricular enhancement (40). However, concomitant bone destruction is quite common in the presence of brain abscess, and CT scanning should therefore be the modality of choice for initial evaluation in most cases.

Treatment

Initial management is dictated by the clinical condition of the patient. Corticosteroids, though they may inhibit host defenses, may effectively lower the intracranial pressure in cases of coma or rapid deterioration. Mannitol may also be useful for this purpose.

Antibiotic therapy should be started as soon as the diagnosis of brain abscess is made. Many authors favor the initial use of high-dose nafcillin or oxacillin and chloramphenicol until culture results are available. When COM is determined to be the cause, long-term coverage with a third generation cephalosporin, an antipseudomonal penicillin, or an aminoglycoside should be considered with metronidazole added for anaerobes.

The management of brain abscess has traditionally involved operative intervention, usually in the form of aspiration or excision of the lesion. Recently, the concept of nonsurgical treatment using antibiotics was introduced by Heineman et al. (41) in a series of six patients with lateralizing signs and lesions localized by electroencephalography. Numerous reports advocating medical management followed, and, using data from these series, Haines et al. (32) assessed the efficacy of such therapy. Including only well-encapsulated lesions on CT or autopsy examination and those with at least 2 weeks of symptoms prior to the start of therapy, they found medical therapy to be successful in 37 of 50 cases (74%) with a mortality of only 4%. These authors, and others (39), concluded that medical therapy may be useful but should be reserved for cases of multiple brain abscesses after a causative organism has been identified by aspiration and for control of cerebritis present in the early stages of the disease or following spillage of abscess contents after drainage. In general, surgery remains the therapy of choice to confirm the diagnosis, identify the causative organism, and decompress the mass lesion. In addition, operative intervention usually reduces the duration of adjunctive antibiotics and shortens the hospital stay.

The primary surgical modalities in the treatment of brain abscess are aspiration and excision. Aspiration is performed through a large-bore needle placed through a bur hole drilled some distance from vital cortical and subcortical structures. Often the cavity is then irrigated, though the efficacy of irrigation in hastening resolution of the abscess is not well documented (39). Reaspiration is indicated for lesions that reaccumulate or do not completely resolve. Excision may be desirable to remove all necrotic and infected tissue. However, the procedure is reserved for encapsulated lesions and should not be performed on those in the early cerebritis stage.

Surgical treatment of brain abscess often results in significant morbidity. In one study, 70% of children showed a postoperative change in school performance and 50% had severe, persistent hemiparesis (42). Seizures occur in 30% to 50% of patients (39). In general, residual neurologic deficits are more profound with excision than with aspiration because surrounding white matter is often removed with the lesion. However, recurrence rates appear to be lower for excised lesions than for aspirated ones (32,39). Mortality rates have been shown to be similar for aspiration, aspiration followed by excision, and primary excision (32). Excision may there-

fore be considered the procedure of choice for abscesses that are superficial and solitary. Aspiration may be more appropriate for lesions that are located in deep or critical areas of the brain, for patients who are too ill for general anesthesia, and for cases involving multiple abscesses.

Antibiotics are continued for several weeks, and the patient is followed closely by serial CT scans. Recurrences require reoperation and have been reported to occur years after initial treatment. Management of the offending ear involves wide-field mastoidectomy with drainage as soon as the patient's neurological condition permits.

Otitic Meningitis

Otitic meningitis is a generalized bacterial infection of the pia and arachnoid with organisms identifiable in the CSF. It remains the most common intracranial complication of otitis media, although its incidence, severity, and morbidity have declined significantly in the antibiotic era (3). In adults meningitis is more likely to result from chronic infection of the middle ear, whereas in the pediatric age group, acute otitis media is a more common cause of meningitis (3).

Generalized meningitis in COM begins as a localized meningitis or pachymeningitis in association with an extradural abscess or other infectious otogenic focus. Bacteria access the CSF and meninges by direct extension through the dura and arachnoid. In suppurative labyrinthitis, infection may spread through the internal acoustic meatus and the aqueducts of the cochlea and vestibule. The CSF is an excellent culture medium with low concentrations of immunoglobulins and abundant glucose for bacterial growth. Phagocytic cells are impaired by poor CSF opsonic activity, and many organisms possess a polysaccharide capsule that further hinders the activity of these cells.

As a result of the infection, vessel permeability increases, allowing an influx of proteins and leukocytes. Transport of fluid out of the CSF is impaired, causing a rise in intracranial pressure. Lactic acid accumulation causes a fall in pH, and glucose metabolism is impaired. Accumulation of pyogenic exudate in the basal cisterns occludes the ventricular foramina, causing noncommunicating hydrocephalus. When this process obstructs the flow of subarachnoid CSF, a communicating hydrocephalus results.

Patients typically present with high fever, severe generalized headache, photophobia, confusion, and stiff neck. Nausea, vomiting, and anorexia are common. Back pain and myalgia are typically severe, with the patient exhibiting a preference for the fetal position. Temperatures higher than 39°C are the rule, often accompanied by tachycardia. A depressed level of consciousness may be noted. The patient is unable to extend the leg with the thigh flexed (Kernig's sign) and may exhibit flexion of the hip and knee when the head is bent (Brudzinski's sign). Cranial nerves are affected in 10% of patients (43). Palsies of the abducens nerve generally resolve with treatment. In contrast, involvement of the eighth nerve and cochlear ducts may cause irreversible hearing loss

(44). Papilledema is rare except where mass lesions are also present. Sequellae include cerebral edema, seizures, subdural effusion, and shock. Delirium may ensue in the late stages, followed by Cheyne-Stokes breathing, coma, and death.

Diagnosis may be made on examination of CSF. However, the examining physician must be alert for signs of other complications and should consider some form of brain imaging if other diagnoses are entertained. Opening CSF pressure will be high, and analysis will reveal an elevated white cell count with a predominance of leukocytes and an elevated protein concentration. A depressed glucose concentration confirms the diagnosis because no other complication has this effect on the CSF. The offending organism can be cultured in 85% of cases (43), providing antibiotic therapy has not been started prior to lumbar puncture.

Treatment

The management of otitic meningitis consists primarily of high-dose antibiotics capable of CSF penetration. When chronic middle ear disease is the cause, coverage for gram-negative organisms is essential. Current recommendations for first line agents are ceftriaxone or cefotaxime in combination with ampicillin or penicillin G. Chloramphenicol is equally efficacious but may induce severe side effects. These regimens provide excellent coverage for gram-negative organisms, including *H. influenzae* and enterobacteria, as well as gram-positive bacteria such as *Pneumococcus*. When *Pseudomonas* meningitis is suspected, ceftazidime is also an appropriate choice for systemic therapy. Intrathecal administration of gentamicin may be considered for resistant cases but has been noted to induce seizures. Maintenance therapy is adjusted in accordance with CSF cultures. Duration of treatment is 7 to 21 days with the longer antibiotic courses directed at gram-negative and anaerobic infections (20).

Patients are followed closely by repeated lumbar puncture. Cerebrospinal fluid cultures should be negative after 2 to 3 days of therapy, but cell counts and chemistries may be abnormal for several days longer.

Adjunctive therapy is helpful in reducing the morbidity of meningitis. When intracranial pressure is elevated, repeated lumbar puncture may permit decompression and prevent neurologic sequelae. Dexamethasone, which may also be effective for this purpose, has been shown to reduce sensorineural hearing loss and death in children with meningitis (45). Debridement of the ear is useful in treating the focus of the infection, and mastoidectomy is indicated when the patient is neurologically stable.

Subdural Infection

Infection of the subdural space is rare and usually occurs in infants as a result of thrombophlebitic spread in meningitis. Less commonly, COM causes an accumulation of infected fluid between the dura and arachnoid as a result of thrombophlebitic spread across dura or direct extension through the dura by erosion. This fluid collection, termed a subdural effusion, may progress to frank purulence if left untreated. A subdural empyema results when pus collects over a large surface area. Subdural abscess is the entrapment of pus by granulation tissue and fibrous tissue in response to the spreading infection. The morbidity of subdural infections is related to their propensity to cause local cortical compression, to generate multiple small cerebral abscesses by thrombophlebitic spread, and to interfere with the normal flow of CSF. As a result, the mortality rate of these infections remains 27% to 35% (46).

The first description of subdural infection is attributed to Richter (1773, cited by Courville [47]), who described such an infection in a patient with chronic frontal sinusitis. Other early cases have been reported by Schutz, Paulsen, Carver, and MacEwen (cited by Courville [47]). However, the route of spread of this infection was not described until 1944 by Courville (47).

Classically, infection of the subdural space reflects upper respiratory tract flora. Streptococcal infection has been the rule, and anaerobes are isolated in approximately 50% of these cases (18). However, of the group of eight cases of subdural infection reported by Gower and McGuirt (3), all were nonsterile effusions with cultures positive for *H. influenzae* and *S. aureus*. Gram-negative rods have also been isolated.

Clinically, subdural infection is marked by nonspecific central neurologic symptoms. Severe headache and drowsiness are the rule, occasionally leading to frank stupor or coma. Meningeal signs are usually present and may be accompanied by focal cortical signs such as hemiplegia and aphasia. Hemianopsia and deviation of the eyes to the affected side may occur, and focal seizures have been observed in some 60% of these cases (46). As a rule, neurologic findings are more focal than would be found in meningitis and more rapid in onset than would be found in the presence of a brain abscess.

Laboratory studies will reveal an elevated white cell count and sedimentation rate. Lumbar puncture may be dangerous and rarely aids in the diagnosis. When performed, an increased CSF pressure is demonstrated, a mild pleocytosis is present, protein concentration is elevated, and glucose level is normal. Definitive diagnosis is usually made by contrast CT scan, though occasionally these abscesses are quite small and barely detectable radiographically (39).

Treatment

Subdural infection is best managed in conjunction with a neurosurgeon. Surgical therapy consists of bur holes for diagnosis, drainage, and irrigation as necessary. Prodigious doses of the intravenous antibiotics previously mentioned are initially directed against the otitic focus and altered in accordance with culture results. When the patient is stable, mastoidectomy should be performed to treat the otologic source of the infection.

Otitic Hydrocephalus

The development of increased intracranial pressure in the absence of brain abscess has been observed in a subset of patients with acute or chronic otitis media. Termed *otitic hydrocephalus* by Symonds in 1931 (48), the disorder is identical to the entity known as pseudotumor cerebri, originally described by Quincke in 1893 (49). As a result, most authors consider the term *otic hydrocephalus* to be synonymous with pseudotumor cerebri resulting from otitis media, with these cases accounting for some 25% of all cases of pseudotumor (50).

The pathophysiology of otitic hydrocephalus remains unclear, but increased production or decreased resorption of CSF is thought to be responsible (18). Impaired function of the arachnoid villi due to thrombosis of the dural venous sinuses or localized meningitis has been suggested as a cause (51). However, thrombosis is a rare finding on radiographic examination or surgical exploration, and most cases of venous thrombosis do not lead to otitic hydrocephalus.

The condition typically arises in children and adolescents with several weeks of middle ear infection. Patients usually present with protracted headache occasionally associated with diplopia and vomiting. The most reliable findings are bilateral papilledema and ipsilateral sixth nerve paralysis. Focal neurologic signs are absent. Lumbar puncture reveals increased opening pressure, usually greater than 300 mm of water, with no cells and normal concentrations of protein and glucose. Radiographic studies are helpful to rule out the presence of mass lesion.

Treatment

Treatment is directed at lowering the elevated CSF pressure to prevent optic atrophy from persistent papilledema. Serial lumbar punctures or placement of a lumbar drain will diminish CSF pressures over the several weeks usually required for the condition to run its course. In prolonged cases, ventricular shunting or subtemporal decompression may be indicated. Diuretics, steroids, and hyperosmolar dehydrating agents have been suggested as an adjunct to therapy (17). Mastoidectomy should be performed to manage the chronically draining ear.

INTRATEMPORAL COMPLICATIONS

Subperiosteal Abscess

Subperiosteal abscess, in the antibiotic era, is a relatively uncommon sequela of otitis media. It is usually associated with the development of acute mastoiditis following an episode of acute otitis media. Far less commonly, except in some third-world nations (52), subperiosteal abscess may complicate chronic suppurative otitis media.

Bezold and Siebenmann, in their 1908 text (53), describe the primary extracranial routes of spread of mastoid infection. The most common of these is extension through the lateral surface of the mastoid cortex, resulting in a subperiosteal abscess. The infection spreads by traveling through preexisting bony dehiscences and along small vessels or by erosion of bone. Progression of the abscess detaches periosteum superiorly and posteriorly but is limited inferiorly by muscle attachments.

The offending organisms usually reflect those of the otitic infection. *Streptococcus* sp. and *Staphylococcus* sp. are common in acute infections, whereas *Proteus* and *Pseudomonas* are more common in cases due to COM.

Signs and symptoms of subperiosteal abscess are straightforward and usually establish the diagnosis. Patients complain or have evidence of postauricular swelling, tenderness, and occasional fluctuance. As a result of the expanding abscess, the auricle is displaced downward, outward, and forward (Fig. 18.7).

Occasionally, infection breaks through the large, thin-walled cells internal to the digastric groove at the mastoid tip. An abscess may subsequently form beneath the sternocleidomastoid muscle, presenting as a tender, fluctuant mass (Fig. 18.8). This abscess, known as Bezold's abscess, may progress along fascial planes to the larynx, the mediastinum, or the retropharyngeal space.

The last route of spread described by Bezold is through the root of the zygoma. This region may occasionally be pneumatized, and involvement of these cells in patients with mastoiditis may cause elevation of the periosteum under the temporalis muscle. Patients present with pain and swelling in the area of the zygomatic arch. The upper half of the auricle may be raised away from the skull.

In cases in which signs and symptoms alone do not establish the diagnosis of subperiosteal abscess, CT scanning may reveal erosion of the mastoid septae or other bone erosion due to cholesteatoma. CT scanning with contrast enhancement may also be useful in localizing a Bezold's abscess in the neck.

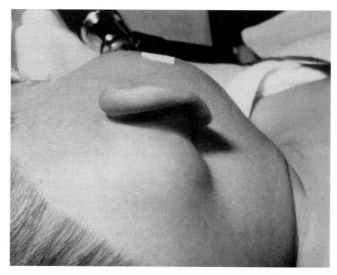

FIG. 18.7 Child with subperiosteal abscess causing downward, outward, and forward displacement of the auricle.

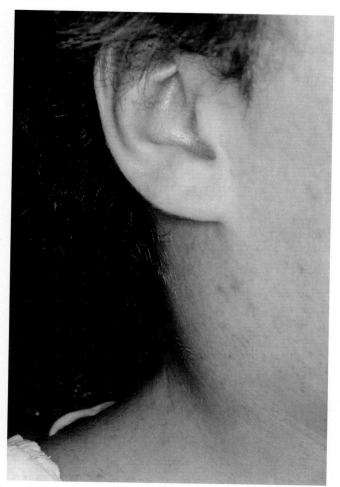

FIG. 18.8 Swelling of the right neck caused by Bezold's abscess beneath sternocleidomastoid muscle.

Facial Paralysis

Facial paralysis may occur as a complication of acute otitis media, COM, or malignant otitis external. In the acute setting, the nerve is usually affected through a dehiscence of the fallopian canal, which is present in some 55% of patients (54). The nerve becomes inflamed and edematous, and neuropraxia results. A direct neurotoxic effect may also contribute to the disorder, but this has not been experimentally confirmed (8). Conservative treatment with antibiotics and myringotomy are usually sufficient to eliminate the infection, and the prognosis for full return of facial function is excellent. Operative decompression of the facial nerve is not indicated unless degeneration of the nerve is suggested by evoked electromyography or electroneuronography.

Facial paralysis due to prolonged acute otitis media (longer than 2 weeks) or to COM usually results from erosion of the bony canal by infection or cholesteatoma (Fig. 18.9). The infectious process compresses the nerve, causing invagination of the nodes of Ranvier and segmental demyelination in the compressed region (8). This process reduces the resistance of the axonal membrane to stretch and may ultimately result in nerve degeneration. Onset is usually slow and progressive, and symptoms may be partial and intermittent. Lacrimal function remains intact unless a concomitant proximal lesion is present. Rarely, facial paralysis is caused by a suppurative labyrinthitis in which a bony sequestrum remains or by chronic osteomyelitis of the petrous pyramid (55).

Etiology is determined by thorough microscopic examination of the ear. CT scanning should be performed to localize cholesteatoma and assess its size. In long-standing facial paralysis, nerve excitability testing, maximal stimulation

Treatment

Treatment of subperiosteal abscess is surgical and consists of incision and drainage of the abscess and culture of its contents, followed by mastoidectomy. The goals of the procedure are to remove diseased tissue and to establish adequate ventilation of the mastoid and middle ear spaces. The minimal operation should be a complete simple mastoidectomy, but more extensive procedures should be performed as indicated in order that these goals be accomplished. Some authors advocate inspection of the posterior and middle cranial fossae to rule out epidural abscess (18). Treatment of a Bezold's abscess requires exploration of the neck as well.

Broad spectrum antibiotic coverage should be started postoperatively and altered when culture results become available. Several days of intravenous therapy in the hospital should be considered prior to discharge on enteral antibiotics. In cases where a diagnosis of osteomyelitis is made, intravenous therapy should be continued for approximately 6 weeks.

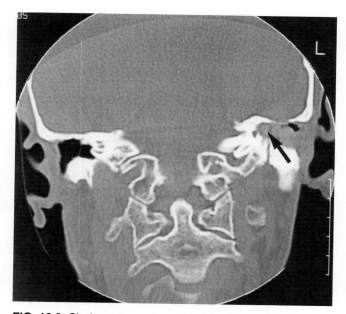

FIG. 18.9 Cholesteatoma invading fallopian canal (*arrow*) in a patient presenting with facial paralysis and chronic otitis media.

testing, electromyography, and electroneurography may help determine the prognosis for recovery of the nerve.

Treatment

Immediate exploration of the middle ear is indicated in all cases of facial paralysis due to COM, in contradistinction to facial paralysis associated with acute otitis media or malignant otitis externa, which is initially treated medically or with a pressure-equalizing tube. In COM-associated paralysis, mastoidectomy is performed and all diseased bone and cholesteatoma are removed. The facial nerve is exposed by removing cholesteatoma matrix but leaving attached granulation tissue to avoid further injury to the nerve. Healthy bone above and below the disease is eggshelled and removed with a Rosen needle to allow the nerve room to swell. Some authors advocate exploration of the fallopian canal from the geniculate ganglion to the stylomastoid foramen (8). In areas where epineurium is violated, the sheath is opened and dehiscences may be repaired by appropriate grafting procedures. Intraoperative cultures are taken to determine appropriate postoperative antibiotic therapy.

Postoperatively, intravenous antibiotics are administered for approximately 1 week. Broad-spectrum coverage is indicated pending culture results. Additional care should include protection and moisturization of the eye. The prognosis for recovery is good if axonal degeneration has not occurred preoperatively.

Petrositis

Just as inflammation and infection of the mastoid air cells may result from infection of the middle ear, so may acute and chronic otitis media affect pneumatized spaces within the petrous temporal bone. When drainage of these spaces is inadequate, the disease process may affect the surrounding structures, causing cranial neuropathies and, in some cases, extension into the middle cranial fossa. This complication of otitis media is known as petrositis and warrants special attention because of the anatomic complexity of the region (Fig. 18.10).

In 1904 Gradenigo (56) described the triad of abducens nerve palsy, severe pain around the eye in the trigeminal distribution, and persistent otorrhea and recognized its associa-

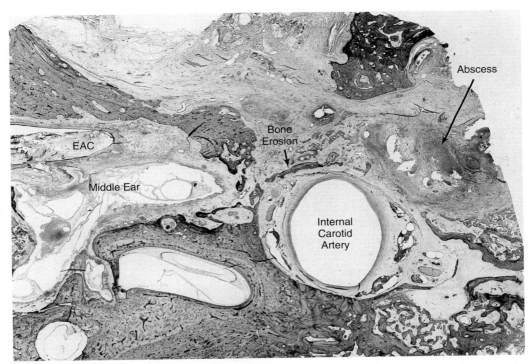

FIG. 18.10 Male, age 76. This man had left recurring suppurative otorrhea for many years. At the age of 76 he complained of left-sided headaches and increased left otorrhea of two months' duration. Examination revealed a malodorous purulent discharge, absence of the tympanic membrane and ossicles, and bulging of the posterior wall of the nasopharynx, all on the left side. On the following day the patient was noted to have palsy of the sixth and tenth cranial nerves, and he died several hours later. Autopsy revealed left chronic suppurative otitis media and mastoiditis, chronic petrous apicitis, abscess in the area of the left eustachian tube, and an extradural abscess in the region of the clivus. Horizontal section: Chronic suppurative otitis media is complicated by resorption osteitis and abscess formation in the peritubal region of the petrous apex. The abscess extended into the retropharyngeal area and was associated with an extradural abscess. 5.8X.

tion with infection of the petrous apex. Subsequently, petrositis was identified as a common, potentially lethal complication of otitis media requiring aggressive treatment. In fact, radical mastoidectomy with labyrinthectomy was the early procedure of choice for treatment of this disorder.

As surgical instrumentation improved and antibiotic therapy reduced the severity of infection in these cases, more conservative approaches to the petrous pyramid were investigated. Eagleton (57) described the first labyrinth-sparing approach beneath the posterior semicircular canal and jugular bulb. Voss, Meltzer, Frenckner, and Lindsay emphasized approaches through various cell tracts connecting the mastoid with the petrous apex (cited by Chole and Donald [58]). Only Ramadier (59) and Lempert (60) advocated a radical approach, exposing the carotid canal through the glenoid fossa.

The surgical anatomy of the petrous apex has been detailed by the histopathologic studies of Lindsay, Eggston and Wolff, and Allam and Schuknecht (cited by Schuknecht and Gulya [61]). A coronal plane through the internal auditory canal divides the air cells of this region into anterior and posterior groups. The posterior air cells, which include the perilabyrinthine cells, as described by Schuknecht and Gulya, are present in 30% of the temporal bones and extend from the epitympanum and antrum around the semicircular canals to the base of the petrous pyramid (61). The anterior or petrous apex air cells are present in 15% of temporal bones and extend from the hypotympanum and tubotympanum around the cochlea to the apex of the pyramid (61). These cells are bordered inferiorly by the carotid canal and superiorly by Meckel's cave and are therefore the least accessible.

The pathogenesis of chronic petrositis is much the same as that of chronic mastoiditis. Offending bacteria include *Pseudomonas* and *Proteus* spp., but mixed infection is common. Organisms may gain access to the petrous apex from the middle ear and mastoid through five separate cell tracts, as described by Schuknecht and Gulya (61). The posteromedial and posterosuperior tracts pass superomedially around the labyrinth and may extend to the anterior cells of the apex. The subarcuate tract, which passes through the arch of the superior semicircular canal, may also reach anteriorly to the apex. The peritubal tract travels a very short distance to the petrous apex in an anteromedial direction around the carotid artery. Finally, the perilabyrinthine tracts extend from the epitympanum to the posterior cells of the perilabyrinthine region. The presence of the bony labyrinth impairs drainage from this area and increases the risk of intracranial extension of disease. Furthermore, the presence of air cells immediately adjacent to bone marrow in nonpneumatized areas of the apex increases the risk of osteomyelitis.

In the antibiotic era, it has become rare for patients with petrositis to present with pure Gradenigo's syndrome. The two most constant symptoms are deep, boring pain and persistent otorrhea following simple mastoidectomy. Occipital, parietal, or temporal pain suggests involvement of the posterior cells, whereas frontal or orbital pain suggests anterior involvement. Diplopia may be present as a result of sixth nerve palsy due to involvement of the abducens as it passes through Dorello's canal beneath the petroclinoid ligament. Patients may also present with low-grade fever, transient facial paralysis, and mild vertigo.

CT with contrast is helpful in confirming the diagnosis. The study may reveal coalescence or bone destruction in the area of the petrous pyramid (Fig. 18.11). Less commonly, an epidural abscess at the apex is found. Gallium and technetium bone scanning may be useful when CT scanning is inconclusive.

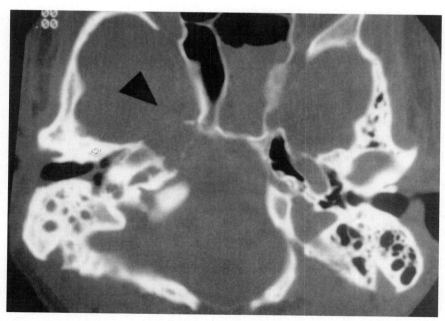

FIG. 18.11 CT scan showing destruction of right petrous apex in a patient with Gradenigo's syndrome.

Treatment

Most cases of acute coalescent petrositis are treated with aggressive intravenous antibiotic therapy in combination with mastoidectomy. However, petrositis due to COM often involves low-grade osteomyelitis of the petrous pyramid and is resistant to conservative therapy. Exploration of the petrous apex is indicated when, despite mastoidectomy, pain remains intractable or symptoms of diplopia, facial weakness, or vertigo are present.

Surgery is directed at removing existing disease, establishing adequate ventilation, and preserving the facial nerve, carotid artery, and labyrinth. Often the choice of a route to the petrous apex is made easier by the presence of purulent drainage or granulation tissue seen at the time of surgery. The initial approach to the petrous apex is through curettage of these tracts extending anteriorly from the mastoid antrum or middle ear. Bone softened due to osteitis is removed and the path of infected cells is followed adjacent to the labyrinthine capsule. In cases of long-standing infection, with this procedure there is some risk of inadvertent entry into a semicircular canal, which will usually result in complete loss of hearing in the affected ear. When osteitic involvement of the labyrinth is severe, a labyrinthectomy may be considered to facilitate access to the apical cells. Osteitis of the fallopian canal may also place the facial nerve at risk.

In cases where fistulous tracts and osteitic bone are not apparent, an exploration of the pneumatized tracts to the apex may be necessary. One popular approach through the infralabyrinthine portion of the perilabyrinthine tract, originally described by Eagleton (62), passes inferior to the posterior canal and internal auditory canal and superior to the jugular bulb. Injury to the jugular bulb may occur through this approach, and bleeding should be controlled with Gelfoam for small rents or with Surgicel and gauze packing if the opening is larger. If an air embolus should occur, the patient should be positioned in Trendelenburg and rolled onto the left side. Preoperative placement of a central venous line may be prudent to facilitate evacuation of an embolus should one occur.

Exploration through the subarcuate tract is an approach popularized by Frenckner (63) but is only possible in the 3% of temporal bones in which the tract is pneumatized (61). Thornvaldt's approach is through the supralabyrinthine portion of the perilabyrinthine tract under the dura. Another operation described by Eagleton (57) for epidural apical abscess requires wide exposure of the middle fossa dura by removing the tegmen, the base of the zygoma, and the temporal squama. The middle fossa dura is elevated as progress is made toward the petrous apex. The procedure is facilitated by use of a lumbar drain, but elevation of the dura from the arcuate eminence is difficult.

More recently, experience has been gained with hypotympanic approaches for the drainage of petrous apex granulomas. Such a procedure requires a transcanal or radical mastoidectomy approach so that the hypotympanum and tubotympanum may be explored for a cell tract leading between the cochlea and the jugular bulb or between the cochlea and the carotid artery. In a well-pneumatized ear, this approach is rather straightforward, especially if a large canalplasty and hypotympanotomy are performed. However, if no cells are located, the radical procedure of Ramadier (59) and Lempert (60) may be the only remaining alternative. In this approach, the anterior canal wall is removed and the mandibular condyle is retracted or removed. The dura of the middle cranial fossa is eggshelled superior to the tensor tympani, and the muscle is removed. The bony carotid canal can now be identified as a rounded prominence medial to the eustachian tube. Superiorly, a triangle of bone separating the middle fossa dura, the cochlea, and the carotid artery overlies the cells of the apex. This bone is removed using a small curet in a posterior direction, away from the artery. Access is thus gained to the entire apex and, after removing the tegmen plate, to the middle and posterior fossa dura.

The Ramadier-Lempert approach is fraught with risks. The bony carotid canal in this area may be dehiscent, and the muscularis media may be thin. Bleeding following injury to the artery cannot be controlled by simple ligation in the neck because of back bleeding from the circle of Willis and requires a craniotomy for central control. In the meantime, the artery must be occluded by compression against the bony canal using cotton pledgets and gauze or by Fogarty catheterization. Neurologic deficits are incurred by 20% to 40% of patients who undergo ligation of the artery, and 10% to 20% of these patients die (58).

Inadvertent entry into the cochlea may result in sensorineural hearing loss. Small violations of the otic capsule may be immediately sealed with bone wax. Other dangers include injury to the facial nerve at or near the geniculate ganglion, entry into the cavernous or superior petrosal sinuses, and tearing of the dura.

Broad spectrum intravenous antibiotics are continued postoperatively. Osteomyelitis of the petrous pyramid requires 6 weeks of therapy with periodic reassessment by bone scanning.

Labyrinthitis

Labyrinthine complications of otitis media arise from the spread of infection into the cochlea and vestibule. Bacteria and inflammatory mediators access the labyrinth through the round window (Fig. 18.12) or oval window or through acquired bony defects (Fig. 18.13). In other cases, the perilymphatic space is violated by advancing cholesteatoma or contaminated by CSF from a preexisting meningitis.

Schuknecht (64) has classified the labyrinthine complications into four types based on the offending noxious agent: (i) acute serous (toxic) labyrinthitis due to bacterial toxins or other mediators of inflammation; (ii) acute suppurative labyrinthitis due to invasion by bacteria; (iii) chronic labyrinthitis due to ingrowth of granulation tissue or cholesteatoma into the labyrinth; and (iv) labyrinthine sclerosis or labyrinthitis ossificans due to replacement of normal

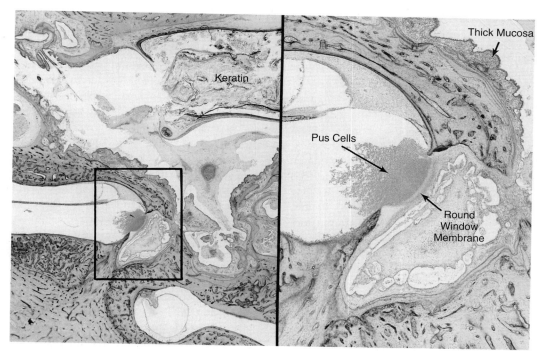

FIG. 18.12 This child developed bilateral otitis media at age 10 months, developed meningitis, and died 3 days later in spite of intensive antibiotic therapy. Both middle ears show pus and thickened mucosa. Of special interest is the accumulation of pus cells on the scala tympani side of the round window niche, suggesting a probable avenue of labyrinth invasion. 6X and 23.6X. (Courtesy of M. Paparella, University of Minnesota.)

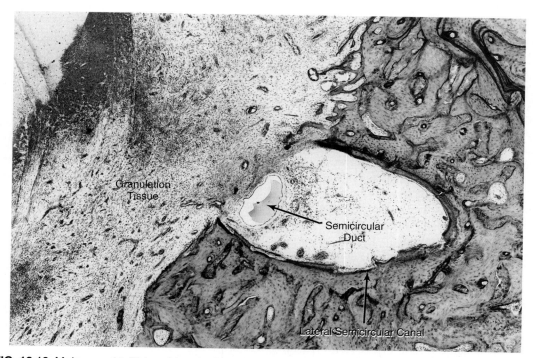

FIG. 18.13 Male, age 15. This subject had bilateral COM and underwent a right radical mastoidectomy in childhood (details unknown). At age 15 he experienced an exacerbation of left otorrhea complicated by meningitis. He was given intensive antibiotic therapy and, although the meningeal signs abated, he developed aphasia and left sixth cranial nerve palsy. Fifteen days after the onset of symptoms a left craniotomy was performed and 70 cc's of pus was evacuated from a large abscess in the posterior part of the temporal lobe. Audiometric study showed a 40-db conductive loss on the left and a profound hearing loss on the right. One month later a left radical mastoidectomy revealed cholesteatoma and granulations in the mastoid with erosion of the tegmen of the middle ear and mastoid. A second craniotomy revealed a still larger temporal lobe abscess. The patient died the following day. Left ear, vertical section. There is erosion and fistulization of the lateral semicircular canal. The endolymphatic duct is intact and surrounded by fibrous tissue infiltrated with polymorphonuclear leukocytes and small round cells. A thick layer of granulation tissue lines the actively eroding walls of the mastoid cavity. 36X.

labyrinthine structures by fibrous tissue and bone. Ludman (17) has observed that the distinction between serous and suppurative labyrinthitis is made in retrospect, depending on if cochlear and vestibular function return, and therefore minimizes its clinical significance. Nevertheless, this classification illustrates the correlation of pathogenesis with clinical outcome.

Serous labyrinthitis is believed to be the most common complication of otitis media. Paparella and Sugiura (65) found evidence of this condition in 83% of cases of acute suppurative otitis media in histopathologic autopsy studies. Serous labyrinthitis develops when the inflammatory process extends from the middle ear to the internal auditory meatus, cochlear aqueduct, or vestibular aqueduct via preformed pathways or from the passage of infected CSF. It is common in cases of labyrinthine fistula but may occur in the presence of any perilabyrinthine infection. Typically, a dilation of labyrinthine blood vessels is followed by movement of inflammatory cells across the round window membrane into the perilymph. A serofibrinous exudate then accumulates in the perilymphatic compartment around the portal of entry and may spread throughout the labyrinth. Over time, the exudate resorbs and is usually replaced by fibrosis in the perilymphatic space.

Acute suppurative labyrinthitis occurs less commonly than acute serous labyrinthitis. The incidence of suppurative labyrinthitis of meningogenic origin is uncertain. Tympanogenic suppurative labyrinthitis in the antibiotic era is estimated at less than 1% (65). The route of bacterial spread through the labyrinth is similar to that of inflammatory cells in serous labyrinthitis, but the destruction of tissue is permanent and more severe. The penetration of the basilar membrane by bacteria and inflammatory cells places the organ of Corti at significant risk. The resistance of Reissner's membrane to cellular penetration creates an osmotic pressure differential between endolymph and perilymph, resulting in endolymphatic hydrops. Spread of infection to the meninges from the labyrinth is an unusual but very morbid occurrence.

Chronic labyrinthitis most often occurs in association with osteitic or cholesteatomatous fistulas through which soft tissue has grown into the labyrinth. The incidence of chronic labyrinthitis is unknown, but cholesteatomatous fistulas are thought to occur in 10% of cases of chronic mastoiditis (66,67). Seventy-five percent of cases involve the horizontal semicircular canal (8), but the oval window footplate may also be eroded by cholesteatoma or granulation tissue. These fistulas are often clinically silent and are discovered unexpectedly at surgery. In most cases they remain covered by cholesteatoma matrix, which prevents inflammatory and suppurative processes from affecting the labyrinth. Loss of this protection due to progression of the fistula permits bacterial invasion and ingrowth of granulation tissue, ultimately leading to loss of labyrinthine function.

Jang and Merchant (68) recently reviewed seven temporal bones with COM and bony labyrinthine fistula. They concluded that such fistulas were caused not only by chole-steatoma but also by granuloma without cholesteatoma. Two predominant mechanisms of bony erosion are thought to exist. First, chronic infection leads to inflammatory cascades, culminating in osteoclastic resorption of bone. This resorption osteitis, which occurs with or without cholesteatoma, occurs at the border between granulation tissue and the bony otic capsule. Second, cholesteatoma matrix may cause noninflammatory osteolysis, either through direct pressure or by production of chemical factors.

Bony fistula is most commonly associated with chronic labyrinthitis with only local soft tissue extending into the labyrinth. In these cases, minimal changes will occur to the inner ear sense organs. In some cases, however, an associated serous or even suppurative process will extend into the labyrinth or vestibule through the fistula (68).

The replacement of labyrinthine structures by fibrous or osseous tissue constitutes labyrinthine sclerosis, or labyrinthitis ossificans. Classically, this process occurs as an end-stage sequela of bacterial meningitis but may also follow suppurative labyrinthitis. By examining animal and human temporal bones, Paparella and Sugiura categorized the events leading from suppuration to ossification within the labyrinth into three stages. The first stage, or acute stage, is marked by the entry of bacteria and leukocytes into the perilymph. In the second stage, or fibrous stage, granulation tissue forms, promoting angiogenesis and fibrotic change. The final ossification stage is characterized by the formation of newly created disorganized osteoid. As disease progresses, mineralization continues and the osteoid is calcified, leading to lamellar bone filling the entire inner ear (65). A recent study used fluorochrome labels in the gerbil to investigate the sequence of events in the development of labyrinthitis ossificans. It was found that, through dynamic bone resorption and remodeling, initial disorganized bone was replaced with lamellar bone which eventually fills the cochlear lumen (69). Although the exact cells of origin in ossification are not known, undifferentiated mesenchymal cells that line the bony cochlea, pericytes surrounding blood vessels, and modiolar and spiral ligament fibroblasts all likely play critical roles (65,70).

In general, suppurative labyrinthitis follows a more fulminant course than serous labyrinthitis. Symptoms of chronic labyrinthitis are usually slowly progressive. Vestibular and cochlear symptoms in labyrinthitis often occur together, but vestibular symptoms may appear first in cases of cholesteatomatous fistula involving a semicircular canal. Spontaneous nystagmus begins as an irritative nystagmus, with the quick phase beating toward the infected ear, but evolves into a paralytic nystagmus beating toward the opposite ear (17). Vertigo, ataxia, and past pointing may accompany the ocular symptoms. Hearing loss is usually of the high frequency sensorineural type. Onset is usually sudden and severe in suppurative labyrinthitis but may be progressive or fluctuating in serous or chronic labyrinthitis. Diplacusis and distortion of sound may also be present.

Patients in whom labyrinthitis is suspected should undergo neurologic evaluation to rule out meningeal involvement prior to otologic testing. Caloric testing, if possible, will usually demonstrate some residual function in serous labyrinthitis, but loss of function may occur in more advanced stages of the disease. Detection and localization of labyrinthine fistulas have been discussed in detail by McCabe (66). Positive and negative pressures are applied to the ear canal through a pneumatic otoscope. A positive fistula test causes transient vertigo and, with positive pressure, conjugate deviation of the eyes and nystagmus toward the opposite ear are noted.

High resolution CT scanning may be useful in preoperative detection of labyrinthine fistulas and labyrinthine erosion by cholesteatoma (see Chapter 4, Fig. 4.6C). In one series (67), 50 patients with chronic suppurative otitis media underwent CT scanning preoperatively. Four of five labyrinthine fistulas discovered at surgery were predicted by the preoperative scans. The only undiagnosed erosion was less than 2 mm.

Treatment

Treatment of labyrinthitis due to otitis media begins with culture of the purulent material and establishment of drainage. In acute infections, myringotomy and insertion of a tympanostomy tube are useful for these purposes. In chronic suppurative otitis media, mastoidectomy is indicated, though some authors advocate delaying surgery until acute symptoms have subsided to avoid the risk of spreading infection (17). Appropriate antibiotic therapy is administered, and the patient is placed on strict bed rest with minimal head movement. Antiemetics are given to control vomiting, and intravenous hydration is ordered to replace losses due to emesis. If hearing loss becomes total and vertigo is intractable, meningitis is considered imminent. Lumbar puncture should be performed and antibiotic therapy is modified to achieve adequate CSF levels.

Conservative management of labyrinthine fistulas is critical to the preservation of auditory and vestibular function. Fistulas involving the vestibule and cochlea place the inner ear at high risk. Consequently, some advocate that the disease involving these lesions should remain undisturbed and exteriorized (8). Similarly, attempts to clear large or deep fistulas carry significant risk (71). In fact, most authors believe that it is safe to leave cholesteatoma matrix over the fistula in an open cavity or staged in a closed cavity procedure as long as there is no infected granulation tissue deep to it. Growth of new bone will close the defect over time. In cases where the nature of the underlying tissue is uncertain, McCabe (66) has advocated biopsy and frozen section examination. In these cases, cholesteatoma is removed with careful preservation of the endosteum. If cholesteatoma matrix is left in an intact canal wall procedure, reexploration in 6 to 12 months is indicated to remove any remaining epithelial pearl (72).

In the antibiotic era, indications for opening the labyrinth for drainage are exceedingly few. Labyrinthectomy should be considered only when the disease process has caused a total loss of function or when meningitis develops despite aggressive antibiotic therapy.

In the presence of labyrinthitis ossificans, intervention is most likely to succeed if administered early. The placement of cochlear implants prior to ossification is optimal. Interventional trials aimed at preventing the various stages leading to ossification are underway. At this point, once ossification with sensorineural hearing loss (SNHL) has occurred, little else can be done other than drilling out the cochlea in anticipation of cochlear implantation. Poorer results have been reported with more advanced ossification (73).

SENSORINEURAL HEARING LOSS

The notion that a causal relationship between COM and SNHL exists is controversial. Although some clinical studies refute this association, most studies in the literature support it. One review of 67 patients who underwent surgery for adhesive otitis found SNHL exceeding 10-db hearing loss (HL) in at least one frequency in 76% of patients (74). Blakeley and Kim reported a highly significant association between COM and SNHL. The deficit was mild, with a mean hearing loss of 5 db, and was more likely to occur in the presence of purulent infection. Severity of the infection was found not to be positively correlated to the presence of SNHL (75). Others have implicated severity and duration as being important predictors of SNHL (76,77).

Animal studies have been conducted to investigate the possible mechanism of how chronic infection could cause SNHL. Proposed mechanisms have included several possible factors, including endotoxins, variable bacterial pathogenicity, circulatory factors, and mechanical factors. Diffusion of endotoxin into guinea pig perilymphatic space produced inner ear histologic changes and SNHL (78). Other studies report that streptococcal pneumonia in middle ear infections caused significant SNHL, whereas *E. coli* did not (79). Another theory postulates that middle ear inflammatory changes cause impairment of round window blood flow and thereby decrease oxygen diffusion from the middle ear to the inner ear, resulting in inner ear damage.

As yet, it is not certain if treatment of infection can prevent the development of SNHL. Furthermore, there is no known reliable treatment of SNHL following COM.

HIV AND AIDS

The spread of HIV and AIDS has led to the emergence of many opportunistic infections previously not found in immunocompetent hosts. To date, there are no reports in the literature to show that COM is more prevalent in HIV and AIDS patients. However, cases of atypical pathogens have been isolated in the middle ear and mastoid in these populations. In particular, *Pneumocystis carinii* otitis media and mastoiditis have been reported in recent years (80–82). Clinical presentation is variable but is often marked by the

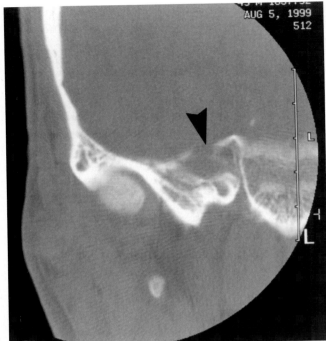

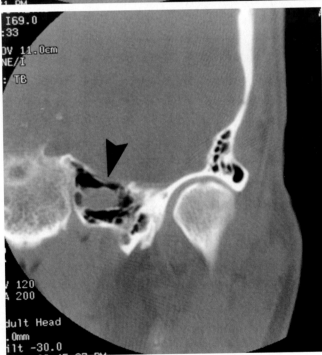

FIG. 18.14 This subject is a 49-year-old AIDS patient with a history of several months of headaches and right ear pain. Serial examinations revealed worsening edema and erythema of the external ear canal skin and tympanic membrane without granulation tissue. After failure of topical drops, the ear canal skin was biopsied and found to contain *Pneumocystis carinii*. The CT scan reveals erosion and remodeling of the anteromedial aspect of the temporal bone in the region of the roof of the carotid canal (*arrow*, **A**). The opposite ear had bony dehiscence of the carotid canal but no surrounding inflammation and fluid (*arrow*, **B**). The patient improved clinically on Septra and intravenous pentamidine. The patient did not have any significant neurologic deficits at any time.

presence of external and middle ear polyps, which stain positive for *P. carinii* when treated with Grocott-Gomori methenamine–silver nitrate stain. Symptoms include otalgia, mixed hearing loss, otorrhea, and tinnitus. The route of spread may be lymphatic or hematogenous, although Gherman et al. advocate retrograde spread through the eustachian tube (80). In the few reported cases in the literature, successful treatment regimens have included 21 days of oral Septra (82), Septra and Dapsone (83), and intravenous pentamidine (81).

Kaposi's sarcoma is a progressive mesenchymal tumor characterized by red-purple plaques and nodules in skin and mucosa. This malignancy is seen in much higher frequency in AIDS patients. Kaposi's sarcoma has been reported in the nasopharynx and external ear, predisposing to middle ear infection (84). Recently, the first case of Kaposi's sarcoma of the mastoid was reported in a 33-year-old HIV-positive male patient who presented with meningitis and purulent otorrhea. Mastoidectomy was performed with histopathology of the mastoid granulation tissue, revealing Kaposi's sarcoma (85).

Although malignant or necrotizing external otitis is a separate clinical entity from COM, such cases are characterized by skull base osteomyelitis, which may extend through the temporal bone surrounding the middle ear, mastoid, and petrous apex. Classically, this disease usually occurs in elderly diabetic patients. However, several cases have been reported in HIV and AIDS patients without diabetes (86,87). In contrast to the classical presentation of necrotizing external otitis, AIDS patients with this disease generally do not present with granulation tissue in the external auditory canal, but the disease is typically more severe and with a poorer outcome. One series of AIDS patients with necrotizing external otitis revealed a 42% (3 out of 7) mortality rate despite aggressive antibiotic therapy (86). Although *Pseudomonas* is still the most common pathogen, several cases of *Aspergillus* necrotizing external otitis have been reported in the AIDS population.

HIV and AIDS have forced clinicians to change the way they view opportunistic infection. As in other organ systems, these diseases have led to the emergence of unusual otologic complications. This requires that otologists be vigilant for the presence of atypical manifestations in their immunocompromised patients with ear disease (Fig. 18.14).

REFERENCES

1. Morand SF. *Opuscules de Chirurgie*. Paris: G Desprez et P.A. Le Prieur, 1762–1772;161.
2. Kafka MM. Mortality of mastoiditis and cerebral complications with review of 3225 cases of mastoiditis with complications. *Laryngoscope* 1935;45:790–822.
3. Gower D, McGuirt WF. Intracranial complications of acute and chronic infectious ear disease: a problem still with us. *Laryngoscope* 1983;93:1028–1033.
4. Courville CB. Symposium: Intracranial complications of otitis media and mastoiditis in the antibiotic era. I. Modification of the pathology of otitic intracranial lesions by antibiotic preparations. *Laryngoscope* 1955;65:31–46.

5. Prellner K, Rydell R. Acute mastoiditis. Influence of antibiotic treatment on the bacterial spectrum. *Acta Otolaryngol (Stockh)* 1986;102:52–56.

6. Ballenger JJ. Complications of ear disease. In: Ballenger JJ, ed. *Diseases of the nose, throat, ear, head, and neck,* 13th ed. Philadelphia: Lea & Febiger, 1985;1170–1196.

7. Glasscock ME III, Shambaugh GE Jr. Intracranial complications of otitis media. In: Glasscock ME III, Shambaugh GE Jr, eds. *Surgery of the ear,* 4th ed. Philadelphia: WB Saunders, 1990;249–275.

8. Neely JG. Complications of temporal bone infection. In: Cummings CW, Fredrickson JM, Harker LA, Krause CJ, Schuller DE, eds. *Otolaryngology—head and neck surgery,* 4th ed. St Louis: Mosby, 1986;2988–3015.

9. Harker LA, Koontz FP. The bacteriology of cholesteatoma. In: McCabe BF, Sadé J, Abramson M, eds. *Cholesteatoma.* Proceedings of the First International Conference. Birmingham, Alabama: Aesculapius Publishing, 1977.

10. Rupa V, Raman R. Chronic suppurative otitis media: complicated versus uncomplicated disease. *Acta Otolaryngol (Stockh)* 1991;111:530–535.

11. Piccirillo JF, Parnes SM. Ciprofloxacin for the treatment of chronic ear disease. *Laryngoscope* 1989;99:510–513.

12. Giamarellou H, Galanakis N, Dendrinos C, et al. Evaluation of ciprofloxacin in the treatment of *Pseudomonas aeruginosa* infections. *Eur J Clin Microbiol* 1986;5:232–235.

13. Merchant SN, Wang P, Jang CH, et al. Efficacy of tympanomastoid surgery for control of infection in active chronic otitis media. *Laryngoscope* 1997;107:872–877.

14. Samuel J, Fernandes CM, Steinberg JL. Intracranial otogenic complications: a persisting problem. *Laryngoscope* 1986;96:272–278.

15. Lund WS. A review of 50 cases of intracranial complications from otogenic infection between 1961 and 1977. Quoted by Glasscock ME III, Shambaugh GE Jr, eds. *Surgery of the ear,* 4th ed. Philadelphia: WB Saunders, 1990;251.

16. Schwaber MK, Pensak ML, Bartels LJ. The early signs and symptoms of neurotologic complications of chronic suppurative otitis media. *Laryngoscope* 1989;99:373–375.

17. Ludman H. Complications of suppurative otitis media. In: Kerr AG, ed. *Scott-Brown's otolaryngology,* 5th ed. London: Butterworth & Company, 1987;264–291.

18. Snow JB Jr. Cranial and intracranial complications of otitis media. In: English GM, ed. *Otolaryngology.* Philadelphia: JB Lippincott, 1988.

19. Jaisinghani VJ, Paparella MM, Schachern PA, et al. Tympanic membrane/middle ear pathologic correlates in chronic otitis media. *Laryngoscope* 1999;109:712–716.

20. Sanford JP. *Guide to antimicrobial therapy 1990.* West Bethesda: Antimicrobial Therapy, Inc., 1990.

21. Quijano M, Schuknecht HF, Otte J. Temporal bone pathology associated with intracranial abscess. *ORL J Otorhinolaryngol Relat Spec* 1988;50:2–31.

22. Southwick FS, Richardson EP Jr, Swartz MN. Septic thrombosis of the dural venous sinuses. *Medicine* 1986;65:82–106.

23. Tveteras K, Kristensen S, Dommerby H. Septic cavernous and lateral sinus thrombosis: modern diagnostic and therapeutic principles. *J Laryngol Otol* 1988;102:877–882.

24. Meltzer PE. Treatment of thrombosis of the lateral sinus. A summary of the results obtained during twelve years at the Massachusetts Eye and Ear Infirmary. *Arch Otolaryngol* 1935;22:131–142.

25. Garcia RD, Baker AS, Cunningham MJ, et al. Lateral sinus thrombosis associated with otitis media and mastoiditis in children. *Pediatr Infect Dis J* 1995;14:617–623.

26. Seid AB, Sellars SL. The management of otogenic lateral sinus disease at Groote Schuur Hospital. *Laryngoscope* 1973;83:397–403.

27. Karlin RJ, Robinson WA. Septic cavernous sinus thrombosis. *Ann Emerg Med* 1984;13:449–455.

28. Dawes JDK, 1971. Quoted by Alford BR, Cohn AM. Complications of suppurative otitis media and mastoiditis. In: Paparella MM, Shumrick DA, eds. *Otolaryngology,* 2nd ed. Philadelphia: WB Saunders, 1980;1502.

29. Villringer A, Seiderer M, Bauer WM, et al. Diagnosis of superior sagittal sinus thrombosis by three-dimensional magnetic resonance flow imaging. *Lancet* 1989;1:1086–1087.

30. Hawkins DB. Lateral sinus thrombosis: a sometimes unexpected diagnosis. *Laryngoscope* 1985;95:674–677.

31. MacEwen W. *Pyogenic infective diseases of the brain and spinal cord.* Glasgow: J Maclehose & Son, 1893.

32. Haines SJ, Mampalam T, Rosenblum ML, et al. Cranial and intracranial bacterial infections. In: Youmans JR, ed. *Neurological surgery,* 3rd ed. Philadelphia: WB Saunders, 1990;3707–3735.

33. Evans W. The pathology and etiology of brain abscess. *Lancet* 1931;1:1231–1289.

34. Beekhuis GJ, Taylor M. Ear and sinus aspects of intracranial suppurative disease in cranial and intracranial suppuration. In: Gurdjian ES, ed. *Cranial and intracranial suppuration.* Springfield, IL: Charles C Thomas, 1969.

35. Bradley PJ, Manning KP, Shaw MD. Brain abscess secondary to otitis media. *J Laryngol Otol* 1984;98:1185–1191.

36. Ayyagari A, Pancholi VK, Kak VK, et al. Bacteriological spectrum of brain abscess with special reference to anaerobic bacteria. *Indian J Med Res* 1983;77:182–186.

37. Maurice-Williams RS. Open evacuation of pus: a satisfactory surgical approach to the problem of brain abscess? *J Neurol Neurosurg Psychiatry* 1983;46:697–703.

38. Mawson SR. *Diseases of the ear,* 3rd ed. Oxford: Alden & Mowbray Ltd, 1974;17–62.

39. Britt RH. Brain abscess. In: Wilkins RH, Rengachary SS, eds. *Neurosurgery.* New York: McGraw-Hill, 1985;1928–1956.

40. Haines AB, Zimmerman RD, Morgello S, et al. MR imaging of brain abscesses. *Am J Roentgenol* 1989;152:1073–1085.

41. Heineman HS, Braude AI, Osterholm JL. Intracranial suppurative disease. Early presumptive diagnosis and successful treatment without surgery. *JAMA* 1971;218:1542–1547.

42. Carey ME, Chou SN, French LA. Experience with brain abscesses. *J Neurosurg* 1972;36:1–9.

43. Durack DT, Perfect JR. Acute bacterial meningitis. In: Wilkins RH, Rengachary SS, eds. *Neurosurgery.* New York: McGraw-Hill, 1985;1921–1928.

44. Dodge PR, Davis H, Feigin RD, et al. Prospective evaluation of hearing impairment as a sequela of acute bacterial meningitis. *N Engl J Med* 1984;311:869–874.

45. Lebel MH, Freij BJ, Syrogiannopoulos GA, et al. Dexamethasone therapy for bacterial meningitis. Results of two double-blind, placebo-controlled trials. *N Engl J Med* 1988;319:964–971.

46. Renaudin JW. Cranial epidural abscess and subdural empyema. In: Wilkins RH, Rengachary SS, eds. *Neurosurgery.* New York: McGraw-Hill, 1985;1961–1963.

47. Courville CB. Subdural empyema secondary to purulent frontal sinusitis. A clinicopathologic study of forty two-cases verified at autopsy. *Arch Otolaryngol* 1944;39:211–230.

48. Symonds CP. Otitic hydrocephalus. *Brain* 1931;54:55–71.

49. Quincke H. Ueber meningitis serosa: Volkmann's Sammlung klinischer Vortrage. NF 1893, Nr 67, in: Quincke H. Ueber Meningitis serosa und verwandte zustande. *Dtsch Z Nervenheilk* 1897;9:149.

50. Isaacman DJ. Otitic hydrocephalus: an uncommon complication of a common condition. *Ann Emerg Med* 1989;18:684–687.

51. Pfaltz CR, Griesemer C. Complications of acute middle ear infections. *Ann Otol Rhinol Laryngol* 1984;93[Suppl]:133–137.

52. Ibekwe AO, Okoye BC. Subperiosteal mastoid abscesses in chronic suppurative otitis media. *Ann Otol Rhinol Laryngol* 1988;97:373–375.

53. Bezold F, Siebenmann F. *Text-book of otology.* Holinger J, trans. Chicago: EH Colegrove, 1908;179–185.

54. Schuknecht HF, Gulya AJ. *Anatomy of the temporal bone with surgical implications.* Philadelphia: Lea & Febiger, 1986;161–184.

55. Glasscock ME III, Shambaugh GE Jr. Aural complications of otitis media. In: Glasscock ME III, Shambaugh GE Jr, eds. *Surgery of the ear,* 4th ed. Philadelphia: WB Saunders, 1990;277–292.

56. Gradenigo G. Ueber Circumscripte Leptomeningitis mit spinalen Symptomen. *Arch Ohrenheilk* 1904;51:60–62.

57. Eagleton WP. Unlocking of the petrous pyramid for localized bulbar (pontile) meningitis secondary to suppuration of the petrous apex. Report of four cases with recovery in three. *Arch Otolaryngol* 1931;13:386–422.

58. Chole RA, Donald PJ. Petrous apicitis. Clinical considerations. *Ann Otol Rhinol Laryngol* 1983;92:544–551.

59. Ramadier J. Les ostéites petreuses profondes (petrosites). *Otorhinolaryngol Int* 1933;17:816.

60. Lempert J. Complete apicectomy (mastoidotympanoapicectomy). A new technique for the complete exenteration of the apical carotid portion of the petrous pyramid. *Arch Otolaryngol* 1937;25:144–177.

61. Schuknecht HF, Gulya AJ. *Anatomy of the temporal bone with surgical implications.* Philadelphia: Lea & Febiger, 1986;111–128.

62. Eagleton WP. Localized bulbar cisterna (pontine) meningitis, facial pain, and sixth nerve paralysis and their relation to caries of the petrous apex. *Arch Surg* 1930;20:386–420.

63. Frenckner P. Some remarks on the treatment of apicitis (petrositis) with or without Gradenigo's syndrome. *Acta Otolaryngol (Stockh)* 1932;17:97–120.

64. Schuknecht HF. *Pathology of the ear.* Cambridge, MA: Harvard University Press, 1974.

65. Paparella MM, Sugiura S. The pathology of suppurative labyrinthitis. *Ann Otol Rhinol Laryngol* 1967;76:554–586.

66. McCabe BF. Labyrinthine fistula in chronic mastoiditis. *Ann Otol Rhinol Laryngol* 1984;112 [Suppl]:138–141.

67. Bates GJEM, O'Donoghue GM, Anslow P, et al. Can CT detect labyrinthine fistulae pre-operatively? *Acta Otolaryngol (Stockh)* 1988;106:40–45.

68. Jang CJ, Merchant SN. Histopathology of labyrinthine fistulae in chronic otitis media with clinical implications. *Am J Otol* 1997;18:15–25.

69. Nabili V, Brodie HA, Neverov NI, et al. Chronology of labyrinthitis ossificans induced by streptococcus pneumoniae meningitis. *Laryngoscope* 1999;109:931–935.

70. Chen MC, Harris JP, Keithley EM. Immunohistochemical analysis of proliferating cells in a sterile labyrinthitis animal model. *Laryngoscope* 1998;108:651–656.

71. Gacek RR. The surgical management of labyrinthine fistulae in chronic otitis media with cholesteatoma. *Ann Otol Rhinol Laryngol* 1974;83 [Suppl]:1–19.

72. Sheehy JL, Brackmann DE. Cholesteatoma surgery: management of the labyrinthine fistula—a report of 97 cases. *Laryngoscope* 1979;89:78–87.

73. Balkany T, Bird PA, Hodges AV, et al. Surgical technique for implantation of the totally ossified cochlea. *Laryngoscope* 1998;108:988–992.

74. Tos M. Sensorineural hearing loss in acute and chronic middle ear diseases. *Acta Otolaryngol (Stockh)* 1989;457 [Suppl]:87–93.

75. Blakley BW, Kim S. Does chronic otitis media cause sensorineural hearing loss? *J Otolaryngol* 1998;27:17–20.

76. Vartiainen E, Karjalainen S. Factors influencing sensorineural hearing loss in chronic otitis media. *Am J Otolaryngol* 1987;8:13–15.

77. Paparella MM, Brady DR, Hoel R. Sensori-neural hearing loss in chronic otitis media and mastoiditis. *Trans Am Acad Ophthalmol Otolaryngol* 1970;74:108–115.

78. Guo Y, Wu Y, Chen W, et al. Endotoxic damage to the stria vascularis: the pathogenesis of sensorineural hearing loss secondary to otitis media? *J Laryngol Otol* 1994;108:310–313.

79. Morizono T, Giebink GS, Paparella MM, et al. Sensorineural hearing loss in experimental purulent otitis media due to Streptococcus pneumoniae. *Arch Otolaryngol* 1985;111:794–798.

80. Gherman CR, Ward RR, Bassis ML. Pneumocystis carinii otitis media and mastoiditis as the initial manifestation of the acquired immunodeficiency syndrome. *Am J Med* 1988;85:250–252.

81. Park S, Wunderlich H, Goldenberg RA, et al. *Pneumocystis carinii* infection in the middle ear. *Arch Otolaryngol Head Neck Surg* 1992;118:269–270.

82. Sandler ED, Sandler JM, LeBoit PE, et al. *Pneumocystis carinii* otitis media in AIDS: a case report and review of the literature regarding extrapulmonary pneumocystosis. *Otolaryngol Head Neck Surg* 1990;103:817–821.

83. Smith MA, Hirschfield LS, Zahtz G, et al. Pneumocystis carinii otitis media. *Am J Med* 1988;85:745–746.

84. Morris MS, Prasad S. Otologic disease in the acquired immunodeficiency syndrome. *Ear Nose Throat J* 1990;69:451–453.

85. Linstrom CJ, Pincus RL, Leavitt EB, et al. Otologic neurotologic manifestations of HIV-related disease. *Otolaryngol Head Neck Surg* 1993;108:680–687.

86. Ress BD, Luntz M, Telischi FF, et al. Necrotizing external otitis in patients with AIDS. *Laryngoscope* 1997;107:456–460.

87. Hern JD, Almeyda J, Thomas DM, et al. Malignant otitis externa in HIV and AIDS. *J Laryngol Otol* 1996;110:770–775.

CHAPTER 19

Osteoradionecrosis of the Temporal Bone

Joseph B. Nadol, Jr.

Although the effects of radiation on bone have been known for many years (1), its effects on the temporal bone and labyrinth received little attention before 1950. Radiation-induced damage has been described in the external auditory canal, middle ear, ossicular chain, mastoid, petrous apex, and membranous labyrinth. Osteoradionecrosis of the temporal bone may be defined as death and sequestration of the bone following radiation therapy to the temporal bone or surrounding structures, such as the nasopharynx. Ramsden et al. (2) described two distinct clinical forms of osteoradionecrosis: localized, involvement of the tympanic bone that resolves after separation of sequestration; and diffuse, necrosis of the temporal bone resulting in secondary injury to brain, labyrinth, facial nerve, and carotid artery. Clinical signs of osteoradionecrosis may occur many years following administration of radiation.

RADIATION EFFECTS ON THE TEMPORAL BONE

External and Middle Ear

Isolated lesions induced by radiation therapy may be seen in the external ear canal and, less commonly, in the middle ear. Borsanyi (3) described necrosis of the skin of the external ear canal in approximately 10% of 100 patients who received radiation therapy for nasopharyngeal carcinoma and other tumors in the head and neck. In a study of 29 patients with osteoradionecrosis, Ramsden et al. (2) found that the most common manifestation of osteoradionecrosis of the temporal bone was necrosis of tympanic bone of the floor or anterior wall of the external auditory canal. Osteoradionecrosis of the ossicles has also been described (4–6).

Labyrinth

Hearing loss, which may be severe to profound, may occur months or years after radiation therapy to the temporal bone (7,8). The incidence of sensorineural loss may reach 36% of patients who have received a full course of radiation (7), and

in some cases vestibular damage has also been described. The effect of radiation on the membranous labyrinth as studied in an animal model (9) includes delayed degeneration of sensory and supporting cells in the organ of Corti and loss of auditory neurons. In this animal model of radiation labyrinthitis, a linear relationship between radiation dose and the percent of missing outer hair cells and supporting cells was found. In addition, significant loss of myelinated nerve fibers was seen in areas unassociated with hair cell loss, suggesting that degenerative neuropathy may be an additional and primary effect.

Mastoid and Petrous Apex

More diffuse osteoradionecrosis of the temporal bone may occur, resulting in intracranial complications (2). Although this diffuse form is most common in individuals with radiation therapy directed primarily at lesions within the temporal bone (2), diffuse and progressive osteoradionecrosis may occur in cases in which the temporal bone was not the primary focus of radiation (10,11). The incidence of diffuse osteoradionecrosis increases with radiation dose. Cole (12) found clinical evidence of osteoradionecrosis in 19% of 21 patients treated with radiation therapy for glomus jugulare tumors. In a series of 20 patients treated with surgery and postoperative radiation therapy (13), osteoradionecrosis was described in 25%. Wang and Doppke (14) reported that osteoradionecrosis may be minimized by limiting the radiation dose to 2,000 rets (nominal standard dose equivalent to 7,400 rads in 37 fractions at a rate of 5 fractions per week). Nadol and Schuknecht (10) described an incidence of osteoradionecrosis of 42% in cases of squamous cell carcinoma of the temporal bone that were treated with surgery resulting in an open mastoid cavity, followed by full-course radiation therapy, whereas in another group of patients receiving an average dose of 4,610 rads, no osteoradionecrosis occurred despite an open cavity technique, suggesting both a positive correlation with radiation dosage and the possibility of a threshold phenomenon.

RADIOBIOLOGY AND HISTOPATHOLOGY OF OSTEORADIONECROSIS

Ewing (1) described three clinical situations that predisposed to osteoradionecrosis: (i) proximity of bone to the body surface, (ii) superinfection or trauma, and (iii) poor blood supply. The primary response appears to be a vasculitis and inhibition of mitosis. There is evidence of progressive vascular damage over time, including endarteritis, thrombosis, and progressive ischemia (15), with no evidence of spontaneous microvascularization with time. Hence, the risk of osteoradionecrosis increases continuously after radiation therapy.

The histopathologic changes in bone include death of osteocytes resulting in empty bone lacunae, a progressive osteolysis and replacement by fibrillar connective tissue, decrease or cessation of new bone formation, and obliterative endarteritis (Figs. 19.1 and 19.2). Osteolysis may be greatly accelerated by superinfection (1,2,10,16).

CLINICAL PRESENTATION OF OSTEORADIONECROSIS

A wide spectrum of clinical signs and symptoms of osteoradionecrosis may first occur from months to years following radiation therapy (2,11). Localized osteoradionecrosis of the temporal bone may occasionally simulate chronic external otitis. However, chronicity and, particularly, the presence of exposed and necrotic bone with a history of previous radiation therapy to the head and neck should raise the suspicion of early osteoradionecrosis. Exposed bone usually occurs on the floor or anterior wall of the external auditory canal (Fig. 19.3). The bone itself is irregular and necrotic and may have surrounding superinfection. Persistent or intermittent drainage and pain are characteristic. Diffuse osteoradionecrosis may present with profuse otorrhea, deep-seated ear pain, loss of facial nerve function, cochlear and vestibular involvement, and intracranial complications, including meningitis, brain abscess, and thrombosis or rupture of the carotid artery (17).

There is a paucity of published data on radiographic imaging of osteoradionecrosis. By computed tomography (CT) scan (Fig. 19.4), profuse osteoradionecrosis is suggested by an irregular osteolytic lesion and surrounding fibrosis. When there is a superinfection, the radiographic appearance may be identical to that seen in chronic osteomyelitis. In localized osteoradionecrosis manifested by otoscopic identification of exposed necrotic bone in the external auditory canal, findings on CT may be minimal. The utility of bone scanning in osteoradionecrosis of the temporal bone is unknown. T2-weighted magnetic resonance imaging may hold promise in the evaluation of osteoradionecrosis of the temporal bone (18).

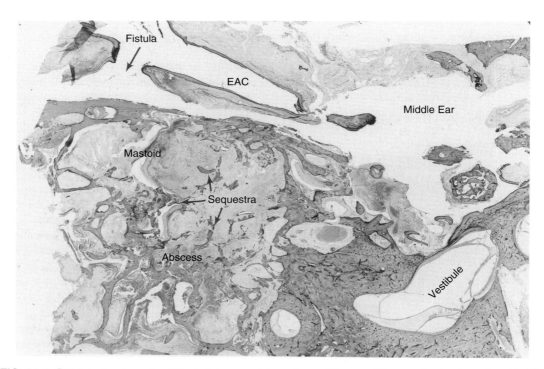

FIG. 19.1 Osteoradionecrosis of the left temporal bone in an 84-year-old man who had received 4,000 rads of external beam radiation over 10 days to a cutaneous squamous cell carcinoma of the preauricular area, completed 9 years before death. There is a fistula between the external auditory canal (EAC) and mastoid. Within the mastoid there is extensive necrosis of bone with bony sequestra embedded in fibrous tissue. There is an abscess in the central mastoid tract. There is no evidence of carcinoma of the mastoid or temporal bone. 5.2X.

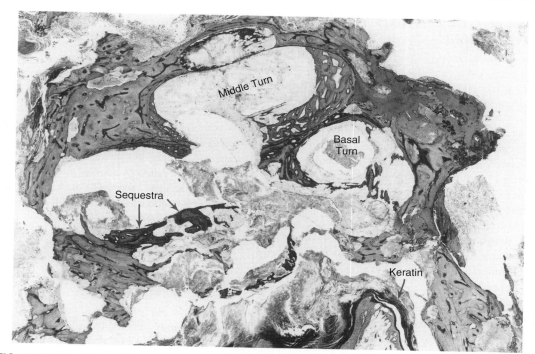

FIG. 19.2 Extensive erosion of the right temporal bone and bony labyrinth in a 58-year-old woman who died of cerebellar abscess complicating osteoradionecrosis. She had received 6,000 rads of external beam radiation to the right temporal bone for epidermoid carcinoma of the mastoid and middle ear with invasion of the labyrinth 2 years prior to death. Nonmalignant squamous cell epithelium has invaded some areas, but islands of viable epidermoid carcinoma are also seen. 15.2X.

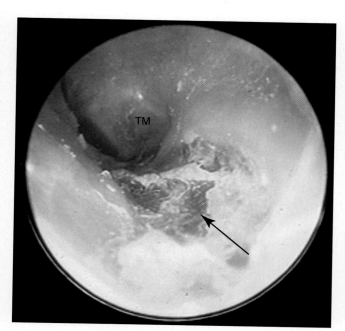

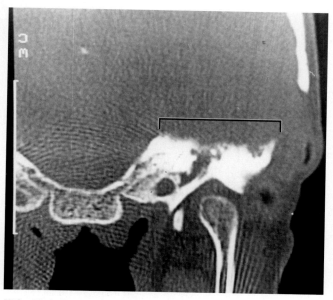

FIG. 19.3 A localized osteoradionecrosis of the left external auditory canal. Nonviable bone *(arrow)* is visible on the floor of the canal. The tympanic membrane (TM) is intact. The patient had received a full course of radiation therapy for nasopharyngeal carcinoma approximately 6 years before the onset of bilateral localized osteoradionecrosis of the temporal bone.

FIG. 19.4 Coronal CT scan of the right temporal bone in a 35-year-old woman who developed purulent drainage from the right ear canal approximately 1 year following 6,000 rads of external beam radiation for a low-grade astrocytoma of the right temporal lobe. There is soft tissue density within the mastoid air cell system and erosion of the tegmen mastoidea *(bracket)* due to osteoradionecrosis of the mastoid.

TREATMENT OF OSTEORADIONECROSIS OF THE TEMPORAL BONE

Prevention

It is clear that there is increasing risk of osteoradionecrosis with an increased dose of radiation therapy and also with larger fractions of therapy. Osteoradionecrosis may be minimized by limiting radiation dosage to no more than 2,000 rets (14). Despite careful attention to radiation dosage, osteoradionecrosis may occur. Preparation of the temporal bone for radiation therapy will significantly decrease the incidence of osteoradionecrosis. In 29 cases of squamous cell carcinoma, lateral temporal bone resection or extended radical mastoidectomy followed by thick soft tissue coverage of exposed bone by tympanomastoid obliteration significantly decreased the incidence of osteoradionecrosis (19). The surgical technique is similar to that described in Chapter 15 (total tympanomastoid obliteration).

Treatment of Established Osteoradionecrosis

Osteoradionecrosis of the temporal bone may occur following radiation to primary and metastatic lesions adjacent to the temporal bone, such as the nasopharynx or temporal lobe. In such cases, preparation of the temporal bone for ra-

diation therapy is impractical, and despite careful dosimetry, osteoradionecrosis may occur.

Localized Osteoradionecrosis

Localized osteoradionecrosis may be managed expectantly. Superinfection of the external canal may be treated with otic drops and oral, and occasionally, parenteral antibiotics. Osteonecrotic and sequestering bone may be exposed within the external auditory canal for months to years and usually does not require surgical intervention. Recurrent or chronic infection of localized osteonecrotic bone is treated by surgical debridement and coverage of the bony margins of resection with vascularized soft tissue pedicles.

Progressive Diffuse Osteoradionecrosis

Progressive diffuse osteoradionecrosis of the temporal bone may result in increasing pain, uncontrolled purulent drainage, facial nerve paralysis, and intracranial complication, and demands treatment. Wide surgical debridement of involved bone followed by generous soft tissue coverage of the bony defect has been shown to be successful in such cases (10,11) (Chapter 15). The temporoparietal fascial flap (Fig. 19.5) provides a reliable source of well-vascularized

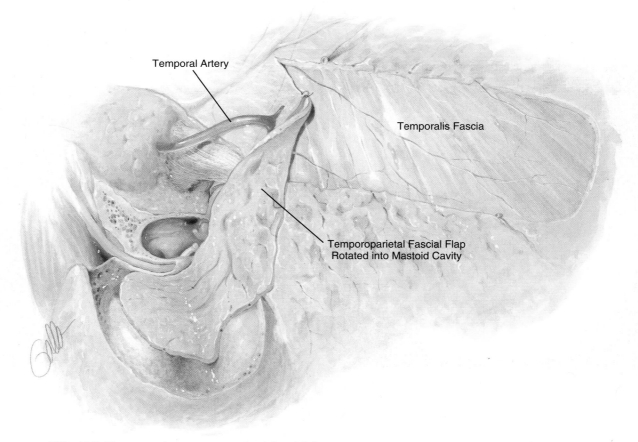

FIG. 19.5 The use of a temporoparietal fascial flap to provide a well-vascularized pedicle following canal wall–down mastoidectomy for osteoradionecrosis of the temporal bone.

tissue for the purpose of bony coverage or obliteration of the surgical defect (17). Intraoperative and postoperative parenteral antibiotics based on culture and sensitivity may be required, particularly when there is radiologic evidence of osteolysis. Preoperative administration of tetracycline to help identify the margins of vascularized bone (6) may prove a useful adjunct in delineating the extent of required bony debridement. Hyperbaric oxygen therapy may produce an angiogenic response in irradiated bone and hence provide a useful preoperative adjunct to debridement of osteoradionecrotic bone (6,15,20).

REFERENCES

1. Ewing J. Radiation osteitis. *Acta Radiol* 1926;6:399–412.
2. Ramsden RT, Bulman CH, Lorigan BP. Osteoradionecrosis of the temporal bone. *J Laryngol Otol* 1975;89:941–955.
3. Borsanyi S. The effects of radiation therapy on the ear. *South Med J* 1962;55:740–743.
4. Gyorkey J, Pollock FJ. Radiation necrosis of the ossicles. *Arch Otolaryngol* 1960;71:793–796.
5. Keleman G. Radiation and ear: experimental studies. *Acta Otolaryngol (Stock/i)* 1963;[Suppl 184]:1–48.
6. Kveton JF. Surgical management of osteoradionecrosis of the temporal bone. *Otolaryngol Head Neck Surg* 1988;98:231–234.
7. Leach W. Irradiation of the ear. *J Laryngol Otol* 1965;79:870–880.
8. Moretti JA. Sensorineural hearing loss following radiotherapy to the nasopharynx. *Laryngoscope* 1976;86:598–602.
9. Bohne BA, Marks JE, Glasgow GP. Delayed effects of ionizing radiation on the ear. *Laryngoscope* 1985;95:818–828.
10. Nadol JB Jr, Schuknecht HF. Obliteration of the mastoid in the treatment of tumors of the temporal bone. *Ann Otol Rhinol Laryngol* 1984;93:6–12.
11. Wurster CF, Krespi YP, Curtis AW. Osteoradionecrosis of the temporal bone. *Otolaryngol Head Neck Surg* 1982;90:126–129.
12. Cole JM. Glomus jugulare tumor. *Laryngoscope* 1977;87:1244–1258.
13. Wang CC. Radiation therapy in the management of carcinoma of the external auditory canal, middle ear, or mastoid. *Radiology* 1975;16: 713–715.
14. Wang CC, Doppke K. Osteoradionecrosis of the temporal bone: consideration of nominal standard dose. *J Radiat Oncol Biol Phys* 1976;1: 881–883.
15. Marx RE, Johnson RP. Studies in the radiobiology of osteoradionecrosis and their clinical significance. *Oral Surg Oral Med Oral Pathol* 1987;64:379–390.
16. Schuknecht HF, Karmody CS. Radionecrosis of the temporal bone. *Laryngoscope* 1966;76:1416–1428.
17. Guida RA, Finn DG, Buchalter IH, et al. Radiation injury to the temporal bone. *Am J Otol* 1990; 11:6–11.
18. Nishimura R, Baba Y, Murakami R, et al. MR evaluation of radiation otomastoiditis. *Tnt J Rad Oncol Biol Phys* 1997;1:55–60.
19. Cheney ML, Megerian CA, Brown MT, et al. The use of the temporoparietal fascial flap in temporal bone reconstruction. *Am J Otol* 1996;17:137–142.
20. Ashamalla HL, Thone SR, Goldwein JW. Hyperbaric oxygen therapy for the treatment of radiation-induced sequelae in children. The University of Pennsylvania experience. *Cancer* 1996;77:2407–2412.

CHAPTER 20

Malignant External Otitis

Marlene L. Durand

Malignant otitis externa (MOE) is an invasive bacterial infection of the external auditory canal and skull base. It involves the soft tissues adjacent to the skull base and often progresses to osteomyelitis of the skull base. It occurs primarily in elderly patients with diabetes mellitus and is nearly always due to *Pseudomonas aeruginosa*. Patients typically present with weeks to months of unilateral ear pain and drainage. Cranial neuropathies may be present; a facial nerve palsy is the most common. Patients are usually afebrile and appear nontoxic. Physical examination may be normal except for the finding of granulation tissue in the mid–external auditory canal. Computed tomography (CT) or magnetic resonance imaging (MRI) may demonstrate bony erosion of the skull base. Cultures of purulent drainage and of the granulation tissue in the ear canal should be taken prior to starting antibiotics. Treatment consists of prolonged (at least 6 weeks) systemic antibiotic therapy; surgical debridement is almost never necessary.

The disease was first described by Meltzer and Kelemen in 1959 (1). In 1968, however, Chandler was the first to name it "malignant otitis externa" when he described 13 patients with the infection, seven of whom died (2). Since then, the disease has also been labeled "necrotizing," "progressive," and "invasive" otitis externa (3–5), although "malignant" remains the most commonly used adjective.

PATHOGENESIS

Pseudomonas is not a normal colonizer of the ear canal in either diabetic or nondiabetic patients (6). It is a water-loving organism, however, and can be cultured from sinks and faucets, as well as lake and tap water. It is not clear why this organism is the predominant cause of otitis externa and MOE, although its predilection for warm, moist environments may be a partial explanation.

Pseudomonas bacteria in the ear canal are thought to invade through the fissures of Santorini into deeper soft tissues, temporal bone, and then skull base (Fig. 20.1). The facial nerve becomes involved as the infection spreads through the stylomastoid foramen. Cranial nerves (CN) IX, X, and XI may be affected if the infection spreads to the jugular foramen and CN XII as the infection extends to the hypoglossal canal. Infection of the petrous apex may involve CN VI and less often CN V. Extension into the temporomandibular joint may cause a destructive osteomyelitis (7).

Most patients with MOE are diabetic, but hyperglycemia per se is probably not a factor in pathogenesis of MOE (8). Rather, the microangiopathy caused by diabetes most likely leads to hypoperfusion in the skin of the temporal bone and increased local susceptibility to infection (5). A histopathologic study of two patients who died from MOE revealed thickening of periodic acid-Schiff–positive material in the subendothelial basement membrane of the capillaries in skin overlying the temporal bones (5). Most patients with MOE are over age 60, and blood vessel changes occur with aging as well.

RISK FACTORS

Diabetes mellitus is the major risk factor for MOE; in most series, diabetic patients account for more than 90% of cases (5,8). Unlike diabetic patients with mucormycosis, ketoacidosis in patients presenting with MOE is very rare and diabetes is often mild. Combining data on 35 diabetic patients in three recent series of MOE studies where specific diabetic status was reported, 20% were diet controlled, 40% used oral hypoglycemics, and only 40% were insulin dependent (9–11).

Irrigation of the external ear canal to remove cerumen may be a risk factor for MOE. Rubin and colleagues reported that nearly two thirds of their patients with MOE had a history of aural irrigation with tap water within a few days prior to the onset of symptoms (12), and others have also noted this association (13,14).

Older age is also a risk factor for MOE, and the average age of patients in several series was 67 or older (8). Malignant otitis externa is rare in children, and those who develop the disease usually do not have diabetes but are immunocompromised (e.g., malignancy, chemotherapy) (15,16).

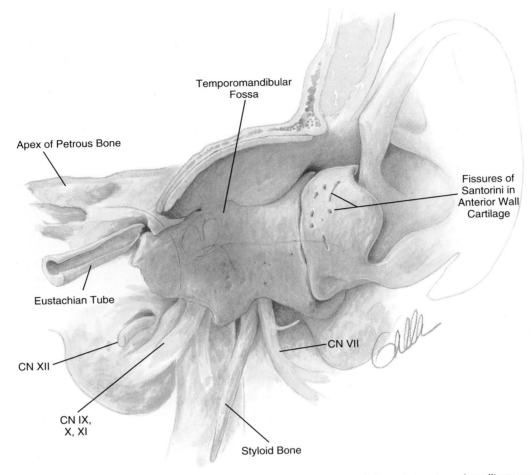

FIG. 20.1 Malignant otitis externa. Bacteria (usually *Pseudomonas*) from the external auditory canal invades through the fissures of Santorini into deeper soft tissues and bone. Infection usually spreads inferiorly first and may progressively involve the stylomastoid foramen and cranial nerve VII, followed by involvement of cranial nerves IX and X and occasionally XI in the jugular foramen. Further spread inferiorly may lead to cranial nerve XII palsy. Infection also may spread from the auditory canal anteriorly to involve the temporomandibular joint or medially into the petrous apex to involve cranial nerve VI.

Nondiabetic adults may also develop MOE, and many such patients are immunocompromised. Although nondiabetics generally account for fewer than 10% of patients, two groups from Israel have reported that 22% (5 of 23) (9) and 30% (9 of 30) (17) of their MOE patients had no risk factors other than age (all older than 65 years).

Nondiabetic patients with acquired immunodeficiency syndrome (AIDS) may develop MOE, although few such patients have been reported. *Aspergillus* was the pathogen in two AIDS patients with MOE, *Pseudomonas* in four others (18).

CLINICAL PRESENTATION

Most patients with MOE have chronic otorrhea and otalgia. Duration of symptoms prior to diagnosis is usually weeks to months, even in recent series (10). Patients may develop otorrhea prior to the onset of pain. The amount of drainage is variable. When ear pain develops, it initially may be mild, gradually increasing over several weeks to a deep, aching, persistent pain. It is often worse at night, awakening the patient from sleep (19). Patients may complain of headache, especially temporal and parietal on the affected side. Temporomandibular joint pain and tenderness may occur, and pain may be so severe that patients avoid chewing (8). One third of patients complain of hearing loss (5). Patients usually have no systemic symptoms of infection, such as fever, chills, or night sweats.

Facial nerve palsy was found on presentation in approximately one third of patients in older series (5) and generally developed after at least 2 months of symptoms (20). Rarely facial palsy appears as early as 1 week after onset of illness. Other cranial neuropathies develop after the appearance of facial palsy and have been a poor prognostic sign (5). Cranial nerves IX, X, XI, and XII are more often involved than V and VI. Only one patient has been described with documented cranial nerve II involvement (21). This patient developed unilateral blindness from optic nerve invasion by *Pseudomonas* after a 2-year course of refractory MOE involving multiple cranial nerves (VI, VII, IX, X, XII). Cranial nerve III palsy had developed in the affected eye 2 weeks earlier. It should be emphasized, however, that cranial neuropathies are usually late findings in MOE. In a recent series of 23 patients diagnosed soon (1 to 6 weeks) after onset of symptoms, no patient presented with cranial neuropathies (22).

The classic finding on physical examination is granulation tissue in the inferior portion of the ear canal, at the bony cartilaginous junction. The canal is often edematous and erythematous. A purulent discharge is nearly always present. The tympanic membrane is often obscured by granulation tissue, but when visible it is often intact (5). There may be periauricular tenderness and pain with movement of the pinna. Tenderness is often present in the lateral aspect of the infratemporal fossa and may be elicited by digital pressure between the mandible and mastoid tip. Hearing loss may be evident in the affected ear. Facial palsy and other cranial neuropathies may be present, as noted earlier. The remainder of the physical examination is usually unremarkable.

LABORATORY FINDINGS

Routine chemistry studies are normal aside from an elevated glucose level in diabetic patients. The white blood cell count is usually normal or minimally elevated. The cardinal laboratory abnormality in MOE is the erythrocyte sedimentation rate (ESR), which is elevated in nearly every patient. It is often markedly elevated (more than 50 mm/hour) and is one of the few nonrheumatologic conditions that cause elevation greater than 100. One group reported that the ESR was elevated in all 25 of their MOE patients, with mean value of 87 mm/hour (8). The ESR decreases over several weeks with appropriate therapy. Relapse of infection after apparently successful therapy is often heralded by renewed ESR elevation.

Patients with known diabetes usually have elevated glucose levels, but as noted previously, ketoacidosis is very rare (15,23). Patients who present with MOE but have no history of diabetes should have fasting glucose and hemoglobin A_1C levels tested.

BACTERIOLOGY

P. aeruginosa, an aerobic gram-negative bacillus, is the cause of nearly all cases of MOE. However, cultures of purulent drainage and granulation tissue should be obtained prior to starting systemic antibiotics in all patients for two reasons. First, it is important to determine antibiotic susceptibility of the *Pseudomonas* strain prior to starting prolonged

therapy, and second, rare cases of MOE may be due to other organisms. If cultures are only obtained after starting systemic antibiotics, a culture that doesn't grow *Pseudomonas* may be discounted as falsely negative.

Fewer than 10 cases of MOE due to bacteria other than *Pseudomonas* have been reported. These include three cases of *Staphylococcus aureus* (24–26), two cases of *Proteus mirabilis (26,27), and two cases of Klebsiella* (one also grew *Enterobacter*) (9). Three of these patients had diabetes, two had AIDS, one was an infant, and one was not further identified. An additional case of *S. aureus* in a healthy 25-year-old man was characterized by bilateral erosion of the ear canal skin and may not be MOE (28). Two cases of classic MOE in which cultures grew primarily *S. epidermidis* have been reported, although causality is hard to prove with this ear canal colonizer (29,30).

Approximately 20 cases due to fungi have been reported (18,31–33). All but one were due to *Aspergillus* (*A. fumigatus* more often than *A. flavus*); one was due to *Malassezia sympodialis* (34). Nearly all patients had hematologic malignancies or AIDS, although two cases occurred in elderly diabetics, and two in patients who were elderly (over 80 years old) but not diabetic or immunocompromised (31,35).

RADIOLOGIC STUDIES

The CT scan is the most helpful radiologic study in diagnosing and following MOE (Fig. 20.2). The ability of CT to delineate normal fat planes in the area inferior to the temporal bone makes it particularly useful in this disease (36). A study analyzing 33 sequential CT scans in 11 patients with MOE found that soft tissue in the external auditory canal and fluid in the mastoid or middle ear were found in nearly all patients (37). Other findings included abnormal soft tissue around the eustachian tube (7 of 11, 64%), mass effect in nasopharynx (54%), subtemporal extension (54%), parapharyngeal space involvement (54%), and disease in the masticator space (27%). In all cases, clinical cure occurred before radiologic improvement, and areas of bone destruction on CT did not return to normal. Findings on CT that did improve or resolve slowly with successful therapy included fluid in the mastoid or middle ear and soft tissue abnormalities beneath temporal bone and skull base.

MRI is much less sensitive than CT for demonstrating cortical bone erosion, however, so CT is the preferred study at initial diagnosis (38). A study that compared CT and MRI at diagnosis and follow-up in seven patients with MOE found that subtemporal soft tissue abnormalities were seen with both modalities in all patients but were better appreciated with MRI (38). This study concluded that MRI may also be better than CT for evaluation and follow-up of meningeal enhancement and changes within the osseous medullary cavity.

The usefulness of nuclear medicine studies in MOE is not clear. Technetium-99 bone scanning and gallium-67 scanning are both very sensitive (90% to 100%) in detecting

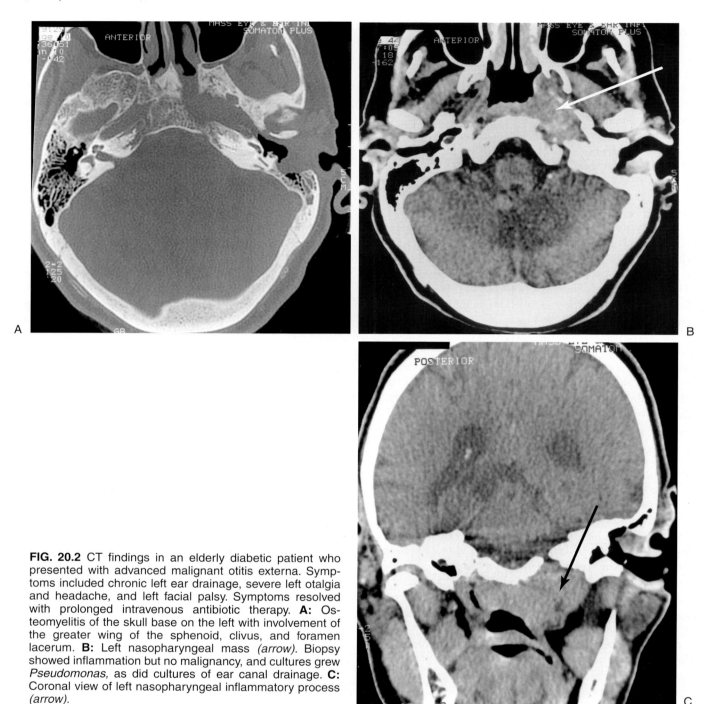

FIG. 20.2 CT findings in an elderly diabetic patient who presented with advanced malignant otitis externa. Symptoms included chronic left ear drainage, severe left otalgia and headache, and left facial palsy. Symptoms resolved with prolonged intravenous antibiotic therapy. **A:** Osteomyelitis of the skull base on the left with involvement of the greater wing of the sphenoid, clivus, and foramen lacerum. **B:** Left nasopharyngeal mass *(arrow)*. Biopsy showed inflammation but no malignancy, and cultures grew *Pseudomonas,* as did cultures of ear canal drainage. **C:** Coronal view of left nasopharyngeal inflammatory process *(arrow).*

early MOE but have low specificity. A positive bone scan may be seen in any condition of the head and neck that causes inflammation, including simple external otitis or carcinoma (8). Gallium scanning is also positive in nearly all patients with MOE and has been recommended by some authors as a means of following clinical improvement (39). However, one study described two patients who had recurrence of disease despite a negative gallium study (40).

DIFFERENTIAL DIAGNOSIS

Although MOE may be mistaken for simple otitis externa, the latter diagnosis should be suspect in an elderly diabetic patient with findings that typify MOE (e.g., persistent deep pain, canal granulation tissue, elevated ESR, CT abnormalities). Benign necrotizing osteitis of the external canal is a rare condition that occurs in nondiabetic patients (41). Patients present with chronic otorrhea but not typically pain, and a sequestrum is seen in the external meatus. The absence of pain and the ear canal findings would distinguish this condition from MOE.

Carcinoma of the temporal bone cannot be differentiated from MOE by radiologic studies, and in rare cases the clinical presentation may be similar. The finding of *Pseudomonas* on culture of the external canal is not pathognomonic for MOE, because it may be present as part of a simple external otitis in a patient with underlying carcinoma. In addition, two patients have been described who had both MOE and squamous cell carcinoma of the temporal bone (42,43). In each case, the patient underwent a second biopsy because of failure to respond to antibiotic therapy and the diagnosis of carcinoma was made histologically.

Patients with skull base involvement from MOE may have unilateral retropharyngeal swelling on CT that is indistinguishable from nasopharyngeal carcinoma, and the converse is true. Biopsy of the nasopharyngeal mass in MOE, however, reveals only inflammation, and cultures are positive for *Pseudomonas* (44).

TREATMENT

Antibiotics

Appropriate antibiotic therapy alone will cure most cases of MOE. At least 6 weeks of antibiotics are required. If infection has recurred, 8 to 12 weeks are indicated. Because nearly all cases are due to *P. aeruginosa*, therapy directed against this organism should be started as soon as cultures are obtained. Antibiotics should be adjusted once sensitivity results are known.

Serious *Pseudomonas* infections are usually treated with combination therapy using agents from two different classes of antibiotics. Older articles proposed use of combination therapy with an antipseudomonal beta-lactam plus an aminoglycoside (e.g., ticarcillin plus tobramycin). However, aminoglycoside therapy given for more than 2 weeks is likely to have significant nephrotoxicity and ototoxicity. Prolonged aminoglycoside therapy should be avoided, especially in elderly diabetics. Quinolones are preferred over aminoglycosides because of their lack of toxicity, excellent tissue penetration, and good bioavailability from oral dosing. Ciprofloxacin is the quinolone of choice because it has the greatest activity against *Pseudomonas*.

Many authors have reported success in treating MOE with ciprofloxacin alone. Although many of these cases had early disease (9), some had extensive disease that had failed to respond to conventional combination therapy but responded to ciprofloxacin (10,11,45). Of concern with ciprofloxacin monotherapy for *Pseudomonas*, however, is the development of resistance during therapy. A report of patients treated with 6 to 14 weeks of ciprofloxacin for chronic *Pseudomonas* osteomyelitis of long bones or sternum found that partial or complete resistance developed in 31% (4 of 13 patients) (46). In MOE, there have been few reports of failure due to documented ciprofloxacin resistance. One patient

with *Pseudomonas* MOE initially responded but then worsened after 8 weeks of ciprofloxacin therapy. Repeat cultures showed that the same *Pseudomonas* phage type was still present but was now resistant to ciprofloxacin (47).

Another report found that 9% of 58 patients with MOE treated with ofloxacin or pefloxacin developed resistant *Pseudomonas* (48). These agents are less active against *Pseudomonas* than ciprofloxacin, however, and the rate of development of resistance during ciprofloxacin therapy for MOE is unknown.

There are no trials comparing success with combination therapy versus ciprofloxacin alone in treating MOE. However, because of the risk of resistance developing during monotherapy, we favor combination therapy with ciprofloxacin plus a second agent for sensitive strains of *Pseudomonas*. No synergy studies are available, but it seems reasonable to use ceftazidime (or ticarcillin or piperacillin) as the second agent. Intravenous ceftazidime 2 g q8h requires less frequent administration than ticarcillin or piperacillin, so it is easier as a home intravenous antibiotic agent. Oral ciprofloxacin 750 mg bid will give blood levels equal to intravenous ciprofloxacin 400 mg bid if absorption is normal; divalent cations, such as calcium and magnesium found in antacids, will decrease quinolone absorption and should be avoided. For sick patients with advanced disease and uncertain absorption, intravenous ciprofloxacin may be indicated initially. For a patient with advanced disease in whom a highly resistant *Pseudomonas* is likely, empiric therapy with imipenem plus amikacin may be indicated until culture results are available because resistance to these agents is very rare.

Surgery

The role of surgery is limited to superficial local debridement (e.g., aural polypectomy). Most patients in early series underwent a major surgical procedure (e.g., deep debridement, mastoidectomy, facial nerve decompression) in an attempt to control the infection, but mortality in these series was 50% (2). It should be noted that until 1969, the only antipseudomonal agents available were aminoglycosides, which have poor tissue penetration, and systemic colistin or polymixin, which are very toxic. With the advent of antipseudomonal beta-lactams in 1969 (initially carbenicillin and later ticarcillin, piperacillin, ceftazidime) and their use in combination with aminoglycosides, mortality decreased to approximately 20% (49). Experience in recognizing and treating this disease, plus the availability of quinolones in the 1990s, has decreased mortality to less than 10% (8). Medical therapy is the treatment of choice, and major surgical debridement is no longer advocated. Indeed, some authors believe that temporal bone surgery is contraindicated in MOE because it will open up new planes for the spread of infection (10).

Hyperbaric Oxygen

The role of hyperbaric oxygen is unclear, but this therapy should be considered in patients for whom appropriate antibiotic therapy is unsuccessful. Rare cases of MOE with extensive disease, worsening despite antibiotic therapy, have improved rapidly once hyperbaric oxygen was added (50,51).

OUTCOME

Clinical Response

Patients who are responding to therapy typically have a steady decline in their otalgia, usually within the first week of effective therapy. In one series, otalgia responded an average of 6 days after starting therapy (11); in another, relief of pain occurred an average of 18 days after starting therapy (9). Patients whose symptoms continue to improve should have a follow-up CT scan at the end of therapy to serve as a baseline should subsequent relapse occur. The bony changes seen on CT are unlikely to improve despite cure. Soft tissue abnormalities seen on CT or MRI will slowly improve, although radiologic improvement typically lags behind clinical cure.

Persistent or worsening pain usually signals progression of disease and should prompt further evaluation. This should include repeat ear cultures, ESR, radiologic studies (CT and MRI), and possibly biopsy for deeper cultures and to exclude carcinoma. Patients with progressive disease should have change in antibiotic therapy, particularly if they were receiving ciprofloxacin alone. Two potent "reserve" antipseudomonal antibiotics (e.g., imipenem plus amikacin) should be chosen while awaiting repeat culture results, then modified based on sensitivities.

Relapse

Relapse of infection after apparently successful therapy may occur in up to 20% of patients. The first sign of relapse is usually recurrent otalgia, and this should prompt repeat examination, cultures, CT scan, and ESR. The ESR, which almost always decreases with appropriate therapy, is elevated once again. Relapse may occur many months after therapy is completed, although usually occurs within 3 months.

Mortality

A review of 95 cases published through 1979 reported an overall mortality rate of 36% (5) but a higher rate with cranial nerve involvement. Mortality was only 14% in patients with no cranial neuropathies or other central nervous system deficits, 53% with facial nerve palsy, and 60% if additional neurologic deficits were present. All cases were due to *Pseudomonas*.

Mortality is clearly related to extent of disease at diagnosis. Recent series have reported mortality rates of 10% or less, and this may be partly due to earlier recognition and treatment of disease. In one recent series of 23 patients, no patient died from progression of MOE, and overall mortality

was 4% (9). However, patients had very early disease at presentation with an average of only 3 weeks of symptoms. Lower mortality may also be due to better antibiotic therapy. A series of 10 consecutive patients who received prolonged ciprofloxacin therapy were cured, including 6 with evidence of extensive infection (10). Conventional combination therapy is highly effective as well; a series of 40 patients treated from 1978 to 1985 with a semi-synthetic penicillin plus an aminoglycoside had an attributable mortality rate of only 5% (25).

CONCLUSION

Malignant external otitis is still a disease most commonly seen in elderly diabetic patients. *P. aeruginosa* causes nearly all cases; fewer than 30 exceptions have been reported. Surgery is not indicated except for local debridement of the ear canal. Treatment should be with systemic antibiotics (e.g., ciprofloxacin plus ceftazidime) for at least 6 weeks. Current overall mortality rates are 5% to 10%. With early diagnosis, this is no longer a "malignant" disease.

REFERENCES

1. Meltzer PE, Kelemen G. Pyocyaneous osteomyelitis of the temporal bone, mandible and zygoma. *Laryngoscope* 1959;69:1300–1316.
2. Chandler JR. Malignant external otitis. *Laryngoscope* 1968;78:1257–1294.
3. Evans IT, Richards SH. Malignant (necrotising) otitis externa. *J Laryngol Otol* 1973;87:13–20.
4. Cohn AM. Progressive necrotizing otitis. Malignant external otitis. *Arch Otolaryngol* 1974;99:136–139.
5. Doroghazi RM, Nadol JB, Hyslop NE, et al. Invasive external otitis. Report of 21 cases and review of the literature. *Am J Med* 1981;71:603–614.
6. Salit IE, Miller B, Wigmore M, et al. Bacterial flora of the external canal in diabetics and nondiabetics. *Laryngoscope* 1982;92:672–673.
7. Midwinter KI, Gill KS, Spencer JA, et al. Osteomyelitis of the temporomandibular joint in patients with malignant otitis externa. *J Laryngol Otol* 1999;113:451–453.
8. Rubin J, Yu VL. Malignant external otitis: insights into pathogenesis, clinical manifestations, diagnosis, and therapy. *Am J Med* 1988;85:391–398.
9. Lang R, Goshen S, Kitzes-Cohen R, et al. Successful treatment of malignant external otitis with oral ciprofloxacin: report of experience with 23 patients. *J Infect Dis* 1990;161:537–540.
10. Levenson MJ, Parisier SC, Dolitsky J, et al. Ciprofloxacin: drug of choice in the treatment of malignant external otitis (MEO). *Laryngoscope* 1991;101:821–824.
11. Rubin J, Stoehr G, Yu VL, et al. Efficacy of oral ciprofloxacin plus rifampin for treatment of malignant external otitis. *Arch Otolaryngol Head Neck Surg* 1989;115:1063–1069.
12. Rubin J, Yu VL, Kamerer DB, et al. Aural irrigation with water: a potential pathogenic mechanism for inducing malignant external otitis? *Ann Otol Rhinol Laryngol* 1990;99:117–119.
13. Zikk D, Rapoport Y, Himelfarb MZ. Invasive external otitis after removal of impacted cerumen by irrigation [letter]. *N Engl J Med* 1991;325:969–970.
14. Ford GR, Courteney-Harris RG. Another hazard of ear syringing: malignant external otitis. *J Laryngol Otol* 1990;104:709–710.
15. Sobie S, Brodsky L, Stanievich JF. Necrotizing external otitis in children: report of two cases and review of the literature. *Laryngoscope* 1987;97:598–601.
16. Rubinstein E, Ostfeld E, Ben-Zaray S, et al. Necrotizing external otitis. *Pediatrics* 1980;66:618–620.
17. Shpitzer T, Stern Y, Cohen 0, et al. Malignant external otitis in nondiabetic patients. *Ann Otol Rhinol Laryngol* 1993;102:870–872.

18. Weinroth SE, Schessel D, Tuazon CU. Malignant otitis externa in AIDS patients: case report and review of the literature. *Ear Nose Throat J* 1994;73:772–778.
19. Chandler JR. Malignant external otitis and facial paralysis. *Otolaryngol Clin North Am* 1974;7:375–383.
20. Corey JP, Levandowski RA, Panwalker AP. Prognostic implications of therapy for necrotizing external otitis. *Am J Otol* 1985;6:353–358.
21. Holder CD, Gurucharri M, Bartels LJ, et al. Malignant external otitis with optic neuritis. *Laryngoscope* 1986;96:1021–1023.
22. Sade J, Lang R, Goshen S, et al. Ciprofloxacin treatment of malignant external otitis. *Am J Med* 1989;87(5A):138S–141S.
23. Merritt WT, Bass JW, Bruhn FW. Malignant external otitis in an adolescent with diabetes. *J Pediatr* 1980;96:872–873.
24. Bayardelle P, Jolivet-Granger M, Larochelle D. Staphylococcal malignant external otitis. *Can Med Assoc J* 1982;126:155–156.
25. Babiatzki A, Sade J. Malignant external otitis. *J Laryngol Otol* 1987;101:205–210.
26. Ress BD, Luntz M, Telischi FF, et al. Necrotizing external otitis in patients with AIDS. *Laryngoscope* 1997;107:456–460.
27. Coser PL, Stamm AE, Lobo RC, et al. Malignant external otitis in infants. *Laryngoscope* 1980;90:312–316.
28. Keay DG, Murray JA. Malignant otitis externa due to *Staphylococcus* infection. *J Laryngol Otol* 1988;102:926–927.
29. Soldati D, Mudry A, Monnier P. Necrotizing otitis externa caused by *Staphylococcus* epidermidis. *Eur Arch Otorhinolaryngol* 1999;256:439–441.
30. Barrow HN, Levenson MJ. Necrotizing "malignant" external otitis caused by *Staphylococcus* epidermidis. *Arch Otolaryngol Head Neck Surg* 1992;118:94–96.
31. Gordon G, Giddings NA. Invasive otitis externa due to *Aspergillus* species: case report and review. *Clin Infect Dis* 1994;19:866–870.
32. Hern JD, Almeyda J, Thomas DM, et al. Malignant otitis externa in HIV and AIDS. *J Laryngol Otol* 1996;110:770–775.
33. Munoz A, Martinez-Chamorro E. Necrotizing external otitis caused by *Aspergillus* fumigatus: computed tomography and high resolution magnetic resonance imaging in an AIDS patient. *J Laryngol Otol* 1998;112:98–102.
34. Chai FC, Auret K, Christiansen K, et al. Malignant otitis externa caused by Malassezia sympodialis. *Head Neck* 2000;22:87–89.
35. Cunningham M, Yu VL, Turner J, et al. Necrotizing otitis externa due to *Aspergillus* in an immunocompetent patient. *Arch Otolaryngol Head Neck Surg* 1988;114:554–556.
36. Curtin HD, Wolfe P, May M. Malignant external otitis: CT evaluation. *Radiology* 1982;145:383–388.
37. Rubin J, Curtin HD, Yu VL, et al. Malignant external otitis: utility of CT in diagnosis and follow-up. *Radiology* 1990;174:391–394.
38. Grandis JR, Curtin HD, Yu VL. Necrotizing (malignant) external otitis: prospective comparison of CT and MR imaging in diagnosis and follow-up. *Radiology* 1995;196:499–504.
39. Parisier SC, Lucente FE, Som PM, et al. Nuclear scanning in necrotizing progressive "malignant" external otitis. *Laryngoscope* 1982;92:1016–1019.
40. Gherini SG, Brackmann DE, Bradley WG. Magnetic resonance imaging and computerized tomography in malignant external otitis. *Laryngoscope* 1986;96:542–548.
41. Kumar BN, Walsh RM, Sinha A, et al. Benign necrotizing osteitis of the external auditory meatus. *J Laryngol Otol* 1997;111:269–270.
42. Mattucci KF, Setzen M, Galantich P. Necrotizing otitis externa occurring concurrently with epidermoid carcinoma. *Laryngoscope* 1986;96:264–266.
43. Grandis JR, Hirsch BE, Yu VL. Simultaneous presentation of malignant external otitis and temporal bone cancer. *Arch Otolaryngol Head Neck Surg* 1993;119:687–689.
44. Chandler JR, Grobman L, Quencer R, et al. Osteomyelitis of the base of the skull. *Laryngoscope* 1986;96:245–251.
45. Morrison GA, Bailey CM. Relapsing malignant otitis externa successfully treated with ciprofloxacin. *J Laryngol Otol* 1988;102:872–876.
46. Gilbert DN, Tice AD, Marsh PK, et al. Oral ciprofloxacin therapy for chronic contiguous osteomyelitis caused by aerobic gram-negative bacilli. *Am J Med* 1987;82:254–258.
47. Cooper MA, Andrews JM, Wise R. Ciprofloxacin resistance developing during treatment of malignant otitis externa. *J Antimicrob Chemother* 1993;32:163–164.
48. Giamarellou H. Malignant otitis externa: the therapeutic evolution of a lethal infection. *J Antimicrob Chemother* 1992;30:745–751.
49. Chandler JR. Pathogenesis and treatment of facial paralysis due to malignant external otitis. *Ann Otol Rhinol Laryngol* 1972;81:648–658.
50. Davis JC, Gates GA, Lerner C, et al. Adjuvant hyperbaric oxygen in malignant external otitis. *Arch Otolaryngol Head Neck Surg* 1992;118:89–93.
51. Shupak A, Greenberg E, Hardoff R, et al. Hyperbaric oxygen for necrotizing (malignant) otitis externa. *Arch Otolaryngol Head Neck Surg* 1989;115:1470–1475.

PART V

Surgery for Conductive Hearing Loss

CHAPTER 21

Otitis Media with Effusion

Michael J. Cunningham and Roland D. Eavey

Otitis media is the most common diagnosis made by physicians who care for children. Eighty percent of children have experienced at least one episode of otitis media by 3 years of age (1). In contrast to acute otitis media (AOM), otitis media with effusion (OME) defines a collection of fluid in the tympanomastoid compartment without the signs and symptoms of acute inflammation. This term includes and replaces other synonyms for this condition, such as secretory otitis media, nonsuppurative otitis media, catarrhal otitis media, and glue ear.

Although the term *OME* implies chronicity, a chronic middle ear effusion is specifically defined as one documented to be present longer than 8 weeks. Subacute OME is the proper designation for a documented effusion of 21 days' to 8 weeks' duration. Any effusion present less than 3 weeks is arbitrarily referred to as acute (2).

The prevalence of OME in the pediatric population in this country has only recently been established. Monthly examinations of children 2 through 6 years of age in a day care setting in Pittsburgh, Pennsylvania revealed that 53% of the children in the first year of the study and 61% of the children in the second year demonstrated OME (3). Otitis media with effusion was far more prevalent in these children during the fall and winter months and was significantly associated with viral upper respiratory tract infections.

PATHOGENESIS OF OTITIS MEDIA WITH EFFUSION

Abnormal eustachian tube function appears to be the most important factor in the pathogenesis of OME, particularly in children without a history of recent acute otitis. Noninfectious OME is believed to be a sequela of persistently high negative middle ear pressure resulting from functional or mechanical eustachian tube obstruction (4). Functional eustachian tube obstruction is defined as persistent eustachian tube collapse due to increased tubal compliance, an inactive opening mechanism, or both. Such functional eustachian tube obstruction most probably accounts for the age-dependent predisposition of infants and young children to OME (5); it has been attributed to anatomic differences in

the length, width, and angle of the eustachian tube (6). Similar anatomic-physiologic mechanisms also account for racial and familial differences in predisposition to OME (7). This correlation of anatomic abnormality, physiologic eustachian tube dysfunction, and increased predisposition to OME is most clearly demonstrated by the cleft palate population (8,9). Similarly, children with Down syndrome and other congenital craniofacial anomalies are high-risk groups for the development of OME (10).

Mechanical eustachian tube obstruction can be of an intrinsic or extrinsic nature. Intrinsic mechanical obstruction is typically attributed to tubal inflammation and secondary edema. Potential inflammatory provocateurs include infectious upper respiratory tract viruses (11), inhalant allergens in atopic individuals (12), household cigarette smoke exposure (13), and radiation therapy (14). Extrinsic mechanical obstruction has most often been attributed to adenoid hypertrophy. Less commonly, congenital nasopharyngeal cysts, juvenile angiofibroma, or nasopharyngeal malignancies in the adolescent and adult populations may play a similar obstructive role.

The exact role of enlarged adenoid tissue in the pathogenesis of OME most probably entails several mechanisms in addition to physical blockage of the nasopharyngeal end of the eustachian tube (15–17). A large adenoid or equivalent mass may obstruct the posterior choanae, contributing directly to increased nasopharyngeal pressure during swallowing and indirectly to nasopharyngeal–middle ear reflux. Adenoidal lymphoid tissue may also serve as a bacterial reservoir from which middle ear reinfection can occur (18).

Systemic factors may also predispose certain individuals toward the development or persistence of OME. Immunosuppression/immunodeficiency (19) and the immotile cilia syndromes (20) are two examples.

DIAGNOSIS OF OTITIS MEDIA WITH EFFUSION

Otitis media with effusion has also been called silent otitis because of its common asymptomatic presentation. This is particularly true in infants and young children (21). The absence of fever and constitutional symptoms in such cases often delays the diagnosis, and the effusions tend to be truly chronic in duration.

Children with chronic OME are often brought to the attention of their primary care physicians due to suspected hearing loss, often in association with speech delay. Older children may complain of ear pain or fullness; younger children may manifest this symptom by ear tugging. Occasionally children with OME present with balance difficulties.

An earlier diagnosis of OME in a subacute phase is often made in children following a recent AOM episode. Up to 40% of children have persistent middle ear effusion 4 weeks following a bout of AOM, and this middle ear fluid persists in 20% and 10% of children at 2 and 3 months' status after diagnosis, respectively (22). Such persistent, postinfectious OME is particularly likely to occur in children under 6 years of age (23).

Children with chronic OME are also more prone to develop recurrent AOM than children whose middle ears are free of effusion (24). This interrelationship of AOM and OME accounts for the common presentation in young children of both recurrent and persistent middle ear disease.

The physical diagnosis of OME is made by otoscopic inspection of tympanic membrane translucency, color, position, and mobility. The pathognomonic appearance of trapped air within the effusion appearing as bubbles or an air-fluid level is only occasionally seen. More often, decreased translucency of the tympanic membrane results in a relative inability to visualize commonly seen middle ear landmarks such as the incudostapedial joint, promontory, and round window niche.

The color of the eardrum is variable. Both serous and mucoid effusions may impart an amber hue. Purulent effusions may appear white with associated increased vascularity of the pars tensa. Effusions of a mixed character with a nondescript dull gray tympanic membrane appearance are common.

Although any tympanic membrane position is possible, mild retraction of the eardrum indicative of negative middle ear pressure, as well as effusion, is often observed. The short process of the malleus appears more prominent and the manubrium foreshortened in such circumstances.

The presence of effusion with or without associated high negative pressure can significantly impede the movement of the eardrum in response to pneumatic otoscopy. The normal inward movement of the tympanic membrane with slight external canal positive pressure and outward movement with negative pressure is dampened or eliminated in characteristic fashion depending on both the contents and pressure of the middle ear (25). In experienced hands pneumatic otoscopy is both a sensitive and specific diagnostic tool (26).

Diagnostic accuracy can be further enhanced by the use of acoustic impedance measurements, particularly tympanometry. Measurements made with the electroacoustic impedance bridge provide an objective assessment of middle ear pressure and tympanic membrane compliance, and tympa-

nometric tracings can be used to predict the presence or absence of middle ear effusion with a considerable degree of certainty (27). The accuracy of the diagnosis of OME is highest when pneumatic otoscopic and tympanometric findings are used in combination; sensitivity is 97% and specificity is 90% under such circumstances (28).

Acoustic reflectometry is an additional technique that shows promise as a means of detecting OME, particularly as a screening device in unskilled hands (29). The acoustic otoscope is a handheld instrument that contains both an 80-dB sound source and a microphone that measures both transmitted and reflected sound. The operating principle is that a sound wave within the external ear canal will be reflected from an intact tympanic membrane; the more sound reflected, the greater the likelihood of an effusion being present.

Finally, the documentation or confirmation of a mild conductive hearing loss may be the initial clue indicating the presence of otherwise asymptomatic OME in children. However, for reasons to be discussed, the assessment of hearing alone is not an accurate screening method for identifying the presence of middle ear effusion.

COMPLICATIONS OF OTITIS MEDIA WITH EFFUSION

Hearing loss is the most common complication and sequela of OME. The loss is typically conductive and mild. Children ages 2 to 12 years with OME demonstrate mean three-frequency pure-tone averages and speech reception thresholds of 24.5- and 22.7-dB hearing level (HL), respectively; comparative mean bone-conduction scores average 3-dB HL (30). Less of an effect on hearing sensitivity is noted at 2,000 Hz in comparison to a slightly greater impairment in the 500- to 1,000-Hz lower frequency range.

The effect of OME on infant hearing levels is less easily discernible due to the limitations of sound-field behavioral audiometry. Testing for the better ear, average speech awareness threshold in infants ages 6 to 24 months with OME have been ascertained at 24.6-dB HL (31). More recent studies have utilized auditory brainstem response (ABR) testing to provide ear-specific data in this age group. Mild to moderately elevated ABR thresholds in the presence of middle ear effusion are documented (32).

The hearing loss associated with OME does fluctuate. The composite data from several studies indicate that, within the speech frequency range, approximately 90% of patients with OME exhibit a conductive hearing loss between 16- and 40-dB HL; however, at any one time, 49% of patients with OME would pass a hearing evaluation utilizing a 20-dB hearing threshold (33). This fluctuating nature of the hearing loss associated with OME is the reason the assessment of hearing is not an absolutely accurate screening method for this disorder.

The potential effect of the fluctuating mild to moderate hearing loss associated with OME on linguistic and intellectual development remains controversial. Three comprehensive reviews of previously published studies show an association between OME in infancy and early childhood and later language delays and decreased learning skills (34–36). Clear documentation that the OME is the sole reason for the retarded development in such cases, however, is lacking. It is postulated that in young children the hearing impairment of OME, even when fluctuating and mild, has an adverse effect because it occurs during a critical period of language acquisition. This handicapping effect may be further augmented by disruption of normal parent-child interactions by the otitis disease process, and it may be particularly disabling in children with other educational impediments such as visual impairment, mental retardation, learning disorders, and neurosensory hearing losses.

The majority of the intratemporal and intracranial complications of otitis media occur secondary to AOM and chronic suppurative otitis media (Chapter 18); such complications are infrequently associated with OME. Exceptions to this rule include tympanosclerosis and tympanic membrane atelectasis with or without cholesteatoma formation.

Tympanosclerosis, more appropriately termed *myringosclerosis* when limited to the tympanic membrane, is characterized by the formation of white plaques in the eardrum or nodular deposits in the submucosa of the middle ear. Such plaques and nodules represent calcified hyalinized debris believed to be the end product of a chronic inflammatory or traumatic process (37). Although found more commonly in children who have had tubes, tympanosclerosis is reported in 10% to 20% of patients with bilateral OME in the nonintubated ear (38,39).

Displacement of the eardrum from its normal position toward the promontory is termed *retraction* or *atelectasis.* Several authors attribute such drum displacement to an inflammatory process occurring in underventilated ears, the atelectatic ear being viewed as representative of a more severe manifestation of eustachian tube dysfunction following OME (40,41). When thickening of the mucous membrane of the middle ear occurs in association with tympanic membrane atelectasis, the term *adhesive otitis media* is often applied. Such a proliferation of fibrous tissue may fix the ossicles, resulting in a conductive hearing loss. Osteitis with ossicular erosion, particularly of the long process of the incus, may also occur. In the presence of severe localized tympanic membrane atelectasis, a retraction pocket or even perforation may develop. Such retraction pockets, particularly in the posterosuperior quadrant, may be associated with both ossicular erosion and cholesteatoma formation.

Chronic OME in infancy and early childhood is additionally believed to result in reduced mastoid pneumatization, the functional significance of which, other than its association with tympanic membrane atelectasis, is uncertain (42).

Neurosensory hearing loss is a rare complication of otitis media, being more associated with labyrinthitis or possibly AOM than OME. The sudden development or progression of sensorineural hearing loss in a child with OME should raise suspicion of a congenital perilymphatic fistula (43).

MANAGEMENT OF OTITIS MEDIA WITH EFFUSION

Danish cohort studies have demonstrated a tremendous variability in the clinical course of untreated OME. Whereas 60% of children have one or more OME episodes that clear spontaneously within 1 to 3 months' duration, 30% have much longer lasting episodes of 3 to 9 months' duration, and 10% have extremely prolonged episodes persisting for 1 or more years (44). Otitis media with effusion, in the majority of children, appears to be a benign disease that will disappear, even without treatment, over a short period. A significant proportion of children, however, develop one or more episodes of chronic OME with the potential complications and sequelae thereof. These children and their adult counterparts with chronic OME are the principal patient groups for whom medical and surgical management become necessary.

MEDICAL MANAGEMENT OF OTITIS MEDIA WITH EFFUSION

Several nonsurgical options exist for the treatment of OME. One or more of these methods may be appropriate in the initial management of the child or adult with OME prior to embarking on surgical intervention.

Inflation of the middle ear has been purported to have a beneficial effect in the treatment of OME since the days of Politzer. Theoretically, air insufflated into the middle ear displaces middle ear effusion; repetitive insufflation should enhance middle ear drainage. Multiple methods of middle ear inflation by autoinflation or politzerization have been reported in the literature with variable results (45,46). The most recently described method of autoinflation, based on a modified Valsalva technique, utilizes an anesthesia mask attached to a flow meter allowing for quantitative control (47). These authors also report a new method of documenting eustachian tube opening during autoinflation using a combination of tympanometry and frequency spectrum analysis of ear canal sounds called sonotubometry. When these new techniques were applied in a randomized control study to 41 children with chronic OME unresponsive to antibiotic therapy, no therapeutic efficacy of sustained middle ear autoinflation was demonstrable.

The most common drug treatment of OME in children and adults had been the oral administration of systemic decongestant-antihistamine medications. A 1982 survey of American Academy of Otolaryngology members revealed that 91% of otolaryngologists considered such oral medications efficacious in the treatment of OME (48). A subsequent, double-blind, randomized, clinical trial was published in 1983 in which a 4-week course of an antihistamine-decongestant combination was compared with placebo in 553 children ages 7 months through 12 years with chronic OME (49). The study failed to show any beneficial drug effect. The rate of clearance of middle ear effusion, both unilateral and bilateral, was identical in both treatment groups.

A similarly designed study published in 1987 demonstrated the addition of an antihistamine-decongestant combination to amoxicillin or placebo to provide no additional advantage in OME resolution in the 518 children so compared (50).

Mucolytic agents such as guaifenesin and bromhexine have recently been investigated in animal studies and in limited observation trials in adults with OME (51,52). Although theoretically promising, no clinical role has yet been established for these agents.

Both systemic and topical corticosteroids have been suggested for use in the treatment of OME; clinical trials to date have only been performed with the former. The conclusions of the better designed of these studies assessing the efficacy of short-term systemic steroid use in treating OME have been conflicting. Schwartz et al. (53), using a double-blind, crossover study, reported 70% of children had cleared their middle ear effusions after a 1-week course of prednisone plus sulfonamide, compared with only 5% of those treated with sulfonamide alone. Although criticized due to the short duration of documented effusion in their study of children prior to treatment, the difference in clearance rates between the steroid and placebo groups is impressive. Macknin and Jones (54) found no difference between the use of dexamethasone or placebo in clearing middle ear effusions in children with well-documented chronic OME. However, their overall rate of effusion resolution was a very low 6%. Subtherapeutic steroid dosages and the absence of an antibiotic treatment baseline are criticisms of this study. Lambert (55), in prospective, double-blind, crossover fashion, assessed 60 children with chronic OME documented by combined pneumatoscopy and tympanometry. Concomitant amoxicillin was administered to both steroid and placebo groups. Prednisone plus amoxicillin proved no more effective than amoxicillin alone in resolving chronic OME. Overall, 60% of patients cleared their effusions. The results of the study actually supported a beneficial effect of antibiotic as opposed to steroid therapy.

Otitis media with effusion had been assumed to be sterile until microbiologic studies in the late 1970s revealed that approximately 50% of middle ear aspirates from children with chronic effusions demonstrated bacteria (56). Up to one fourth of the effusions demonstrated bacteria (56). Up to one fourth of the effusions grew pathogenic organisms, including *Haemophilus influenzae, Branhamella catarrhalis, Streptococcus pneumoniae, Staphylococcus aureus,* and *Streptococcus pyogenes,* in order of frequency. Later studies revealed beta-lactamase production to be common among the *H. influenzae, B. catarrhalis,* and *S. aureus* isolates (57). These microbiologic findings indicate that OME, despite its absence of acute signs and symptoms, may represent a low-grade infection in a substantial proportion of patients.

A trial of antibiotic therapy is highly desirable in previously untreated patients with OME. The antibiotics chosen and duration of therapy recommended are the same as those used in children with AOM. A number of small, nonblinded studies have reported trimethoprimsulfamethoxazole and erythromycin to be efficacious in the treatment of OME (58–60). Mandel et al. (50) showed in a randomized, double-blind, placebo-controlled study that a 14-day course of amoxicillin resulted in a significantly higher effusion-free rate at 2 and 4 weeks in the drug-treated group. However, a 50% recurrence rate was found when children who were effusion-free at 4 weeks were followed up for an additional 3 months. Thomsen et al. (61) demonstrated a more impressive resolution of middle ear effusion at 4 weeks following 1 month of amoxicillin-clavulanate potassium therapy (61%) compared with placebo (30%). The tympanometric-documented improvement in their antibiotic-treated children also persisted for a longer period, up to 8 months' status after treatment.

Antibiotic therapy, perhaps with a beta-lactamase–resistant antibiotic, appears to be a worthwhile consideration in the initial management of OME. Even when successful, posttherapeutic surveillance is recommended due to a high anticipated rate of otitis recurrence.

Final mention under medical management must include those 25% to 30% of allergic children and adults who demonstrate serous OME as part of their overall upper respiratory tract presentation. In addition to the pharmacologic agents already mentioned, their total management often requires environmental controls, hyposensitization treatments, and dietary manipulation in some patients (62).

SURGICAL MANAGEMENT OF OTITIS MEDIA WITH EFFUSION

Patients who have persistent OME unresponsive to medical management, especially if present for at least 3 months, are reasonable candidates for surgical intervention. This is particularly true in patients with bilateral OME and associated hearing loss or patients with unilateral OME and secondary nonaudiologic middle ear complications.

MYRINGOTOMY WITH AND WITHOUT TYMPANOSTOMY TUBES

The ideal otologic treatment of uncomplicated serous otitis media should achieve removal of the effusion, correct secondary hearing loss, and prevent recurrence through the provision of middle ear ventilation. Myringotomy with aspiration temporarily achieves the first two of these three goals. Myringotomy with aspiration is a reasonable initial treatment in adults and children who do not require general anesthesia for the procedure to be performed and who do not appear to have an underlying systemic condition that would suggest the need for sustained middle ear ventilation. In children of the age where the need for general anesthesia precludes the performance of repeated middle ear aspirations or in patients of any age with suspected chronic OME predisposition, the placement of tympanostomy tubes at the time of initial myringotomy is favored.

Four studies have compared the efficacy of myringotomy with aspiration alone versus myringotomy accompanied by tube placement in the absence of adenoidectomy or adenotonsillectomy surgery (38,63–65). All four studies found a significant difference in the length of the effusion-free period and in the duration of improved hearing favoring the intubated as opposed to nonintubated ears. Gates et al. (64), in particular, documented a 170-day difference in the average effusion-free interval in the tympanostomy tube versus myringotomy group. This difference was primarily accounted for by the average duration of tube function, which approximated 154 days.

Neel et al. (66) have hypothesized that the creation and maintenance of ambient pressure in the middle ear by way of ventilation tubes allows mucosal recovery and aeration of the middle ear–mastoid air cell system. The children in the Gates et al. study (64) are continuing to be followed from the time of tympanic membrane closure after tube extrusion in order to assess whether the prolonged middle ear ventilation afforded by the tubes does yield any long-term benefits.

TYMPANOSTOMY TUBES

Historical Development and Operative Considerations

The need to maintain the patency of the myringotomy site for sustained drainage and ventilation was recognized as far back as the nineteenth century. The writings of Politzer and Dalby (cited by Alberti [67]) describe the unsuccessful use of various materials, including catgut, fish bones, lead wires, silver cannulas, and gold rings. Politzer himself devised a hard rubber eyelit containing grooves to fit the tympanic membrane. Limited success combined with a high rate of associated infection eventually led to the abandonment of this procedure, until Armstrong (68) reintroduced the idea of sustained middle ear ventilation in 1954.

Armstrong used a 1.5-mm diameter, straight shaft, polyethylene tube to relieve a nonresolving middle ear effusion in an adult ear that had been refractory to medical management and previous myringotomy. The tube was designed to remain in place 2 to 3 weeks.

Subsequent modifications in tube shape were made by Armstrong and others to promote longer tube duration within the tympanic membrane. House (69) devised a polyethylene tube with one flared end to fit behind the eardrum; Sheehy (70) introduced the short double-flared collar-button tube, and Lindeman and Silverstein (71) followed soon thereafter with the arrow tube design.

Tube composition materials also changed with the theoretical goal of enhancing biocompatibility. Teflon, Silastic, and stainless steel grommets all were introduced in the 1960s (72–74). Gold-plated silver and titanium alloy tubes appeared later in the 1980s (75). Clinical studies have failed to document any significant differences among these various tube materials from a functional standpoint (76,77).

Further diversification in tube design occurred in response to refinement of the surgical indications for myringotomy with tympanostomy tube placement. The distinction in the need for short- versus long-term ventilation dictates different tube requirements. For the initial treatment of serous otitis media in otherwise healthy children and adults, short-term ventilation is often warranted. Ideally the tubes chosen for this purpose should remain within the eardrum at least 6 to 12 months, and complete tympanic membrane healing should follow after their desired spontaneous extrusion. Armstrong, Shephard, and Reuter-Bobbin tubes have been shown to be suitable for such ventilation purposes. Leopold and McCabe (78) found long polyethylene and Shephard tubes to remain functional for at least 6 months; Reuter-Bobbin tubes demonstrated a slightly better functional performance. More recently, Weigel et al. (79) demonstrated 2-year postinsertion extrusion rates of 94%, 80%, and 66% for Shephard, Armstrong, and Reuter-Bobbin tubes, respectively. Small flange tubes of similar design would be expected to be equally efficacious for short-term ventilation purposes.

Patients with serous otitis media refractory to previous short-term ventilation management become candidates for long-term ventilation. Long-term ventilation should also be initially considered in adults and children with anticipated chronic OME problems. Included in this group are patients with cleft palates and other craniofacial abnormalities associated with chronic eustachian tube dysfunction, as well as pharyngeal tumor patients treated by palatal resection or irradiation.

The initial long-term ventilation tubes were designed to clip over the malleus for retention purposes (80,81). Incisions both anterior and posterior to the malleus were required, and placement proved cumbersome. Most long-term tubes utilized today incorporate a large medial flange and are made of pliable, principally Silastic, materials to allow for easier placement. The Per-Lee (82) tube, for example, incorporates a wide circular flange and a large-diameter stem. The Goode T-tube (83) is longer and of narrower stem diameter. In both these tubes the medial flange and shaft can be shortened to facilitate insertion. Other short-term tube prototypes have also been modified with a T-tube design to enhance their duration of ventilation.

Spontaneous extrusion of long-term ventilation tubes is quite infrequent. Only 31% of T-tubes had spontaneously extruded by 2 years in one comparative study (79); the incidence for Per-Lee tubes is even less, approximating 5% (82). Elective removal of long-term ventilation tubes is typically required. The average longevity of T-tubes and Per-Lee tubes at elective removal is 33 and 51 months, respectively (82,83). The T-tube shape is designed to promote easy removability; this can often be done as an office procedure in cooperative children and adults. This is less true of Per-Lee tubes. Young children may require a general anesthetic for tube removal. This possible need for a second operative removal procedure should be strongly considered prior to the placement of long-term ventilation tubes in the pediatric population.

The duration even a short-term tube remains within the tympanic membrane can be enhanced by selective placement. Van Baarle and Wentges (84) established the rate of tube extrusion to be, in part, a function of epithelial migration across the tympanic membrane. These authors' sentiments that an anterosuperior tympanic membrane placement favored tube longevity were further echoed by Armstrong (85), who additionally advocated a snug placement up against the fibrous annulus for tube retention. This issue of tube longevity versus quadrant of insertion was critically assessed by Leopold and McCabe (78). They found no significant difference in extrusion rates among three short-term tubes—Shephard, long polyethylene with flange, and Reuter-Bobbin types—for the three quadrants of insertion (anterosuperior, anteroinferior, posteroinferior) utilized. They did, however, note some tube-specific patterns of preference. Shephard tubes, for example, were found to remain longer when placed in the anterosuperior quadrant, whereas the inferior quadrants proved best for Reuter-Bobbin tubes.

Operative Procedure

The insertion of tympanostomy tubes can be performed under local or general anesthesia, the latter often being necessary in children or uncooperative adult patients. The operating microscope is typically utilized both for its provision of magnification and binocular vision. The basic instrumentation required includes any of a variety of ear specula of different sizes (we prefer the bell-shaped Gruber speculum in children); a ring or wire loop curette for cerumen removal; a straight or angled myringotomy knife (we prefer the latter); suction tubes of 3, 5, and 7 French size; a toothed or smooth-jawed otologic forceps for holding the tube; and an ear dressing forceps for postoperative wick placement. We additionally use a straight or slightly curved Rosen pick to aid in tube insertion. A small ear hook is also kept available for possible tube retrieval.

Controversy exists over the degree of sterility required during myringotomy with tympanostomy tube placement. Practices vary from complete operating room precautions utilizing gowns and gloves, microscope draping, and canal sterilization to ambulatory settings with the use of gloves alone, limited patient draping, and no canal preparation.

The location and type of myringotomy incision performed also varies. Preferences among otolaryngologists regarding the site of tympanostomy tube placement reveal favored sites to be posteroinferior (53%), anteroinferior (38%), and anterosuperior (5%) (86). Insertion into the posterosuperior quadrant is not advised due to the possibility of ossicular disruption (Fig. 21.1A), as well as increased concern of the development of tympanic membrane atrophy with subsequent retraction pocket and/or perforation in this region. An anteroinferior or posteroinferior position is generally favored, taking care to avoid insertion directly over the promontory (Fig. 21.1B). In the presence of generalized atelectasis, the anterosuperior portion of the middle ear adjacent to the eustachian tube orifice may be the only area with enough space to allow tube placement. An anterior placement does appear to improve visualization of the os of the tube on postoperative otoscopic examination.

Whereas large circumferential incisions are utilized when myringotomy alone is being performed to enhance middle ear drainage (Fig. 21.2A), such incisions often prove too large to adequately secure most tympanostomy tubes. Smaller incisions, in a radial orientation for reasons to be discussed, are preferred (Fig. 21.2B). The incision must be large enough, however, to allow evacuation of any middle ear effusion present. A thick middle ear effusion may require a second counterincision to be made (Fig. 21.2C). This provision of two incisions allows air to enter the middle ear space on suctioning, facilitating the removal of tenacious fluid (Fig. 21.2D). We prefer to apply the suction to the counterincision in such cases, decreasing trauma to the planned intubation site.

The technique of tube placement or intubation varies greatly with the type of tympanostomy tube chosen (Fig. 21.3). The Baxter beveled button grommet (Microtek Medical Inc.) that we use in our practice has a circular flange, the leading edge of which can be easily placed into the myringotomy incision site (Fig. 21.4A). A fine suction or pick can then be used to exert pressure on the still external edge if the alligators cannot complete the insertion, tucking the flange behind the incision in buttonhole-like fashion (Fig. 21.4B). The os of the tube is carefully suctioned to ensure patency following final placement (Fig. 21.4C).

Perioperative systemic antibiotics are not routinely used unless the child demonstrates acute inflammatory otitis media. The use of topical antibiotic otic solutions immediately postoperatively varies with the preferences of the individual surgeon. The potential benefit of such solutions in preventing postoperative complications is discussed in the following section.

Adverse Outcomes

The performance of myringotomy with tympanostomy tube placement is not without its limitations. Although typically a simple and straightforward operation, intraoperative problems are possible.

Inadequate local anesthesia may result in pain. General anesthesia risks are similar to other otologic procedures, being both anesthetic and patient specific. Stenotic or otherwise distorted external ear canals, including simply age-related narrowing, can limit access to the tympanic membrane. Smaller diameter variations in tympanostomy tube size have been of help in this respect, enabling placement through equally small specula. Middle ear pathology, especially severe tympanic membrane atelectasis, can further increase the difficulty of both myringotomy and intubation. Retracted, flaccid tympanic membranes tend to tear easily, and reduced intratympanic distances may dictate changes in tube choice or quadrant of insertion.

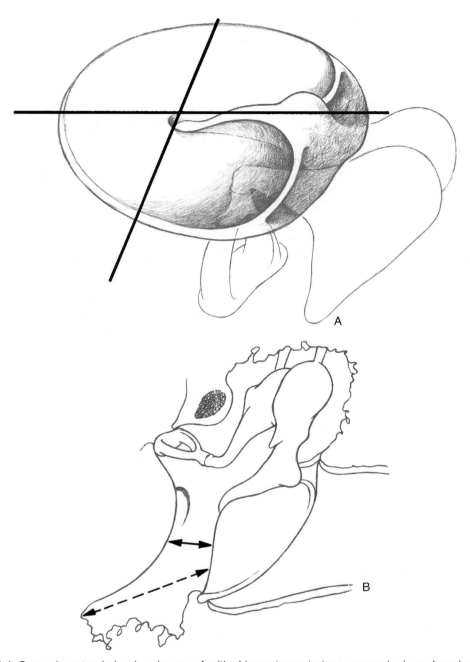

FIG. 21.1 Several anatomic landmarks are of critical importance to tympanocentesis and myringotomy with tube placement. **A:** Instrumentation in the posterosuperior quadrant *(shaded)* is contraindicated due to the possibility of ossicular disruption. **B:** Tube placement in the inferior portion of the tympanic membrane is generally favored due to the greater depth of the middle ear space toward the hypotympanum *(dashed arrow)*. Note the limited intratympanic distance between the eardrum and promontory; middle ear mucosal trauma may result from too deep a myringotomy incision in this region *(solid arrow)*.

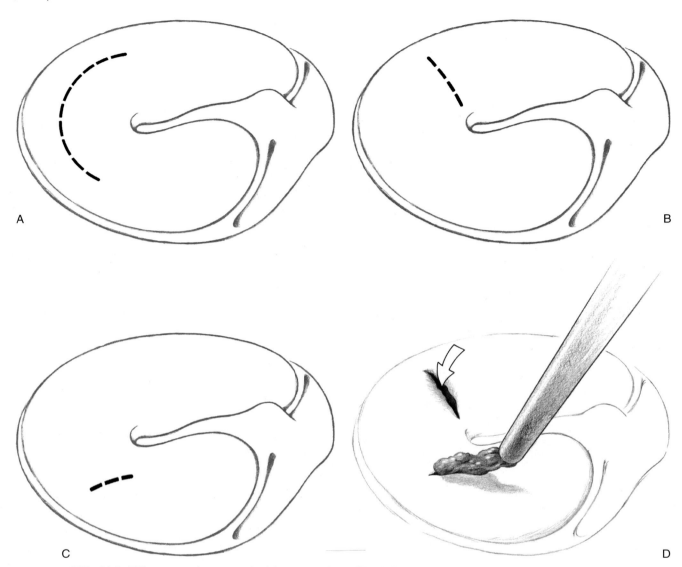

FIG. 21.2 Different myringotomy incisions may be utilized depending on the clinical indication. **A:** A wide curvilinear incision is useful for drainage purposes alone or when Per-Lee tube placement is planned. **B:** A short linear incision in a radial direction allows for adequate removal of most middle ear effusions, as well as tube securement. **C:** Aspiration of a thick mucoid effusion from the middle ear may require the creation of a second counterincision. **D:** Air entry through one incision, as suction is applied to the other, facilitates mucoid effusion removal.

Both small external canals and atelectatic middle ears increase the likelihood of bleeding from skin or mucous membrane disruption by instrument manipulation. Bleeding is also a common occurrence in acutely inflamed ears; avoiding obvious blood vessels on the eardrum surface with a radial incision at the time of myringotomy can decrease this complication. The temporary placement of a wick or cotton ball soaked in local vasoconstrictor solution may be necessary for hemorrhage control in some cases.

Too small an incision may make intubation difficult, and too large an incision may not properly hold the tube. Temporary loss of the tympanostomy tube through the incision into the middle ear space dictates attempted retrieval. A small

hook or suction device may prove helpful; sometimes a second myringotomy incision is necessary. Ossicular continuity should not be placed in jeopardy if the tube migrates. In such cases, a second tube should be initially secured; a later tympanotomy can be performed, if necessary, to retrieve the first tube.

Ossicular chain disruption can potentially occur if instrumentation is performed in the posterosuperior quadrant. A deep posteroinferior myringotomy could theoretically cause round window disruption and secondary sensorineural hearing loss. A dehiscent facial nerve could possibly be injured in similar fashion. Middle ear vascular abnormalities, specifically a high jugular bulb or glomus tympanicum,

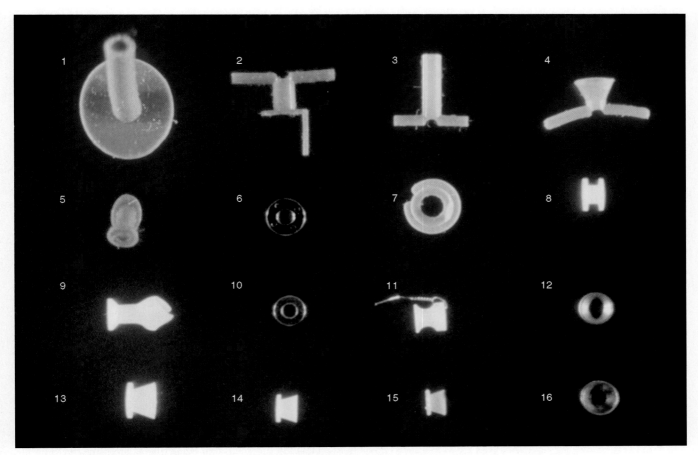

FIG. 21.3 Well over 100 tympanostomy tubes are available for use incorporating different designs and composite materials. A few are illustrated here. The tubes on the *top* line (from *left* to *right,* no. 1 through no. 4) are generally regarded as long-term ventilation tubes due principally to their larger base or flange, which promotes tube retention. The bottom three lines depict an array of short-term ventilation tubes. *(1)* Silicone Per-Lee tube, *(2)* silicone T-grommet, *(3)* silicone modified Goode T-tube, *(4)* silicone Baxter beveled T-tube, *(5)* Teflon modified Armstrong beveled grommet, *(6)* stainless steel Reuter-Bobbin tube, *(7)* silicone Paparella type 1 tube, *(8)* Teflon collar-button tube, *(9)* Teflon Lindeman-Silverstein arrow tube, *(10)* gold collar-button tube, *(11)* Teflon Shephard grommet with stainless steel wire, *(12)* platinum V Bobbin tube, *(13)* Teflon Baxter beveled button, *(14)* Teflon mini-Baxter beveled button, *(15)* silicone mini-Baxter beveled button, *(16)* gold Baxter beveled button.

could result in significant hemorrhage if not preoperatively recognized. Packing the middle ear and canal usually achieves temporary control of bleeding in such cases.

Postoperatively, the obstruction of tympanostomy tubes by blood, cerumen, and inspissated secretions is quite a common problem. Leopold and McCabe (78) noted a 2-month period between tube nonfunction and tube extrusion. Lumen obstruction with secondary tube nonfunction can become an indication for tube removal when refractory to medical therapy. Tube obstruction is especially troublesome when it occurs secondary to bleeding in the immediate perioperative period. Per-Lee (82) documented bleeding in 11% of his long-term ventilation tube placements; in 30% of these cases, tube removal proved necessary. The incidence of intraluminal obstruction by blood in short-term ventila-

tion tube placement has been established to be 4.7% (87); the lesser degree of manipulation required in the placement of these tubes most probably accounts for this comparatively decreased incidence. Various intraoperative methods are practiced to prevent tube clotting, including the instillation of drops and ointments or the placement of wicks or obturators into the tube lumen (87,88). The efficacy of these methods is unproven.

The treatment of intraluminal obstruction of tympanostomy tubes to date has been more art than science. Topical otic drop preparations have been used to occasionally open a tube lumen blocked by inspissated secretions; their efficacy in dissolving a hard cast of obstructing dry blood is less dependable. Otomicroscopic suctioning or instrumental manipulation is often necessary in an attempt to reestablish tubal patency.

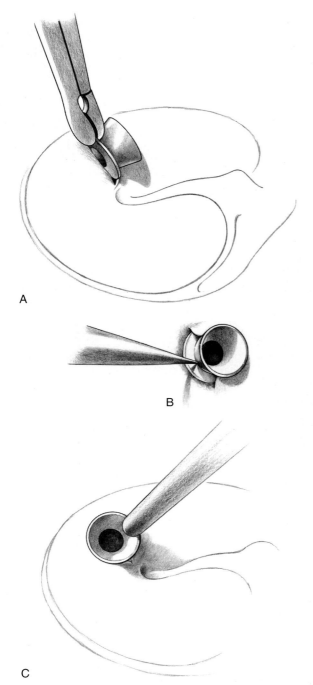

A

B

C

FIG. 21.4 Our technique of tympanostomy tube placement is illustrated. **A:** The leading edge of the circular flange of the Baxter beveled button tube is placed into the incision site. **B:** A pick or fine suction is used to exert pressure on the still-exposed opposite side, tucking the entire flange behind the eardrum in buttonhole-like fashion. **C:** The os of the tube is suctioned to ensure patency and to test securement of placement.

Aside from premature extrusion and tube obstruction, the most common complication associated with tube placement is postintubation otorrhea. The duration of ventilation, which principally relates to the type of tympanostomy tube chosen, greatly influences otorrhea rates. The reported incidence of this problem ranges from 15% to 34% with short-term ventilation tubes; figures increase to as high as 41% to 74% in long-term ventilation tube studies (79,82,89–98).

An important distinction needs to be made between immediate-onset and delayed-onset drainage. Immediate onset drainage is typically defined as otorrhea noted between intubation and the time of the first postoperative visit, a period varying, depending on the study, from 7 days to 7 weeks. The incidence of immediate-onset otorrhea has similarly varied from 5.5% to 19%, higher rates being associated in part with longer follow-up periods (91,94,97,98). Early-onset otorrhea is believed to be secondary principally to middle ear infection or contamination at the time of surgery. The incidence of postoperative otorrhea is higher in children with purulent as opposed to mucoid or serous effusions (97,98) and is also higher in patients with a history of prior tube placement (92). Ear canal sterilization and perioperative topical or systemic antibiotic use appears to have significantly decreased the incidence of immediate-onset otorrhea in some studies (94,97) but has had no demonstrable beneficial effect in others (98). Recommendations regarding sterility precautions and external ear canal preparation at the time of surgery remain uncertain.

Delayed otorrhea, that occurring at any time between the first postoperative visit and tube extrusion, has many potential causes. Recurrent bouts of otitis media will obviously produce drainage. The presence of a patent tympanostomy tube may also facilitate the reflux of nasopharyngeal secretions into the middle ear. The work of Gates et al. (93) would suggest that such intrinsic causes may play a comparatively less important role in the pathogenesis of delayed onset postoperative otorrhea than extrinsic factors. They documented a predominance of postoperative otorrhea during the summer months when water contamination from summer swimming activities would be most common, as well as a lower otorrhea rate during the winter months when the rate of new episodes of recurrent intrinsic otitis would be expected to be higher. Many other authors have implicated external water-borne contamination as a major factor in the development of postintubation otorrhea. A variety of water protection mechanisms have arisen in response, ranging from complete avoidance of swimming activities to postoperative topical antibiotic use after each water exposure (99). Canal occlusion during bathing or swimming is a common choice (100). Cotton balls or lamb's wool coated with petrolatum, as well as a variety of commercial and custom-made water precaution molds, have been utilized.

One of the more novel approaches to this problem of water contamination was the development of tympanostomy tubes with a gas-porous but water-resistant membrane. Theoretically such semipermeable membrane tubes would not only obviate the need for water protection but would decrease the likelihood of nasopharyngeal reflux by maintenance of the middle ear cushion. The clinical use of such tubes has yielded mixed results. Cantekin et al. (101) abandoned the use of these tubes due to an 85% incidence of tube nonfunction with recurrent middle ear effusions or acute otitis episodes. Subsequent studies have reported a much lower incidence of tube failure and complications in only 10% to 15% of patients (102–104). An increase in the membrane pore size from 0.5 to 1.0 microns is believed to be partially responsible for these improved results. Of greater apparent importance is adherence to an operative technique, including complete suction evacuation of all middle ear effusion contents, avoidance of membrane contact with blood or cerumen, and perioperative systemic antibiotic coverage. The role of topical antibiotic drop preparations in ears ventilated with semipermeable membrane tubes has not been addressed.

The treatment of postintubation otorrhea in patients with standard nonmembrane tubes is typically empiric. Topical antibiotic or antibiotic-steroid drop combinations, with or without accompanying systemic antibiotics, are often utilized. The efficacy of this practice relative to the bacteriologic characteristics of otorrhea from tympanostomy tubes was assessed by Schneider (105). In children younger than 3 years of age, the organisms cultured are similar to those found in AOM, and systemic antibiotic therapy suitable for AOM should suffice. In children older than 3 years of age, staphylococcal species and *Pseudomonas aeruginosa* are the predominant cultured organisms. Because *P. aeruginosa* is insensitive to oral antimicrobials, with the exception of ciprofloxacin hydrochloride, the only satisfactory nonparenteral therapy in children is the use of topical drops containing agents useful against these organisms. A trial of oral ciprofloxacin can be safely used in the adolescent and adult populations.

A small subset of patients, between 2% to 5%, may develop persistent otorrhea after intubation despite standard treatment measures, including culture-specific antimicrobial therapy (89,90). In such cases, especially if unilateral, removal of the tube may prove necessary. The development of granulation tissue surrounding tympanostomy tubes is an infrequent but not rare occurrence. The work of Hawke and Keene (106) suggests that the pathogenesis of granulation tissue around ventilation tubes may be more of a foreign body granuloma reaction to trapped squamous epithelium than a true reaction to the tube itself. Long-term Silastic tubes, in particular, have been associated with the peritubal development of granulation tissue (82,83). Persistent bilateral postintubation otorrhea, especially if recurrent after tube change, should prompt a search for an underlying occult predisposition to middle ear disease, such as nasopharyngeal obstruction or, less commonly, immunodeficiency or ciliary disorders.

Tympanic membrane perforation after tube extrusion is an additional complication of tympanostomy tube placement. The incidence of postintubation perforation most clearly relates to the type of tympanostomy tube utilized. The incidence following extrusion of short-term ventilation tubes varies between 0% and 2% (79,90,107). In contrast, the risk following spontaneous extrusion or planned removal of long-term ventilation tubes is much higher. Goode (83) originally claimed a 3% incidence of perforation with the T-tube; more recent studies suggest an incidence as high as 12% (79). Per-Lee (82) reports a 25% perforation rate with his tube; this figure has been confirmed by other investigators even after trimming of the tube's wide circular flange. Such perforations following the extrusion or removal of long-term ventilation tubes may not always be an adverse outcome. In specific patients with a chronic OME predisposition, such "permanent" middle ear ventilation may actually be desirable.

The etiology of postintubation tympanic membrane perforations most likely occurs secondary to peritubal drum atrophy (108,109). Per-Lee (82) noted peritubal tympanic membrane atrophy in 29 of 248 intubated ears, 14 of which eventually developed persistent perforations. Thin flaccid areas at the site of intubation, even after short-term ventilation, are commonly observed. Armstrong (85) suggested that linear incisions in a radial direction would spare the maximum number of fibers in the middle tympanic membrane layer and minimize this complication. The functional significance of these so-called monomeric or dimeric membranes in the absence of a perforation or localized retraction pocket is believed negligible.

Another common change observed in the tympanic membrane and often attributed to previous intubation is myringosclerosis. Myringosclerosis most probably represents the end stage of an inflammatory process characterized by degeneration of collagenous tissues, hyalinization, and eventual calcification into a pathognomonic, firm, white plaque (37). Myringosclerosis is a complication of both treated and untreated OME patients but is found more often in children who have tubes (38,39). Distinguishing the effects of the underlying disease process itself from those of intubation can be difficult. From a functional standpoint, the hearing loss attributed to myringosclerosis is less than 0.5 dB when evaluated by pure-tone testing at 250, 1,000, and 4,000 Hz (110). This is an insignificant degree of impairment.

Of perhaps greatest concern among tympanostomy tube complications is the risk of cholesteatoma. Most series from this country give an incidence of less than 1% (95,107); reported rates are slightly higher in the European literature (92,111). The etiology of postintubation cholesteatomas appears to be secondary to either shedding of epithelial cells onto a denuded promontory at the time of tube placement or from complications of a postextrusion atrophic tympanic membrane retraction pocket. Histopathologic studies have failed to show skin growing around the tube margin as a potential source of future entrapment (112). The issue of postintubation cholesteatoma appears to be of limited importance. Cholesteatoma obviously occurs much more often in the absence of tubes. Many patients, in fact, have probably been spared the development of a cholesteatoma within a retracted tympanic membrane due to tubal ventilation.

Rarely, tympanostomy tubes may fall into the middle ear. This occurred once in 838 tube tympanostomies in a study by Hughes et al. (107) and in far less than 1% of cases in as yet unpublished data by Cunningham et al. (113). Wide myringotomy and extraction are recommended in such circumstances; rarely an exploratory tympanotomy may be necessary for tube retrieval.

A final, not uncommon problem associated with the use of tympanostomy tubes is the need for removal when spontaneous extrusion has not occurred. As previously indicated, this happens more often with long-term as opposed to short-term ventilation tubes and poses a greater dilemma in children in whom the use of general anesthesia may be required. In children in whom tympanostomy tubes have been inserted bilaterally and in whom only one tube spontaneously extrudes, the remaining tube can usually be removed if the opposite middle ear remains free of middle ear effusion for at least 1 year after documented tympanic membrane closure (114). This method of management is based on the observation that eustachian tube function in children is usually symmetrical bilaterally.

Older children and adults with prolonged retention of bilateral tympanostomy tubes may be assessed by means of the modified inflation-deflation eustachian tube function test. Such testing can also be applied to adults with unilateral tube retention. The modified inflation-deflation test assesses passive and active eustachian tube function (115). Documentation of adequate eustachian tube function may be helpful in predicting successful tube removal and eventual tympanic membrane closure. Studies correlating success of tympanoplasty surgery with the results of preoperative inflation-deflation tests are supportive in this regard (116).

ALTERNATIVE METHODS OF SUSTAINED MIDDLE EAR VENTILATION

Both cautery and laser myringotomies have been performed in an attempt to create long-lasting perforations to promote sustained middle ear ventilation and obviate the need for tympanostomy tubes (117,118). Such thermal myringotomies have demonstrated a patency rate ranging from 1 to 4 weeks. Saito et al. (119), by means of cautery, created larger perforations of a size equivalent to one fourth of the eardrum. These large openings did remain patent longer; an average of 3 months is reported. No mention is made, however, of the incidence of permanent perforation with this method.

Kent (120) critically assessed the use of thermal myringotomy in comparison to tympanostomy tube placement in the pediatric population. The 1- × 2-mm tympanic membrane perforations he created typically healed in 3 to 5 weeks; all closed by 8 weeks. Children had significantly more pain symptoms in their thermal myringotomy ears, and there was a recurrence of middle ear effusion in 40% of the children within 6 months on the thermal myringotomy side. No advantages of this technique over tube insertion for sustained middle ear drainage were demonstrated.

An alternative to transtympanic ventilation of the middle ear was proposed by Wright and Wright in 1977 (121). Their Silastic eustachian tube prosthesis was initially designed to improve eustachian tube function at the time of tympanoplasty. The indications for its use were expanded by Lesinski et al. (122) to improve middle ear ventilation in children and adults with chronic eustachian tube dysfunction and secondary OME. In 13 such patients the Silastic eustachian tube prosthesis was placed through an anterior myringotomy incision into the eustachian tube orifice. All patients developed recurrent OME postoperatively, and there was a very high rate of spontaneous Silastic eustachian tube prosthesis extrusion. The ineffectiveness of this technique in treating children with chronic OME was also confirmed by Wright et al. in a later publication (123).

Prolonged middle ear ventilation is also the goal of the Silverstein permanent aeration tube (124). Available in two lengths of uniform 1.1-mm diameter, this flanged silicone rubber tube is designed for transosseous placement in adult patients with chronic OME or eustachian tube dysfunction. It is stated to be particularly useful in patients with atelectatic tympanic membranes in whom the placement of a transtympanic tympanostomy tube may be undesirable. Although initially reported as an adjunctive procedure in children with chronic OME undergoing ossicular reconstruction (125), it is not presently recommended for use in children or in patients of any age at the time of middle ear–mastoid surgery (126).

Transosseous placement of the Silverstein permanent aeration tube entails the elevation of a tympanomeatal flap and the drilling of a 1.5-mm hole through the bony annulus into the facial recess at the level of the round window. A trough is created in the adjacent osseous external canal wall. The Silverstein permanent aeration tube is inserted through the drill hole in the bony annulus; it is anchored in position by a combination of the overlying bony bridge of the annulus, the tympanomeatal flap, and the adjacent trough in the external canal wall. Irrigation of the Silverstein permanent aeration tube with both an antibiotic otic and heparin-saline solution is recommended at the time of placement.

The most common operative problem reported with this technique is failure to adequately secure the Silverstein permanent aeration tube due to creation of a shallow external canal trough or destruction of the bony bridge at the annulus. There also exists the potential for damage to either the facial nerve posteriorly or chorda tympani nerve anteriorly during the drilling phase of the procedure. The careful identification of anatomic landmarks, together with the use of intraoperative facial nerve monitoring, are recommended to significantly decrease the possibility of neural injury (127).

The Silverstein permanent aeration tube is subject to the same postoperative complications described for tympanostomy tubes with a 44% incidence of obstruction and a 23% incidence of delayed otorrhea (126). An average length of intubation of 51 months is reported for the Silverstein permanent aeration tube (126), a figure interestingly identical to that reported for the long-term transtympanic Per-Lee ventilation tube (82).

ADENOIDECTOMY

The most common nonotologic surgical procedure undertaken to reduce the occurrence of otitis media in the pediatric population is adenoidectomy. The potential etiologic role of enlarged adenoid tissue in the pathogenesis of OME has been discussed previously. The efficacy of this procedure in the treatment and prevention of OME has been argued with conflicting results for many years (17,128). Two recently published, well-controlled clinical studies, however, do establish a significant benefit of adenoidectomy in the treatment of this disease (129,130).

Gates et al. (129) focused on children ages 4 to 8 years old with well-documented, long-standing, middle ear effusions refractory to medical management. Children were randomized to one of four treatment groups: bilateral myringotomies alone, myringotomy with tubes, adenoidectomy with myringotomies, or adenoidectomy with placement of tympanostomy tubes. Children who received adenoidectomy combined with myringotomy or with tube placement demonstrated better 2-year outcomes in terms of several measurement factors (time with effusion, time with abnormal hearing, time to first recurrence of effusion, and number of surgical retreatments) than children who received myringotomy or tube placement alone. This beneficial effect was not influenced to any appreciable degree by the size of the adenoid tissue as judged by preoperative radiographs. In fact, the surgical technique employed by the otolaryngologists in this study did not entail routine curettage of the fossae of Rosenmüller. These two observations raise interesting questions regarding the pathogenic role of adenoid enlargement in this disease entity.

The Gates et al. study (129) additionally documented a lower incidence of complications in the adenoidectomy with myringotomy group in terms of such patients remaining largely free of the postoperative otorrhea and need for water precautions characteristic of the children in their tympanostomy tube groups. This comparatively decreased morbidity prompted the authors to recommend adenoidectomy with myringotomy alone as the first-line surgical management of chronic OME in children 4 years of age and older.

The more recently published Paradise et al. study (130) similarly involved children with well-documented chronic middle ear effusions. The children in this study ranged from 1 to 15 years of age. They had failed not only prior medical otitis management but prior surgical intervention as well. All had developed recurrent AOM or OME following extrusion of at least one set of previously placed tympanostomy tubes. Such children were therefore felt to be at higher risk for recurrent/persistent middle ear disease.

Treatment assignments in this study initially included adenoidectomy versus medical management alone, with tympanostomy tube placement being performed in patients with middle ear effusion(s) refractory to the aforementioned methods. The primary outcome measure was the proportion of time with otitis media; additional secondary outcome measures such as the number of secondary episodes of otorrhea and number of tympanostomy tube procedures required were also investigated. Adenoidectomy routinely entailed curettage of the fossae of Rosenmüller in patients so treated. Statistically significant differences were found in the adenoidectomy group compared with the control group in terms of less time spent with otitis media over the first 2 years of the study. Results were similar for both the randomized study group and for a nonrandomized group of children whose initial treatment was chosen on a basis of parental preference. The authors felt their results substantiated the use of adenoidectomy in the treatment of children with OME who had failed prior tympanostomy tube placements.

Previous studies have established that the addition of tonsillectomy to adenoidectomy has no more beneficial effect than adenoidectomy alone in the treatment of middle ear disease (131,132). Associated indications for surgery, however, such as obstructive airway symptoms or recurrent pharyngeal infection, may dictate the performance of a joint adenotonsillectomy in children with OME.

TYMPANOMASTOIDECTOMY

A tympanomastoidectomy procedure may be required in the treatment of chronic OME when all other medical and standard surgical methods of management, including long-term middle ear ventilation and adenoidectomy, have failed. This may be particularly true in patients with a systemic predisposition to infectious or inflammatory disease. A previously unsuspected pathologic middle ear–mastoid process such as cholesterol granuloma or cholesteatoma may be discovered in such cases. The more common finding, however, is a middle ear and mastoid cavity containing hyperplastic, sometimes polypoid, mucosa (133). Reversal of disease in such situations requires maintained aeration of the middle ear–mastoid air cell system in addition to definitive surgery; the concurrent placement of a long-term ventilation tube may be necessary depending upon the type of tympanomastoidectomy procedure performed.

AMPLIFICATION

As a final note, in children or adults with bilateral OME and associated hearing loss in whom medical and surgical intervention proves ineffectual or cannot be appropriately performed, the fitting of hearing aids should be considered (134). This is especially true in young children at an age critical for speech and language acquisition in whom an intercurrent illness will delay surgery for a prolonged period.

REFERENCES

1. Teele DW, Klein JO, Rosner B. Epidemiology of otitis media during the first seven years of life in children in greater Boston: a prospective, cohort study. *J Infect Dis* 1989;160:83–94.
2. Bluestone CD. State of the art: definitions and classification. In: Lim DJ, Bluestone CD, Klein JO, Nelson JD, eds. *Recent advances in otitis media with effusion.* Philadelphia: BC Decker Inc, 1984;1–4.
3. Casselbrant ML, Brostoff LM, Cantekin EI, et al. Otitis media with effusion in preschool children. *Laryngoscope* 1985;95:428–436.
4. Bluestone CD, Klein JO. Otitis media, atelectasis and eustachian tube dysfunction. In: Bluestone CD, Stool SE, eds. *Pediatric otolaryngology.* Philadelphia: WB Saunders, 1990;341–372.
5. Bluestone CD, Beery QC. Concepts on the pathogenesis of middle ear effusions. *Ann Otol Rhinol Laryngol* 1976;85[Suppl 25]:182–186.
6. Sadler-Kimes D, Siegel MI, Todhunter JS. Age-related morphologic differences in the components of the eustachian tube/middle ear system. *Ann Otol Rhinol Laryngol* 1989;98:854–858.
7. Beery QC, Doyle WJ, Cantekin EI, et al. Eustachian tube function in an American Indian population. *Ann Otol Rhinol Laryngol* 1980;89[Suppl 68]:28–33.
8. Bluestone CD. Eustachian tube obstruction in the infant with cleft palate. *Ann Otol Rhinol Laryngol* 1971;80[Suppl 2]:1–30.
9. Doyle WJ, Reilly JS, Stool SE, et al. Eustachian tube function in children with unrepaired cleft palates. In: Lim DJ, Bluestone CD, Klein JO, et al, eds. *Recent advances in otitis media with effusion.* Philadelphia: BC Decker, 1984;59–62.
10. White BL, Doyle WJ, Bluestone CD. Eustachian tube function in infants and children with Down's syndrome. In: Lim DJ, Bluestone CD, Klein JO, et al, eds. *Recent advances in otitis media with effusion.* Philadelphia: BC Decker, 1984;62–66.
11. McBride TP, Doyle WJ, Hayden FG, et al. Alterations of the eustachian tube, middle ear, and nose in rhinovirus infection. *Arch Otolaryngol Head Neck Surg* 1989;115:1054–1059.
12. Doyle WJ, Friedman R, Fireman P, et al. Eustachian tube obstruction after provocative nasal antigen challenge. *Arch Otolaryngol* 1984;110:508–511.
13. Kraemer MJ, Richardson MA, Weiss NS, et al. Risk factors for persistent middle-ear effusions. Otitis media, catarrh, cigarette smoke exposure, and atopy. *JAMA* 1983;249:1022–1025.
14. Myers EN, Beery QC, Bluestone CD, et al. Effect of certain head and neck tumors and their management on the ventilatory function of the eustachian tube. *Ann Otol Rhinol Laryngol* 1984;93[Suppl 114]:3–16.
15. Bluestone CD, Wittel RA, Paradise JL, et al. Eustachian tube function as related to adenoidectomy for otitis media. *Trans Am Acad Ophthalmol Otolaryngol* 1972;76:1325–1339.
16. Bluestone CD, Cantekin EI, Beery QC. Certain effects of adenoidectomy on eustachian tube ventilatory function. *Laryngoscope* 1975;85:113–127.
17. Gates GA, Avery CA, Cooper JC Jr, et al. Chronic secretory otitis media: effects of surgical management. *Ann Otol Rhinol Laryngol* 1989;98[Suppl 138]:2–32.
18. Pillsbury HC III, Kveton JF, Sasaki CT, Frazier W. Quantitative bacteriology in adenoid tissue. *Otolaryngol Head Neck Surg* 1981;89:355–363.
19. Pelton SI, Teele DW, Reimer CB, et al. Immunologic characteristics of children with frequent recurrences of otitis media. In: Lim DJ, Bluestone CD, Klein JO, et al, eds. *Recent advances in otitis media.* Philadelphia: BC Decker, 1988;143–146.
20. Jahrsdoerfer R, Feldman PS, Rubel EW, et al. Otitis media and the immotile cilia syndrome. *Laryngoscope* 1979;89:769–778.
21. Marchant CD, Shurin PA, Tutihasi MA, et al. Detection of asymptomatic otitis media in early infancy. In: Lim DJ, Bluestone CD, Klein JO, et al, eds. *Recent advances in otitis media with effusion.* Philadelphia: BC Decker, 1984;32–33.
22. Teele DW, Klein JO, Rosner BA. Epidemiology of otitis media in children. *Ann Otol Rhinol Laryngol* 1980;89[Suppl 68]:5–6.
23. Kaneko Y, Okitsu T, Sakuma M, et al. Incidence of secretory otitis media after acute inflammation of the middle ear cleft and the upper respiratory tract. In: Lim DJ, Bluestone CD, Klein JO, et al, eds. *Recent advances in otitis media with effusion.* Philadelphia: BC Decker, 1984;34–36.
24. Stangerup SE, Tos M. Etiologic role of acute suppurative otitis media in chronic secretory otitis. *Am J Otol* 1985;6:126–131.
25. Bluestone CD, Klein JO. Methods of examination: clinical examination. In: Bluestone CD, Stool SE, eds. *Pediatric otolaryngology.* Philadelphia: WB Saunders, 1990;111–124.
26. Paradise JL, Smith CG, Bluestone CD. Tympanometric detection of middle ear effusion in infants and young children. *Pediatrics* 1976;58:198–210.
27. Gates GA, Avery C, Cooper JC, et al. Predictive value of tympanometry in middle ear effusion. *Ann Otol Rhinol Laryngol* 1986;95:46–50.
28. Cantekin EI, Bluestone CD, Fria TJ, et al. Identification of otitis media with effusion in children. *Ann Otol Rhinol Laryngol* 1980;89[Suppl 68]:190–195.
29. Oyiborhoro JM, Olaniyan SO, Newman CW, et al. Efficacy of acoustic otoscope in detecting middle ear effusion in children. *Laryngoscope* 1987;97:495–498.
30. Fria TJ, Cantekin EI, Eichler JA. Hearing acuity of children with otitis media with effusion. *Arch Otolaryngol* 1985;111:10–16.
31. Nozza RJ. Effects of otitis media with effusion on infant auditory function. *Ann Otol Rhinol Laryngol* 1988;97[Suppl 133]:64.
32. Roland PS, Finitzo T, Friel-Patti S, et al. Otitis media. Incidence, duration, and hearing status. *Arch Otolaryngol Head Neck Surg* 1989;115:1049–1053.
33. Bess FH. Hearing loss associated with middle ear effusion. Workshop on effects of otitis media on the child. *Pediatrics* 1983;71:640–641.
34. Ventry IM. Effects of conductive hearing loss: fact or fiction. *J Speech Hear Disord* 1980;45:143–156.
35. Paradise JL. Otitis media during early life: how hazardous to development? A critical review of the evidence. *Pediatrics* 1981;68:869–873.
36. Ruben RJ, Bagger-Sjoback D, Downs MP, et al. Recent advances in otitis media. Complications and sequelae. *Ann Otol Rhinol Laryngol* 1989;98[Suppl 139]:46–55.
37. Schiff M, Poliquin JF, Catanzaro A, et al. Tympanosclerosis. A theory of pathogenesis. *Ann Otol Rhinol Laryngol* 1980;89[Suppl 70]:1–16.
38. Kilby D, Richards SH, Hart G. Grommets and glue ears: two-year results. *J Laryngol Otol* 1972;86:881–888.
39. Tos M, Bonding P, Poulsen G. Tympanosclerosis of the drum in secretory otitis after insertion of grommets. A prospective, comparative study. *J Laryngol Otol* 1983;97:489–496.
40. Sadé J, Berco E. Atelectasis and secretory otitis media. *Ann Otol Rhinol Laryngol* 1976;85[Suppl 25]:66–72.
41. Bluestone CD, Cantekin EI, Beery QC, et al. Functional eustachian tube obstruction in acquired cholesteatoma and related conditions. In: McCabe BF, Sadé J, Abramson M, eds. *Cholesteatoma. First International Conference.* Birmingham, AL: Aesculapius Publishing, 1977;325–335.
42. Tos M, Stangerup SE. Mastoid pneumatization in secretory otitis. Further support for the environmental theory. *Acta Otolaryngol (Stockh)* 1984;98:110–118.
43. Bluestone CD. Otitis media and congenital perilymphatic fistula as a cause of sensorineural hearing loss in children. *Pediatr Infect Dis J Suppl* 1988;7:S141–145.
44. Fiellau-Nikolajsen M. Frequency and course of the disease. Danish approach to the treatment of secretory otitis media. *Ann Otol Rhinol Laryngol* 1990;99[Suppl 146]:7.
45. Shea JJ. Autoinflation treatment of serous otitis media in children. *J Laryngol Otol* 1971;85:1254–1258.
46. Schwartz DM, Schwartz RH, Redfield NP. Treatment of negative middle ear pressure and serous otitis media with Politzer's technique. An old procedure revisited. *Arch Otolaryngol* 1978;104:487–490.
47. Chan KH, Bluestone CD. Lack of efficacy of middle ear inflation: treatment of otitis media with effusion in children. *Otolaryngol Head Neck Surg* 1989;100:317–323.
48. American Academy of Otolaryngology—Head and Neck Surgery. Results of 1981 drug survey. *The Bulletin* 1982;1:1–4.
49. Cantekin EI, Mandel EM, Bluestone CD, et al. Lack of efficacy of a decongestant-antihistamine combination for otitis media with effusion ("secretory" otitis media) in children. *N Engl J Med* 1983;308:297–301.

50. Mandel EM, Rockette HE, Bluestone CD, et al. Efficacy of amoxicillin with and without decongestant-antihistamine for otitis media with effusion in children. *N Engl J Med* 1987;316:432–437.

51. Hori F, Kawauchi H, Suzuki M, et al. Pharmaceutical treatment of experimental otitis media with effusion. In: Lim DJ, Bluestone CD, Klein JO, et al, eds. *Recent advances in otitis media.* Philadelphia: BC Decker, 1988;254–258.

52. Roydhouse N. Bromhexine in the treatment of otitis media with effusion. In: Lim DJ, Bluestone CD, Klein JO, et al, eds. *Recent advances in otitis media with effusion.* Philadelphia: BC Decker, 1984;266–268.

53. Schwartz RH, Puglese J, Schwartz DM. Use of a short course of prednisone for treating middle ear effusion. A double-blind crossover study. *Ann Otol Rhinol Laryngol* 1980;89[Suppl 68]:296–300.

54. Macknin ML, Jones PK. Oral dexamethasone for treatment of persistent middle ear effusion. *Pediatrics* 1985;75:329–335.

55. Lambert PR. Oral steroid therapy for chronic middle ear perfusion: a double-blind crossover study. *Otolaryngol Head Neck Surg* 1986;95: 193–199.

56. Riding KH, Bluestone CD, Michaels RH, et al. Microbiology of recurrent and chronic otitis media with effusion. *J Pediatr* 1978;93: 739–743.

57. Lim DJ, Lewis DM, Schram JL, et al. Antibiotic-resistant bacteria in otitis media with effusion. *Ann Otol Rhinol Laryngol* 1980;89[Suppl 68]:278–280.

58. Marks NJ, Mills RP, Shaheen OH. A controlled trial of cotrimoxazole therapy in serous otitis media. *J Laryngol Otol* 1981;95:1003–1009.

59. Healy GB. Antimicrobial therapy of chronic otitis media with effusion. *Int J Pediatr Otorhinolaryngol* 1984;8:13–17.

60. Sundberg L. Antibiotic treatment of secretory otitis media. *Acta Otolaryngol (Stockh)* 1984;[Suppl 407]:26–29.

61. Thomsen J, Sederberg-Olsen J, Balle V, et al. Antibiotic treatment of children with secretory otitis media. A randomized, double-blind, placebo-controlled study. *Arch Otolaryngol Head Neck Surg* 1989;115: 447–451.

62. Hurst DS. Allergy management of refractory serous otitis media. *Otolaryngol Head Neck Surg* 1990;102:664–669.

63. Smyth GD, Patterson CC, Hall S. Tympanostomy tubes: do they significantly benefit the patient? *Otolaryngol Head Neck Surg* 1982;90: 783–786.

64. Gates GA, Wachtendorf C, Hearne EM, et al. Treatment of chronic otitis media with effusion: results of tympanostomy tubes. *Am J Otolaryngol* 1985;6:249–253.

65. Mandel EM, Rockette HE, Bluestone CD, et al. Myringotomy with and without tympanostomy tubes for chronic otitis media with effusion. *Arch Otolaryngol Head Neck Surg* 1989;115:1217–1224.

66. Neel HB III, Keating LW, McDonald TJ. Ventilation in secretory otitis media: effects on middle ear volume and eustachian tube function. *Arch Otolaryngol* 1977;103:228–231.

67. Alberti PW. Myringotomy and ventilating tubes in the 19th century. *Laryngoscope* 1974;84:805–815.

68. Armstrong BW. A new treatment for chronic secretory otitis media. *Arch Otolaryngol* 1954;59:653–654.

69. House HP. Polyethylene in middle ear surgery. *Arch Otolaryngol* 1960;71:926–931.

70. Sheehy JL. Collar button tube for chronic serous otitis. *Trans Am Acad Ophthalmol Otolaryngol* 1964;68:888–889.

71. Lindeman RC, Silverstein H. The "arrow tube." *Arch Otolaryngol* 1964;80:473.

72. Pappas JJ. Middle ear ventilation tubes. *Laryngoscope* 1974;84: 1098–1117.

73. Per-Lee JH. Experiences with a "permanent" wide flange middle ear ventilation tube. *Laryngoscope* 1969;79:581–591.

74. Reuter SH. The stainless steel bobbin middle ear ventilation tube. *Trans Am Acad Ophthalmol Otolaryngol* 1968;72:121–122.

75. Heumann H, Steinback E, Seuffer R. Über die Anwendbarkeit von Paukenröhrchen aus Edelmetall. *Laryngol Rhinol Otol* 1982;61:17–19.

76. Tami TA, Kennedy KS, Harley E. A clinical evaluation of gold-plated tubes for middle-ear ventilation. *Arch Otolaryngol Head Neck Surg* 1987;113:979–980.

77. Handler SD, Miller L, Potsic WP, et al. A prospective study of titanium ventilation tubes. *Int J Pediatr Otorhinolaryngol* 1988;16:55–60.

78. Leopold DA, McCabe BF. Factors influencing tympanostomy tube function and extrusion: a study of 1,127 ears. *Otolaryngol Head Neck Surg* 1980;88:447–454.

79. Weigel MT, Parker MY, Goldsmith MM, et al. A prospective randomized study of four commonly used tympanostomy tubes. *Laryngoscope* 1989;99:252–256.

80. Silverstein H. Malleus clip tube for long-term equalization of middle ear pressure. *Trans Am Acad Ophthalmol Otolaryngol* 1966;70: 640–642.

81. Turner JL. Myringostomy by use of a fixed prosthesis. *Laryngoscope* 1967;77:524–533.

82. Per-Lee JH. Long-term middle ear ventilation. *Laryngoscope* 1981; 91:1063–1073.

83. Goode RL. Advantages of the T-tube for short and long-term middle ear ventilation. *Laryngoscope* 1983;93:376–378.

84. Van Baarle PW, Wentges RT. Extrusion of transtympanic ventilating tubes, relative to the site of insertion. *ORL J Otorhinolaryngol Relat Spec* 1975;37:35–40.

85. Armstrong BW. Prolonged middle ear ventilation: the right tube in the right place. *Ann Otol Rhinol Laryngol* 1983;92:582–586.

86. Armstrong BW. What your colleagues think of tympanostomy tubes. *Laryngoscope* 1968;78:1303–1313.

87. Cunningham MJ, Harley EH Jr. Preventing perioperative obstruction of tympanostomy tubes: a prospective trial of a simple method. *Int J Pediatr Otorhinolaryngol* 1991;21:15–20.

88. Friedberg J. Removable ventilating tube obturator—how to save a ventilating tube. *Int J Pediatr Otorhinolaryngol* 1987;13:227–229.

89. McLelland CA. Incidence of complications from use of tympanostomy tubes. *Arch Otolaryngol* 1980;106:97–99.

90. Luxford WM, Sheehy JL. Myringotomy and ventilation tubes: a report of 1,568 ears. *Laryngoscope* 1982;92:1293–1297.

91. Herzon FS. Tympanostomy tubes. Infectious complications. *Arch Otolaryngol* 1980;106:645–647.

92. Draf W, Schulz P. Insertion of ventilation tubes into the middle ear: results and complications. A seven-year review. *Ann Otol Rhinol Laryngol* 1980;89[Suppl 68]:303–307.

93. Gates GA, Avery C, Prihoda TJ, et al. Delayed onset post-tympanotomy otorrhea. *Otolaryngol Head Neck Surg* 1988;98:111–115.

94. Gates GA, Avery C, Prihoda TG, et al. Post-tympanostomy otorrhea. *Laryngoscope* 1986;96:630–634.

95. Holt JJ, Harner SG. Effects of large-bore middle ear ventilation tubes. *Otolaryngol Head Neck Surg* 1980;88:581–585.

96. Meyerhoff WL. Use of tympanostomy tubes in otitis media. *Ann Otol Rhinol Laryngol* 1981;90:537–542.

97. Balkany TJ, Barkin RM, Suzuki BH, et al. A prospective study of infection following tympanostomy and tube insertion. *Am J Otol* 1983;4:288–291.

98. Baldwin RL, Aland J. The effects of povidone-iodine preparation on the incidence of post-tympanostomy otorrhea. *Otolaryngol Head Neck Surg* 1990;102:631–634.

99. Jaffe BF. Are water and tympanotomy tubes compatible? *Laryngoscope* 1981;91:563–564.

100. Johnson DW, Mathog RH, Maisel RH. Tympanostomy tube protection with ear plugs. *Arch Otolaryngol* 1977;103:377–380.

101. Cantekin EI, Bluestone CD, Rood SR. Evaluation of the polytetrafluoroethylene-membrane ventilation tube. *Laryngoscope* 1977;87: 1951–1960.

102. Bailey Q. The Castelli membrane in the treatment of glue ear. *J Laryngol Otol* 1980;94:377–382.

103. Plotkin RP. Middle ear ventilation with the Castelli membrane tube. *Laryngoscope* 1981;91:1173–1175.

104. Levinson SR, Gill AJ, Teich L. Semipermeable membrane tubes: a prospective study. *Otolaryngol Head Neck Surg* 1982;90:622–628.

105. Schneider ML. Bacteriology of otorrhea from tympanostomy tubes. *Arch Otolaryngol Head Neck Surg* 1989;115:1225–1226.

106. Hawke M, Keene M. Artificial eustachian tube-induced keratin foreign-body granuloma. *Arch Otolaryngol* 1981;107:581–583.

107. Hughes LA, Warder FR, Hudson WR. Complications of tympanostomy tubes. *Arch Otolaryngol* 1974;100:151–154.

108. Harell M, Shea JJ. Hazards of ventilation tubes. *Adv Otorhinolaryngol* 1978;23:22–28.

109. Barfoed C, Rosborg J. Secretory otitis media. Long-term observations after treatment with grommets. *Arch Otolaryngol* 1980;106:553–556.

110. Tos M, Stangerup SE. Hearing loss in tympanosclerosis caused by grommets. *Arch Otolaryngol Head Neck Surg* 1989;115:931–935.

111. Gundersen T, Tonning F-M. Ventilating tubes in the middle ear. Long-term observations. *Arch Otolaryngol* 1976;102:198–199.

112. Bingham BJ, Milroy CM. The histological appearance of the tympanic edge in contact with an indwelling ventilation tube (grommet). *Clin Otolaryngol* 1989;14:297–303.

113. Cunningham MJ, Eavey RD, Krouse JH, et al. Middle ear ventilation tubes: experience with removal. Laryngoscope 1993;103:659–662.

114. Bluestone CD, Klein JO. *Otitis media in infants and children.* Philadelphia: WB Saunders, 1988;179–180.

115. Cantekin EI, Bluestone CD, Parkin LP. Eustachian tube ventilatory function in children. *Ann Otol Rhinol Laryngol* 1976;85[Suppl 25]:171–177.

116. Bluestone CD, Cantekin EI, Douglas GS. Eustachian tube function related to the results of tympanoplasty in children. *Laryngoscope* 1979;89:450–458.

117. Goode RL, Schulz W. Heat myringotomy for the treatment of serous otitis media. *Otolaryngol Head Neck Surg* 1982;90:764–766.

118. Lau P, Shelton C, Goode RL. Heat myringotomy. *Laryngoscope* 1985;95:38–42.

119. Saito H, Miyamoto K, Kishimoto S, et al. Burn perforation as a method of middle ear ventilation. *Arch Otolaryngol* 1978;104:79–81.

120. Kent SE. Thermal myringotomy versus grommets in the management of secretory otitis media. *Int J Pediatr Otorhinolaryngol* 1989;17:31–35.

121. Wright JW Jr, Wright JW III. Preliminary results with use of an eustachian tube prosthesis. *Laryngoscope* 1977;87:207–214.

122. Lesinski SG, Fox JM, Seid AB, et al. Does the silastic eustachian tube prosthesis improve eustachian tube function? *Laryngoscope* 1980;90:1413–1428.

123. Wright JW III, Wright JW Jr, Hicks GW. The eustachian tube revisited. *Otolaryngol Head Neck Surg* 1978;86:834–837.

124. Silverstein H. Permanent middle ear aeration. *Arch Otolaryngol* 1970;91:313–318.

125. Silverstein H. Ossicular reconstruction in chronic seromucinous otitis media. *Arch Otolaryngol* 1971;93:42–45.

126. Haberkamp TJ, Silverstein HL. Permanent middle ear aeration: long-term follow-up of transosseous ventilating tubes. *Laryngoscope* 1987;97:1145–1148.

127. Silverstein H, Smouha E, Jones R. Routine identification of the facial nerve using electrical stimulation during otological and neurotological surgery. *Laryngoscope* 1988;98:726–730.

128. Paradise JL, Bluestone CD, Rogers KD, et al. Efficacy of adenoidectomy in recurrent otitis media. Historical overview and preliminary results from a randomized, controlled trial. *Ann Otol Rhinol Laryngol* 1980;89[Suppl 68]:319–321.

129. Gates GA, Avery CA, Prihoda TJ, et al. Effectiveness of adenoidectomy and tympanostomy tubes in the treatment of chronic otitis media with effusion. *N Engl J Med* 1987;317:1444–1451.

130. Paradise JL, Bluestone CD, Rogers KD, et al. Efficacy of adenoidectomy for recurrent otitis media in children previously treated with tympanostomy-tube placement. Results of parallel randomized and nonrandomized trials. *JAMA* 1990;263:2066–2073.

131. Maw AR. Chronic otitis media with effusion and adenotonsillectomy: a prospective randomized controlled study. In: Lim DJ, Bluestone CD, Klein JO, et al, eds. *Recent advances in otitis media with effusion.* Philadelphia: BC Decker, 1984;299–302.

132. Maw AR. Age and adenoid size in relation to adenoidectomy in otitis media with effusion. *Am J Otolaryngol* 1985;6:245–248.

133. Holmquist J, Jarlstedt J, Tjellstrom A. Surgery of the mastoid in ears with middle ear effusion. *Ann Otol Rhinol Laryngol* 1980;89[Suppl 68]:322–323.

134. Bluestone CD, Klein JO. *Otitis media in infants and children.* Philadelphia: WB Saunders, 1988;189.

CHAPTER 22

Surgery for Otosclerosis and Fixation of the Stapes

Joseph B. Nadol, Jr., and Harold F. Schuknecht

There are more than 20 genetically determined disorders that produce a conductive hearing loss that involves stapes fixation (1). In addition, there are numerous acquired disorders, including tympanosclerosis and trauma, which may result in significant conductive hearing loss due to fixation of the stapes. Nevertheless, the most common disorder causing fixation of the stapes is otosclerosis, an autosomal dominantly inherited bony dysplasia that seems to affect only the otic capsule and only in man (2). In addition to its known genetic predisposition, chronic viral infection of bone may also play a role in the pathogenesis of otosclerosis (3). Otosclerosis may cause conductive hearing loss in one or both ears in up to 1% of the Caucasian population.

HISTORICAL PERSPECTIVE

When the first attempts were made to improve hearing by surgical approaches to the oval window (4–9), otosclerosis had not yet been recognized as a pathologic entity. These early efforts were unsuccessful because of inadequate instrumentation and the lack of adequate magnification. Then, after an exciting and moderately successful 20 years of fenestration surgery introduced by Sourdille (10) and Lempert (11), and a short-lived experience with stapes mobilization begun by Rosen (12), the era of stapedectomy began. Although Hall and Rytzner (13) had some success with stapedectomy, it was Shea's technique (14) of substituting a vein graft and polyethylene tube for the stapes that gave the first consistently successful results.

The nomenclature of contemporary stapedectomy procedures is somewhat confusing. Thus some would call the creation of a small fenestra in the footplate a *stapedotomy,* whereas others would call this a *partial stapedectomy.* At a most fundamental level, there are three principal types of stapes procedures in contemporary usage designed to overcome conductive hearing loss (Table 22.1).

The fundamental differences in technique involve two steps of the procedure. The first is the management of the oval window and footplate and the second is the technique of interposition to reestablish continuity of the ossicular chain with the oval window. Bone removal at the oval window may include total or partial removal of the footplate. Partial removal may include fractional removal, such as removal of the posterior third or half of the footplate. In the small fenestra technique, a circular opening is made in the central footplate either with a laser or with a microdrill. Some authors have recommended sectioning of the footplate to allow partial remobilization of the posterior half. Thus Silverstein (15) has recommended a laser STAMP procedure in which ossicular chain is separated from the fixed anterior footplate by removal of the anterior crus and transverse sectioning of the footplate with a laser to allow reestablishment of mobility through the posterior crus and newly mobilized posterior segment.

Numerous prostheses have been developed to reestablish continuity between the ossicular chain and the oval window, including a variety of pistons of varying diameters and materials, combinations of prosthetic materials and tissue

TABLE 22.1 *Nomenclature for contemporary stapes surgery*

I. Management of oval window and footplate
  A. Total removal of footplate
  B. Partial removal of footplate
    1. Fractional removal
    2. Small fenestra
  C. Sectioning footplate without removal ("partial mobilization")
II. Reestablishment of continuity between ossicular chain and oval window
  A. Incus to oval window
    1. Piston
    2. Maintenance of posterior crus ("physiologic stapedectomy")
    3. Fat-wire
  B. Malleus to oval window
    1. Piston
    2. Fat-wire

TABLE 22.2 *Algorithm and nomenclature for planning and describing stapes surgery*

Elements of procedure	Incision and approach	Exposure of middle ear	Management of oval window and fixed footplate	Method for reestablishing continuity between ossicular chain and oval window Incus to oval window
Examples	Transcanal Endaural Postauricular	Anteriorly based tympanomeatal flap	Total removal of stapes footplate Partial removal of footplate, posterior half, small fenestra drill-out Drill-out with small fenestra	Piston with tissue graft without tissue graft Fat-wire prosthesis Vein graft with preservation of posterior crus Malleus to oval window piston or fat-wire prosthesis

grafts such as the fat-wire prosthesis, and reestablishment of continuity using the posterior crus, as championed by Hough (16). In conformance with the algorithm for describing surgical procedures described in Chapter 11, we recommend the nomenclature illustrated in Table 22.2. Notice that the term *stapedotomy* has been deliberately avoided, because it means a small-fenestra partial stapedectomy to some authors and sectioning of the footplate without creating a fenestra to others.

On the basis of animal experiments in which several different types of tissue and prostheses were tested in cats, Schuknecht et al. (17) devised the fat-wire technique in conjunction with total stapes removal. In the search for simpler surgical techniques and for improvement in results, new methods were proposed by many surgeons. Among these were partial stapedectomy (18), vein graft and Teflon strut (19), wire loop prosthesis (20), Teflon-wire piston (21,22), Gelfoam-wire prefabricated prosthesis (23), and stainless steel piston (24,25). In 1969 Schuknecht and Applebaum (26) reported that consistent excellent hearing gains could be achieved by introducing a small diameter (0.6-mm) Teflon-wire piston through a small fenestra in the footplate. Small fenestra stapedectomy has virtually eliminated many of the complications of total stapedectomy, such as postoperative vertigo, reparative granuloma, and fibrous fixation of the lenticular process to the promontory, and is our procedure of choice for stapes fixation caused by otosclerosis and other causes.

INDICATIONS/CONTRAINDICATIONS AND INFORMED CONSENT FOR STAPEDECTOMY SURGERY

Indications

In general, there should be a conductive loss of at least 25 db in frequencies 250 to 1 kHz or higher as determined by audiometry and the presence of a negative Rinne using a 512 cps tuning fork. The presence of a concomitant sensorineural hearing loss does not necessarily contraindicate stapes surgery. Thus if a hearing aid will still be required even after successful stapedectomy, the procedure may well be worthwhile to improve auditory performance using amplification. This is particularly relevant in a patient with a

profound mixed hearing loss in whom, after stapedectomy, a high gain amplifier may be beneficial. Only one ear is operated on at a time. The ear with the higher pure-tone average is generally selected. Following successful stapedectomy on one side, an interval of 8 to 12 months is generally allowed to pass to be sure the results are stable before recommending surgery in the opposite ear.

Contraindications

Elective stapedectomy on an only hearing ear is almost always contraindicated. One exception may be a case of a profound mixed loss in which a conventional hearing aid provides no auditory improvement and in which cochlear implantation would be indicated if stapedectomy does not allow the use of a conventional hearing aid. Stapedectomy is contraindicated in cases with active infection either of the middle ear or external auditory canal or in the case of perforation of the tympanic membrane. Patients with unstable medical conditions, as determined by a medical consultant, may be better advised to continue to use a hearing aid rather than undergo elective surgery. Patients in whom vestibular function is absolutely critical for their employment may be better advised to avoid stapedectomy rather than risk postoperative vestibular symptoms. In general, elective stapedectomy should not be done if the operative or nonoperative ear is unstable. Thus ipsilateral Meniere's disease or immune-mediated sensorineural loss is a relevant contraindication to surgery. Likewise the presence of contralateral chronic active otitis media, Meniere's disease, or immune-mediated sensorineural loss is also a relative contraindication.

Informed Consent for Stapedectomy

Insofar as possible, the surgeon should advise his patient on the broad outline of the procedure plan, as described in Table 22.2. Thus most patients will be advised that their surgery is to be done by a transcanal route, that a laser may be employed during the procedure, and that, for example, a piston prosthesis is planned. However, it is important for the patient to recognize and accept the fact that the surgical procedure may have to be modified depending on findings at the time of the procedure. The risks of surgery include failure of surgery to improve hearing by virtue of residual conductive hearing loss; creation of a sensorineural loss, either partial or complete; vestibular dysfunction; perforation of the tympanic membrane; facial nerve dysfunction (either motor or sensory); and late failure of the procedure or development of a perilymph fistula. The patient should certainly be aware of the nonoperative option of the use of a hearing aid.

The entire spectrum of stapes surgery will not be covered in this chapter. Rather, the preferred methodology as practiced at the Massachusetts Eye and Ear Infirmary will be discussed. During the course of this description, alternative methodology for the specific portion of the procedure will be included.

METHOD OF PERFORMING PRIMARY STAPEDECTOMY*

Anesthesia

The patient is offered either a local or general anesthesia. Local anesthesia certainly has the advantage of allowing monitoring of vestibular symptoms at the time of fenestration of the footplate and insertion of the prosthesis. This is of particular advantage in revision surgery, where the origi-

---

*Earlier descriptions and reviews (27–29) will provide additional details.

nal prosthesis may be attached by adhesions to the contents of the vestibule. On the other hand, general anesthesia provides assurance, both to the patient and the surgeon, of absolute control of head motion and prevention of pain. In general, approximately 50% of patients will select a general anesthesia. For patients who are particularly nervous or claustrophobic or who otherwise have difficulty maintaining the surgical position, general anesthesia is preferentially recommended.

Surgical Procedure

Positioning

Proper positioning of the patient will facilitate exposure. The patient is placed in a supine head-hanging position and the head rotated slightly to the opposite shoulder to place the tympanic membrane approximately in the horizontal plane and to open the angle between the auricle and the ipsilateral shoulder (Fig. 22.1A). A headrest that is separable from the remainder of the operating table is preferred to facilitate appropriate positioning. The headrest is fitted with a fastening mechanism for a self-retaining speculum holder with sufficient degrees of freedom to allow proper positioning of the speculum and to accommodate varying degrees of head-hanging and rotation (Fig. 22.1B).

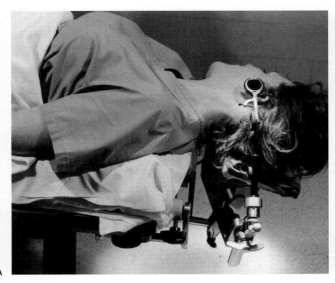

A

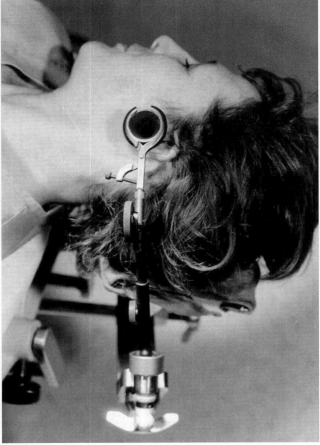

B

FIG. 22.1 A: The proper position for stapes surgery includes a slight head-hanging position with the chin turned to the opposite shoulder to open the angle between the ear and ipsilateral shoulder. **B:** A speculum holder is attached to the head rest and has sufficient degrees of freedom to allow easy adjustment of the angulation of the speculum during the procedure.

With either monitored intravenous anesthesia or general anesthesia, a local anesthetic block of the external auditory canal is performed using a combination of Xylocaine and epinephrine.

Exposure

A small triangular tympanomeatal flap is elevated (Fig. 22.2) and the bony tympanic annulus is curetted to provide surgical access to the oval window (Fig. 22.3). Curettage is complete when the bony pyramidal eminence is visible posteriorly and the facial nerve is visible superiorly. At this point, the middle ear should be inspected and patency of the round window, mobility of the incus and malleus, and fixation of the stapes should be confirmed. The incudostapedial joint is separated (Fig. 22.4). Using a scissors or the argon laser, the stapedius tendon is sectioned (Fig. 22.5). A posterior crurotomy is accomplished (Fig. 22.6). If visible, an anterior crurotomy may also be done to separate the superstructure from the footplate (Fig. 22.7). The remaining superstructure is fractured toward the promontory.

Fenestration

If the mucous membrane of the footplate is thin, it is not disturbed; if it is thick, it is elevated from the footplate but only in the area to be fenestrated or coagulated with a laser (Fig. 22.8). Using a motor-driven, sharp cutting bur or diamond-surfaced bur measuring 0.7 mm in diameter (Fig. 22.9A) or a laser (Fig. 22.9B), an opening is made in the thinnest part of the footplate. Lasers in the visible range (argon and KTP-532) and invisible range (CO_2) are used for stapes surgery.

The advantages of visible laser include the fact that the aiming and treatment beams are identical and can be delivered through a fiber-optic handheld bundle. However, visible lasers are only partially absorbed by the white bone of the stapes footplate and theoretically pass through an open vestibule and are absorbed by a pigmented tissue within the inner ear. Significant temperature elevation at the level of the saccule and utricle has been reported using the visible lasers (30). However Marquet (31), Perkins (32), DiBartolomeo (33), McGee (34), and Horn et al. (35) have all used the argon or KTP-532 lasers with success.

Optical delivery systems now provide the precision to allow the CO_2 to be applied to middle ear surgery. The CO_2 laser has the advantage of no significant penetration or caloric effect on the perilymph (36). However, it has the disadvantage of not being deliverable through a fiber-optic bundle and hence must be attached to the operating microscope with a separate coaxial aiming beam.

Clear advantages of the laser include (i) its hemostatic properties; (ii) precision that far exceeds other handheld instruments; (iii) the ability to vaporize the thicker posterior crus, therefore reducing the chance of a floating footplate; (iv) the ability to create a precise fenestra in the footplate without excessive footplate or perilymph motion, thus minimizing the risk of acoustic trauma; and (v) the ability to fenestrate a floating footplate without risk of depressing the footplate into the vestibule as is inherent in other fenestration techniques.

Because the argon laser is delivered through a fiber-optic bundle, it becomes defocused very rapidly after leaving the end of the probe. Thus the probe is withdrawn a few millimeters, the cutting action is lost, and the laser becomes an

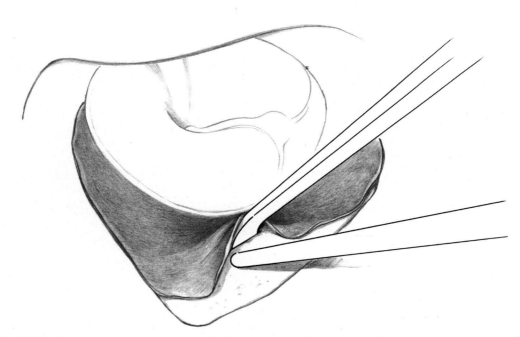

FIG. 22.2 A triangular segment of meatal skin is incised with a roller knife and is elevated to the tympanic annulus to create an anteriorly based tympanomeatal flap.

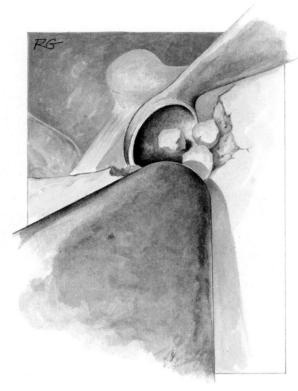

FIG. 22.3 The posterior bony annulus is curetted to allow visualization of the facial nerve superiorly, the pyramidal eminence posteriorly, and the entire circumference of the oval window.

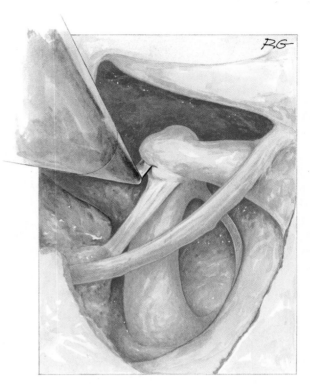

FIG. 22.4 The incudostapedial joint is separated with a joint knife.

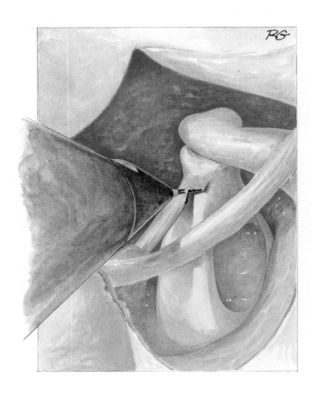

FIG. 22.5 The tendon of the stapedius muscle is separated using an argon laser.

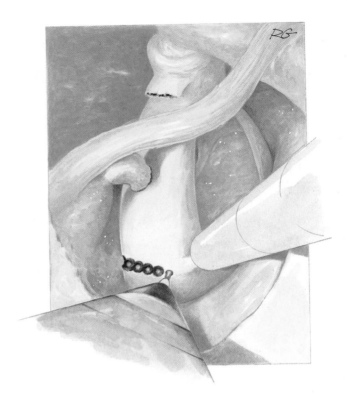

FIG. 22.6 A posterior crurotomy is done using the argon laser.

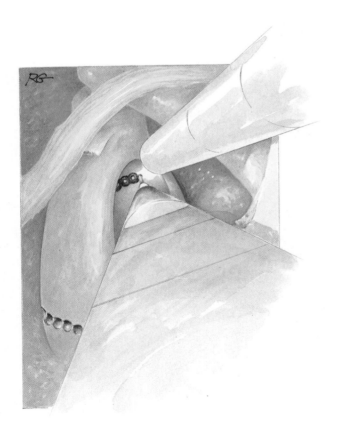

FIG. 22.7 If visible, an anterior crurotomy with laser is done.

excellent coagulator of small mucosal vessels which are common in the area of the otosclerotic focus anteriorly. Using the argon laser (typical setting 1.8 watts, 0.1 second), a rosette is created in the center of the footplate (Fig. 22.9B). Because the fiber-optic bundle delivers a spot size of approximately 200 microns, a rosette 3 to 4 diameters wide should result in a circular fenestra in the footplate measuring approximately 0.7 mm, which is sufficient to accommodate a 0.6-mm diameter piston. To avoid development of heat at the footplate level, 2 to 3 seconds is allowed to pass between each laser pulse. Once the "black char" of the laser spot has been created, absorption of subsequent pulses is made easier by overlapping the laser spots, taking advantage of the fact that the visible laser is better absorbed by a dark color. The typical appearance of a single lasered spot on the footplate will be a black char measuring approximately 200 microns in diameter, a more central white char, consisting of vaporized bone, and a central "pinhole" where the perilymph has been exposed (Fig. 22.9B).

When a sufficient rosette has been created, a fenestra is completed using the side of a straight pick or a rasp while suctioning at the edge of the stapes footplate but never over the fenestra (Fig. 22.10). In case of a thick footplate, a laser may be used at the beginning of the fenestration to devascularize the mucosa overlying the footplate, followed by a microdrill to quickly thin the footplate. The final fenestration may be done with the laser.

Measuring the Length of the Prosthesis

A measuring rod having a diameter of 0.6 mm and calibrated for length is used to determine simultaneously the adequacy of the size of the fenestra and the appropriate length of the piston prosthesis to be used (Fig. 22.11A, B).

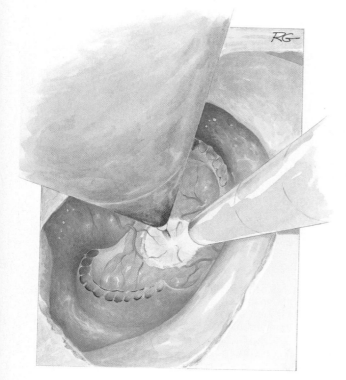

FIG. 22.8 By withdrawing the argon laser from the footplate approximately 1 mm the laser beam becomes an effective coagulator for mucosal vessels on the lateral surface of the footplate.

Placement and Attachment of the Prosthesis

The Schuknecht Teflon-wire piston consists of a cylindrical piston head made of Teflon (polytetrafluoroethylene) and a malleable piston rod made of 38-gauge (0.004 inch; 0.10 mm) SMO-316 nonmagnetic stainless steel wire. The piston head is 2.5 mm in length and is available in 0.6- and 0.8-mm diameters. One end of the rod is firmly set in the Teflon piston and the other is shaped into an open loop for attachment to the long process of the incus. The prostheses are available from several instrument suppliers in 3.25- to 4.75-mm lengths in increments of 0.25 mm. The combined length of the piston head and rod (exclusive of the loop) is used to identify the length of the prosthesis (Fig. 22.12).

A piston using platinum wire and ribbon has also been developed (Fig. 22.13). It is fashioned after the Schuknecht stainless steel wire Teflon piston and has the advantage of platinum wire shaft and a platinum ribbon loop. The wire allows easy alteration of the angulation once the prosthesis is in place, and the platinum loop provides a wider purchase on the incus. In addition, platinum is also somewhat easier to crimp because it does not have the metallic "memory" of stainless steel.

The prosthesis is grasped at an appropriate angle (Fig. 22.14A, B) and set in place so that the piston enters the fenestra and the wire loop engages the long process of incus in one maneuver. In general, the long axis of the smooth alligator and the prosthesis should be approximately the same. During insertion, if a different angle is required, it can be easily achieved by loosening slightly the grasp on the prosthesis and tapping the prosthesis gently against either the annulus posteriorly or incus anterior to achieve the desired angle. Before the loop is tightened, the mobility of the prosthesis is tested by gently depressing the incus. With this maneuver the prosthesis should move freely within the fenestra. If the patient notices vertigo when this is done, the prosthesis should be removed and replaced with one of a shorter length or modified by cutting off a small segment of the distal part of the piston with scissors. The piston should extend about 0.25 mm into the vestibule.

The loop is then crimped to the incus with sufficient firmness to create a stable linkage (Fig. 22.15). The loop should be securely wrapped around the long process. The posterior blade of the crimping forceps should be parallel to the shaft of the prosthesis. Posterior angulation of the crimping device will result in bending of the straight portion of the wire shaft. Angulating the crimping forceps slightly either superiorly or inferiorly (Fig. 22.16) will allow the operator to monitor the crimping process looking between the two blades of a crimping forceps (Fig. 22.17A, B). Improper closure of the loop (Fig. 22.18A, B) can result in a residual conductive hearing loss or bone erosion from friction caused by a loose prosthesis. After the loop is secured, adjustments may be made in the angle of the prosthesis by bending the wire portion of shaft with a right-angle hook to achieve optimal functional orientation within the fenestra. The success of this maneuver should be monitored by gently elevating the long process of the malleus while watching the motion of the prosthesis. If there is differential motion between the wire loop and incus, friction between the Teflon shaft and the margins of the fenestra should be assumed and a modification of the angle made to achieve smooth motion. A small pledget of Gelfoam soaked

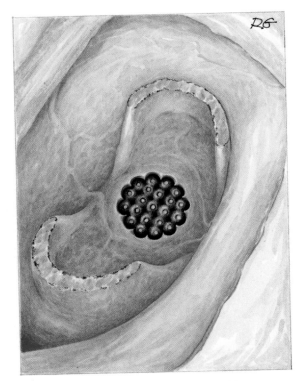

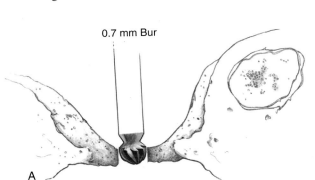

0.7 mm Bur

A

B

FIG. 22.9 A: As one method of fenestration, a microdrill using a 0.7-mm cutting and then diamond bur is used to fenestrate the footplate. **B:** As an alternate to microbur fenestration (Fig. 22.8), the argon laser may be used to fenestrate the footplate. A rosette of laser burns is created in the center of the footplate. Because the diameter of the argon laser fiber-optic bundle is 200 microns, 4 or 5 laser burn diameters are adequate to create a 0.7-mm fenestra. Each burn is characterized by black periphery representing charred bone. A more central white circle represents vaporized bone and a pin hole at the very center represents complete fenestration, through which small droplets of perilymph may be seen.

in normal saline is placed around the piston (Fig. 22.19). Alternatively, especially if the fenestra is somewhat larger than planned, a tissue graft (e.g., lobular fat or perichondrium) may be used to seal the oval window. The tympanomeatal flap is returned to its anatomic position and held in place with silk strips, soaked in normal saline, and a piece of synthetic sponge or cotton. Antibiotic prophylaxis begun intraoperatively is generally continued for 1 week postoperatively while the rosebud packing is in place. The patient is discharged from the hospital in most cases on the day of surgery or as soon thereafter as the patient's condition allows.

Should part or all of the footplate become mobile, that part can be removed and a larger piston with a tissue seal placed in the oval window. If the footplate is mobile but stable, a fenestra may still be made in its central portion using the otologic laser.

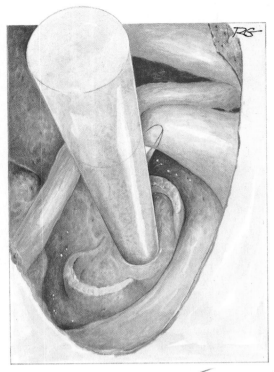

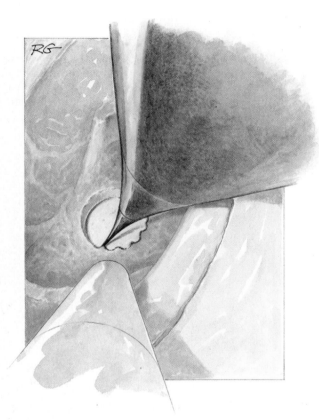

FIG. 22.10 With a 24 F-gauge section near the fenestra but never over it, the fenestra is completed with a straight pick and a footplate rasp if necessary.

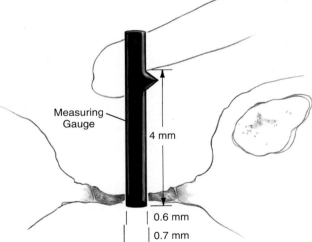

FIG. 22.11 **A:** A measuring stick with a diameter of 0.6 mm is placed to determine proper diameter of the fenestra and to measure the prosthesis length. **B:** The measuring stick (0.6 mm in diameter) should easily pass the fenestra. The top of a lateral projection from the measuring stick is at 4 mm from the end of the stick. An additional 0.25 mm is added to allow sufficient penetration of the vestibule. Thus in the example shown here, a prosthesis of 4.25 mm by 0.6 mm would be employed.

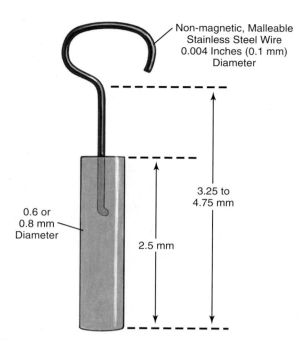

Non-magnetic, Malleable
Stainless Steel Wire
0.004 Inches (0.1 mm)
Diameter

3.25 to
4.75 mm

0.6 or
0.8 mm
Diameter

2.5 mm

FIG. 22.12 Teflon stainless steel wire piston (designed in 1960 by H.F. Schuknecht and H. Treace) is available from several commercial suppliers. The stainless steel wire is non-magnetic and is therefore not affected by magnetic resonance imaging.

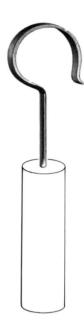

FIG. 22.13 The "MEEI prosthesis" is fashioned after the Schuknecht prosthesis. The wire is platinum flattened to a ribbon at the loop to allow more secure grasp on the incus. The vertical shaft of the wire remains cylindrical to allow angulation of the prosthesis if necessary.

FIG. 22.14 Grasping the prosthesis. Before introducing the prosthesis in the ear, the surgeon views the surgical field to determine the angle at which the prosthesis should be grasped to permit simultaneous introduction of the piston into the fenestra and engagement of a wire loop onto the long process of the incus. **A:** In general, the proper angle of grasp will place the long axis of the smooth forceps nearly parallel to the long axis of the piston. **B:** Left view. The position of the grasp is correct, but the angle is too acute (as compared with Fig. 22-14**A**). Right view. Incorrect grasp of prosthesis. The grasp is on the loop of the prosthesis, which will interfere with engagement of the loop onto the incus.

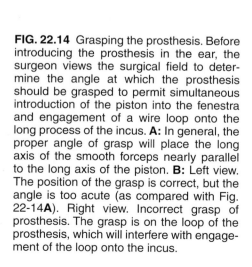

A

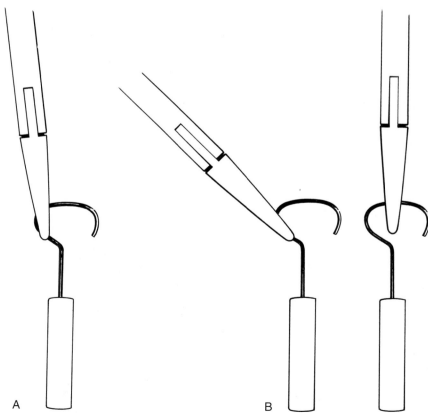

B

Total Footplate Removal

There are conditions in which a total footplate removal is unavoidable. The most common of these conditions include a floating footplate, comminuted fracture of the footplate, and conditions resulting from previous unsuccessful stapes surgery. Also, in some medical settings the equipment for the small fenestra technique, such as lasers or microdrills and prefabricated prostheses, are not available. Under these conditions, the footplate can be removed in its entirety and replaced with a tissue graft and prosthesis (Figs. 22.20 to 22.23). The authors' technique utilizes either a fat-wire prosthesis fabricated on a wire-bending die or a Teflon-wire piston prosthesis with fat grafts placed around the piston. In the latter method, the piston extends into the vestibule for 0.25 mm and no tissue is interposed between it and the fluid of the vestibule.

The footplate should be removed with as little trauma as possible to the mucosa of the oval window niche and with the least possible disturbance of perilymph. Aspiration of perilymph allows plasma from mucosal trauma, blood, and air to enter the vestibule and degrades the fluid environment of the sensory and neural tissues, as well as causing spatial distortion of the vestibular labyrinth. Intraoperative vertigo alerts the surgeon to the fact that the vestibular labyrinth is being traumatized and that a modification in technique is indicated.

FABRICATING THE FAT-WIRE PROSTHESIS

After the stapes has been removed, a small pledget of Gelfoam soaked in balanced salt solution is placed in the oval window while the fat-wire prosthesis is being made. Alternatively, if total footplate removal is planned or anticipated, the fat-wire prosthesis may be made prior to opening the oval window. The maneuvers are described for right-handed persons aided by 10X magnification of the binocular operating microscope:

STEP 1: (Fig. 22.24) A 6-inch length of 0.004-inch diameter (38-gauge) nonmagnetic stainless steel wire (SMO-316) is selected and is formed into a loop with a single overhand knot.

STEP 2: A symmetrical piece of nontraumatized ear lobe adipose tissue that has been cut to measure 2 × 2 × 3 mm is placed on the edge of the platform of the wire-bending die. The wire is grasped and the loop is guided to the tissue graft and partly closed around the graft.

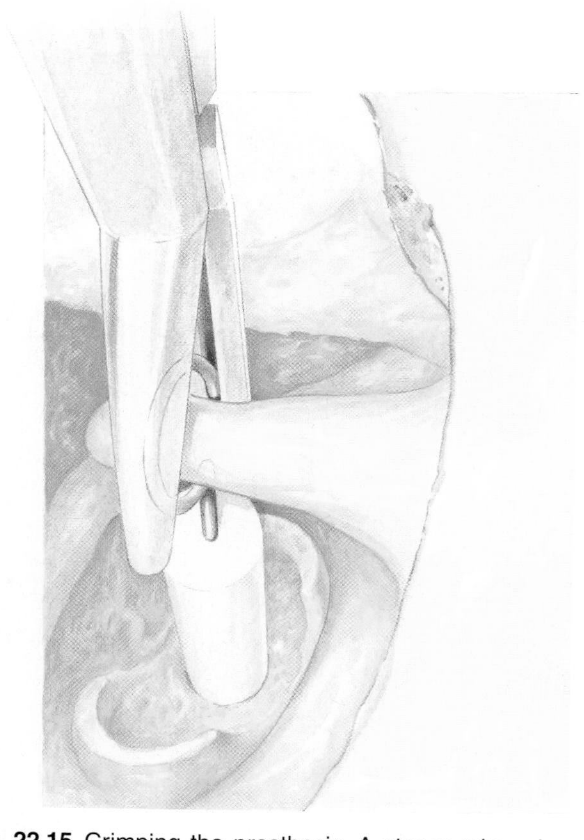

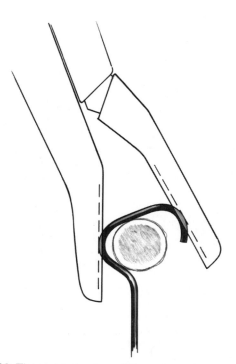

FIG. 22.15 Crimping the prosthesis. A stapes wire crimper simultaneously holds the wire against the shaft of the incus and closes the loop anteriorly.

FIG. 22.16 The posterior jaw of the crimper should be approximately parallel to the wire shaft to avoid bending the shaft during closure. The posterior jaw will simultaneously hold the loop against the incus posteriorly and superiorly, and the loop is closed by the anterior jaw.

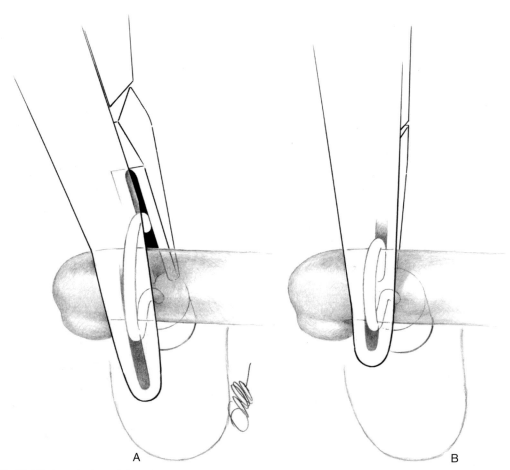

FIG. 22.17 Angulation of the crimper. **A:** Proper angulation allows the loop of the prosthesis to be seen between the jaws. **B:** Improper angulation of the crimper obscures visualization of the loop during the crimping process.

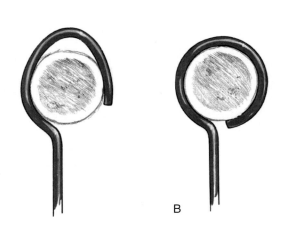

A   B

FIG. 22.18 A: This view shows a poorly crimped loop that is likely to allow differential motion of the prosthesis and the incus, resulting in residual conductive loss and perhaps delayed incus necrosis. Such a loop should now be engaged with a right-angle pick and the prosthesis removed holding the incus in place with the 24-gauge suction tube. The prosthesis is then replaced. A common cause for this problem is crimping of the loop when it is located near the end of the long process of the incus, in which case the open end of the loop strikes the lenticular process. Alternatively, it may occur if the posterior jaw of the crimper is not used to gently hold the prosthesis against the shaft of the incus during loop closure. **B:** This view shows a properly crimped loop that contours to the shaft of the incus.

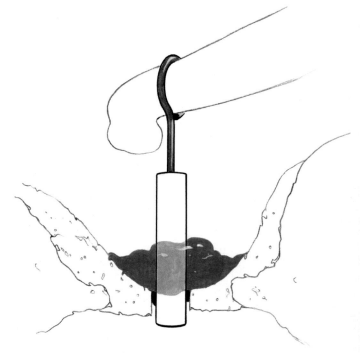

FIG. 22.19 The piston extends approximately 0.25 mm into the perilymphatic fluid of the vestibule. A small pledget of saline-soaked Gelfoam is placed around the piston. Alternatively a tissue seal may be achieved using tragal perichondrium or lobular fat.

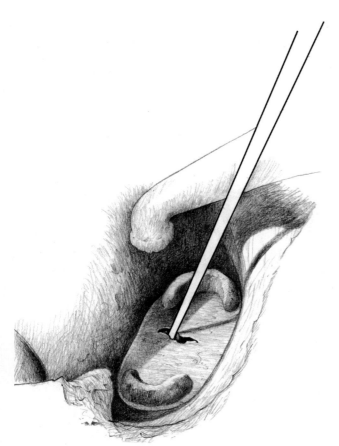

FIG. 22.20 A total stapedectomy begins by removing the crura, fracturing the footplate in the thinnest area using a straight pick. Alternately, if a unintended fracture occurs, a small angulated pick may be used to insert into the fracture line and elevate the footplate fragments.

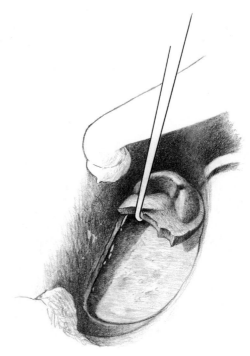

FIG. 22.21 Using an angulated hook, the anterior portion of the footplate remnant is removed.

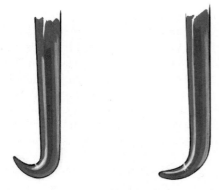

FIG. 22.22 These views show a satisfactory hook on the left damaged and a splayed hook on the right. Such seemingly insignificant factors may become critical in this exacting surgery. The surgeon should routinely monitor all instruments for damage.

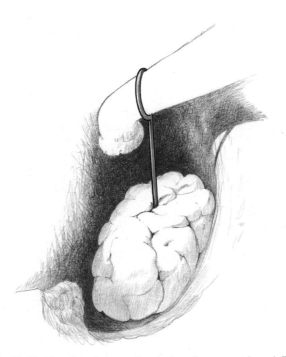

FIG. 22.23 The fat-wire prosthesis has been employed. The fat graft fills the oval window and overlaps the window margins by about 0.25 to 0.5 mm. The medial surface of the fat graft is at the level of the previous footplate. The shaft of the prosthesis is centered both in the fat graft and in the oval window.

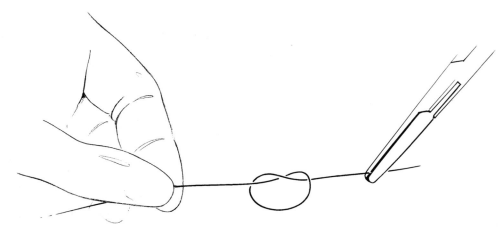

FIG. 22.24 The first step in the fabrication of a fat-wire prosthesis is to create a single overhand knot with a 6-inch (15-mm) piece of 0.004-inch (0.1-mm) diameter SMO-316 stainless suture wire.

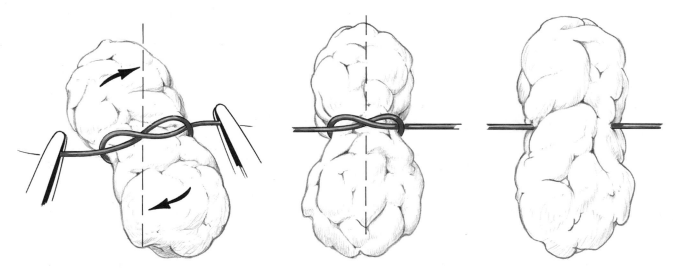

FIG. 22.25 The fat graft trimmed to measure 2 × 3 mm that rests overlapping the edge of a shelf of a prosthesis jig is engaged by the wire loop at its center.

STEP 3: (Fig. 22.25) The position of the graft is manipulated within the loop so that it is centered on the knot with the long axis of the graft perpendicular to the wire. As it is tightened, the knot settles into the center of the tissue graft.

STEP 4: (Fig. 22.26) The platform of the wire-bending die is positioned with the small post nearest the surgeon. While keeping the wire taut (between finger grip on the left and forceps grip on the right), the wire to the right of the graft is looped around the large post of the wire-bending die. While pulling slightly to the right, the wire then is lowered so that it assumes a position between the large and small posts. Keeping the long axis of the graft in the horizontal plane, the wire is drawn farther to the right until the graft has reached the proper position on the scale of the wire-bending die. For the average ear, the left edge

of the tissue graft is brought even with the 4-mm mark (4 mm from the center of the large post). While always keeping the wire taut, the end that is held by the left hand is brought toward the surgeon to a position perpendicular to the long axis of the platform of the wire-bending die. The forceps is released from the wire and used to gently nudge the wire from the die.

STEP 5: (Fig. 22.27A) A sharp, pointed wire-cutting scissors is used to cut the loop near the shaft to preserve a nearly complete circular loop.

STEP 6: (Fig. 22.27B) While continuing to hold the prosthesis in the gloved fingers of the left hand, the loop is opened with a small forceps (alligator type with smooth jaws). The opening should measure about 1 mm so that it will readily pass over the long process of the incus.

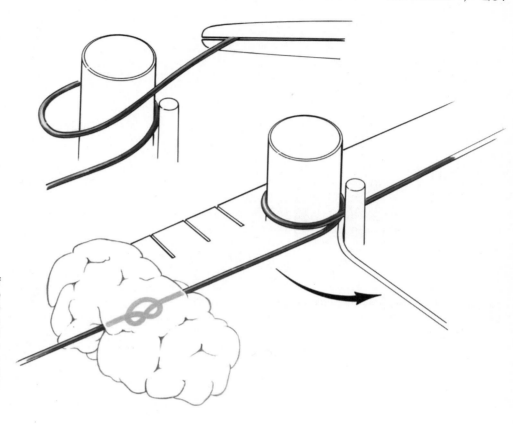

FIG. 22.26 With the long axis of the fat graft parallel to the plane of the platform of the jig, the wire is wrapped around the large post and pulled to the right until the left surface of the graft is located at the 4-mm mark on the scale of the platform. The shaft of the prosthesis is now moved to the right to form the loop.

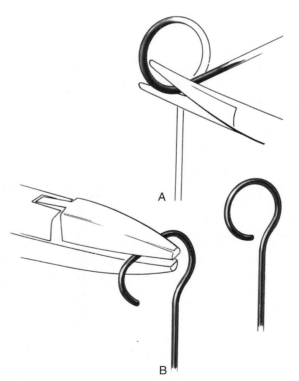

STEP 7: While continuing to hold the wire with the left hand, a sharp-pointed tissue scissors (such as Iris or fine plastic scissors) is used to further trim the tissue graft as required to achieve proper size and symmetry.

STEP 8: (Fig. 22.28) As the wire is cut next to the knot, the tissue prosthesis will adhere to the blades of the wire-cutting scissors. It is transferred to the platform of the wire-bending die and kept moist with saline solution. The Gelfoam pledget is removed from the oval window, and the prosthesis is introduced without allowing it to touch the speculum or ear canal. The fat graft (2 × 2 × 3 mm) should comfortably fill the oval window niche. The knot of the wire prosthesis should be located in the center of the fat graft (Figs. 22.29 and 22.30), and it will now be located slightly lateral to the plane where the footplate was previously located.

FIG. 22.27 After removing the prosthesis from the wire-bending die, the loop is cut (**A**) and opened (**B**) using a smooth jawed micro-alligator.

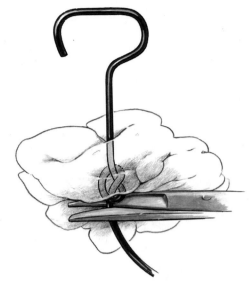

FIG. 22.28 The jaws of a wire-cutting scissors are slid along the wire until the knot is felt, and the wire is then cut.

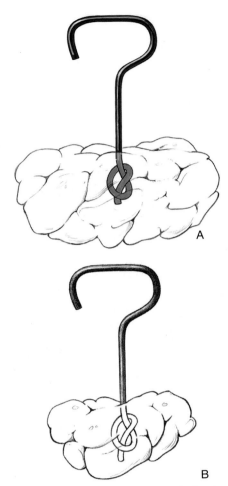

FIG. 22.29 A: When properly fabricated, the knot is small and centered and is entirely contained within the fat graft. **B:** A fat graft that is too small to seal the oval window.

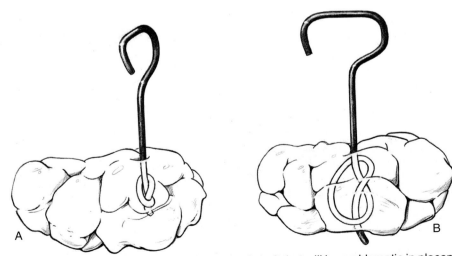

FIG. 22.30 A: This view shows an eccentrically located shaft that will be problematic in placement of the prosthesis. **B:** Here the loop has not been adequately tightened, resulting in a large knot that may either overlap a bony margin of the oval window or may result in part of the wire protruding into the vestibule.

PROBLEMS ENCOUNTERED DURING AND AFTER STAPES SURGERY

Intraoperative Problems and Complications

Exostoses of the External Auditory Canal

Small exostoses usually do not impair access to the mesotympanum and may be left intact. Even moderately sized exostoses that are limited to the anterior canal wall usually do not interfere with the surgical approach. The trauma of removal of large exostoses contraindicates the simultaneous performance of stapes surgery. In such cases it is prudent to first remove the exostoses and to delay stapedectomy until healing is complete.

Tears in the Tympanomeatal Flap

Tears of the tympanomeatal flap may occur in the following locations: (i) A linear tear or buttonhole perforation may occur in the skin flap. Usually these tears require no repair; however, when replacing the flap at the conclusion of the procedure, care must be taken to avoid infolding the margins of the tear. (ii) The skin flap may separate from the tympanic annulus. This usually occurs in an inferior location and is due to failure to elevate the tympanic annulus from its sulcus. Another cause for tears of this type is "undermining," that is, elevating the midportion of the flap without simultaneous elevation at the incisional margins. Usually no repair is required if the separation occurs inferiorly; however, if it occurs superiorly, grafting may be necessary. Such small tears near the annulus but central to the tympanomeatal flap may be repaired at the end of the procedure by placing a small saline-soaked pledget of Gelfoam in the middle ear near the annulus and then advancing the posterior aspect of the tympanomeatal flap slightly in an anterior direction to closely approximate the torn edges. (iii) Tears of the pars tensa are less common and usually occur in thin replacement membranes.

When grafts are necessary most tears can be satisfactorily repaired with fatty connective tissue from the ear lobe. A flat piece of tissue of suitable size is introduced into the perforation with the bulk of the graft on the medial surface. The margins of the perforation are approximated as closely as possible. These grafts will adhere to the medial surface of the area being repaired and need not be held in place with supportive Gelfoam. Tears of the pars flaccida usually are caused by a misdirected superior incision; fortunately they heal spontaneously without the formation of cholesteatomas.

High Jugular Bulb

A superiorly located jugular bulb may come into juxtaposition with the tympanic annulus and in this position is vulnerable to injury during elevation of the tympanomeatal flap (Fig. 22.31). For this reason the elevation of the tympanic annulus inferiorly should not be performed blindly. Tears of the jugular bulb result in profuse bleeding and constitute an alarming, although not serious, complication. The bleeding can be controlled by elevating the head of the operating table and packing the area with Gelfoam, Surgicel, Oxycel, or similar hemostatic agent. Modest pressure over the

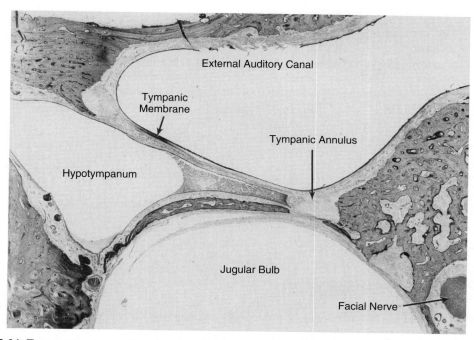

FIG. 22.31 Temporal bone section showing a high jugular bulb that abuts the tympanic annulus without bony separation. In such a situation, the jugular bulb may be inadvertently opened during the process of elevating the tympanomeatal flap (14X).

Gelfoam for a few minutes will generally result in cessation of bleeding. If the bleeding is readily controlled, the operation may continue, but if the tear is large and the bleeding is difficult to control, the procedure should be terminated.

Disarticulation of the Incus

The incus may be inadvertently dislocated during curetting of the bony annulus or during manipulations in the oval window area. Subluxation of the incus implies a partial tear of the capsule of the incudomalleal articulation. In this situation there is usually sufficient remaining intact capsule to hold the incus in its normal anatomic position. Although the long process of the incus will be excessively mobile, the operation can be completed and the functional result is usually satisfactory. Dislocation of the incus, on the other hand, implies a complete disruption of the incudomalleal articulation; this accident usually requires removal of the incus and use of a malleus-grip prosthesis. Attempts to replace and maintain the dislocated incus in its normal position until healing of the capsule occurs are rarely successful.

Fracture of the Long Process of the Incus

This is an unusual complication, but it may happen during the wire-tightening procedure. In fractures near the tip of the long process, the stump may be long enough to accommodate the wire loop. If this is not possible, a malleus-grip prosthesis must be used. When the lenticular process is fractured during removal of the stapes, it may be grasped with a cupped forceps and removed. When the lenticular process is particularly long and close to the promontory, it should be fractured and removed to prevent a fibrous adhesion to the promontory. A pneumatized incus, although rare, may predispose to fracture (Fig. 22.32).

Overhanging Facial Nerve

The location of the facial nerve should be determined as soon as the oval window area is exposed. Normally, the nerve lies encased in the fallopian canal immediately superior to the oval window and poses no problem in stapes surgery. If the facial nerve overhangs the superior part of the oval window, it should be gently palpated to determine if there are dehiscences in its bony canal. It is common for the nerve to protrude from such dehiscences (Fig. 22.33). Thickened mucosa caused by an active underlying otosclerotic lesion may obscure a protruding facial nerve. Rarely the facial nerve may lie inferior to the oval window or split into two bundles that pass superior and inferior to the oval window. In some cases the nerve completely obscures the footplate and the crura protrude through a small slit between the nerve and promontory. After removing the crura, if any part of the footplate can be visualized, it is usually possible to complete a stapedotomy procedure. During the fenestration, caution should be exercised to avoid trauma with either laser or microdrill to

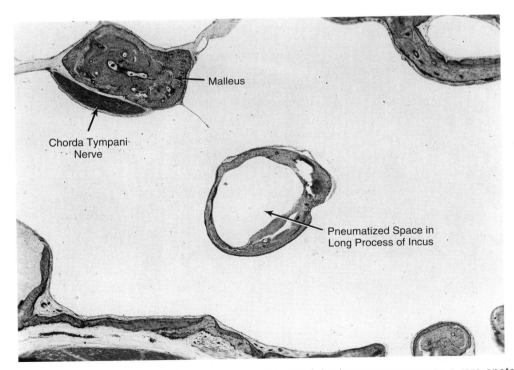

FIG. 22.32 Pneumatization of the long process and body of the incus may occur as a rare anatomic variant. Pneumatization occurs through a small opening on the anteromedial surface of the long process. This condition is present in approximately 3 of 1,500 ears in the temporal bone collection of the Massachusetts Eye and Ear Infirmary. It is obvious that this condition renders the long process susceptible to fracture during the crimping procedure (25.5X).

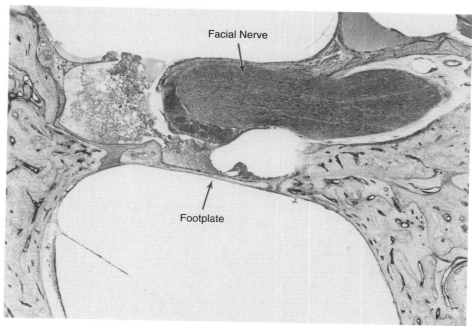

FIG. 22.33 Overhanging facial nerve. Often the fallopian canal is dehiscent in the area of the oval window. In such cases the facial nerve may protrude through the dehiscence to overlap part of the oval window. Any soft tissue in the area of the oval window niche must be considered the facial nerve until proven otherwise (22.1X).

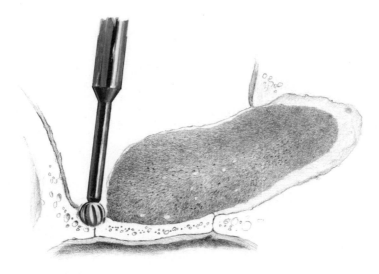

FIG. 22.34 If the footplate is not totally obscured by the dehiscent facial nerve, a fenestra is still possible by using a microbur of 0.7 mm in diameter. The fenestration may occur in the footplate or at the stapediovestibular joint, overlapping the cochlear side no more than 0.7 mm to avoid injury of the membranous labyrinth.

the dehiscent facial nerve. The creation of a fenestra using the space provided by a combination of a marginal burr hole and the exposed portion of the footplate (Fig. 22.34) may be necessary to accommodate a 0.6-mm diameter prosthesis.

Facial Palsy

Facial palsy occurring intraoperatively is the result of either direct injury to the nerve trunk in the region of the oval window or injection of local anesthetic agent near the nerve as it passes through the parotid gland anterior to the external auditory canal or directly into middle ear. Direct injury most often results from mistaking the nerve for thickened mucous membrane. If nerve fibers have been transected, dyskinesis of facial motor function is a certain clinical sequela. In the case of inadvertent exposure of the nerve to anesthetic agent, complete recovery of function can be expected within a few hours.

Obliterative Otosclerosis of the Oval Window

Obliterative otosclerosis of the oval window is of three types: (i) massive thickening of the footplate that virtually fills the oval window niche, (ii) massive overgrowth of the margins of the oval window obliterating the niche and obscuring the footplate, and (iii) a combination of footplate thickening and marginal overgrowth (Fig. 22.35). Experience has shown that the appropriate surgical approach is saucerization of the oval window with bone removal burs (Fig. 22.36) followed by the standard small fenestra technique using a drill or laser. In general the fenestra should be somewhat larger than a small fenestra of a footplate because some new bone formation can be expected after a "drill out." A total stapedectomy is contraindicated in these cases because of an unacceptably high incidence of surgically induced sensorineural hearing loss.

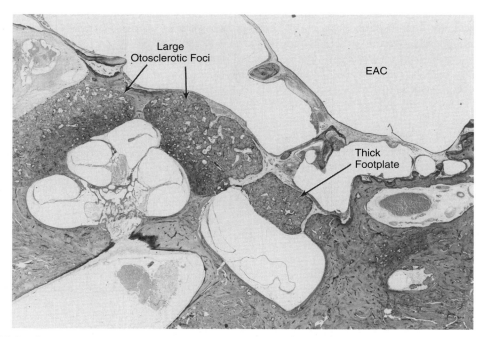

FIG. 22.35 Obliterative otosclerosis. This temporal bone section shows obliteration of the oval window niche by a thick otosclerotic focus. In such cases, total stapedectomy is contraindicated and even a carefully performed stapedectomy often meets with limited success (7.9X).

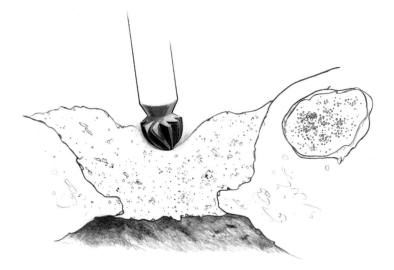

FIG. 22.36 Saucerization of the obliterative otosclerotic focus is done with a microdrill. The final fenestration may be done with a microdrill or laser. The final fenestration should be approximately 0.8 mm for a 0.6-mm diameter piston because some reparative bony regrowth may occur.

Round Window Otosclerosis

Complete obliteration of the round window niche with otosclerosis is a cause of residual conductive hearing loss following stapedectomy. For this reason, in every case the round window niche should be inspected intraoperatively and its condition recorded in the operative note as either normal, narrowed, possibly obliterated, or definitely obliterated. It is often impossible to be certain whether the round window is totally obliterated. Therefore, if there is a reasonable chance that the round window niche is patent to the middle ear, the stapes procedure should proceed. Exploration or removal of the bone from the round window niche is contraindicated because of a high risk of postoperative sensorineural loss. In addition, as shown in Fig. 22.37 obliterative otosclerosis in the round window niche may extend into the intracochlear space.

Persistent Stapedial Artery

A persistent stapedial artery has been reported to be present in about 1 in 5,000 to 1 in 10,000 ears (37). It presents as a pulsating artery that traverses the anterior part of the obturator foramen of the stapes (Fig. 22.38). The artery measures about 1.5 mm in diameter, leaving sufficient space posterior to it to complete the stapedotomy procedure. A small artery traversing the footplate is a normal finding and is not to be confused with a persistent stapedial artery. Coagulation of the persistent stapedial artery is contraindicated. If in the judgment of the operating surgeon, there is inadequate room to perform a stapedectomy or too high a risk of injury to the artery, then the procedure should be abandoned and the hearing loss rehabilitated using a hearing aid.

Malleus Ankylosis

Idiopathic malleus ankylosis has no clinical or pathologic relationship to otosclerosis or any other otologic disorder. Presumably it occurs as either a congenital anomaly or an acquired condition of unknown cause. The condition is present in 8 of 1,400 ears (0.57%; 5.7 per 1,000) from adult subjects in the temporal bone collection at the Massachusetts Eye and Ear Infirmary (Fig. 22.39). Presumably either the head of malleus fails to completely separate from the walls of the epitympanum during embryogenesis or the bony spurs that normally approximate the head of malleus hypertrophy and fuse to the malleus. About a 15- to 20-db hearing loss is attributable to malleus fixation and is additive when associated with stapes fixation. The diagnosis is readily made preoperatively by either pressure otoscopy or palpation of the manubrium. Malleus mobility should be assessed both preoperatively and intraoperatively to aid in the assessment of postoperative results. The operation record should contain a notation as to the mobility of the malleus. Corrective surgery for a fixed malleus requires removal of the incus and head of the malleus and the use of a malleus-grip prosthesis.

It is very rare for the incus to be fixed, but in this case, after removal of the incus, a malleus-grip technique is also required.

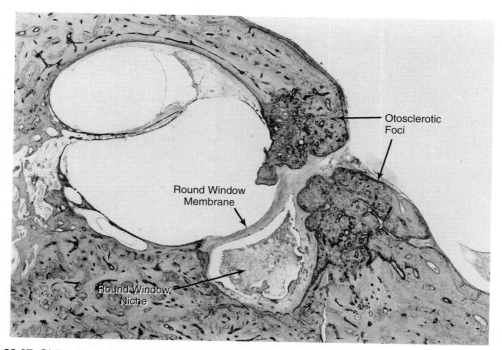

FIG. 22.37 Obliteration of the round window by otosclerosis. This 55-year-old woman had undergone a right stapedectomy at age 41 without improvement in hearing. Histologic study demonstrated obliteration of the round window by otosclerosis (22.1X).

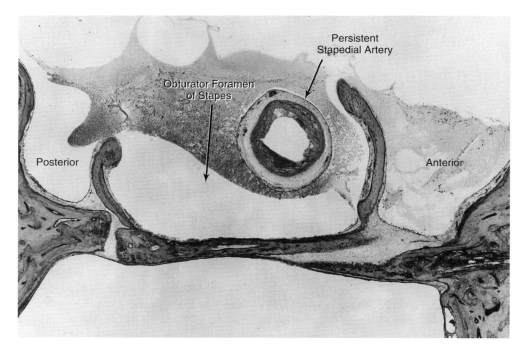

FIG. 22.38 Persistent stapedial artery. This temporal bone section shows a persistent stapedial artery in its usual location in the anterior part of the obturator foramen (intercrural space). If there is sufficient room, stapedotomy can be performed posterior to the artery (34.1X).

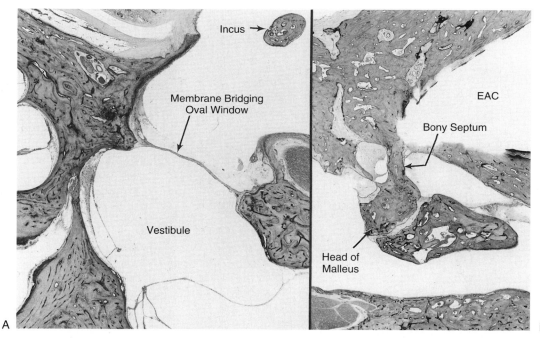

FIG. 22.39 Malleus fixation. This 81-year-old woman had undergone a right stapedectomy at the age of 70 for 25-db conductive hearing loss. The entire stapes was removed and replaced by a Gelfoam-wire prosthesis. However, hearing was not improved postoperatively and 1 year prior to death there was a 30-db air-bone gap. **A:** Histologic study of the temporal bone showed the prosthesis to be well placed and functional. The oval window was bridged by a thin neomembrane. No otosclerosis was seen at the margin. It is possible but improbable that otosclerosis was present in the footplate and therefore removed entirely. However, it is more likely that the conductive hearing loss was entirely explained by malleus fixation (10.4X). **B:** The head of the malleus is seen ankylosed to the anterolateral wall of the epitympanum by a bony septum (8.3X).

Gushers and Oozers

A flow of cerebrospinal fluid (CSF) immediately following fenestration of the footplate occurs often enough to have generated the common parlance of *gusher* for a pouring, jet-like outflow and *oozer* for a milder, persistent flow.

It has been established that the gusher is a consequence of a defect in the cribrose area at the fundus of the internal auditory canal, which creates a confluence of the subarachnoid space with the perilymphatic space of the vestibule (38). These defects measure 1 to 2 mm in diameter. Gushers are known to occur principally in ears with congenital fixation of the footplate. Plester (personal communication) believes that a gusher is always an indication that the fixed footplate is of congenital etiology. If a gusher is suspected as a possibility on clinical or radiographic grounds, preparation for the potential need to lower spinal fluid pressure may be done by (i) placement of an indwelling lumbar subarachnoid drain; or (ii) placement of a urinary catheter to allow administration of a rapid-acting diuretic intraoperatively if necessary. If a gusher is unanticipated, if possible, the stapes procedure may be completed always using a tissue seal at the oval window area (e.g., fat-wire prosthesis or piston plus perichondrial graft). A lumbar subarachnoid spinal catheter may be then used to lower the spinal fluid pressure to allow healing at the oval window. If it is impossible to complete the stapes procedure because of the profuseness of spinal fluid flow, as a last resort a tissue graft may be placed over the oval window and the middle ear packed, leaving the tympanomeatal flap reflected (39) (Fig. 22.40). Packing is removed 4 or 5 days later and the tympanomeatal flap returned to the posterior canal wall. After an interval of several months to allow healing at the oval window and to reestablish a sterile middle ear environment, reconstruction may be done. However, care should be taken to avoid reopening of the fenestra.

The oozer is caused by the presence of a large patent cochlear aqueduct and is a common occurrence in stapes surgery for otosclerosis. The largest patent cochlear aqueduct found in the temporal bone collection at the Massachusetts Eye and Ear Infirmary is 0.2 mm in diameter at its narrowest point. The stapes surgery need not be altered, as the ooze of CSF is self-limiting; however, fluid may be present in the middle ear for several days postoperatively, during which time prophylactic antibiotics are indicated.

Bleeding

Bleeding from the incisional areas of the ear canal should be controlled before the middle ear is entered. This is accomplished by infiltrating the skin of the posterior bony canal wall with small volume of 1% lidocaine (Xylocaine) containing 1:50,000 epinephrine (MIVA anesthesia) or 1:100,000

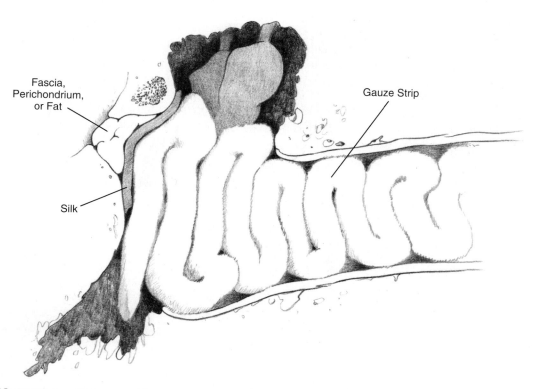

FIG. 22.40 As a last resort, if a tissue graft attached to an incus cannot be achieved, a CSF gusher may be controlled by placing fascia in the oval window held with packing. After 5 days, the packing is removed and the tympanomeatal flap returned to its anatomic position. A revision ossiculoplasty can be done at a later time without fenestrating the neomembrane over the oval window.

epinephrine (general anesthesia). Cotton pledgets are used to compress bleeding points, and bleeding vessels are coagulated with a high-frequency coagulation unit (Hyfrecator). Small bleeding points may alternatively be coagulated using the handheld argon laser held a few millimeters away from the bleeding site to take advantage of the coagulation ability of the defocused Argon beam. When the crural arch is fracture-dislocated, there may be bleeding from the mucosa of the footplate and at the disrupted incudostapedial articulation. This bleeding is self-limiting but can be reduced by gentle pressure with epinephrine-soaked cotton pledgets. The vestibule is not opened until all bleeding has been controlled. In the unlikely event that blood enters the vestibule, for example in total footplate removal, a clot is allowed to form and, when the bleeding has been controlled, the clot is gently lifted from the vestibule with a 24-gauge suction cannula.

Floating or Depressed Footplate

The floating footplate problem usually occurs in an ear with minimal stapes fixation when the attempt is made to fracture the crural arch. If the crura and stapes remain intact, the entire stapes is removed. If the crural arch has fractured, it is removed and an inferior marginal bur hole is made that permits a small pick to be introduced to engage the undersurface of the footplate and extract it (Fig. 22.41). Alternately, if the footplate is mobile but not subluxed and the stapediovestibular ligament seems intact and stable, a small fenestra may be created with a otologic laser. This should not be attempted with an otologic drill because pressure applied to the mobilized footplate may cause its subluxation and depression.

There is no good surgical solution for the depressed footplate, that is, a footplate that has settled down into the vestibule. It is a near certainty that the patient will suffer immediate and protracted vertigo. A footplate depressed in a trapdoor or tilted configuration can sometimes be removed by engaging the nondepressed margin with a small hook at a crural remnant. No attempts should be made to remove a to-tally depressed footplate. A tissue graft with prosthesis (e.g., fatwire) can be introduced in the usual manner. The hearing results are unpredictable, varying from total loss to excellent improvement, and vertigo of varying severity and duration is a virtual certainty. Although instrumentation of the vestibule should be avoided, retrieval of a mobile and partially depressed segment may be facilitated by the injection of freshly drawn venous blood from the patient into the oval window niche and allowing this to coagulate. At that time, gentle aspiration of the coagulum using a 24 French suction cannula may elevate or extract the fragment.

Clinical experience has shown that it is not necessary to remove small pieces of footplate, bone dust from drilling, or broken bits of metal picks from the vestibule. Animal and human studies have shown that these foreign bodies become attached to the walls of the vestibule or membranous labyrinth and become encapsulated in a fibrous tissue.

Early Postoperative Complications

Otitis Media

Despite the use of prophylactic antibiotics, acute bacterial infection occurring within the first few days after surgery is a rare but serious complication. The principal symptoms are persistent pain and fever. The packing should be removed and intravenous antibiotic therapy instituted at once. The risk, of course, is possible spread to the inner ear and CSF. After full healing of the tympanic membrane and middle ear has occurred (approximately 6 weeks), acute suppurative otitis media in an ear with a stapes prosthesis may be treated in the usual fashion with oral antibiotics.

Vertigo

Vertigo occurring intraoperatively or immediately after surgery is a clear indication of a traumatic surgical procedure (40). The trauma may take the form of a direct contact injury

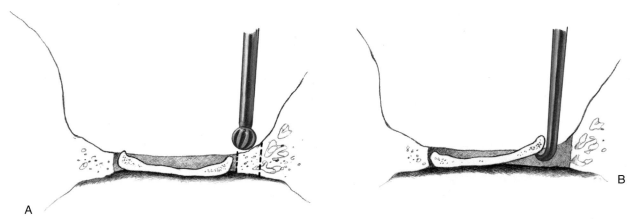

A

B

FIG. 22.41 Technique of using a marginal bur hole to correct floating or subluxed footplate. **A:** An inferior marginal bur hole overlapping the cochlear side of the stapediovestibular joint. No more than 0.7 mm is created to allow entry into the vestibule of a 0.3-mm angulated hook (**B**).

to the membranous labyrinth, particularly the utricular macula, which has a close anatomic relationship to the oval window (Fig. 22.42). Other causes for immediate vertigo are aspiration of perilymph, resulting in pneumolabyrinth and causing anatomic distortion of the sense organs, and hemolabyrinth, causing biochemical degradation of the perilymph. Vestibular suppressant drugs and bed rest are useful forms of therapy. Following direct trauma to the labyrinth, the duration of vertigo may be prolonged (weeks); however, following pneumolabyrinth or hemolabyrinth, the duration of vertigo is usually short (days).

Reparative Granuloma

This exuberant granulomatous reaction is a host response to trauma of the middle ear mucosa. The symptoms usually are noted between the fifth and fifteenth postoperative days and consist of the onset of unsteadiness, tinnitus, and hearing loss after an initial hearing gain. Otoscopy reveals an edematous hypervascular skin flap and a reddish discoloration of the posterior part of the tympanic membrane. Audiometry shows a mixed hearing loss worse for the high frequencies and a decreased speech discrimination score. Spontaneous nystagmus occurs toward the opposite side. It seems quite clear that the perilymph undergoes biochemical degradation by the proteinaceous exudate of the granuloma, and surgical removal of the granuloma as an emergency procedure is indicated. When this is done, about one-half of the cases experience recovery of hearing and the remainder have varying degrees of permanent sensorineural hearing loss. The vertigo gradually subsides over a period of weeks to months. The postoperative reparative granuloma is primarily a complication of a traumatic stapedectomy and is almost nonexistent as a complication of a well-executed small fenestra technique.

Perforation of the Tympanic Membrane

Perforations are usually the result of direct intraoperative trauma; however, postoperative otitis media is also a cause. Areas of dimeric membrane (without a lamina propria) are particularly susceptible to injury or ischemic necrosis and may result in a perforation in the early postoperative period.

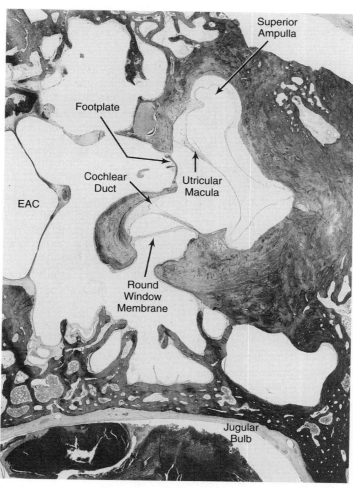

FIG. 22.42 This vertical section of a temporal bone shows the normal anatomic relationship of the utricle and cochlear duct to the oval window (4.7X).

If the perforation is small, a fat-graft repair as an office procedure may suffice. Perforations that persist will require myringoplasty.

Delayed Facial Palsy

The onset of facial palsy several days following stapes surgery is caused by mild direct intraoperative trauma. Presumably delayed edema results in temporary dysfunction of neural excitation (neuropraxia). Although the surgeon may have been unaware of any encounter with the nerve, it is virtually certain that direct contact was made. Recovery of facial movement occurs within a few days to a few weeks. No therapy is indicated except to protect the cornea from desiccation. A rapidly tapered oral administration of steroids may shorten the period of paresis.

Sensorineural Hearing Loss

Sensorineural hearing loss occurring in the immediate postoperative period may be attributed to direct trauma to the membranous labyrinth (e.g., rupture of the cochlear duct), degeneration of tissue grafts with contamination of the perilymphatic fluid by the products of tissue decay (40), or, later in the postoperative period (10 to 14 days), the formation of a reparative granuloma. These early complications of surgery may cause mild to profound hearing losses. When the loss is partial, it is usually worse for high frequencies and often is associated with a significant loss of word discrimination. High-tone hearing losses that peak at 4 kHz can be attributed to acoustic trauma caused by excessive manipulations of the footplate or prosthesis. No reliable treatment exists for sensorineural loss that occurs immediately following surgery. However, if there is a documented deterioration of hearing following an initial improvement, either a perilymph fistula or reparative granuloma should be considered.

Conductive Hearing Loss

Unexpected conductive hearing losses that persist in the early postoperative period are usually caused by one or more of the following conditions: (i) malfunction of the prosthesis (e.g., too short, eccentrically located in the oval window [Fig. 22.43], loose attachment to the incus); (ii) fibrous adhesions (e.g., fibrous tissue proliferation in the oval window, fibrous fixation of the lenticular process to the promontory); (iii) pathology of the tympanic membrane (e.g., perforation, laxity and retraction of the posterior part); (iv) failure to recognize malleus fixation; (v) failure to recognize round window obliteration; or (vi) temporary effusion or hemotympanum.

Exploratory tympanotomy can be performed to identify the cause of the hearing loss, after which appropriate corrective measures can be applied when feasible. Corrective surgery for the various pathologies might include replacing a malfunctioning prosthesis, introducing a Teflon disc to eliminate adhesion of the lenticular process to the promontory (Fig.

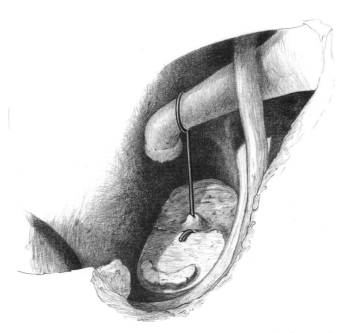

FIG. 22.43 Impingement or overlap of the prosthesis (in this case a fat-wire prosthesis) upon remnants of the fixed footplate or oval window will cause a residual conductive hearing loss.

22.44), myringoplasty for perforation of the tympanic membrane, and removal of a fixed head of the malleus and use of a malleus-grip prosthesis. In general, a delay of several months between primary and revision surgery is indicated.

Late Postoperative Complications

Perilymph Fistula

The development of a perilymph fistula is a very real and potentially serious complication of stapes surgery. The classical symptoms are fluctuating sensorineural hearing loss and mild to moderate episodic unsteadiness. A sudden, severe loss of hearing and severe vertigo can occur but are unusual. Deaths from bacterial labyrinthitis and meningitis have been reported. Pressure otoscopy commonly reveals a positive Hennebert's sign (fistula sign), which is probably caused by movement of an air bubble in the vestibule. The Hallpike maneuver with the affected ear downward may induce mild positional unsteadiness and nystagmus. Exploratory tympanotomy is indicated when a perilymph fistula is suspected. Corrective surgery requires an appropriate tissue graft and replacement of the prosthesis. Perilymph fistulas are primarily a complication of total stapedectomy techniques and are rare with the small fenestra technique.

Sensorineural Hearing Loss

A sudden and severe sensorineural loss may occur after an initial hearing improvement as a late complication of stapes surgery. When it is associated with immediate postoperative

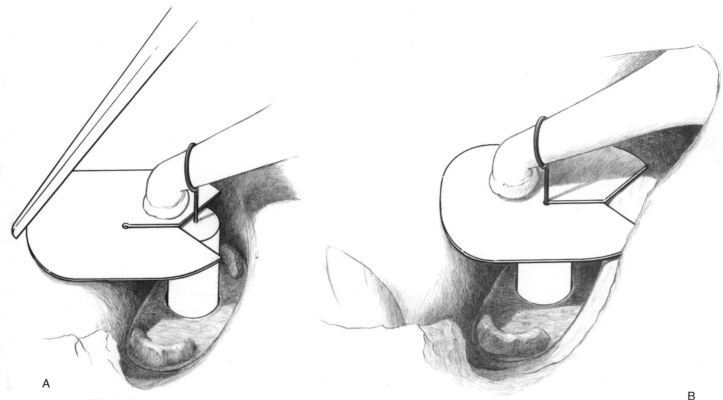

A

B

FIG. 22.44 A Teflon disc is used when there is a risk for postoperative fibrous adhesions between the incus and the promontory or facial nerve. **A:** The beveled leading edge centers the disc on the shaft as it is pushed superiorly. **B:** The disc rides over the fallopian canal as the shaft of the prosthesis reaches its final resting position in the center of the disc. The disc should not impinge on the cochleariformis process. This technique may be used for primary procedures where the mucosa has been traumatized or in revision cases where abundant adhesions between the incus and promontory or facial nerve are encountered.

severe vertigo, the sudden hearing loss may be attributable to intraoperative trauma. However, sudden hearing loss may also occur after uneventful and atraumatic surgery. The etiology remains unknown.

Trauma to the structures of the vestibule can also result in collapse of the saccule or reuniting duct, which interferes with the longitudinal flow of endolymph. This injury leads to subsequent cochlear endolymphatic hydrops and the symptoms of episodic vertigo and fluctuating hearing loss (40). These types of inner ear pathologies cannot be clearly differentiated from perilymph fistula; therefore surgical exploration is necessary either as an emergent procedure for the sudden losses or as a planned procedure for the cases with chronic episodic symptoms.

Delayed Onset Conductive Hearing Loss

Revision surgery has revealed the following causes for delayed onset conductive hearing losses: (i) resorptive osteitis of incus; (ii) in the case of the gel-wire technique that has been used with total stapedectomy, migration of the wire prosthesis to the edge of the oval window, causing diminished sound transmission; (iii) continuing or recurring otosclerotic bone or other new bone formation that narrows the

oval window niche and restricts the movement of the prosthesis; (iv) continuing growth of otosclerotic bone that obliterates the round window months or years following a successful stapes operation; and (v) fixation of the head of the malleus after an initially successful stapedectomy. Presumably the surgical manipulations of the malleus cause abrasive trauma between the head of malleus and bony spurs in the epitympanum and lead to ankylosis.

Resorptive Osteitis of the Incus

This complication is the result of a foreign-body reaction either to the prosthesis, as occurred with the polyethylene struts, or to an unstable linkage at the site of attachment of the prosthesis to the incus. A loosely attached prosthesis causes focal resorptive osteitis that can result in destruction of the long process of the incus distal to the attachment (Fig. 22.45). Another less common physical cause for osteitis occurs in total stapedectomies when a piston prosthesis is placed on a tissue graft rather than into the vestibule. Under these conditions, the tissue graft, with its advantageous position under the prosthesis, can force it laterally. This causes pressure erosion of the long process at the site of linkage with the prosthesis and leads to discontinuity and extrusion

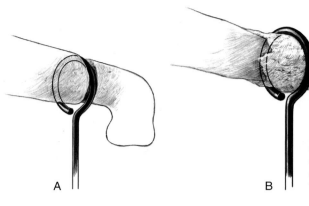

FIG. 22.45 Rarefying osteitis of the incus (incus resorption) may occur with any type of stapes prosthesis. **A:** Resorption of part of the incus leads to a loose linkage between the prosthesis and incus. **B:** The entire distal end of the incus has been resorbed. The prosthesis may then migrate laterally or more rarely medially.

of the prosthesis. Another possible cause for incus necrosis is differential motion of the stapes prosthesis and incus. For example, if movement of the shaft of the piston is impeded by fibrous adhesion or friction at the margins of the fenestra in the oval window, differential motion between the prosthesis and the incus may occur, which over time may lead to resorptive osteitis.

The symptoms of resorptive osteitis begin with a fluctuation of hearing related to the state of inflation of the middle ear, and at this stage it is common for patients to perform the Valsalva maneuver repeatedly throughout the day to improve sound transmission. Some patients also note that hearing is improved in certain positions of the head, as when stooping over. Total discontinuity may occur suddenly when sneezing, blowing the nose, or bumping the head or may simply progress slowly. The typical end result of discontinuity is a large bone-air gap.

Corrective surgical measures require removal of the prosthesis and attachment of a new prosthesis of appropriate length to either the stump of the long process of the incus or to the manubrium. When reattaching to the incus, the stump should be grooved on both anterior and posterior surfaces to create a linkage that will not slip. The platinum ribbon prosthesis (Fig. 22.13) may allow a more secure attachment to the incudal remnant. A manubrium attachment requires a wraparound technique.

An eccentric wire prosthesis should be replaced by a piston prosthesis that extends through an opening into the vestibule rather than placing it on the surface of an oval window membrane. A prosthesis that is fixed by regrowth of bone should be removed, an adequate opening made into the vestibule, and a piston introduced that extends into the vestibule. Fixation of the head of the malleus is corrected by removing the head of the malleus and introducing a malleus-grip prosthesis.

In most revision stapes operations a Teflon disc should be introduced to prevent adhesions forming between the lenticular process and promontory.

THE MALLEUS-GRIP PROSTHESIS

Ears with conductive hearing loss caused by multiple ossicular pathologies present a special surgical challenge. The malleus-grip prosthesis (41) was designed for the management of ears having fixation, fracture, luxation, or anomaly of the stapes in association with disease of the malleus or incus.

The approach is the same as for incus attachment stapedectomy. A tympanomeatal flap is elevated and the bony annulus is removed sufficiently to expose the oval window area. The plica mallearis (Fig. 22.46) is incised, and the tympanic membrane is freed from the manubrium in the area between its lateral process and the umbo.

Initially the pathology of each ossicle is determined by inspection and gentle manipulation. Inadvertent mobilization of a fixed ossicle by excessive pressure should be avoided. If the head of the malleus is fixed, the incus is removed and the head of the malleus is amputated with a guillotine malleus nipper and removed. Separation of the tympanic membrane from the malleus and initial fixation of the prosthesis to the malleus handle is facilitated by performing these two maneuvers prior to nipping and removing the head of the malleus. Final positioning of the malleus grip prosthesis into the oval window follows amputation and removal of the head. If only the incus is fixed, which is rare, it alone is removed. A prerequisite condition for this type of surgery is that the stapes be fixed, fractured, luxated, or anomalous. The management of the stapes will consist of either stapedectomy, in which case a fat-wire prosthesis can be used, or small fenestra technique, which will accommodate a Teflon-wire piston. The malleus-grip procedure is contraindicated, however, if the footplate of the stapes is mobile; in this case an interpositioning procedure is preferred so as to avoid the risks inherent in opening the inner ear.

The cross-sectional oval configuration of the manubrium introduces an important consideration in the design of the hook of the prosthesis. Thus the loop must be larger than the one commonly used for the round cross-sectional configuration of the long process of the incus. The fabrication of the

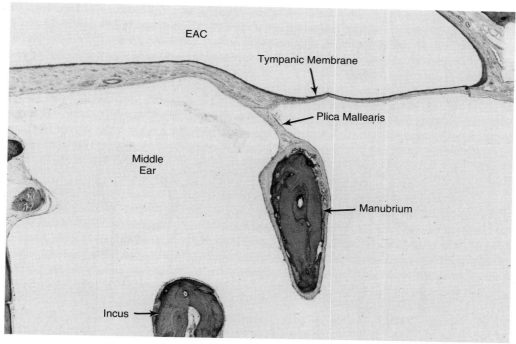

FIG. 22.46 The plica mallearis is the fold of mucous membrane that lies between the manubrium and the tympanic membrane. It is widest midway between the lateral process of the malleus and the umbo, and it is in this area that the malleus grip prosthesis should be placed (21.4X).

malleus-grip fat-wire prosthesis is done on the wire-bending die described for the incus-attachment prosthesis. Alternatively, Teflon-wire pistons in several lengths are available from commercial suppliers. The length of the prosthesis is about 5 to 5.5 mm, and the loop is larger than for incus attachment (Fig. 22.47). The determination of the proper length of the prosthesis for each ear is accomplished in part by the use of a measuring stick but more importantly by the process of repeated placements and adjustments.

As in the incus attachment technique, the fat graft that measures 2 × 2 × 3 mm should comfortably fill the oval window niche. The piston technique requires that the piston extend slightly into the vestibule through a fenestra opening in the footplate. If inward displacement of the prosthesis causes vertigo, it is shortened. The capability of monitoring for subjective vertigo is a strong argument for the use of local anesthesia rather than general anesthesia in these cases. A small piece of autogenous tissue or Gelfoam may be placed around the piston.

The loop is crimped to the manubrium in a wraparound manner. This is accomplished by partly closing the loop with a crimper and then completing the closure by pulling the free end of the wire with a hook while stabilizing the shaft in the grip of a forceps (Fig. 22.48). Experience has shown that this attachment must be tight, as a loose one promotes resorption osteitis of the manubrium, which may lead to extrusion of the prosthesis. The shaft of the prosthesis can then be adjusted to bring the prosthesis into a right angle with the plane of the footplate (Fig. 22.49) and finally insertion of the piston into the oval window fenestra.

Functional success is enhanced and complications are fewer if the following tenets are observed:

1. Select for surgery only those cases with a normal (or near normal) tympanic membrane. Perforations, atrophy, retraction, and neomembranes are contraindications to this method. Very few fenestrated ears are suitable for this procedure because extensive removal of the bony tympanic annulus has resulted in medial displacement of the tympanic membrane. The membrane should be normally tense to ensure restriction of displacements associated with changes in middle ear pressures.
2. Select for surgery only those cases with a plica mallearis, thus avoiding excessive contact of the prosthesis with the tympanic membrane, possibly causing erosion and crusting, which in turn may lead to osteitis of the manubrium and extrusion of the prosthesis. High power otoscopy will identify those ears in which the tympanic membrane is adherent to the entire manubrium, thus obliterating the plica mallearis.
3. Take special care to ensure that the length of the prosthesis is appropriate. After setting the prosthesis in place and before crimping, manipulate the manubrium and determine that the location and movement of the prosthesis at the oval window is appropriate.
4. Crimp the prosthesis to the manubrium in a tight wraparound manner, because a loose prosthesis causes frictional irritation and resorption osteitis at the site of contact with the bone. The end result is disengagement and extrusion of the prosthesis.

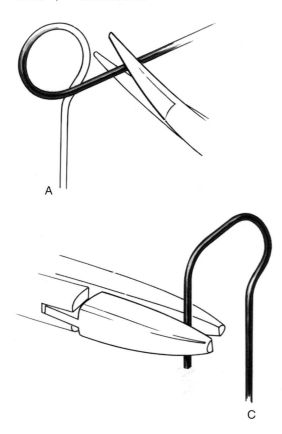

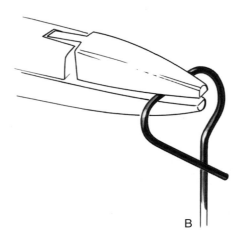

FIG. 22.47 A custom-made malleus-grip fat-wire prosthesis, made on the wire bending die, is generally 1 mm longer (5 mm) and has a longer free end of the loop than the standard incus attachment fat-wire prosthesis. **A:** The wire is cut outside the intersection between loop and shaft to allow a longer free end. **B:** The loop is open with a smooth jawed microforceps. **C:** The free end of the loop is straightened to accommodate the manubrium.

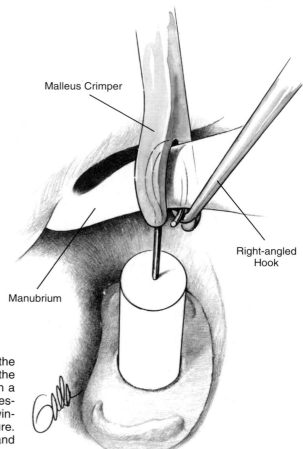

Malleus Crimper

Right-angled Hook

Manubrium

FIG. 22.48 After placing the prosthesis, the loop is closed over the manubrium in a wraparound fashion. This is done by partially closing the loop with a crimper and wrapping around the free end of the loop with a right-angled hook. This may be done with the shaft entered into the fenestra or may be done with the Teflon shaft directed posterior to the oval window to prevent trauma to the vestibule during the wraparound procedure. The shaft of the prosthesis then may be bent to properly angulate it and place it into the fenestra.

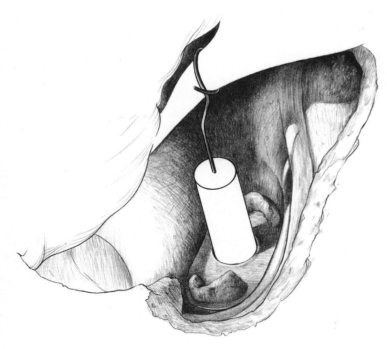

FIG. 22.49 A proper angulation and centering of the prosthesis using a Teflon wire malleus attachment. Because the malleus is anterior to the oval window, angulation of the prosthesis is necessary to allow a perpendicular entry of the shaft of the prosthesis into the oval window. The final length of the prosthesis may also be modified using this angulation. Malleus attachment prostheses are commercially available in 4.5- to 6.5-mm lengths and diameters of 0.6 and 0.8 mm.

REFERENCES

1. Nadol JB Jr. Pathoembryology of the middle ear. *Birth Defects* 1980;26:181–209.
2. Wang P-C, Merchant SN, McKenna MJ, et al. Does otosclerosis occur only in the temporal bone? *Am J Otol* 1999;20:162–165.
3. McKenna MJ, Kristiansen AG, Haines J. Polymerase chain reaction amplification of a measles virus sequence from human temporal bone sections with active otosclerosis. *Am J Otol* 1996;17:827–830.
4. Kessel J. Über das Ausschneiden des Trommelfelles und Mobilisieren des Steibügels. *Arch Ohrenheilk* 1876;11:99.
5. Boucheron E. La mobilisation de l'etrier et son proceed operatoire. *Un Med* (Paris) 1888;46:412.
6. Miot C. De la mobilisation de l'etrier. *Rev Laryngol (Bord)* 1890;10:113;145:200.
7. Moure EJ. De la mobilisation de l'etrier. *Rev Laryngol (Bord)* 1890;10:225–233.
8. Blake CJ. Stapedectomy and other middle ear operations. *Trans Am Otol Soc* 1893;5:464–473.
9. Jack FL. Remarkable improvement in hearing by removal of the stapes. *Trans Am Otol Soc* 1893;5:284–305;474–487.
10. Sourdille M. New technique in the surgical treatment of severe and progressive deafness from otosclerosis. *Bull N Y Acad Med* 1937;13:673–691.
11. Lempert J. Fenestra nov-ovalis: a new oval window for the improvement of hearing in cases of otosclerosis. *Arch Otolaryngol* 1941;34:880–912.
12. Rosen S. Mobilization of the stapes to restore hearing in otosclerosis. *New York J Med* 1953;53:2650–2653.
13. Hall A, Rytzner C. Stapedectomy and autotransplantation of ossicles. *Acta Otolaryngol (Stockh)* 1957;47:318–324.
14. Shea JJ Jr. Fenestration of the oval window. *Ann Otol Rhinol Laryngol* 1958;67:932–951.
15. Silverstein H. Laser stapedotomy minus prosthesis (laser STAMP): a minimally invasive procedure. *Am J Otol* 1998;19:277–282.
16. Hough JVD. Partial stapedectomy. *Ann Otol Rhinol Laryngol* 1960;69:571–596.
17. Schuknecht HF, McGee TM, Colman BH. Stapedectomy. *Ann Otol Rhinol Laryngol* 1960;69:597–609.
18. Hough JVD. Partial stapedectomy. *Trans Am Otol Soc* 1960;48:170–195.
19. Shea JJ, Sanabria F, Smyth GDL. Teflon piston operation for otosclerosis. *Arch Otolaryngol* 1962;76:516–521.
20. House HP. Experiences with stapes surgery. In: Schuknecht HF, ed. *Otosclerosis.* Boston: Little, Brown, 1962;447–456.
21. Scheer AA. Stapedectomy as a definitive procedure. *Arch Otolaryngol* 1962;76:522–531.
22. Guilford F. Panel on techniques and results of stapes surgery. *Arch Otolaryngol* 1963;78:546–573.
23. Schuknecht HF. A new stapedectomy prosthesis. *Arch Otolaryngol* 1964;80:474.
24. McGee TM. The stainless steel piston: surgical indications and results. *Arch Otolaryngol* 1965;81:34–40.
25. Robinson M. A four-year study of the stainless steel stapes. *Arch Otolaryngol* 1965;82:217–235.
26. Schuknecht HF, Applebaum EL. Surgery for hearing loss. *N Engl J Med* 1969;280:1154–1160.
27. Schuknecht HF. *Stapedectomy.* Boston: Little, Brown, 1971.
28. Schuknecht HF. Current method of stapes surgery. *Adv Otorhinolaryngol* 1987;37:101–103.
29. Schuknecht HF, Bentkover SH. Partial stapedectomy and piston prosthesis. In: Snow JB Jr, ed. *Controversy in otolaryngology.* Philadelphia: WB Saunders, 1980;281–291.
30. Lesinski SG. Lasers for otosclerosis. *Laryngoscope* 1989;99[Suppl 46]:1–24.
31. Marquet J. Small hole stapedectomy. *Proceedings of the Sixth Shambaugh International Workshop on Otomicrosurgery and Third Shea Fluctuating Hearing Loss Symposium.* Huntsville, AL: Strode Publishers Inc, 1980.
32. Perkins RC. Laser stapedotomy for otosclerosis. *Laryngoscope* 1980;90:228–241.
33. DiBartolomeo JR. A versatile argon microsurgical laser. *Otolaryngol Head Neck Surg* 1982;90:139–141.
34. McGee TM. The argon laser in surgery for chronic ear disease and otosclerosis. *Laryngoscope* 1983;93:1177–1182.
35. Horn KL, Gherini S, Griffin GM Jr. Argon laser stapedectomy using an endo-otoprobe system. *Otolaryngol Head Neck Surg* 1990;102:193–198.
36. Lesinski SG, Stein JA. CO_2 laser stapedotomy. *Laryngoscope* 1989;99[Suppl 46]:20–24.
37. House HP, Patterson MD. Persistent stapedial artery. A report of two cases. *Trans Am Acad Ophthalmol Otolaryngol* 1964;68:644–646.
38. Schuknecht HF, Reisser C. The morphologic basis for perilymphatic gushers and oozers. *Adv Otorhinolaryngol* 1988;39:1–12.
39. Schuknecht HF. Mondini dysplasia. A clinical and pathological study. *Ann Otol Rhinol Laryngol* 1980;89[Suppl 55]:1–23.
40. Schuknecht HF, Mendoza AM. Cochlear pathology after stapedectomy. *Am J Otolaryngol* 1981;2:173–187.
41. Schuknecht HF, Bartley MB. Malleus grip prosthesis. *Ann Otol Rhinol Laryngol* 1979;95:531–534.

CHAPTER 23

Ossiculoplasty and Tympanoplasty in Chronic Otitis Media

Saumil N. Merchant

Chronic suppurative otitis media (COM) is a chronic inflammatory disease of the middle ear and mastoid that often results in partial or total loss of the tympanic membrane and ossicles, leading to conductive hearing losses that can range in severity up to 60 to 70 dB. Chronic otitis media is a common condition, affecting 0.5% to 30% of any community (1). Therefore a conservative estimate of the number of people in the world suffering from COM is more than 120 million. The mainstay of therapy for COM is surgical, with the main goals being eradication of disease, prevention of recurrence, and preservation or improvement of hearing. Mastoidectomy is designed to eradicate disease in the mastoid and middle ear, whereas tympanoplasty is an operation designed to reconstruct the middle ear hearing mechanism (2). In the United States, more than 70,000 tympanoplasty and mastoidectomy procedures are performed annually (3).

Selection of surgical approaches for COM is discussed in Chapters 9 and 11. Surgery for repair of tympanic membrane perforations is discussed in Chapter 14, and mastoidectomy procedures are described in Chapter 17. This chapter focuses on the rationale for and the surgical techniques used to restore hearing after eradicating disease in the tympanomastoid compartment.

CLASSIFICATION OF TYMPANOPLASTY

The modern era of tympanoplasty was ushered in by Wullstein (4) and Zöllner (5). Subsequently, many other otologic surgeons contributed to the development and refinement of tympanoplasty techniques. Wullstein classified the operations as types I through V, based on the concepts of sound transformation at the oval window and sound protection of the round window. A modified version of Wullstein's classification is presented and used in this chapter.

This work was supported in part by research grants from the National Institute on Deafness and Other Communication Disorders of the National Institutes of Health.

Type I

Type I tympanoplasty refers to repair of the tympanic membrane without altering the ossicular system. The procedure includes exploration of the middle ear to inspect and ensure normality of the ossicles. *Myringoplasty* refers to repair of the tympanic membrane alone without inspection of the ossicular chain.

Type II

Type II tympanoplasty refers to repair of the tympanic membrane and ossicular system with restoration of the lever mechanism, which is a normal function of the malleus and incus. The most common condition leading to type II tympanoplasty is osteitic resorption of the lenticular process of the incus, which is repaired with a bone graft or synthetic prosthesis.

Type III

Type III tympanoplasty restores sound conduction to the oval window by one of the following three types of columella reconstruction: (i) A stapes columella consists of placing the tympanic membrane or graft onto an intact stapes. (ii) A minor columella consists of placing an ossicle graft from the stapes capitulum to the tympanic membrane or manubrium. A synthetic prosthesis of this type is termed a *partial ossicular replacement prosthesis (PORP)*. (iii) A major columella, performed when the stapes crura are missing, consists of an ossicle graft placed from the footplate to the tympanic membrane or manubrium. Such a synthetic prosthesis is termed a *total ossicular replacement prosthesis (TORP)*.

Type IV

In type IV tympanoplasty, the stapes footplate is allowed to remain directly exposed to incoming sound from the ear canal and a tissue graft is placed to acoustically shield the round window membrane from sound. The air space enclosed between the acoustic shield and the round window is called the cavum minor. The cavum minor is aerated via the eustachian tube.

Type V

The type V operation is used to bypass an ankylosed stapes footplate and is performed as a second-stage procedure after eradication of active disease. There are two subtypes: (i) Type Va tympanoplasty is the original Wullstein type V and consists of fenestration of the lateral semicircular canal to bypass the ankylosed stapes footplate. (ii) A type Vb is similar to a type IV, but the stapes footplate is removed and the oval window is sealed by a tissue graft (6). Type Va procedures are rarely performed, having been largely supplanted by type Vb operations.

PHYSIOLOGIC PRINCIPLES OF TYMPANOPLASTY

The goals of tympanoplasty are to restore sound pressure transformation at the oval window by coupling an intact tympanic membrane with a mobile stapes footplate via an intact or reconstructed ossicular chain and to provide sound protection for the round window membrane by means of a closed, air-containing, mucosa-lined middle ear (4).

In the normal ear, most of the middle ear gain is provided by the area ratio; that is, the tympanic membrane gathers force over its surface and then couples the gathered force to the smaller footplate of the stapes. It is pertinent to note that the mean gain provided by the normal human middle ear is only approximately 20 dB between 250 and 1,000 Hz, and the gain decreases by 6 to 8 dB per octave at frequencies above 1,000 Hz (7). Consequently, a mechanically mobile but suboptimal tympanoplasty combined with adequate middle ear aeration and round window protection can result in no middle ear gain but still produce a relatively good hearing result. For example, a tympanoplasty that gives a middle ear gain of 5 dB but leaves the middle ear aerated and allows round window motion will result in an air-bone gap of only 15 dB.

Because the cochlea responds to a *difference* in sound pressure between the oval and round windows, it is important to understand how this difference depends on the relative *magnitude* and *phase* of the two sound pressures. In the normal ear and after successful tympanoplasty, the magnitude of sound pressure at the oval window is significantly greater than that at the round window, and under these circumstances, differences in phase have little effect on determining the window pressure difference (7). Therefore the goal of tympanoplasty should be to increase the magnitude of sound pressure at the oval window relative to the round window, without regard to phase.

PATHOLOGIC CONSIDERATIONS

A number of pathologic changes can occur in the middle ear and mastoid as a result of COM (8). These tissue responses can compromise sound transmission, leading to conductive hearing loss, and they can also play an important role in determining the success or failure of tympanoplasty. In addition, the host response to ossicular implants and grafts is an important determinant of the long-term efficacy of ossicular reconstruction (9,10). Insight into these pathologic factors can help a surgeon to make more rational decisions regarding selection of cases and surgical techniques to optimize both control of disease and restoration of hearing.

Pathology of Chronic Otitis Media

Active COM, both with and without cholesteatoma, may lead to resorptive osteitis of the ossicular chain (Fig. 23.1). The lenticular process of the incus is the most commonly affected part of the chain, leading to discontinuity at the incudostapedial joint or its replacement with a fibrous band. Resorption can also involve the stapes crura, body of incus, and manubrium, in that order of frequency.

Chronic otitis media may lead to ankylosis or fixation of an ossicle as a result of proliferation of fibrous tissue, deposition of tympanosclerosis, or neoosteogenesis. Tympanosclerotic fixation may involve one, two, or all three ossicles. Common sites of fixation are the malleus head in the epitympanum (Fig. 23.2) and the stapes footplate at the oval window (Fig. 23.3). Ossicular fixation may occur in association with tympanic membrane perforation and ossicular resorption, and failure to recognize fixation may lead to an unsatisfactory surgical result.

Some cases of healed, inactive COM result in end-stage pathology, characterized by fibrosis and cyst formation (fibrocystic sclerosis), that obliterates large portions of the tympanomastoid compartment (Fig. 23.4). The cystic spaces are lined by mucosal epithelium that has been overrun by proliferation of fibrous tissue. Often there is deposition of new bone in the mastoid antrum and central mastoid cell tract (fibroosseous sclerosis). Another example of inactive COM is *epidermization,* which refers to keratinizing squamous epithelium lining areas of the middle ear but without retention of keratin (Fig. 23.5). Fibrocystic or fibroosseous sclerosis and epidermization represent nonprogressive, end-stage pathology that is a contraindication to tympanoplasty surgery, because it is very difficult to restore middle ear aeration in such cases.

Pathology of Middle Ear Grafts and Implants

Tympanic membrane perforations can be successfully repaired using a variety of graft materials. Autologous tissue such as temporalis fascia, tragal cartilage perichondrium, and earlobe adipose tissue are all adequate grafting materi-

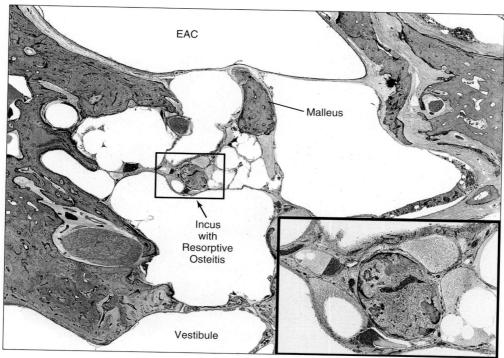

FIG. 23.1 Ossicular resorption. Horizontal section from an ear with COM without cholesteatoma. A small focus of chronic inflammation has resulted in osseous resorption and fibrous replacement of the inferior part of the long process of the incus (12X). The inset shows a higher power view of the incus. EAC, external auditory canal (63X).

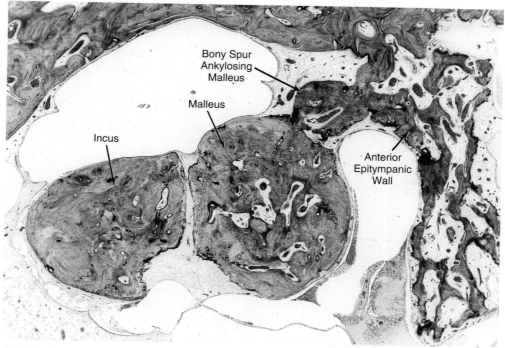

FIG. 23.2 Ossicular fixation. Epitympanum of left ear showing bony ankylosis of the head of the malleus to the anterior epitympanic wall. It is presumed that this osteogenetic reaction occurred in response to a previous acute or subacute otitis media.

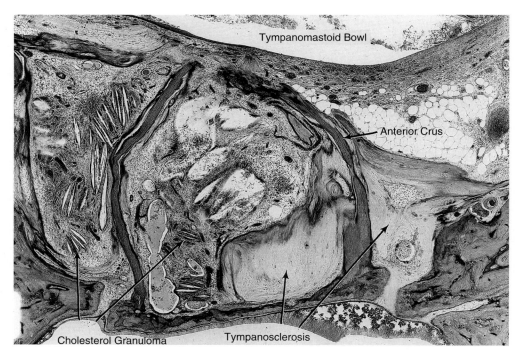

FIG. 23.3 Ossicular fixation. Oval window niche in an ear with a healed radical tympanomastoidectomy cavity. A fibroproliferative reaction and tympanosclerotic deposits have fixed the stapes. The capitulum of the stapes has been resorbed, and crura appear devitalized.

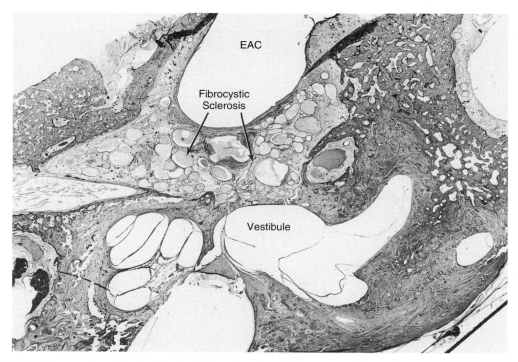

FIG. 23.4 Fibrocystic sclerosis. Horizontal section from right temporal bone showing healed COM. The middle ear is obliterated with fibrous tissue and cystic spaces. The mastoid shows osseous sclerosis. This type of nonprogressive, end-stage pathology is a contraindication to tympanoplasty surgery (6X). EAC, external auditory canal.

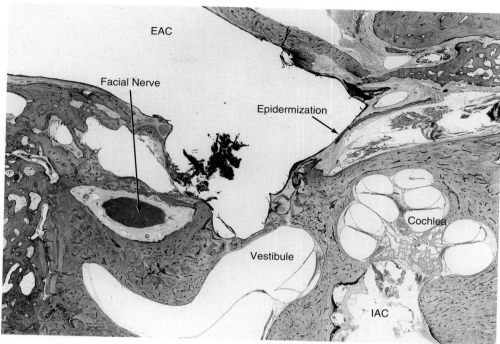

FIG. 23.5 Epidermization. Horizontal section from left temporal bone with inactive COM showing squamous epithelium lining the middle ear, but there is no retention of keratin. The auditory and vestibular sense organs and nerves appear normal. Epidermization is also a contraindication to tympanoplasty surgery. EAC, external auditory canal; IAC, internal auditory canal (10X).

als with ease of availability near the surgical site and uniformly high take rates in excess of 90%.

Ossicular grafts and prostheses are different in many ways when compared with implants placed elsewhere in the body. Ossicular implants must couple well at their ends to bone or soft tissue but must remain suspended in air elsewhere to avoid unwanted ankylosis (e.g., to the promontory or facial nerve canal). They must maintain not only their shape and size but also their acoustic transmission properties over long periods. For example, changes in mechanical properties of an implant, such as stiffness, can lead to changes in middle ear sound transmission. Furthermore, the recipient middle ear milieu in COM is potentially hostile as a result of active or arrested inflammatory disease or because of inadequate eustachian tube function. Persistent or recurrent infection can predispose to breakdown and resorption of an implant, and tubal insufficiency can accelerate implant extrusion. Also, homograft and synthetic ossicular implants are potentially subject to immune-mediated rejection.

A variety of autograft, homograft, and synthetic materials have been used for reconstructing the ossicular chain. *Autologous ossicle grafts* (incus or head of malleus), when available, constitute the material of choice (Fig. 23.6). They maintain their morphologic contour, size, shape, and physical integrity for long periods, more than 20 years. They do not incite formation of new bone nor do they undergo resorption (in the absence of infection). They undergo slow replacement of nonviable bone by new bone formation through a process of "creeping substitution." It is critical to avoid thermal injury when sculpturing such grafts (Fig. 23.7), and the generous use of irrigation is recommended. The general availability, low cost, ease of handling, and time-tested functional results make autologous ossicles a good first choice for ossiculoplasty.

Cortical bone grafts are readily obtained from the mastoid cortex through a postauricular or endaural incision. A 2-mm bur is used to create troughs around a segment of bone that will roughly meet the requirements for length, thickness, and contour. The strut is then separated from the mastoid cortex with an osteotome and then further sculpted with drills, using liberal irrigation to prevent thermal injury. The behavior of autologous cortical bone struts is histologically similar to that of ossicular bone grafts (Fig. 23.8), and cortical bone is a useful and viable alternative for ossiculoplasty.

Homologous human ossicles are also well tolerated histologically. Creeping substitution occurs less rapidly than with autologous ossicles. There are no overt features of immune-mediated rejection. Ossicle grafts made of *cartilage* often develop chondromalacia with loss of stiffness and a tendency to become resorbed over time. Hence, cartilage grafts are not optimal for ossicular reconstruction, although they are probably adequate as a buffer between prosthesis and the tympanic membrane.

A variety of *synthetic ossicular implants* are currently available. Those made of porous high-density polyethylene (Plastipore) have been shown to elicit an intense foreign-

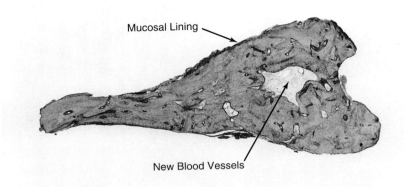

FIG. 23.6 Incus autograft implanted for 1 year. The graft has maintained its shape and is covered by middle ear mucosa. There are no areas of active bone resorption or exuberant new bone formation. New blood vessels are evident in the core of the implant (42X).

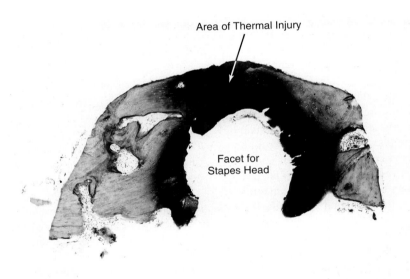

FIG. 23.7 Incus autograft implanted for 1 year, 7 months. There is intense basophilic staining of the area where a bur had been used to create a facet for the stapes head. This presumably resulted from thermal injury. In an adjacent section (not shown), this necrotic bone had undergone full-thickness resorption and replacement by fibrous tissue (45X).

body giant cell reaction that becomes well established within a few weeks and probably continues for the duration of the implant. Microdegradation of the plastic material occurs and appears to increase with time, eventually leading to implant failure in many cases (Fig. 23.9). More recently, many other synthetic materials have been used for ossiculoplasty, including bioactive glasses (Bioglass, Ceravital), aluminum oxide ceramic, carbon, hydroxylapatite, gold, titanium, hydroxylapatite-polyethylene (Hapex), and others.

The histological fate of these other synthetic materials in the human middle ear needs further study. Although these materials may work well in an animal model, results in an animal model cannot always be extrapolated to humans because of species differences and many unique human factors such as chronic inflammation and eustachian tube dysfunction. The extrusion rate of synthetic implants is significantly higher than for autologous tissues. Placement of a cartilage buffer between a synthetic prosthesis and the tympanic membrane

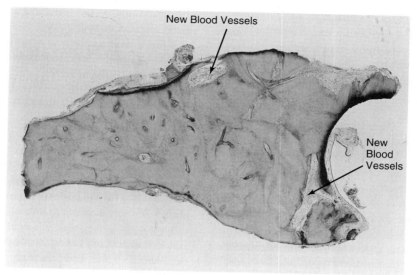

FIG. 23.8 Autograft cortical bone strut in place for 7 months. Its structure is intact without active resorption or new bone formation. Revascularization is evident at its periphery. Areas of thermal injury from the bur are seen on the surface as basophilic staining (31X).

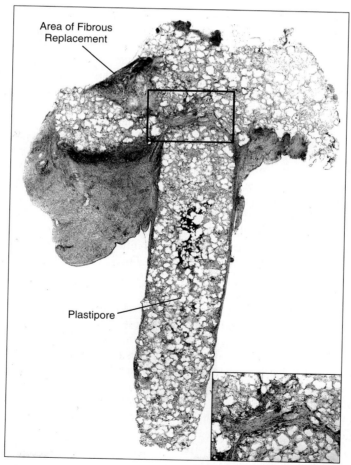

FIG. 23.9 TORP in place for 4 years, 4 months. The porous spaces of the implant have been extensively invaded by fibroblasts, plasma cells, macrophages, and foreign-body giant cells. There has been partial resorption of the platform of the TORP with replacement by fibrous tissue (27X). Inset shows a higher power view of outlined area demonstrating the foreign-body giant cell response within the TORP (150X).

has decreased the rate of extrusion, although it has not eliminated the problem. Long-term studies examining biocompatibility, extrusion potential, and functional results are needed before one can determine the place of synthetic implants in otologic surgery.

SELECTION OF CASES

Tympanoplasty should be considered when there is a conductive hearing loss of 30 dB or greater in an ear with COM that has good cochlear function. Tympanoplasty is contraindicated in a dead ear or in an ear with poor cochlear function. Tympanoplasty is not advisable in an ear with fibrocystic sclerosis because of high propensity for postoperative nonaeration of the middle ear and recurrent fibrosis. Similarly, epidermization is a contraindication because of the risks of nonaeration, prosthesis extrusion, and iatrogenic cholesteatoma.

Tympanoplasty carries a small risk of inducing a sensorineural hearing loss. Therefore it is important that cochlear function in the contralateral ear be at an adequate level, and an only hearing ear or much better hearing ear is a contraindication for tympanoplasty.

Children younger than 5 years are poor candidates for tympanoplasty because of risk of subsequent failure from otitis media and poor eustachian tube function. For the elderly, and for adults with serious medical problems, one has to determine whether the benefits of surgery outweigh the risks of anesthesia.

It is important to determine whether the COM in the ear under consideration is active or inactive (Chapter 17). *Active COM with cholesteatoma* necessitates surgical treatment to remove cholesteatoma (mastoidectomy or atticotomy) in conjunction with tympanoplasty. *Active COM without cholesteatoma* should be treated medically to control infection and eliminate otorrhea, thus converting the process to inactive COM. Expectant observation for 6 months is recommended, and if the ear remains dry, then elective tympanoplasty may be performed. Failure of medical management in active COM without cholesteatoma generally indicates the need for combining mastoidectomy with tympanoplasty. Ears that drain intermittently and do not have cholesteatoma (*inactive COM with frequent reactivation*) need attention to obvious inciting events such as water exposure to control otorrhea. If there are no obvious predisposing events, then mastoidectomy is recommended in conjunction with tympanoplasty to eliminate infection and granulation in the mastoid tracts, antrum, and epitympanum.

In patients with bilateral COM, determining which ear to operate on first depends on the type of COM and the severity of conductive hearing loss. In general, the ear with more active disease should be chosen first. With bilateral inactive disease, the poorer hearing ear should be operated on first, similar to the selection process for patients with otosclerosis. An exception to this rule may involve patients with bilateral air-bone gaps with a small difference in the hearing level between the two ears and a better chance for hearing gain in the better hearing ear.

Patients with a history of multiple failed tympanoplasties are likely to have insurmountable hurdles, including nonfunctioning eustachian tubes, middle ear fibrosis, tendency for failures of tympanic membrane grafts, and extrusion of prostheses. In such patients, the goal of chronic ear surgery should be to make the ear safe and dry, and hearing improvement should be achieved by amplification rather than by additional tympanoplasty surgery.

It is sometimes difficult to assess whether tympanoplasty surgery will result in a hearing gain that will be subjectively perceived by the patient to be an improvement in hearing ability. Overall, hearing includes the ability to detect speech in both quiet and in noise, as well as the ability to localize sound. The hearing benefit perceived by a given patient after tympanoplasty depends not only on the magnitude of improvement in air-bone gap but also on the level of cochlear function in the operated ear, the hearing level in the contralateral ear, the symmetry of hearing levels between the two ears, the level of central auditory processing, and the patient's lifestyle (11). For example, a patient with a bilateral 50-dB conductive hearing loss who undergoes a successful tympanoplasty in one ear is likely to report more benefit than a patient with a unilateral 50-dB conductive loss who also undergoes a successful tympanoplasty, although in technical terms both operations were equally successful. Patients may express disappointment that their hearing has not improved as much as they had expected. The following initial conditions seem most likely to result in patients being dissatisfied with their hearing improvement: (i) excellent hearing in one ear and a moderate-to-severe mixed type hearing loss in the surgical ear, (ii) longstanding unilateral loss, (iii) a postoperative hearing level that still requires a hearing aid in spite of successful surgery, and (iv) a conductive hearing loss as shown by audiometry but with a positive Rinne test at 256 Hz and 512 Hz (12). Patients with these conditions should not necessarily be excluded from surgical treatment, but the degree of expected improvement must be fully discussed with them to ensure that they have a realistic expectation of what can be achieved.

It must be emphasized that the surgical decision making for tympanoplasty in a patient with COM must be individualized. As discussed earlier, several factors should be considered, including hearing levels in the diseased and contralateral ear, pathology and activity of COM, age, and the general health and medical condition of the patient. These factors must be modified by the experience and talent of the otologic surgeon.

PREOPERATIVE EVALUATION

An otologic history, examination, and audiometric evaluation are done to determine if tympanoplasty surgery is indicated. The clinician must proceed in a logical manner and must quantify the conductive hearing loss, assess cochlear reserve, gain some insight into the probable ossicular pathology, assess the activity of COM, assess eustachian tube function, assess the contralateral ear, and eliminate potential contraindications. Having decided to proceed with surgery, the surgeon should formulate a preoperative plan, including the type of anesthesia, surgical approach, and type of tympanoplasty. The plan should be flexible to allow for intraoperative revision and modification as necessary.

A history of otorrhea in a patient without cholesteatoma warrants further attention to determine its etiology. As discussed in Chapter 17, medical management may convert the process to inactive COM, and if the ear remains dry for several months, elective tympanoplasty can be considered. Recurrent otorrhea can sometimes be secondary to lack of water precautions or secondary to hearing aid usage, which produces a moist environment. Persistent or recurrent otorrhea despite attention to these factors usually signifies the need for mastoid exploration in addition to tympanoplasty.

Careful otoscopic evaluation using the monocular 6X otoscope or binocular otomicroscope can provide a wealth of useful information to the trained eye. The size and shape of a perforation should be noted, which in conjunction with the extent of anterior canal wall convexity will help to determine the surgical approach. Areas of the tympanic membrane that are dimeric or atrophic may necrose after elevation of a tympanomeatal flap and should be reinforced by grafting. The presence of chronic middle ear effusion, fibrocystic sclerosis of the middle ear, and epidermization are all indicative of eustachian tube dysfunction and constitute contraindications to tympanoplasty. A retraction pocket of the pars flaccida or tensa with retention of keratin debris signifies a cholesteatoma. Signs of infection may be obvious, such as pooling of pus in the middle ear, or subtle, such as minute granulations at the margins of a perforation or an inflamed and edematous middle ear mucosa.

One should assess the integrity of the ossicular chain. Mobility of the malleus can be evaluated by pressure otoscopy if the tympanic membrane is intact or by gentle instrumental manipulation if the drum is perforated. A perforation may allow for inspection of the incus and stapes. Common areas of resorptive osteitis are the long process of the incus and the stapes crura. Chalky white tympanosclerotic plaques around the oval window may signify fixation of the footplate, in which case a second stage stapedectomy may be necessary. If the stapes is visible through a perforation, its mobility may be assessed by observing the superstructure and stapes tendon using otomicroscopy while eliciting the crossed stapedial reflex using a Barany noise box to stimulate the contralateral ear.

A functioning eustachian tube is critical to the success of tympanoplasty surgery; however, tests of eustachian tube function that can be used preoperatively as a reliable predictor of surgical success do not exist (13,14). Autoinflation of the ear by the Valsalva maneuver can be of diagnostic value in some patients. It may help to determine the extent of retraction and mobility of the tympanic membrane or a retraction pocket. In the presence of a perforation, simultaneous autoinflation and auscultation can demonstrate the anatomic patency of the tube. However, forced inflation is unphysiologic and is therefore not a valid test of eustachian tube function. Indirect indicators for poor eustachian tube function include bilateral chronic otitis media, chronic serous otitis media in the contralateral ear, uncontrolled rhinosinusitis, cleft palate, and other skull base anomalies.

A careful review of the audiometric profile in conjunction with otoscopy can often help the clinician to anticipate ossicular chain pathology, which in turn can help in preoperative planning and patient counseling. Perforations of the tympanic membrane result in a predominantly low frequency air-bone gap that is roughly proportional to the size of the perforation. A subtotal or total perforation results in a conductive loss of approximately 40 to 50 dB. An air-bone gap that is disproportionately large for the size of a perforation should suggest ossicular discontinuity or fixation. The paper patch test maneuver can be used to predict the probable hearing level that can be achieved by closure of a tympanic membrane perforation. A piece of cigarette paper or Gelfilm coated with ointment is placed over the perforation, and the hearing is assessed before and after application of the patch. Lack of hearing improvement after placing the patch suggests an additional ossicular lesion such as fixation or discontinuity.

Ossicular discontinuity in the presence of an intact tympanic membrane results in a relatively flat 60-dB conductive hearing loss. Ossicular discontinuity with a tympanic membrane perforation gives a somewhat smaller conductive loss of approximately 40 to 50 dB. Resorption of the incudostapedial joint and replacement by a fibrous band often results in a fluctuating conductive hearing loss with better hearing thresholds when the ear is autoinflated. (Lateral displacement of the tympanic membrane and incus by autoinflation causes the fibrous band to become taut, improving sound transmission.) Such ears also tend to demonstrate an air-bone gap that is somewhat greater for higher frequencies than for the lower frequencies. A conductive hearing loss in a patient with an intact, healthy tympanic membrane and an aerated middle ear usually indicates ossicular fixation. Stapes fixation because of tympanosclerosis or otosclerosis can result in a conductive hearing loss up to 50 dB. In contrast, isolated fixation of the malleus head rarely results in an air-bone gap greater than 15 to 25 dB.

SURGICAL TECHNIQUES

This section focuses on details of the various tympanoplasty procedures with and without ossicular linkage. The reader is referred to other chapters for details regarding incisions and approaches (Chapter 9), skin grafting (Chapter 10), canaloplasty (Chapter 13), and mastoidectomy (Chapter 17).

Type I Tympanoplasty

Type I tympanoplasty involves replacement of part or all of the tympanic membrane with a tissue graft, usually temporalis fascia, perichondrium, or earlobe adipose tissue. The procedure is indicated when there is a perforation or retraction of the tympanic membrane but the ossicular chain is intact and mobile. Type I tympanoplasty may be elective or performed in conjunction with a mastoidectomy. Details of tympanic membrane repair are described in Chapters 14 and 15.

Type II Tympanoplasty

In type II tympanoplasty, the tympanic membrane and ossicular chain are repaired such that the lever mechanism, which is a normal function of the malleus and incus, is restored (Fig. 23.10). In practice, this procedure is performed for osteitic resorption of the lenticular process or capitulum of the stapes. Often, the area of resorption is replaced by a fibrous band. The fibrous band should be first removed with scissors or a laser. Continuity of the ossicular chain can be restored in one of several ways, including a bone strut, a synthetic prosthesis, or otologic cement. If there is any doubt about the stability or adequacy of mechanical coupling of the reconstruction, the surgeon should remove the incus and convert to a type III, minor columella tympanoplasty.

Type III Tympanoplasty

Stapes Columella

A stapes columella reconstruction involves placing the tympanic graft or tympanic membrane directly on the capitulum of the stapes (Fig. 23.11). The procedure is usually done in association with canal wall–down mastoidectomy for active COM. The posterior bony canal wall should be removed to the level of the facial nerve. The new tympanic cavity (cavum major) is limited superiorly by the tensor tympani semicanal and tympanic segment of the facial nerve and posteriorly by the mastoid segment of the facial nerve. The mastoid cavity and epitympanum are usually obliterated with pedicled or free muscle-fascial grafts supplemented with bone paté, and all raw surfaces are skin grafted. A crescent of Teflon or Silastic is often placed in the tympanic cavity to prevent adhesions of the tympanic graft to the medial wall of the middle ear and to facilitate epithelialization of the tympanic cavity.

Minor Columella

A minor columella is suitable for reconstructing an ear with an intact posterior canal wall and mobile stapes superstructure (Fig. 23.12). A minor columella may be the only procedure, as in an elective tympanoplasty for inactive COM, or may be combined with a canal wall–up mastoidectomy for active COM. As discussed earlier, autologous ossicles are preferred as reconstructive material. The incus can be removed by first dislocating it with a right-angle hook, followed by grasping the long process and removing the body from the epitympanum with a twisting rotatory motion. The malleus head can also serve as a source of autologous material and is removed after first transecting the neck with a guillotine-like nipper.

The unsculptured ossicle graft should be placed into the middle ear and a decision made as to the size, position, and

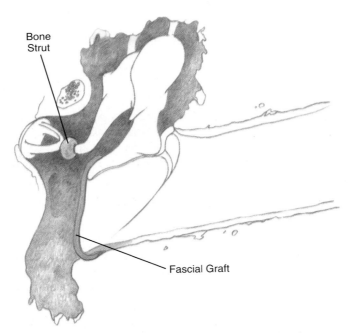

Bone Strut

Fascial Graft

FIG. 23.10 Type II tympanoplasty. This sketch shows a small bone strut interposed between the long process of incus and stapes in association with a medial onlay fascial graft repair of a tympanic membrane perforation. Type II tympanoplasty implies reestablishing the lever mechanism of the sound transmission system.

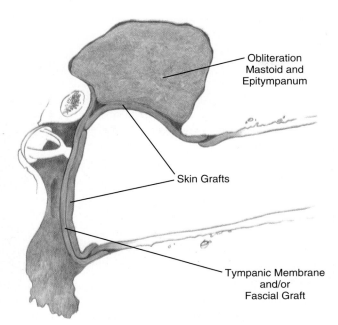

FIG. 23.11 Type III tympanoplasty, stapes columella. This sketch is representative of the canal wall–down type III tympanoplasty. The fascial graft bridges the middle ear and is placed in direct contact with the stapes head. The epitympanum and mastoid cavity are obliterated with pedicled or free muscle-fascial grafts supplemented with bone paté, and all unepithelialized surfaces are skin grafted.

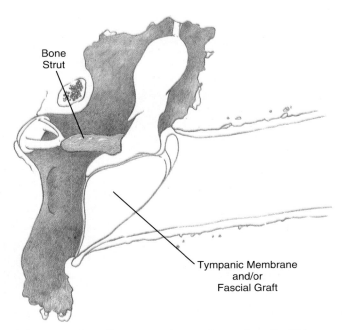

FIG. 23.12 Type III tympanoplasty, minor columella. This approach is commonly used in canal wall–up procedures and consists of interposing a sculptured bone strut (or PORP) between the stapes head and the manubrium or tympanic membrane.

shape of the strut for sculpturing. The graft is then removed and sculpted to suitable dimensions under an operating microscope using small burs and liberal saline irrigation to avoid thermal injury. A facet is drilled into the graft to accommodate the stapes capitulum, and a groove is created on the opposite side to accept the manubrium (Fig. 23.13A). The use of measuring sticks facilitates precise shaping so that the strut fits snugly between the stapes head and the manubrium. Ideally, the graft should lock into place and be held in position without the aid of Gelfoam. If the manubrium is missing or too far anterior for a stable assembly, then the strut is brought from the stapes head to the tympanic graft or tympanic membrane (Fig. 23.13B). The graft should be sufficiently long to produce a slight bulge in the tympanic membrane but not too close to the bony tympanic annulus to risk subsequent fixation. Gelfoam may be placed around it for stabilization. After sculpturing the minor columella to suitable dimensions, the tympanic membrane is grafted, if necessary. The tympanomeatal flap, including the tympanic graft, is then raised once again, the sculpted ossicle graft is placed in the middle ear, and the tympanomeatal flap is put back onto the canal wall. Alternative materials for minor columella reconstruction include cortical bone struts, homograft ossicles, and a variety of synthetic PORPs. A buffer of cartilage is often interposed between a PORP and the tympanic membrane to decrease the potential for extrusion.

If the manubrium has been medially retracted by unopposed pull of the tensor tympani muscle, the tensor tendon is cut and the manubrium is elevated with gentle pressure to lateralize it. Even if the manubrium is excluded from the direct sound-conducting system, retaining the manubrium helps to maintain the shape of the tympanic membrane that might otherwise collapse.

Major Columella

A major columella is interposed between the stapes footplate and tympanic membrane or manubrium in cases where the stapes crura are missing and the footplate is intact and mobile (Fig. 23.14). A major columella reconstruction can be combined with a canal wall–up or canal wall–down mastoidectomy. An ossicular or cortical bone strut has a risk of delayed ankylosis of the strut to the fallopian canal or promontory, and better results may be achieved with an inert synthetic material (i.e., a TORP).

Careful manipulation and sizing is critical to prevent excessive pressure and cracking of the footplate. Ideally, the TORP should be placed at the center of the footplate and made to couple to the manubrium. Proper length is important such that the TORP locks in place with just enough tension between the manubrium and the footplate to provide proper sound transmission, as well as mechanical stability to hold it in place without the use of Gelfoam. If the manubrium is ab-

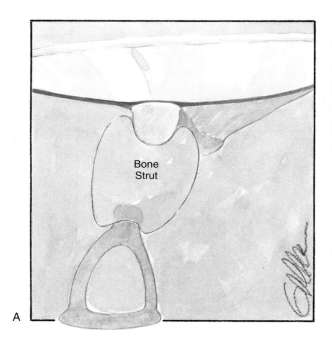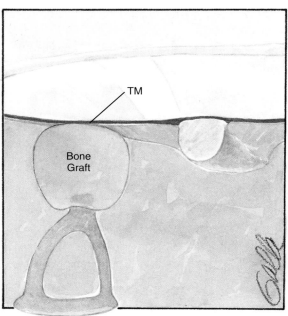

A   B

FIG. 23.13 Type III tympanoplasty, minor columella. **A:** The anatomic relationships are favorable for interpositioning the bone strut between the stapes capitulum and the manubrium. **B:** The manubrium is too far anterior for a stable assembly between the stapes head and the manubrium. Hence, the bone strut is brought from the stapes head to the tympanic membrane or fascial graft. The columella graft should be sufficiently long to produce a slight bulge at the tympanic membrane but not too close to the bony tympanic annulus to risk subsequent fixation. TM, tympanic membrane.

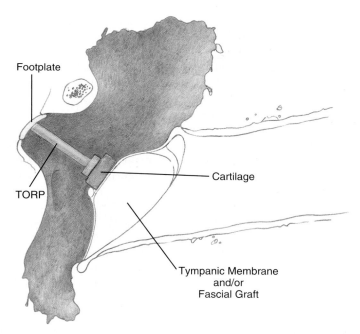

FIG. 23.14 Type III tympanoplasty, major columella. A major columella implies bridging the space from the footplate to the tympanic membrane, fascial graft, or manubrium. TORPs are available in several types of alloplastic material and are generally preferable to bone struts, which have a tendency to ankylose to the walls of the oval window niche. A cartilage buffer is placed between the TORP and tympanic membrane, fascial graft, or manubrium.

sent or in an anatomically unfavorable situation, the TORP should be brought to the tympanic graft or tympanic membrane and surrounded by Gelfoam to stabilize it. It is important to shorten the length of the TORP to prevent it from tenting the tympanic membrane, especially in a canal wall–down mastoid cavity. Tenting of the drum or tympanic graft by the TORP often leads to extrusion. Placement of a cartilage buffer cap between the TORP and the tympanic graft is also used to decrease the chance of extrusion.

Type IV Tympanoplasty

The type IV procedure is suitable when there is a canal wall–down mastoidectomy and the tympanic membrane, malleus, incus, and stapes superstructure are missing, but the footplate is mobile (Figs. 23.15 and 23.16). The principles of a type IV tympanoplasty are to exteriorize the footplate, acoustically separate the oval window from the round window, and shield the round window with a sufficiently stiff tissue graft. The type IV procedure is a simple yet robust alternative to using a TORP in that it avoids problems of TORP extrusion, rejection, and displacement, and the results of a type IV are no worse than those of TORPs.

Mucosa around the oval window niche is removed and bone is exposed to allow the tissue graft to adhere to the margins of the oval window niche (Fig. 23.16A). A small piece of temporalis fascia is placed in the sinus tympani between the two windows to help in acoustically isolating the round window from the oval window. The round window is then acoustically shielded by a crescent-shaped piece of tragal or meatal cartilage (or a piece of 1-mm thick Silastic) (Fig. 23.16B). A large piece of temporalis fascia is then placed superficial to the cartilage graft, and a U-shaped aperture is cut in the fascia to keep the oval window niche exposed (Fig. 23.16C). The footplate is covered by a very thin, split-thickness skin graft that is invaginated into the oval window niche (Fig. 23.16D). The skin graft must overlap the fascia graft anteriorly and inferiorly. The skin is maintained in proper position by a small cotton plug soaked in saline or antibiotic solution that will remain in place for at least 3 weeks under the deep packing.

When the oval window niche is too narrow or too deep for skin survival or the footplate is fixed, a type V tympanoplasty can be contemplated as a second stage procedure after complete healing has occurred. In anticipation of this later, staged procedure, the oval window niche is filled with an adipose tissue plug. Adipose tissue has the tendency to preserve its structure and to inhibit formation of adhesions and fibrous tissue.

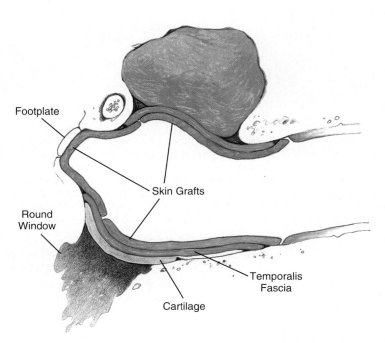

FIG. 23.15 Type IV tympanoplasty. This procedure requires a canal wall–down tympanomastoidectomy. The sketch shows a fascial graft reinforced with a piece of cartilage bridging the hypotympanum to create a cavum minor that is aerated by the eustachian tube. The graft acoustically insulates the round window membrane from the external auditory canal. A thin, split-thickness skin graft lines the oval window niche. The epitympanum and mastoid cavity have been obliterated with pedicled or free muscle-fascial grafts supplemented with bone paté. All unepithelialized surfaces are skin grafted.

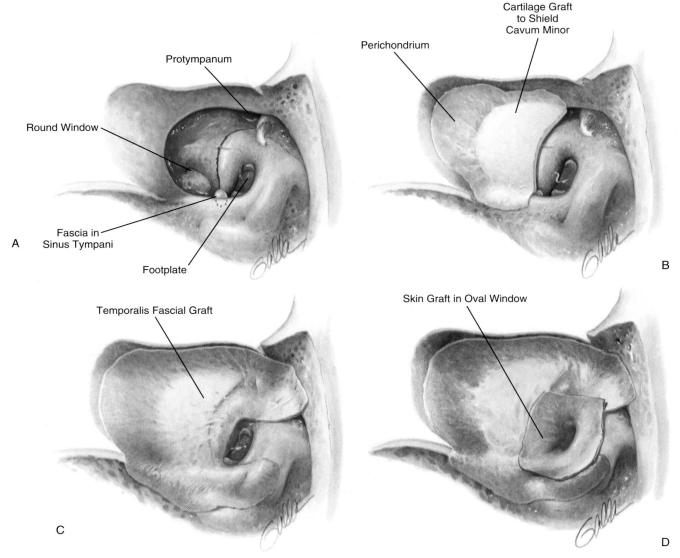

FIG. 23.16 Type IV tympanoplasty. **A:** Mucosa around the oval window niche has been removed, and a small piece of fascia is placed in the sinus tympani between the two windows. **B:** The round window is acoustically shielded by a crescent-shaped piece of cartilage, whose perichondrium is reflected and placed onto the canal wall for stabilization of the cartilage. **C:** A piece of temporalis fascia is placed superficial to the cartilage graft, and a U-shaped aperture is cut in the fascia to expose the oval window niche. **D:** The footplate is covered by a very thin, split-thickness skin graft invaginated into the oval window niche and held in place by a small cotton ball. The skin graft must overlap the fascia graft.

Type Vb Tympanoplasty

Type Vb tympanoplasty can be performed under certain conditions as a second stage procedure after canal wall–down type III or IV tympanomastoidectomy (Fig. 23.17). The conditions are: (i) a clean, dry tympanomastoid cavity with no evidence of infection or recurrent disease; (ii) an aerated cavum minor with the round window membrane acoustically isolated from the footplate and ear canal by a healthy, intact tissue graft; (iii) an air-bone gap greater than 35 dB; and (iv) a fixed footplate.

A flap is elevated to expose the footplate, a stapedectomy is performed to remove the fixed footplate, the oval window niche is filled with an adipose graft, and the overlying flap is thinned or replaced with a split-thickness skin graft to cover the adipose tissue. In general, hearing results after type V procedures are superior to those after type IV tympanoplasty (7).

Surgical Packing

In canal wall–down mastoidectomy combined with type III or IV tympanoplasty, the mastoid cavity is obliterated with pedicled or free muscle-fascial grafts or bone paté and covered with a pedicled flap of mastoid periosteum or a piece of temporalis fascia. The skin of the posterior canal wall is

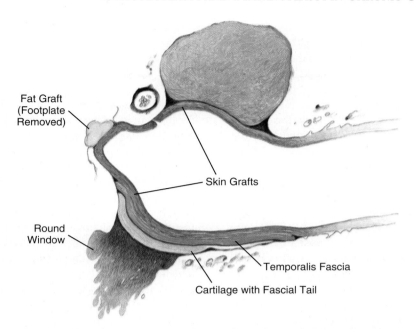

Fat Graft
(Footplate
Removed)

Skin Grafts

Round
Window

Temporalis Fascia

Cartilage with Fascial Tail

FIG. 23.17 Type Vb tympanoplasty. This procedure implies a two-stage approach. In the first stage, a type IV tympanoplasty is performed. If a fixed footplate is identified at this time, a second stage may be contemplated after complete healing and a dry ear with an aerated cavum minor has been achieved. In the second stage, a skin flap is elevated, the footplate is removed, an adipose tissue graft is placed in the oval window, and the skin flap is replaced.

prepared as a laterally based pedicled (Koerner) flap and placed on the anterior surface of the grafts used for mastoid obliteration. Split-thickness skin grafts are used to cover all remaining unepithelialized surfaces. The packing (rosebud dressing) consists of strips of silk or rayon cloth placed on all surfaces in the form of a rosette filled with cotton soaked in saline or antibiotic solution. The distal ends of the silk strips are folded over the cotton to avoid any contact between the cotton and the tissues. The external auditory canal is then packed with gauze and antibiotic ointment. The wound is closed in one or two layers, and a rubber drain is left in place in the infraauricular area for 24 hours.

In elective tympanoplasty or in tympanoplasty combined with canal wall–up mastoidectomy, the unepithelialized surfaces of the ear canal and tympanic graft are covered with skin grafts and held in place with a rosebud dressing. The incision is closed in layers, and the external auditory canal is packed with gauze and antibiotic ointment.

SPECIAL CONSIDERATIONS

Tympanosclerosis Involving the Tympanic Membrane and Ossicles

The chalky, white, avascular deposits of tympanosclerosis generally occur only in ears with healed, inactive COM (8). Small areas of tympanosclerosis within the pars tensa do not impede sound transmission and can, in fact, be used to the

surgeon's advantage because they impart mechanical strength to the tympanic membrane, preventing its retraction in the face of chronic negative middle ear static pressure. However, a large plaque of tympanosclerosis extending to the annulus or the manubrium, especially in the anterior-superior quadrant, can immobilize the tympanic membrane and malleus, in which case the plaque has to be removed. This maneuver may result in a perforation, which then needs to be repaired with temporalis fascia or similar graft.

When tympanosclerosis causes fixation of the ossicles, simple mobilization of ossicles will generally fail to provide long-term hearing improvement. The point or points of ossicular fixation should be determined by gentle manipulation of the individual ossicles. Common areas of fixation are the epitympanum and stapes footplate. Epitympanic fixation is managed by removing the incus, nipping the head of the malleus, and using the incus or malleus head as a minor columellar strut. The nipped head of the malleus should be removed or distracted from the manubrium to prevent refixation of the cut ends.

Tympanosclerotic fixation of the stapes crura or footplate can be managed in some cases by removing the plaques layer by layer, and good long-term mobility can be achieved. Extensive tympanosclerosis involving the oval window requires either a stapedectomy or a retreat from surgery. The risk of sensorineural hearing loss from mobilization or stapedectomy has been reported to vary from 0% to 10%, and the variation in risk is most easily explained on a technical basis, related to the type of procedure and to surgical skill (15). If a decision is made to proceed with stapedectomy, the following guidelines should be followed.

In the presence of a tympanic membrane perforation or active tympanomastoid disease, a two-stage procedure is mandatory. The first stage consists of repair of the tympanic membrane and elimination of suppuration. The second stage, which includes the stapedectomy, is performed several months later, provided the ear is stable and free from disease and the tympanic cavity is well aerated. In an ear with an intact canal wall the following procedures are indicated: (i) If the malleus and incus are both mobile, a conventional stapedectomy is performed. (ii) If the malleus and/or incus are fixed in the epitympanum, the incus is removed, the malleus head is nipped, a stapedotomy or stapedectomy is done, and a malleus–to–oval window prosthesis is introduced. Details are described in Chapter 22. Alternatively, a stapedectomy with a TORP resting on a fascial graft, as described later, can be done. (iii) If the manubrium is missing or anatomically unfavorable (for a malleus–to–oval window prosthesis), then the stapes is removed and a TORP is placed on a temporalis fascia or perichondrial graft that invaginates into the oval window niche and overlaps all margins by 2 to 3 mm (Fig. 23.18). Thus the shaft of the TORP is firmly wedged into the niche and will not enter the vestibule. A cartilage cap is placed on the umbrella end of the TORP, which is brought to the level of the tympanic membrane graft. In cases with a canal wall–down mastoidectomy and an anky-

losed stapes footplate, it is best to convert to a type Vb tympanoplasty at a second stage, as described earlier.

Staging

Staging the operation in tympanoplasty can be considered for the following three different indications: (i) A two-stage procedure is almost always indicated when the stapes is fixed, as discussed in the previous section. (ii) A planned second stage procedure is also performed when there is a high risk of residual cholesteatoma; for example, after an intact canal wall procedure. (iii) A two-stage operation has also been advocated in patients with extensive mucous membrane destruction of the tympanic cavity (16). The first stage consists of eliminating disease, sealing the middle ear with a tissue graft, and placing plastic sheeting over the denuded middle ear. The objective of the first stage is to obtain a well-healed ear with a mucosa-lined, aerated middle ear cleft so that ossicular reconstruction may be performed later at the second stage under ideal circumstances. Considerable difference of opinion exists among experienced otologists in regard to staging for this particular indication (16). The philosophy at the Massachusetts Eye and Ear Infirmary is to try to do the entire procedure in one stage. Every effort is made to eliminate disease and maximize hearing results at the first operation. Should the hearing results be unsatisfactory and if the postoperative status regarding the aeration of the middle

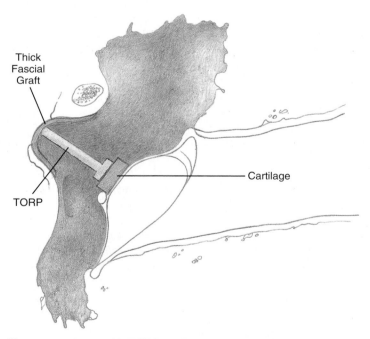

FIG. 23.18 Type III tympanoplasty with TORP and stapedectomy. This procedure implies a two-stage approach. The first stage consists of repair of a tympanic membrane perforation and a canal wall–up mastoidectomy, if necessary. The second stage may be contemplated after complete healing and a dry ear with an aerated tympanic cavity. In the second stage, a tympanomeatal flap is elevated, a stapedectomy is performed, a fascia or perichondrial graft is used to seal the oval window, and a TORP is placed from the oval window to the tympanic membrane or manubrium. A cartilage buffer is placed between the TORP and the tympanic membrane, fascial graft, or manubrium.

ear and control of suppuration is satisfactory, a revision operation for hearing can be done. In many cases, revisions are not necessary and therefore the staging procedure is avoided. Even total drum replacement and a major columella ossiculoplasty in combination with a mastoidectomy, although major technical accomplishments, are successful often enough to challenge the wisdom of planned staging.

POSTOPERATIVE CARE

Prophylactic antibiotic coverage is usually given during surgery and continued for 7 to 10 days postoperatively. The patient is usually discharged from the hospital on the day of surgery or the following morning. The rosebud packing is removed 2 weeks later. Further treatment consists of cleaning and removing debris and applying antiseptic or antibiotic drops until complete healing and epithelialization has taken place. Follow-up visits every 6 months are advisable for early detection and prevention of skin infection, crusting, recurrent disease, or prosthesis extrusion.

COMPLICATIONS

Intraoperative

The reported risk of partial or total sensorineural hearing loss after tympanoplasty ranges from 1% to 5% (17–19). Sensorineural hearing loss can be induced by avulsion or subluxation of the stapes footplate, laceration of the round window membrane, or acoustic trauma due to instrumentation of the ossicles. Manipulation of the stapes footplate should be done gently and with care. The use of a laser to remove disease on or around the footplate may help to minimize iatrogenic trauma to the stapes. In the event of stapes subluxation or dislocation, removal of the footplate and immediate closure with fascia or earlobe adipose tissue decreases the risk of labyrinthitis and loss of cochleovestibular function. High-dose corticosteroids should also be administered parenterally in addition to antibiotics to diminish the risk of sensorineural hearing loss.

Lesions of the facial nerve occur most often at the level of the oval window. Abnormal dehiscence of the nerve can be expected in up to 25% of cases with COM. Avoidance of aggressive manipulations or dissection in the oval window niche area is therefore important. It might be safer to leave residual disease and abstain from trying to improve hearing than to risk a facial palsy.

Postoperative

Frank hematomas of the mastoid or temporal areas are rare, but when they occur, they should be evacuated promptly. An infrequent complication is the development of severe vertigo and sensorineural hearing loss. This situation, which may indicate displacement of a strut medially into the vestibule, warrants immediate exploration. Immediate postoperative

facial palsy generally requires prompt reexploration, as discussed in Chapter 17.

Stenosis of the external auditory canal or meatus caused by excessive scarring can occur during the first postoperative weeks or months. This is often preceded by the formation of granulation tissue, and the risk of stenosis is higher in children than adults. Careful and periodic postoperative follow-up at 2- to 3-week intervals after removal of the rosebud packing can often alert the clinician to the development of granulation tissue, which should be removed and cauterized. If exuberant or recurrent granulation persists, a delayed split-thickness skin graft will usually avoid the occurrence of meatal or canal stenosis.

In cases of partial tympanic graft necrosis with recurring perforation, the application of antibiotic ointment can sometimes induce scar formation and spontaneous closure. A persistent small perforation can sometimes be also closed by adding a graft of earlobe adipose tissue as an outpatient procedure (20).

RESULTS

Tympanomastoid surgery is quite successful in controlling infection and preventing recurrent disease, with success rates in excess of 80% to 90% (21,22). Postoperative hearing results vary widely, depending on the extent of tympanic membrane and ossicular lesions, mucosal disease, cholesteatoma, and eustachian tube function. Patients with inactive COM undergoing type I tympanoplasty have a greater than 90% chance for complete graft take and an 85% to 90% chance for an air-bone gap 20 dB or less (21,23). Hearing results are less satisfactory with advanced lesions of the ossicular chain, extensive mucosal disease, atelectatic ears, and poor eustachian tube function. When the ossicular chain has to be reconstructed (types II to V tympanoplasty), long-term closure of the air-bone gap to less than 20 dB occurs in 40% to 70% of cases in which the stapes is intact and in only 20% to 55% in which the stapes superstructure is missing (21–28).

FACTORS INFLUENCING OUTCOME OF TYMPANOPLASTY

Tympanoplasty surgery is unique compared with surgery elsewhere in the body because of the constraints imposed by a combination of factors, including the pathology of COM, the vagaries of wound healing, and the need for a functioning tympanoossicular system. Otologists routinely place tympanic membrane and ossicular grafts in a recipient middle ear milieu that is hostile as a result of active or arrested inflammatory disease. Tympanic membrane grafts have to be in contact with air over a relatively large portion of their surface areas and must derive nourishment and blood supply from small parts of the graft in contact with the canal wall. Ossicular grafts and prostheses must couple well at their ends to bone or soft tissue but must remain suspended in air elsewhere to transmit sound effectively. Functional success after tympanoplasty is determined in part by the surgeon's technical skill. Other factors also play a significant role, including the mechanics and acoustics of the reconstruction and the biology and pathology of chronic ear disease. An understanding of these factors can provide insight into some of the reasons for failure of tympanoplasty and may pose challenges for future research.

Mechanics and Acoustics of the Middle Ear

Current techniques of tympanoplasty have generally evolved empirically as a result of trial and error. Otologic surgeons have a good general appreciation of various anatomic and pathologic reasons for failure of tympanoplasty, such as nonaeration of the middle ear, abnormalities of the reconstructed tympanic membrane, and inefficient sound transmission via the reconstructed ossicular chain. However, a quantitative understanding of the acoustic consequences of structural variations of a reconstructed ear is generally lacking. Clinical observations indicate that in many instances the anatomic differences between a good and poor hearing result are seemingly minor. For example, minor changes in prosthesis position on the order of 0.5 to 1.0 mm can have relatively large effects on hearing of up to 20 dB (29). In other words, small changes in structure have the capacity to have large effects on function.

Types I, II, and III Tympanoplasty

For types I, II, and III tympanoplasty, the final hearing results depend on three factors: the efficacy of the reconstructed tympanic membrane, the efficacy of the ossicular reconstruction, and the adequacy of middle ear aeration and its static pressure. The tympanic membrane is the major transducer of the middle ear. Motion of the normal tympanic membrane is complex (30): At frequencies below 1,000 Hz, the entire drum moves in phase but the magnitude of motion varies with location. At higher frequencies, different parts of the drum move with varying magnitudes and phases. Although clinical observations suggest that surgical techniques that tend to restore or preserve normal drum anatomy lead to a good hearing result, the acoustic and mechanical properties of reconstructed tympanic membranes are not well understood. Grafted tympanic membranes often lack the conical shape of the normal eardrum, and the thickness and other mechanical properties of reconstructed drums vary widely. How these various properties affect middle ear function remains to be determined.

The acoustic performance of an ossicular prosthesis depends on its *stiffness, position, tension, coupling,* and *mass* (7). The stiffness of most currently used prostheses is adequate. The angle between the stapes and a columellar strut should be 45 degrees or less for optimal sound transmission (31,32). Although it is ideal to attach an ossicular prosthesis to the manubrium, it appears that acceptable results can oc-

cur when the graft is placed against the posterior-superior quadrant of the tympanic membrane as long as 3 to 4 mm of the prosthesis's diameter contacts the eardrum. Tension and length are critical in determining hearing results. The mechanical impedance of biologic structures is inherently nonlinear; the tympanic membrane and annular ligament act as linear elements only over the range of small motions less than 10 μm, associated with physiologic sound levels. The larger displacements created by a prosthesis that is too long will produce stiffening of the annular ligament and tympanic membrane, resulting in excessive tension and hence a poor hearing result. Currently, an assessment of tension cannot be made intraoperatively in an objective fashion, and the otologic surgeon is guided only by his or her intuition; a reliable and objective method to assess tension would be quite useful to the otologic surgeon. *Coupling* refers to how well a prosthesis adheres to the footplate or tympanic membrane, and the degree of coupling will determine whether there is slippage in sound transmission at the end of a prosthesis. Thus a prosthesis will transmit sound effectively only if there is good coupling at both ends. Clinical observations indicate that it is rare to obtain a firm union between a prosthesis and the stapes footplate, and hence, inadequate coupling at the footplate-TORP joint may be a cause of a persistent postoperative air-bone gap. Theoretical and some experimental data indicate that an increase in ossicular mass (e.g., due to a heavy prosthesis) does not cause significant detriment in middle ear sound transmission (33,34).

In the stapes columella type III tympanoplasty (drum graft placed directly on stapes head), when the stapes is mobile and the middle ear is aerated, the average postoperative air-bone gap is 15 to 30 dB, suggesting that there is little middle ear sound pressure gain occurring through the reconstruction (35,36). Experimental and clinical investigations have shown that interposing a thin, flat disc of cartilage (0.3 to 0.5 mm thick and 4 to 6 mm diameter) between the graft and the stapes head improves hearing in such ears by 5 to10 dB (35,36). The cartilage appears to increase the "effective" vibratory area of the graft that is coupled to the stapes, resulting in an increase in the middle ear gain of the reconstructed ear.

A critical parameter for successful tympanoplasty is the presence of an aerated middle ear. Aeration allows the tympanic membrane, the ossicles, and the round window to move. Nonaerated ears have large 45- to 60-dB air-bone gaps (7). How much air is necessary behind a tympanic membrane (i.e., within the middle ear and mastoid)? Currently, available data suggest that reduction of middle ear and mastoid volume from the normal average volume of 6 ml to a volume of 0.4 ml will result in a less than 10-dB conductive hearing loss (34). Volumes smaller than 0.4 ml will lead to progressively larger air-bone gaps, whereas volumes greater than 1.0 ml do not provide additional acoustic benefit. Negative static air pressure in the middle ear space that often occurs in COM has detrimental effects on the mechanics of the tympanic membrane, annular ligament, and suspensory ligaments of the ossicles. For example, a negative middle ear static pressure of –200 mm water is associated with a conductive hearing loss of up to 10 to 15 dB in the lower frequencies below 1,000 Hz (37).

Types IV and V Tympanoplasty

A quantitative model of the type IV procedure has been developed whose predictions match well with clinical results (7,38). The model allows one to explain postoperative hearing results in terms of structural properties of the reconstructed ear. Under optimal conditions of a mobile stapes footplate, an aerated round window niche (cavum minor), and a sufficiently stiff acoustic shield, the theoretically predicted and clinically observed postoperative air-bone gap is approximately 20 dB. Larger air-bone gaps are associated with fibrous or bony stapes fixation, poor aeration of the round window niche, or insufficient stiffness of the acoustic shield. A thin or atrophic tissue graft over the cavum minor may be insufficiently stiff to provide adequate shielding of the round window. The adequacy of such a shield can be determined in an office setting by audiometry before and after covering the shield with a thick layer of ointment. If the audiometric thresholds improve significantly with ointment, more permanent hearing gain may be achieved by surgically reinforcing the shield with a crescent-shaped piece of cartilage or Silastic 1 mm in thickness.

The type V tympanoplasty procedure can also be analyzed quantitatively using the same type IV model (7). Both predicted and observed type V results are superior to the average type IV result (7,39), which is probably related to the lower impedance of adipose tissue within the oval window as compared with the impedance of the normal footplate and annular ligament.

Canal Wall–Up versus Canal Wall–Down Mastoidectomy

From an acoustic and mechanical perspective, a canal wall–down mastoidectomy results in a significant reduction in the size of the residual middle ear air space. However, as long as this air space is greater than 0.4 ml, the acoustic effect of loss of sound transmission should be less than 10 dB, as noted earlier. Because the average volume of the tympanic cavity is 0.5 to 1.0 ml, a canal–wall down procedure should create no significant acoustic detriment, so long as the middle ear is aerated (40). A canal wall–down procedure also results in the creation of a large air space lateral to the tympanic membrane—that is, the air space within the mastoid bowl, including the external auditory canal. This mastoid bowl and ear canal air space generates resonances that can influence middle ear sound transmission favorably or unfavorably (41). The structure-function relationships between the size and shape of a given mastoid cavity and its resonances have not been well defined. An improved understanding of these relationships would help to develop guide-lines for an otologic surgeon to configure a mastoid cavity in ways that could be acoustically beneficial.

Biology and Pathology of Chronic Ear Disease

The biology and pathology of COM can have significant effects on posttympanoplasty hearing results. For example, postoperative mucosal fibrosis, neoosteogenesis, formation of adhesions, and development of negative static pressure in the middle ear can occur over the course of months or years, which in turn can have a detrimental effect on the hearing result. It is instructive to note that the few studies in the literature that assess long-term hearing results show a progressive and systematic decline in initial hearing gain as a function of time. For example, Colleti et al. (27) in a study of 832 ossiculoplasty procedures found that 77% of ears had an air-bone gap 20 dB or less at 6 months, but the same figure decreased to 42% at 5 years.

Proliferation of fibrous tissue and formation of adhesions are significant problems that are more prone to occur when the middle ear mucosa is diseased, removed, or traumatized. Many different materials have been placed in the middle ear in an attempt to prevent formation of adhesions and fibrous tissue. These materials include Gelfoam, hyaluronic acid, Silastic, and Teflon. Gelfoam elicits a host inflammatory response, leading to its resorption. In some cases, this inflammatory response results in adhesions, especially when the middle ear mucosa is deficient. Further, Gelfoam is resorbed within 2 weeks, which is probably insufficient time for mucosal regeneration to occur. Hyaluronic acid is somewhat more difficult to handle than Gelfoam and is also absorbed before mucosal regeneration is likely to be completed. Silastic and Teflon sheeting are relatively inert, but they are not resorbed and can sometimes extrude. On occasion, they become engulfed by fibrous tissue, leading to a nonaerated ear. Hence, none of the currently available spacer materials is ideal. What is needed is a material that will remain in place for several weeks to allow sufficient time for mucosal regeneration and will then undergo degradation and resorption so that the ear can become aerated without fibrosis.

Although rates of successful closure of tympanic membrane perforations are uniformly high, in excess of 90%, a small number of grafted tympanic membranes show undesirable pathologic changes, including proliferation of fibrous tissue and thickening, resorption and excessive thinning, and lack of epithelialization with resulting discharge. The factor or factors controlling such responses are not well understood at present. Histopathologic responses of the ear to various ossicular grafts and prostheses play an important role in determining outcome of tympanoplasty; these have been discussed previously.

Two significant causes for long-term failure of tympanoplasty are total or partial nonaeration of the middle ear and development of negative static pressure. Nonaeration of the middle ear is usually due to eustachian tube dysfunction and results in tympanic membrane graft atelectasis, middle ear effusion, fibrocystic sclerosis of the middle ear, or a combination of these changes. Some postoperative ears that are aerated have a tendency to develop negative static pressure in the middle ear. Over the long term, this negative pressure leads to retraction and atelectasis of the reconstructed tympanic membrane and functional compromise, as well as a predisposition to displacement or extrusion of ossicular prostheses. The negative pressure can also lead to recurrent cholesteatoma. The latter problem is a disadvantage for canal wall–up procedures relative to canal–wall down mastoidectomy.

REFERENCES

1. Sadé J, ed. Prologue. In: *Cholesteatoma and mastoid surgery.* Amsterdam: Kugler Publications, 1982:1–3.
2. Committee on Conservation of Hearing of the American Academy of Ophthalmology and Otolaryngology. Standard classification for surgery of chronic ear infection. *Arch Otolaryngol* 1965;81:204–205.
3. Ruben RJ. The disease in society-evaluation of chronic otitis media in general and cholesteatoma in particular. In: Sadé J, ed. *Cholesteatoma and mastoid surgery.* Amsterdam: Kugler Publications, 1982:111–116.
4. Wullstein H. The restoration of the function of the middle ear in chronic otitis media. *Ann Otol Rhinol Laryngol* 1956;65:1020–1041.
5. Zöllner F. The principles of plastic surgery of the sound-conducting apparatus. *J Laryngol Otol* 1955;69:637–652.
6. Gacek RR. Symposium on tympanoplasty. Results of modified type V tympanoplasty. *Laryngoscope* 1973;83:437–447.
7. Merchant SN, Ravicz ME, Voss SE, et al. Toynbee Memorial Lecture 1997. Middle ear mechanics in normal, diseased and reconstructed ears. *J Laryngol Otol* 1998;112:715–731.
8. Schuknecht HF. *Pathology of the ear,* 2nd ed. Philadelphia: Lea & Febiger, 1993.
9. Schuknecht HF, Shi SR. Surgical pathology of middle ear implants. *Laryngoscope* 1985;95:249–258.
10. Merchant SN, Nadol JB Jr. Histopathology of ossicular implants. *Otolaryngol Clin North Am* 1994;27:813–833.
11. Browning GG. Choice, advice and assessment of patients for ear surgery. *J Roy Soc Med* 1996;89:571–576.
12. Girgis TF, Shambaugh GE Jr. Tuning fork tests: forgotten art. *Am J Otol* 1988;9:64–69.
13. Bluestone CD, Cantekin EI. Current clinical methods, indications and interpretation of eustachian tube function tests. *Ann Otol Rhinol Laryngol* 1981;90:552–562.
14. Sheehy JL. Testing eustachian tube function. *Ann Otol Rhinol Laryngol* 1981;90:562–565.
15. Gibb AG, Pang YT. Surgical treatment of tympanosclerosis. *Eur Arch Otorhinolaryngol* 1995;252:1–10.
16. Sheehy JL, Shelton C. Tympanoplasty: to stage or not to stage. *Otolaryngol Head Neck Surg* 1991;104:399–407.
17. Palva T, Karja J, Palva A. Immediate and short-term complications of chronic ear surgery. *Arch Otolaryngol* 1976;102:137–139.
18. Smyth GD. Sensorineural hearing loss in chronic ear surgery. *Ann Otol Rhinol Laryngol* 1977;86:3–8.
19. Tos M, Lau T, Plate S. Sensorineural hearing loss following chronic ear surgery. *Ann Otol Rhinol Laryngol* 1984;93:403–409.
20. Gross CW, Bassila M, Lazar RH, et al. Adipose plug myringoplasty: an alternative to formal myringoplasty techniques in children. *Otolaryngol Head Neck Surg* 1989;101:617–620.
21. Lee K, Schuknecht HF. Results of tympanoplasty and mastoidectomy at the Massachusetts Eye and Ear Infirmary. *Laryngoscope* 1971;81:529–543.
22. Lau T, Tos M. Long-term results of surgery for granulating otitis. *Am J Otolaryngol* 1986;7:341–345.
23. Wullstein H. Results of tympanoplasty. *Arch Otolaryngol* 1960;71:478–485.
24. Jackson CG, Glasscock ME III, Schwaber MK, et al. Ossicular chain reconstruction: the TORP and PROP in chronic ear disease. *Laryngoscope* 1983;93:981–988.
25. Brackmann DE, Sheehy JL, Luxford WM. TORPs and PORPs in tympanoplasty: review of 1042 operations. *Otolaryngol Head Neck Surg* 1984;92:32–37.
26. Ragheb SM, Gantz BJ, McCabe BF. Hearing results after cholesteatoma surgery: the Iowa experience. *Laryngoscope* 1987;97:1254–1263.
27. Colletti V, Fiorino FG, Sittoni V. Minisculptured ossicle grafts versus implants: long-term results. *Am J Otol* 1987;8:553–559.
28. Goldenberg RA. Hydroxylapatite ossicular replacement prostheses: a four-year experience. *Otolaryngol Head Neck Surg* 1992;106:261–269.
29. Liston SL, Levine SC, Margolis RH, et al. Use of intraoperative auditory brainstem responses to guide prosthesis positioning. *Laryngoscope* 1991;101:1009–1012.
30. Tonndorf J, Khanna SM. Tympanic-membrane vibrations in human cadaver ears studied by time-averaged holography. *J Acoust Soc Am* 1972;52:1221–1233.
31. Vlaming MS, Feenstra L. Studies on the mechanics of the reconstructed human middle ear. *Clin Otolaryngol* 1986;11:411–422.
32. Nishihara S, Goode RL. Experimental study of the acoustic properties of incus replacement prostheses in a human temporal bone model. *Am J Otol* 1994;15:485–494.
33. Gan RZ, Dyer RK, Wood MW, et al. Mass loading on the ossicles and middle ear function. *Ann Otol Rhinol Laryngol* 2001;110:478–485.
34. Rosowski JJ, Merchant SN. Mechanical and acoustic analysis of middle ear reconstruction. *Am J Otol* 1995;16:486–497.
35. Mehta RP, Ravicz ME, Rosowski JJ, et al. Middle-ear mechanics of type III tympanoplasty (stapes columella): I. Experimental studies. *Otol Neurotol* 2003;24:176–185.
36. Merchant SN, McKenna MJ, Mehta RP, et al. Middle-ear mechanics of type III tympanoplasty (stapes columella): II. Clinical studies. *Otol Neurotol* 2003;24:186–194.
37. Murakami S, Gyo K, Goode RL. Effect of middle ear pressure change on middle ear mechanics. *Acta Otolaryngol (Stockh)* 1997;117:390–395.
38. Peake WT, Rosowski JJ, Lynch TJ III. Middle-ear transmission: acoustic versus ossicular coupling in cat and human. *Hear Res* 1992;57:245–268.
39. Montandon P, Chatelain C. Restoration of hearing with type V tympanoplasty. *ORL J Otorhinolaryngol Relat Spec* 1991;53:342–345.
40. Whittemore KR Jr, Merchant SN, Rosowski JJ. Acoustic mechanisms: canal wall-up versus canal wall-down mastoidectomy. *Otolaryngol Head Neck Surg* 1998;118:751–761.
41. Goode RL, Friedrichs R, Falk S. Effect on hearing thresholds of surgical modification of the external ear. *Ann Otol Rhinol Laryngol* 1977;86:441–451.

CHAPTER 24

Congenital Aural Atresia

Antonio De la Cruz and Jose N. Fayad

Congenital aural atresia is characterized by the absence or deformity of the pinna, aplasia, or hypoplasia of the external auditory canal, deformity of the middle ear, and occasional inner ear abnormalities. Aural atresia occurs in 1 in 20,000 live births, with unilateral atresia three times more common than bilateral atresia (1). It occurs more often in males and on the right side. External auditory canal atresia is more often bony than membranous (2,3). In general, a more severe external deformity implies a more severe middle ear abnormality (4,5).

In 1883, Kiesselbach was the first to attempt surgical correction of this malformation (6). More recently, Lascaratos and Assimakopoulos (7) credited the Byzantine physician Paul d'Egine with the use of a straight-sharp-pointed bistouri (scolopomachairon) in the treatment of congenital aural atresia. The attempt by Kiesselbach was, unfortunately, complicated by a facial nerve paralysis. Despite publications by others indicating good functional results, surgery for this disorder did not gain wide acceptance and was considered dangerous (7,8). In 1947, Ombredanne (9) and Pattee (10) reported their hearing improvement results.

In the 1950s, interest in atresiaplasty and tympanoplasty rose with the introduction of the surgical microscope as the teachings of Wullstein and Zöllner carried over into surgery of the congenital ear (6). Ombredanne (11) reported 1,600 cases of major and minor malformations. Gill (12), Crabtree (13), Jahrsdoerfer et al. (14), Marquet et al. (15), Molony and De la Cruz (16), and Bellucci (17) added to the knowledge already available and reported modifications of available surgical techniques and classification of these malformations.

Surgical correction of congenital aural atresia remains a challenging operation despite the improvements in techniques of facial nerve surgery, canalplasty, meatoplasty, tympanoplasty, ossiculoplasty, and tissue grafting. This is a complex surgical problem requiring a thorough knowledge of the anatomy of the facial nerve, oval window footplate variations, and the inner ear. The repair is recommended at age 6 years.

Stringent selection criteria are to be respected if closure of the air-bone gap to within 20 to 30 dB is to be obtained.

Preoperative counseling and long-term postoperative care are essential for optimal results.*

In this chapter we will briefly review the relevant embryology and classification systems and discuss patient evaluation and selection, surgical correction, and postoperative management.

EMBRYOLOGY

Six hillocks derived from the first and second branchial arches fuse to form the auricle. By the end of the third month the primitive auricle is completed. The external auditory meatus develops from the first branchial groove. It takes shape in the sixth month. Its canalization takes place in the seventh month. The subsequent inferior and posterior development of the external auditory meatus carries the middle ear and the facial nerve to their normal positions.

The middle ear cleft develops from the first branchial pouch. The tympanic membrane is formed by the junction between the middle ear cleft and the epithelium of the external auditory canal. The first branchial pouch forms the eustachian tube, tympanic cavity, and mastoid air cells. Meckel's cartilage forms the head of the malleus and body of the incus. Reichert's cartilage forms the remainder of the first two ossicles and the stapes superstructure. The footplate has a dual origin from the otic capsule and the second arch. The ossicles attain their final shape by the fourth month. By the end of the seventh or eighth month, the expanding middle ear cleft surrounds the ossicles and covers them with a mucous membrane (1,20).

The facial nerve is the nerve of the second arch. The membranous portion of the inner ear develops during the third to the sixth week from an auditory placode on the lateral surface of the hindbrain (21,22).

Congenital aural atresia can present in different forms depending on the time of the arrest of intrauterine development. The usual finding of a normal inner ear is explained

---

*References 1, 2, 6, 9, 12, 15, 17–19.

by the fact that the inner ear is already formed by the time the external/middle ear development arrests. Only severe congenital malformations of the external and middle ear are associated with inner ear deformities (23).

CLASSIFICATION

De la Cruz et al. (2) modified Altmann's descriptive system to include practical surgical guidelines. They divided these malformations into minor and major malformations. Minor malformations include (i) normal mastoid pneumatization, (ii) normal oval window footplate, (iii) favorable facial nerve–oval window footplate relationship, and (iv) normal inner ear. Major malformations include poor pneumatization, abnormal or absent oval window footplate, abnormal course of the horizontal portion of the facial nerve, and abnormalities of the inner ear. The clinical importance of this classification is that surgery in cases of minor malformations has the best chance of yielding a good functional result, whereas major malformations are often inoperable.

Jahrsdoerfer et al. (24) developed a point grading system (from 0 to 10) to identify good candidates for surgery. This system takes into consideration mastoid pneumatization, presence of the oval and round windows, course of the facial nerve, status of the ossicles, and external appearance. Allocation of points is based on the results of high resolution computed tomography (CT). They allocate two points for the presence of the stapes and one point for each one of the following parameters: oval window open, middle ear space present, facial nerve course normal, malleus-incus complex present, mastoids well pneumatized, incus-stapes connection present, round window normal, and appearance of the external auditory canal acceptable. A score of eight or better predicts a good surgical result. A score of seven implies a fair chance, six is marginal, and below that the patient becomes a poor candidate for surgery.

In 1955, Altmann (25) developed a widely used classification system that categorizes congenital aural atresia into three groups. Group 1 includes mild deformities; the external auditory canal, although hypoplastic, is present, the tympanic bone is hypoplastic, and the ear drum is small; the tympanic cavity is either normal or hypoplastic. Group 2 includes moderate deformities; the external auditory canal is completely absent, the tympanic cavity is small and its content deformed, and the atresia plate is partially or completely osseous. Group 3 includes severe deformities; the external auditory canal is absent, and the tympanic cavity is markedly hypoplastic or missing.

Schuknecht's system of classification of congenital aural atresia is based on a combination of clinical and surgical observations (26). Type A (meatal) atresia is limited to the fibrocartilaginous part of the external auditory canal and is corrected easily with a meatoplasty. In type B (partial) atresia, there is a narrowing of the cartilaginous and bony external auditory canal. A patent tract allows inspection of the tympanic membrane, which is small and may be partly replaced by a bony septum. Minor ossicular malformations exist, and hearing loss could be mild to severe. Type C (total) atresia includes cases of totally atretic ear canal with a well-pneumatized tympanic cavity. There is a partial or a total atretic plate, the ossicles are fused and most probably not connected to a malformed stapes, and the facial nerve may follow an aberrant course over the oval window. Type D (hypopneumatic total) atresia is a total atresia with poor pneumatization. These patients are poor surgical candidates for hearing improvement.

Chiossone's classification is based on the location of the glenoid fossa (27). In type 1 the fossa is in a normal position, in type II the fossa is slightly displaced, in type III the fossa overlaps the middle ear, and in type IV the fossa overlaps the middle ear and there is poor mastoid pneumatization. Patients with types I and II are ideal surgical candidates, whereas those with type IV are not.

INITIAL EVALUATION AND PATIENT SELECTION

Aural atresia diagnosed in the newborn mandates the search for other abnormalities. When aural atresia is associated with cephalic abnormalities, a full genetic workup is recommended to rule out the possibility of a syndromic child. The most commonly associated syndromes are Treacher Collins, Crouzon's, Klippel-Feil, Pierre Robin, Goldenhar's, drug teratogenicity, and hemifacial microsomia (28). Auditory function is evaluated using auditory brainstem response audiometry during the first few days of life whether the malformation is unilateral or bilateral. In bilateral cases, a bone-conduction hearing aid should be applied as soon as possible. In unilateral cases in which the hearing is normal in the opposite ear, a hearing aid is not indicated.

The incidence of inner ear abnormality associated with congenital aural atresia could be as high as 47% (5). In some unilateral cases, an anacusis may occur on the normal-appearing ear (2,17). It is necessary to counsel the parents and answer their questions regarding the possibility of occurrence of an aural atresia in their subsequent children (no more than the general population), future auricular reconstruction, and daily use of proper amplification. The child should be enrolled in special education at an early age to maximize speech and language acquisition. Radiologic and surgical evaluations are deferred until the child reaches the age of 6 years.

The evaluation includes a hearing test and high resolution CT of the temporal bone in coronal and axial views to assess the degree of the deformities. Auricular reconstruction must be done before hearing reconstruction to avoid interfering with the blood supply to the surrounding soft tissue, which is indispensable for microtia repair.

A patient with congenital atresia may present with a recurrently infected or draining ear or an acute facial palsy. Congenital cholesteatoma is present in 14% of the cases (2).

The priority in these cases is removal of the cholesteatoma and resolution of the infection. The presence of a cholesteatoma necessitates surgery at any age in unilateral and bilateral atresias.

Before undertaking surgery for congenital atresia, two requirements are necessary: the radiologic presence of an inner ear and the audiometric evidence of cochlear function.

TIMING OF AURICULAR RECONSTRUCTION AND ATRESIAPLASTY

In bilateral cases of congenital atresia, auricular reconstruction and atresiaplasty are recommended when the patient is age 6 years. By this time, the costal cartilage has developed sufficiently to allow for harvesting and transfer to the auricle, and the mastoid pneumatization is nearly complete. In unilateral cases, atresiaplasty is indicated only in minor deformities. The microtia repair is done first because of the need of an excellent blood supply to cover the autologous rib graft (29,30). The hearing restoration surgery is performed 2 months after the last step of the microtia repair. Rehabilitation of severe auricular defects can be done using an osseointegrated percutaneous mastoid implant prosthesis, with and without bone-conduction aids, such as a bone-anchored hearing aid (BAHA) (31).

PREOPERATIVE EVALUATION AND PATIENT COUNSELING

Early diagnosis with auditory brainstem response audiometry and bone-conduction hearing aids in bilateral cases should be done in the first weeks of life. Radiologic evaluation can be deferred until age 6 years, using high resolution CT in coronal and axial planes of the temporal bone (Figs. 24.1 to 24.3). Four anatomic parameters as visualized radio-

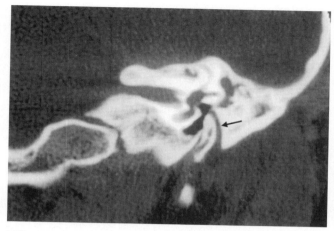

FIG. 24.2 Anteriorly displaced facial nerve (*arrow*) at the level of the oval window and the ampullated end of the lateral semicircular canal.

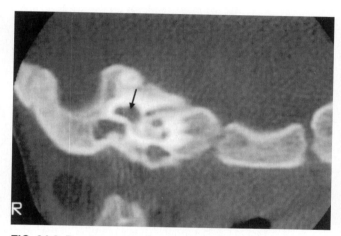

FIG. 24.3 Poorly pneumatized mastoid bone associated with a congenital malformation of the inner ear (*arrow*). The lateral semicircular canal and the vestibule are deformed. The oval window is obliterated. The tegmen is low. This case is inoperable.

graphically are crucial for surgical planning. These include the degree of pneumatization of the mastoid, the course of the facial nerve (both the relationship of the horizontal segment to the oval window and the location of the mastoid segment), the presence or absence of the oval window and stapes footplate, and the status of the inner ear.

Lack of pneumatization is the major cause of inoperability. The most common abnormal course of the facial nerve usually describes a more acute angle (instead of the normal 90 to 120 degrees at the mastoid genu) and lies more anteriorly and more laterally (Fig. 24.4) (32). If the oval window footplate is absent, consider the placement of a hearing aid or the implantation of a BAHA.

The patient is counseled regarding the success of atresiaplasty repair and the chances of a successful hearing improvement. The surgery and postoperative checks are explained to the patient, who will also be counseled regarding

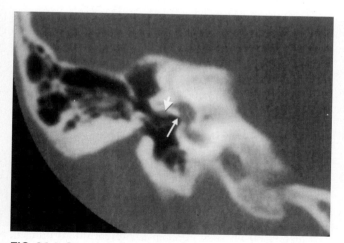

FIG. 24.1 Congenital aural atresia. High resolution CT showing a stenotic ear canal. There is a fused malleus-incus, as would be expected in a case of congenital atresia. The facial nerve is in normal position (*short arrow*), the oval window is patent (*long arrow*), and the mastoid bone is well pneumatized, making this case favorable for surgery.

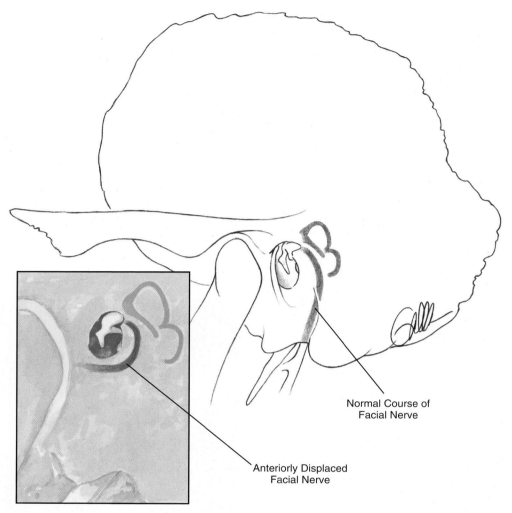

Normal Course of
Facial Nerve

Anteriorly Displaced
Facial Nerve

FIG. 24.4 Schematic representation of the normal facial nerve. Inset: Schematic representation of the facial nerve in congenital atresia.

the possibility of a facial nerve paralysis (1%), total sensorineural hearing loss (2%), high frequency sensorineural hearing loss (5%), and the risk of tympanic membrane graft lateralization (22%). The necessity of postoperative visits for local care to prevent stenosis of the external auditory canal is also explained.

SURGICAL TECHNIQUE

After administration of general endotracheal anesthesia, the patient is placed in the supine position and the head is turned away. Facial nerve monitoring is used on every case. The anesthesiologist is asked to avoid using muscle relaxants. The postauricular and lower abdomen areas are shaved, prepared, and draped. Perioperative antibiotics are administered.

A postauricular incision is made, and care is taken not to expose the costal cartilage graft already in place. Attention is also paid to the mastoid tip, and care is taken not to transect the facial nerve at its exit from the temporal bone. Subcutaneous tissue and mastoid periosteum are elevated anteri-

orly to the level of the temporomandibular joint (Fig. 24.5). Temporalis fascia is harvested and prepared for later grafting. The temporomandibular joint is explored to verify that the facial nerve or the tympanic bone is not lying within it. We will describe the anterior approach, the transmastoid approach, and the modified anterior approach, knowing that there are no distinct boundaries and they complement each other (2,6,17,28).

Anterior Approach

The new ear canal is created at the expense of the mastoid pneumatization. If there is remaining tympanic bone, the new ear canal is created through it or at the level of the mastoid tegmen. If no such remnant is present, the drilling is started at the linea temporalis just posterior to the glenoid fossa. By using cutting and diamond burs, the dissection is carried medially. The mastoid tegmen is followed to the epitympanum, where the fused malleus and incus mass is identified (Fig. 24.6). Care is taken to avoid drilling on the ossic-

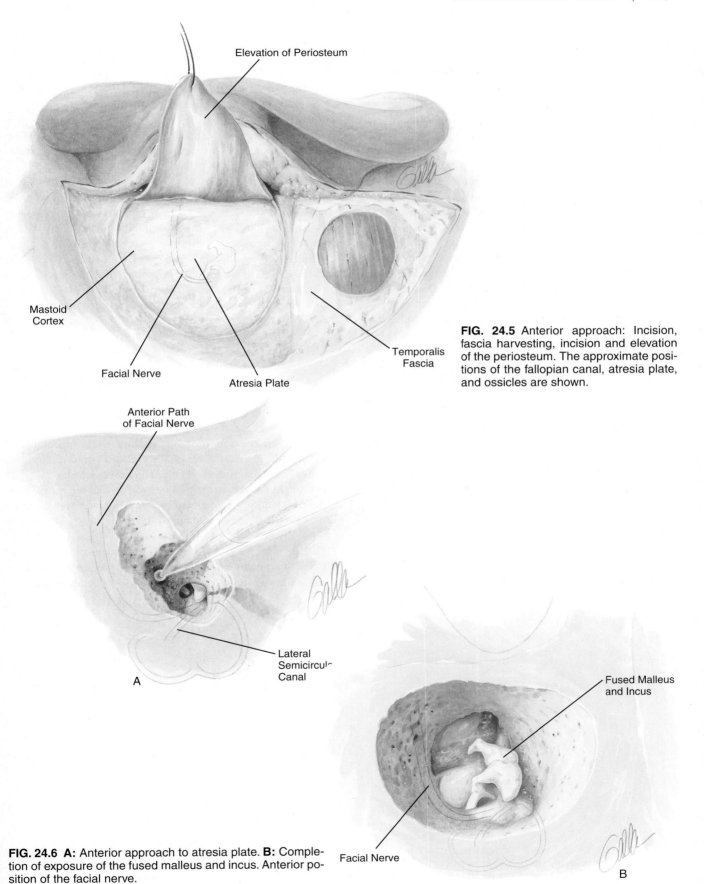

Elevation of Periosteum

Mastoid Cortex

Facial Nerve

Atresia Plate

Temporalis Fascia

FIG. 24.5 Anterior approach: Incision, fascia harvesting, incision and elevation of the periosteum. The approximate positions of the fallopian canal, atresia plate, and ossicles are shown.

Anterior Path of Facial Nerve

Lateral Semicircular Canal

A

Fused Malleus and Incus

Facial Nerve

B

FIG. 24.6 A: Anterior approach to atresia plate. **B:** Completion of exposure of the fused malleus and incus. Anterior position of the facial nerve.

ular mass to prevent high-speed drill energy transmission to the inner ear, which can result in high-frequency sensorineural hearing loss. The epitympanic ossicular mass is dissected free from the atretic bone and is left intact. The facial nerve is identified.

Further removal of the atresia plate is continued using diamond drills and curettes. The goal is to expose completely the ossicular mass (Fig. 24.6B). When dissecting posteriorly and inferiorly, attention is paid to the possibility of an aberrant facial nerve course that is emerging laterally through the atretic bone. Further dissection of adhesions and fibrous ligaments is undertaken using the argon or CO_2 laser. Often the ossicular chain is left in place. Ossicular reconstruction with the patient's own ossicular chain is preferred to the use of a prosthesis. When the ossicular chain is not complete, the reconstruction is done using a cartilage-covered partial or a total ossicular prosthesis, depending on the presence and location of an intact superstructure of the stapes. If access to the oval window footplate is impossible due to a dehiscent facial nerve obliterating the window, hearing reconstruction could be accomplished by fenestration of the lateral semicircular canal or the use of a hearing aid.*

Drilling continues to create an external auditory canal. It must be one and a half times the size of a normal canal (12 mm) to allow for contracture healing in the postoperative period. While creating the external auditory canal, care is taken not to enter the temporomandibular joint or unnecessarily open any mastoid cell.

Using a dermatome, a 0.010-inch thick, 6-cm × 6-cm split-thickness skin graft is obtained from the hypogastric area. Hemostasis at the donor site is obtained using thrombin and a wet gauze containing 1% lidocaine with epinephrine 1:100.000 U solution. A sterile Dermoplast or Op-site is applied to the donor site.

References 6, 9, 16, 18, 33, 34.

The skin graft is then prepared for later grafting. One of the edges is cut in a zigzag fashion to create four or five triangles. The tips of those triangles, as well as the edges on the opposite side of the zigzag, are marked (Fig. 24.7) (35). Marking makes it easier to identify these points later on in the procedure when doing the reconstruction.

Next, the temporalis fascia is prepared. A 20-mm × 15-mm oval piece is cut. Small 3-mm × 6-mm tabs are cut into the anterior and superior parts of the fascia to prevent lateralization of the graft.

The fascia is placed over the ossicular chain medial to the malleus, if present. If the ear is reconstructed using a prosthesis, the fascia is placed over the cartilage covering the prosthesis (Fig. 24.8) (35). The anterior tab is placed into the protympanum in an attempt to prevent lateralization of the graft. Next, the skin graft is placed into position. The zigzag area is directed medially. The skin overlies the fascial graft slightly. The marked tips of the triangles are found and layered over the fascia (6,14). The newly created external auditory canal is completely covered (Fig. 24.9). The reconstruction in the middle ear is stabilized using antibiotic-soaked Gelfoam pledgets. A disk of Gelfilm sheeting is placed over the tympanic membrane to create the anterior tympanomeatal angle. A large Ambrus Merocel wick is placed over the canal packing, and attention is turned to the meatoplasty (Fig. 24.10).

An 11-mm meatus is created, because a third of its diameter will reduce due to normal healing. Skin, subcutaneous tissue, and cartilage are removed in an 11-mm radius core over the newly created meatus. The excess lateral skin graft is brought through the meatoplasty (10), and the ear is stabilized by suturing the periosteum back in place over the mastoid cortex. The lateral edge of the skin graft is attached to the borders of the meatoplasty using 5-0 Ti-Cron sutures. Further absorbable 6-0 fast-absorbing plain gut is used between the previous sutures. The lateral portion of the external auditory canal is packed with a second Ambrus Merocel

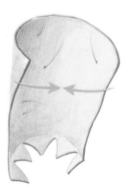

FIG. 24.7 Split-thickness skin graft for lining the external auditory canal. (From De la Cruz A, Chandrasekhar SS. Congenital malformation of the temporal bone. In: Brackmann DE, Shelton C, Arriaga MA, eds. *Otologic surgery.* Philadelphia: WB Saunders, 1994:69–84, with permission.)

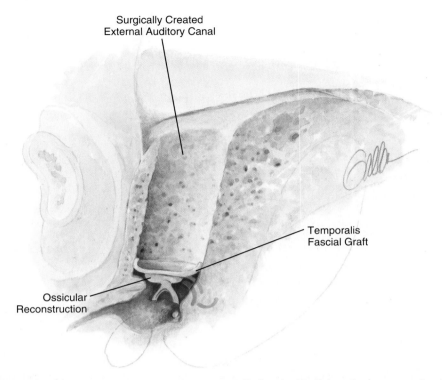

Surgically Created
External Auditory Canal

Temporalis
Fascial Graft

Ossicular
Reconstruction

FIG. 24.8 Tympanic membrane grafting using temporalis fascia. Partial ossicular reconstruction. (From De la Cruz A, Chandrasekhar SS. Congenital malformation of the temporal bone. In: Brackmann DE, Shelton C, Arriaga MA, eds. *Otologic surgery.* Philadelphia: WB Saunders, 1994:69–84, with permission.)

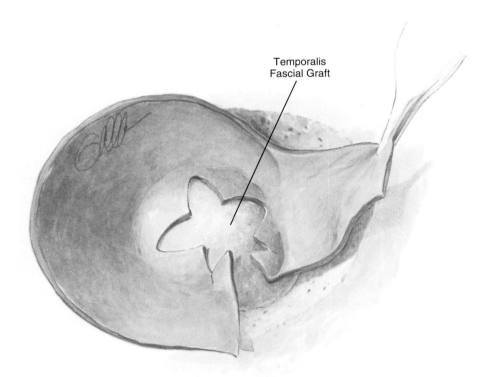

Temporalis
Fascial Graft

FIG. 24.9 Lining of the newly created external auditory canal with split-thickness skin graft.

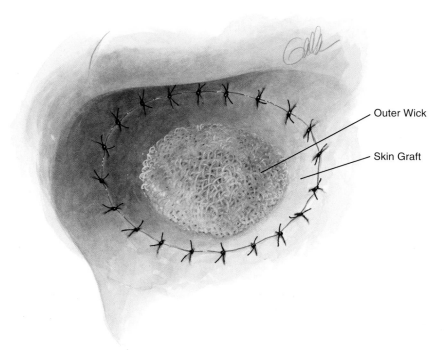

Outer Wick

Skin Graft

FIG. 24.10 Stenting of the external auditory canal. Wicks and sutures in place at the end of the surgery. (From De la Cruz A, Chandrasekhar SS. Congenital malformation of the temporal bone. In: Brackmann DE, Shelton C, Arriaga MA, eds. *Otologic surgery*. Philadelphia: WB Saunders, 1994:69–84, with permission.)

ear wick so that diffuse and constant pressure over the entire meatus is applied, keeping the meatus widely patent (Fig. 24.10). The periosteum is sutured back into position. The postauricular skin incision is closed in layers. Steri-Strips cover the postauricular incision. A mastoid-type dressing is applied, and the patient is awakened from anesthesia.

Transmastoid Approach (Canal Wall–Down Technique)

The transmastoid approach is only of historical importance. It has not been used for many years. In this approach, the drilling starts as posterior as possible from the temporomandibular joint. It starts at the linea temporalis and follows the sinodural angle to the ossicular mass. Mastoid air cell exenteration and lowering of the facial ridge to the facial nerve allows the creation of an external auditory canal with a canal wall–down technique. Bone paté and soft tissue obliteration of the large mastoid cells is performed before undertaking meatoplasty and canal skin grafting.

Modified Anterior Approach

In some patients with thick bony atresia plates and decreased pneumatization, orientation may be difficult for surgeons who infrequently deal with atresia during the medial dissection. Orientation can be achieved by drilling a posterior antrotomy at the sinodural angle to identify the lateral semicircular canal, which will serve as a landmark for the creation of the new external auditory canal. Drilling is done just posterior to the glenoid fossa and carried on as in an intact canal

wall–up canalplasty. Once the canal is created, the reconstruction proceeds in the same way described earlier.

POSTOPERATIVE CARE

The mastoid dressing is removed on the first postoperative day. The Steri-Strips covering the postauricular incision are left in place for 1 week. The patient is asked to keep the operative site dry and to change the cotton ball in the canal meatus as needed. The Dermoplast covering the donor site is left in place for 3 weeks. Epithelialization occurs under the plastic. The patient is given a 5-day course of oral antibiotics.

The patient is then seen 1 week after surgery. The Steri-Strips and the tacking Ti-Cron sutures at the meatus are removed; the donor site is inspected, and the patient is told that the postauricular incision can be washed but that water precautions still apply to the meatus.

The patient is seen again 3 weeks postoperatively. At this time the Ambrus Merocel pack is removed. The meatus is repacked using antibiotic-soaked gelatin sponges, and the patient is asked to apply antibiotic ear drops twice daily to the canal for 8 to 12 weeks.

The first postoperative audiogram is obtained at 6 weeks. Audiograms are then obtained at 6 months, 1 year, and annually thereafter.

PITFALLS

In all cases, we do an anterior approach. Facial nerve monitoring is used at all times, and adequate anesthetic techniques are used to ensure that the facial nerve is not injured during the procedure. In a poorly pneumatized mastoid, the otic capsule may be difficult to distinguish from surrounding bone, so care is taken not to fenestrate the semicircular canals. Postoperative care is very important to achieve proper healing. Patients are counseled preoperatively regarding the importance of postoperative care and the necessity of following the postoperative instructions and keeping postoperatively scheduled appointments. If the meatus is found to be narrowing, usually around the fourth month, it should be dilated every 2 weeks and restented with a large hollowed Merocel Pope wick for 12 to 24 months.

RESULTS

An extensive review of 302 atretic ears in 239 patients from the House Ear Clinic was published in 1985 (2). The De la Cruz classification was used to classify these patients into minor and major categories. Fifty-nine percent of the patients were male, and the right ear was involved in 64% of the unilateral cases. There were 70 bilateral cases. Thirty patients had associated anomalies, including congenital ipsilateral facial anomaly (n = 11), Mondini inner ear deformity (n = 7), Treacher Collins syndrome (n = 6), cleft palate (n = 5), and a stenotic internal auditory canal (n = 1). There were two nonhearing ears before surgery. Of the unilateral patients, five had either nonhearing ears or cholesteatomas in the normal-appearing ear. Nine atretic ears had cholesteatoma, usually lateral to the atretic plate.

Sixty-five ears underwent a primary atresiaplasty. Hearing results were excellent: 16% had a conductive loss of less than 10 dB, 53% under 20 dB, and 73% under 30 dB. Of the patients with poorer auditory outcome, one developed a high-frequency sensorineural hearing loss but preserved the low tones, and one developed a nonhearing ear following an lateral semicircular canal fenestration procedure. In six bilaterally atretic patients, the operated ear was so poorly pneumatized and the deformity so severe that the surgeon aborted the procedure. No patient had postoperative facial palsy. Fourteen percent had cholesteatoma.

Twenty patients needed revision surgery. The most common reason for failure was lateralization of the graft, which occurred in 22% of the patients. Five other patients developed canal stenosis and required reoperation. Persistent drainage may be another reason for revision surgery. The change from full-thickness skin grafts to split-thickness skin grafts has reduced the incidence of canal stenosis. Hearing results following revision surgery have been good. The most recent review was published in 1995 (36). The authors reviewed 92 congenital aural atresiaplasties. Closure of the air-bone gap to less than 30 dB was achieved in 60% of primary surgeries and 54% of revisions.

COMPLICATIONS AND THEIR MANAGEMENT

Complications of atresiaplasty include lateralization of the tympanic membrane in up to 15%, stenosis of the meatus in 12%, total sensorineural hearing loss in 2%, high-frequency sensorineural hearing loss in 5%, and facial nerve palsy in 1%.

Prevention

Care is taken at the time of surgery to help minimize the incidence of lateralization. Modern techniques of tympanoplasty are applied during the reconstruction. The graft is anchored medially to the malleus, and tabs are placed into the protympanum. Use of an accurately sized silicone sheeting disk or Gelfilm helps create an anterior tympanomeatal angle, minimizing blunting and keeping the graft in position. The patient is followed for a long time because lateralization can begin up to 6 months postoperatively.

The incidence of stenosis has been greatly reduced with the use of one-piece split-thickness skin grafts covering all exposed bone. Local care and prevention of infection will prevent graft failure and early restenosis. Careful inspection of the meatus and early restenting with large Merocel wicks can obviate reoperation.

With high resolution CT, the oval window can be identified, and problems due to oval window drill-out can be anticipated. Patients with severe malformations, in whom surgery would be fraught with problems, can be counseled against surgical intervention and fitted with hearing aids. The facial nerve position and trajectory inside the temporal bone can be identified, and, along with facial nerve monitoring, use of this information can further reduce the incidence of facial nerve paralysis.

ALTERNATIVE TECHNIQUES

Patients with bilateral atresia must have early auditory amplification. As soon as possible, newborns receive bone-conduction aids. At age 6 years, if evaluation reveals a high surgical risk or poor predicted outcome, a bone-conduction aid is continued. Implantation of a bone-conduction hearing aid should be considered (31,37–40). These aids can also anchor a synthetic auricular prosthesis.

One type of implantable bone aid available for clinical use is the BAHA, introduced in 1977 in Sweden. The BAHA, utilizing Branemark System implants in combination with the hearing aid, has proved to be a favorable means of providing hearing rehabilitation for certain groups of patients, including those with a congenital ear malformation. The BAHA is a good alternative for a conventional bone hearing aid. Conventional bone hearing aids are usually regarded as a last resort because patients complain of several drawbacks: discomfort because of constant pressure from the steel spring, poor sound quality because of higher-frequency attenuation by the skin, and poor esthetics and insecure positioning of the device. The BAHA works without any pressure on the skin.

Surgery for the BAHA can be performed under local anesthesia and is a one- or a two-stage procedure. To implant the BAHA, a small titanium screw is implanted behind the ear, where it osseointegrates to the mastoid bone. At the same time or after a 3-month healing period, a percutaneous abutment is attached to the screw. The BAHA can then be connected 3 to 5 weeks after the percutaneous abutment is attached.

Audiologic indications for the BAHA include a pure-tone average bone-conduction threshold better than or equal to 45-dB hearing loss (HL) (average 500, 1,000, 2,000, 3,000 Hz). A maximum speech discrimination score better than 60% when using PB word lists is recommended. From an audiologic point of view, the side with the best cochlear function (the best bone-conduction threshold) should be used. Patients with a bone-conduction threshold of 25- to 45-dB HL will be expected to improve but may not achieve levels in the normal range. Patients with a bone-conduction threshold of less than 25-dB HL can be expected to experience hearing improvements that restore hearing levels to normal ranges. Patients must be able to maintain the abutment/skin interface of the BAHA. Careful consideration must be given to the patient's psychologic, physical, emotional, and developmental capabilities to maintain hygiene. Biologic titanium implants can be installed in most patients. Alternative treatments should be considered for patients with a disease state that might jeopardize osseointegration.

The BAHA is not indicated for bilateral implantation or for patients under the age of 18 years. For patients with bilateral hearing loss, the BICROS is an additional microphone that can be used as an accessory to an implanted BAHA fixture and sound processor to overcome the head shadow effect. The accessory microphone is placed in the contralateral ear to the BAHA fixture. The signal is routed from the accessory microphone to the BAHA sound processor via a wire worn behind the neck. It is therefore intended to improve hearing by eliminating the head shadow effect (41).

UNILATERAL ATRETIC EAR

Controversy remains over whether children with unilateral atresia should undergo surgery. In the past, Schuknecht (42), Crabtree (13), and Bellucci (43) have recommended against operating on children with unilateral atresia. These authors argued that the benefit to be gained is minimal in the presence of a contralateral normal hearing ear. Hearing results at that time were unpredictable and often did not approach the 20-dB air-bone gap needed for useful hearing in the atretic ear. Risks of surgery, including facial nerve injury, also precluded operating on the unilateral atretic ear. In a recent review of more than 1,000 operations for aural atresia with and without cholesteatoma, Jahrsdoerfer and Lambert (44) showed that the risk was minimal (1%). The incidence of major complications (total sensorineural hearing loss and facial nerve injury) has decreased over the years, but the incidence of other complications (high-frequency sensorineural loss, tympanic membrane graft lateralization, and restenosis) has essentially remained unchanged. The decision to op-

erate on the unilateral atretic ear must weigh these potential complications along with the possibility of a draining ear. Nevertheless, with excellent preoperative imaging, improved surgical techniques, and advances in technology, we feel the results of atresia surgery are now more predictable. Closure of the air-bone gap to within 30 dB in the properly selected patient can be consistently achieved. A recent review examining long-term stability of hearing results in patients operated on for aural atresia does show some drop-off in hearing thresholds (SRT) over time, however (45). Additional long-term follow-up studies are necessary to document and confirm these hearing results. Jahrsdoerfer (6) and De la Cruz et al. (2) have argued for atresia surgery in selected patients with unilateral atresia. A recent literature review supports this position (46). In the hands of an experienced otologic surgeon with an anatomically favorable patient who (with the parents) understands the risks of potential complications and the need for postoperative care, atresiaplasty in the patient with unilateral atresia is a rewarding operation for both surgeon and patient. Surgical correction of unilateral atresia offers the benefits of a clean, dry ear with binaural hearing, including sound localization and improved hearing in noise.

SUMMARY

The treatment of congenital aural atresia poses a challenge. Early identification by means of auditory brainstem responses, amplification as soon as possible using bone-conduction hearing aids, and speech and language therapy are crucial in bilateral cases. Cooperation with the auricular reconstruction surgeon allows for both esthetic and functional success at age 6 years. Most patients end up with a hearing level between 20 to 30 dB. The risk of facial nerve paralysis is minimal (42). Tympanic membrane graft lateralization and high-frequency sensorineural hearing loss are the challenges of the future. BAHA is a good alternative in otherwise inoperable cases.

REFERENCES

1. Federspil P, Delb W. Treatment of congenital malformations of the external and middle ear. In: Ars B, ed. *Congenital external and middle ear malformations: management.* Amsterdam: Kugler Publications, 1992:47–70.
2. De la Cruz A, Linthicum FH, Jr, Luxford WM. Congenital atresia of the external auditory canal. *Laryngoscope* 1985;95:421–427.
3. Kelemen G. Aural participation in congenital malformations of the organism. *Acta Otolaryngol Suppl* 1974;321:1–35.
4. Harada O, Ishii H. The condition of the auditory ossicles in microtia: findings in 57 middle ear operations. *Plast Reconstr Surg* 1972;50:48–53.
5. Hasso AN, Broadwell RA. Congenital anomalies. In: Som PM, Bergeron RT, eds. *Head and neck imaging,* 2nd ed. St. Louis: Mosby, 1991:960–966.
6. Jahrsdoerfer RA. Congenital atresia of the ear. *Laryngoscope* 1978;88[Suppl 13]:1–48.
7. Lascaratos J, Assimakopoulos D. From the roots of otology: diseases of the ear and their treatment in Byzantine times (324–1453 A.D.). *Am J Otol* 1999;20:397–402.

8. Dean LW, Gittens TR. Report of a case of bilateral, congenital osseous atresia of the external auditory canal with an exceptionally good functional result following operation. *Trans Am Laryngol Rhinol Otol Soc* 1917:296–309.

9. Ombredanne M. Chirurgie de la surdite: fenestration dans les aplasies de l'oreille avec imperforation du conduit. Resultats. *Otorhinolaryngol Int* 1947;31:229–236.

10. Pattee GL. An operation to improve hearing in cases of congenital atresia of the external auditory meatus. *Arch Otolaryngol Head Neck Surg* 1947;45(5):568–580.

11. Ombredanne M. [Surgery of congenital deafness due to ossicular malformations]. *Acta Otorhinolaryngol Belg* 1971;25:837–869.

12. Gill NW. Congenital atresia of the ear. A review of the surgical findings in 83 cases. *J Laryngol Otol* 1969;83:551–587.

13. Crabtree JA. Congenital atresia: case selection, complications, and prevention. *Otolaryngol Clin North Am* 1982;15:755–762.

14. Jahrsdoerfer RA, Cole RR, Gray L. Advances in congenital aural atresia. In: Myers EN, ed. *Advances in otolaryngology head and neck surgery,* vol. 5 Chicago: Mosby, 1991:1–15.

15. Marquet JE, Declau F, De Cock M, et al. Congenital middle ear malformations. *Acta Otorhinolaryngol Belg* 1988;42:117–302.

16. Molony TB, De la Cruz A. Surgical approaches to congenital atresia of the external auditory canal. *Otolaryngol Head Neck Surg* 1990;103:991–1001.

17. Bellucci RJ. Congenital auricular malformations. Indications, contraindications, and timing of middle ear surgery. *Ann Otol Rhinol Laryngol* 1972;81:659–663.

18. Schuknecht HF. Reconstructive procedures for congenital aural atresia. *Arch Otolaryngol* 1975;101:170–172.

19. Linthicum FH, Jr. Surgery of congenital deafness. *Otolaryngol Clin North Am* 1971;4:401–409.

20. Van de Water TR, Maderson PF, Jaskoll TF. The morphogenesis of the middle and external ear. *Birth Defects Orig Artic Ser* 1980;16:147–180.

21. Savic D, Jasovic A, Djeric D. The relations of the mastoid segment of the facial canal to surrounding structures in congenital middle ear malformations. *Int J Pediatr Otorhinolaryngol* 1989;18:13–19.

22. Gill NW. Congenital atresia of the ear. *J Laryngol Otol* 1971;85:1251–1254.

23. Melnick M. The etiology of external ear malformations and its relation to abnormalities of the middle ear, inner ear, and other organ systems. *Birth Defects Orig Artic Ser* 1980;16:303–331.

24. Jahrsdoerfer RA, Yeakley JW, Aguilar EA, et al. Grading system for the selection of patients with congenital aural atresia. *Am J Otol* 1992;13:6–12.

25. Altmann F. Congenital atresia of the ear in man and animals. *Ann Otol Rhinol Laryngol* 1955;64:824–858.

26. Schuknecht HF. Congenital aural atresia and congenital middle ear cholesteatoma. In: Nadol JB, Jr, Schuknecht HF, eds. *Surgery of the ear and temporal bone.* New York: Raven Press, 1993:263–274.

27. Chiossone E. Surgical management of major congenital malformations of the ear. *Am J Otol* 1985;6:237–242.

28. Sando I, Suehiro S, Wood RP, II. Congenital anomalies of the external and middle ear. In: Bluestone CD, Stool SE, eds. *Pediatric otolaryngology.* Philadelphia: WB Saunders, 1983:309–346.

29. Brent B. The correction of microtia with autogenous cartilage grafts: I. The classic deformity. *Plast Reconstr Surg* 1980;66:1–12.

30. Brent B. Auricular repair with autogenous rib cartilage grafts: two decades of experience with 600 cases. *Plast Reconstr Surg* 1992;90:355–374.

31. Hakansson B, Liden G, Tjellstrom A, et al. Ten years of experience with the Swedish bone-anchored hearing system. *Ann Otol Rhinol Laryngol Suppl* 1990;151:1–16.

32. Crabtree JA. The facial nerve in congenital ear surgery. *Otolaryngol Clin North Am* 1974;7:505–510.

33. House HP. Management of congenital ear canal atresia. *Laryngoscope* 1953;63:916–946.

34. Ombredanne M. [Congenital absence of the round window in certain minor aplasias. Further cases]. *Ann Otolaryngol Chir Cervicofac* 1968;85:369–378.

35. De la Cruz A, Chandrasekhar SS. Congenital malformation of the temporal bone. In: Brackmann DE, Shelton C, Arriaga MA, eds. *Otologic surgery.* Philadelphia: WB Saunders, 1994:69–84.

36. Chandrasekhar SS, De la Cruz A, Garrido E. Surgery of congenital aural atresia. *Am J Otol* 1995;16:713–717.

37. Granstrom G, Bergstrom K, Tjellstrom A. The bone-anchored hearing aid and bone-anchored epithesis for congenital ear malformations. *Otolaryngol Head Neck Surg* 1993;109:46–53.

38. Tjellstrom A, Bergstrom K. Bone-anchored hearing aids and prostheses. In: Ars B, ed. *Congenital external and middle ear malformations: management.* Amsterdam: Kugler Publications, 1992:1–9.

39. Niparko JK, Langman AW, Cutler DS, et al. Tissue-integrated prostheses in the rehabilitation of auricular defects: results with percutaneous mastoid implants. *Am J Otol* 1993;14:343–348.

40. Van der Pouw KT, Snik AF, Cremers CW. Audiometric results of bilateral bone-anchored hearing aid application in patients with bilateral congenital aural atresia. *Laryngoscope* 1998;108:548–553.

41. Tjellström A, Håkansson B. The bone-anchored hearing aid. Design principles, indications, and long-term clinical results. *Otolaryngol Clin North Am* 1995;28:53–72.

42. Schuknecht HF. Congenital aural atresia. *Laryngoscope* 1989;99:908–917.

43. Bellucci RJ. Congenital aural malformations: diagnosis and treatment. *Otolaryngol Clin North Am* 1981;14:95–124.

44. Jahrsdoerfer RA, Lambert PR. Facial nerve injury in congenital aural atresia surgery. *Am J Otol* 1998;19:283–287.

45. Lambert PR. Congenital aural atresia: stability of surgical results. *Laryngoscope* 1998;108:1801–1815.

46. Trigg DJ, Applebaum EL. Indications for the surgical repair of unilateral aural atresia in children. *Am J Otol* 1998;19:679–684.

CHAPTER 25

Congenital Cholesteatoma

Trevor J. McGill and Reza Rahbar

Congenital cholesteatoma of the middle ear is a rare clinical entity that classically presents as a white mass in the anterior superior quadrant of the middle ear behind an intact tympanic membrane. This unusual lesion may also occur in other regions of the temporal bone, such as the petrous apex and external canal. Derlacki and Clemis (1) were the first to establish the clinical criteria for diagnosis of congenital cholesteatoma as a white mass medial to the normal tympanic membrane without a prior history of otitis media, ear surgery, perforation, or otorrhea.

It is controversial whether a history of otitis media should be grounds for exclusion because 70% of children have at least one episode of otitis media before age 3 years (2). Congenital cholesteatoma usually occurs as a unilateral white mass, whereas most cases of otitis media are bilateral. Recent clinical and histopathologic studies of congenital cholesteatoma show a normal middle ear mucosa and a normal intact tympanic membrane with 50% of patients younger than age 2 years (3,4). It is unlikely that reversible inflammatory changes could produce an isolated cholesteatoma medial to a perfectly normal tympanic membrane. In 1998 Levenson and colleagues (3) modified the definition of congenital cholesteatoma to include a white mass medial to a normal intact tympanic membrane with no prior history of ear surgery. Thus history of otitis media without otorrhea is not a ground for excluding congenital cholesteatoma.

CLINICAL PRESENTATION

Congenital cholesteatoma is now diagnosed earlier than heretofore. The age at presentation in the most recent series is 1 to 4 years, as opposed to 20 years in the series reported by House and Sheehy (3–5) in 1980. The characteristic appearance is that of a white mass in the anterior superior quadrant of the middle ear behind an intact tympanic membrane (Figs. 25.1 and 25.2).

An apparent increase in the reported incidence of congenital cholesteatoma in recent years may be due, in part, to improvement in diagnostic capabilities, including halogen illumination for otoscopy, pneumatic otoscopy, and routine hearing screening. However, most congenital cholesteatomas present to the otolaryngologist in the setting of a refractory serous otitis media or an abnormality thought to be in the tympanic membrane. The lesion may also be discovered incidentally at the time of a myringotomy.

The incidence of otitis media in patients with congenital cholesteatoma is the same as in the general population. However, a diagnosis of congenital cholesteatoma should be considered in any patient with unilateral middle ear effusion or conductive hearing loss. Although a congenital cholesteatoma limited to the anterior superior quadrant of the middle ear may be entirely asymptomatic, it may cause a unilateral middle ear effusion due to obstruction of the eustachian tube.

Posterior extension toward the incudostapedial joint may cause destruction of the lenticular process of the incus and capitulum of the stapes. Eventually the superstructure of the stapes will be destroyed while the footplate usually remains intact. Progressive growth of congenital cholesteatoma into the attic, aditus ad antrum, and mastoid is similar to acquired middle ear cholesteatoma. At this stage it almost certainly would be complicated by infection or rupture of the tympanic membrane, making it difficult to assume a congenital origin with any degree of certainty.

PATHOGENESIS

Aimi (6) in 1983 postulated that congenital cholesteatoma is caused by migration of ectoderm from the external canal into the middle ear at an early stage of embryonic life. Sobol et al. (7) presented the concept that recurrent otitis media may cause basal cell proliferation in the tympanic membrane, leading to a seemingly congenital cholesteatoma behind an intact tympanic membrane. Northrop and colleagues (8) have proposed that viable amniotic debris within the middle ear of neonates may cause congenital cholesteatoma. Michaels (9) in 1988 theorized that congenital cholesteatoma arises from an epidermoid rest in the developing middle ear. This "epidermoid formation" (4) is present in most fetal ears at the junc-

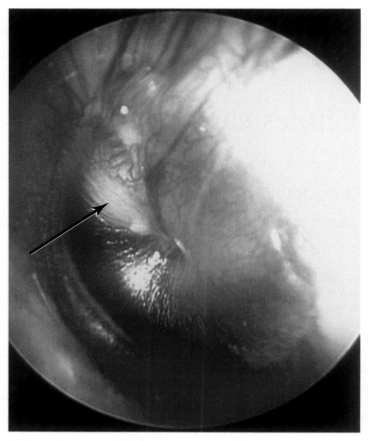

FIG. 25.1 Otoscopic view of a congenital cholesteatoma in the anterior superior segment of the left middle ear (*arrow*).

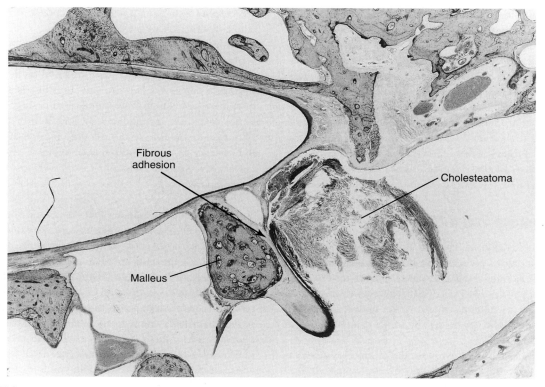

FIG. 25.2 An asymptomatic congenital cholesteatoma in the anterosuperior quadrant of the middle ear. Fibrous adhesion to the anterior aspect of the malleus is seen (18.3X).

tion of the eustachian tube and middle ear near the tympanic ring until 32 weeks' gestation. He postulated that congenital cholesteatoma is caused by persistence and growth of the epidermoid formation. This hypothesis is attractive and explains the propensity of congenital cholesteatoma to appear in the anterosuperior segment of the middle ear. However, conclusive proof awaits the discovery of a lesion of intermediate stage in a temporal bone. Lee et al. (10) in 1998 reinvestigated the role of the epidermoid formation in serial sections of fetal and neonatal temporal bones to assess its relationship to congenital cholesteatoma. Epidermoid formations were found in 88 (42%) of 211 temporal bones from 6 weeks' gestation to 6 months postpartum. The site of the epidermoid formation was an average of 389 microns anterior to the anterior margin of the tympanic membrane. Several epidermoid formations were found on the medial surface of the anterosuperior tympanic membrane. Although the average diameter of an epidermoid formation was 242 microns, some were greater than 1,500 microns in diameter, which approximates the size of a small congenital cholesteatoma. These findings support the concept that the epidermoid formation is a precursor of the common form of closed type of congenital cholesteatoma seen in the anterior superior quadrant of the middle ear.

HISTOPATHOLOGY

Peron and Schuknecht (11) published the first temporal bone histopathologic report of congenital cholesteatoma of the middle ear. McGill et al. (4) presented two further cases for review, and they suggested there are at least two types of congenital middle ear cholesteatoma: (i) A more common "closed" cholesteatoma is located in the anterior superior segment of the middle ear behind an intact tympanic membrane that is present at birth and grows slowly during early infancy (see Fig. 25.2). When confined to the anterior superior quadrant, it is removed in its entirety via a transcanal exploratory tympanotomy. (ii) A rarer "open" form of cholesteatoma occurs where the matrix replaces part of the middle ear mucosa. The matrix may also extend to cover middle ear structures such as the ossicles and intratympanic muscles. Evacuation of the keratin via the eustachian tube may prevent growth of these lesions, and they may remain asymptomatic until they become infected. Surgical management requires a removal of all involved tympanic membrane, ossicles, and mucosa that are covered by cholesteatoma matrix. This open type of congenital cholesteatoma is associated with frequent recurrence.

RADIOLOGIC EVALUATION

Axial and coronal computerized tomography (CT) is useful in ascertaining the location and extension of cholesteatoma within the middle ear. This is not performed in all cases but is advisable where the superior or posterior limit of the middle ear cholesteatoma cannot be visualized by otomicroscopy (Fig. 25.3). Higher resolution CT can also identify erosion of bone of the ossicles, fallopian canal, and scutum.

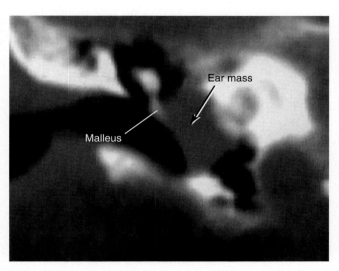

FIG. 25.3 Coronal high resolution CT scan showing a rounded middle ear mass behind an intact tympanic membrane, adjacent to the handle of the malleus.

SURGICAL MANAGEMENT

The management of congenital cholesteatoma is prompt surgical removal. Complete resection via an extended tympanotomy will provide excellent exposure and will permit the removal of an intact cholesteatoma with preservation of normal hearing and with a low incidence of recurrence.

TYMPANOTOMY

Middle ear exploration in children is performed under general anesthesia. Most congenital cholesteatomas can be removed using a transcanal approach. However, a postauricular or endaural approach is sometimes required in children younger than age 2 years or if the cholesteatoma extends into the epitympanum.

Operative Technique

1. If the transcanal approach is selected, local anesthetic ($^1/_2$ lidocaine and 1:200,000 epinephrine) is injected into the soft tissue of the posterior cartilaginous ear canal just lateral to the bony canal.
2. An incision is made in the bony canal with a McCabe knife starting anterior to the lateral process of the malleus and continuing to the posterior inferior portion of the ear canal opposite the umbo. The flap outline should extend 4 mm beyond the osseous tympanic ring (Fig. 25.4). The inferior and superior limbs of this incision can be extended with Bellucci scissors. The flap is elevated with the canal wall elevator until the fibrous annulus is identified.
3. The fibrous annulus is elevated with a straight pick out of its bony sulcus in the region of the chorda tympani nerve. The annulus of the tympanic membrane is ele-

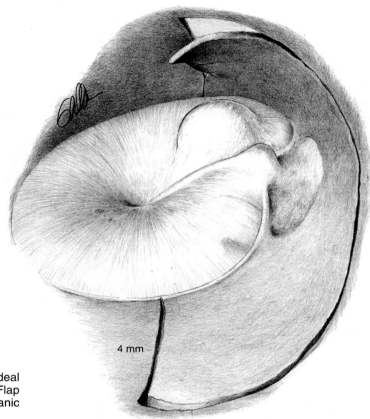

4 mm

FIG. 25.4 An extended superior tympanomeatal flap is ideal for the removal of congenital middle ear cholesteatoma. Flap outline should extend 4 mm beyond the osseus tympanic ring.

vated out of its bony sulcus using an angulated drum elevator.

4. The tympanomeatal flap is reflected anteriorly to expose the contents of the middle ear.

5. Because exposure of the anterior superior segment of the middle ear is needed for excision of congenital cholesteatoma, the tympanic membrane must be elevated from the malleus. Although the tympanic membrane is easily removed from the neck and lateral process of the malleus, it is firmly adherent to the manubrium and umbo. A sickle knife is used to incise the periosteum along the posterior border of the malleus (Fig. 25.5). Thus the layer of periosteum is elevated from the handle of the malleus in continuity with the tympanic membrane. If further exposure is necessary, Bellucci scissors are used to cut the fibrous bands attaching the tympanic membrane to the umbo, thus affording excellent exposure of the entire mesotympanum and ossicular chain (Fig. 25.6).

6. In removing this congenital cholesteatoma confined to the anterior superior quadrant of the middle ear, it is important to avoid penetration of the intact matrix. Dissection using angulated smooth instruments such as a duckbill or whirlybird should be done in the plane between the middle ear mucosa and the perimatrix, thus avoiding contact with the matrix of the congenital

cholesteatoma (Fig. 25.7). Cholesteatoma is usually adherent to the anterior border of the malleus (see Fig. 25.2) and to the promontory. The cholesteatoma is first displaced into the hypotympanum, and then delivered into the external canal. The middle ear may then be inspected with 0-degree and 30-degree ototelescopes. The tympanic membrane is replaced, and a circular disc of Gelfoam is placed on the tympanic membrane to prevent postoperative lateralization of the pars tensa from the manubrium.

7. If the congenital cholesteatoma has extended superiorly into the anterior epitympanum, complete removal may require an atticotomy or tympanomastoidectomy. The open form of congenital cholesteatoma usually presents in the anterior half of the pars tensa, with its matrix forming part of the middle ear mucosa. The matrix may extend to cover the ossicles, intratympanic muscles, and other middle ear structures. Surgical treatment requires removal of all portions of the middle ear covered by this matrix to prevent recurrence (Fig. 25.8). Depending on the nature and extent of the open type of congenital cholesteatoma, surgical approaches may include simple atticotomy, cortical mastoidectomy, and posterior tympanotomy or tympanomastoidectomy with removal of ossicles, and subsequent ossicular reconstruction.

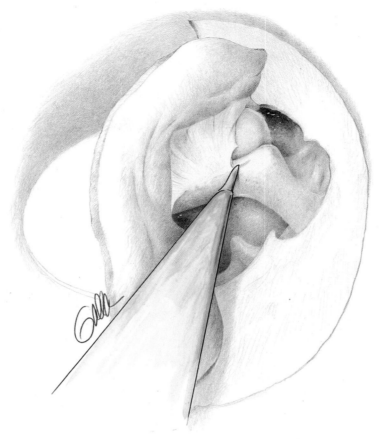

FIG. 25.5 A sickle knife is used to make an incision in the periosteum along the full length of the posterior surface of the malleus. The periosteum is then released from the malleus until the anterior superior quadrant is visualized.

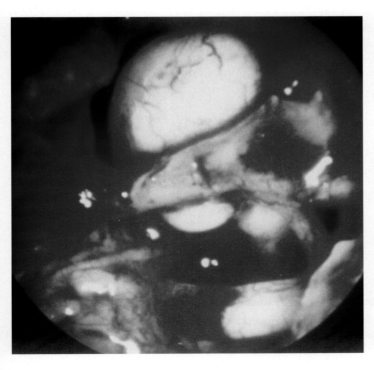

FIG. 25.6 Surgical view of the left middle ear via an extended superior tympanomeatal flap. Note that the closed congenital cholesteatoma in the anterior superior mesotympanum is extending medial to the malleus.

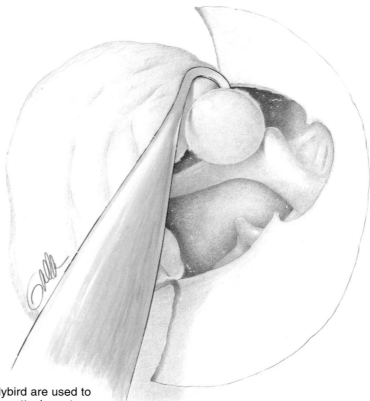

FIG. 25.7 Smooth angulated instruments such as a whirlybird are used to dissect the cholesteatoma from the surrounding middle ear attachments.

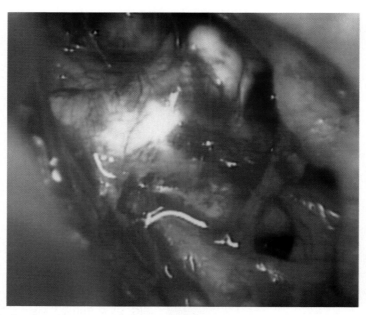

A

FIG. 25.8 A: Otomicroscopic view of the middle ear showing an extensive closed congenital cholesteatoma extending medial to both the malleus and incus.

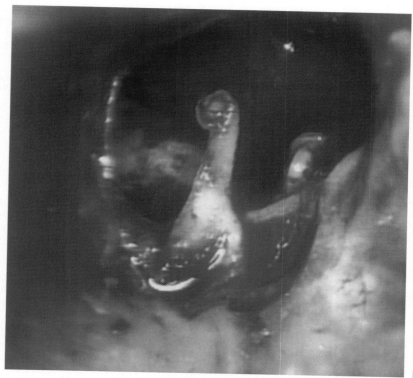

FIG. 25.8, cont'd. B: Otomicroscopic view of the middle ear following surgical removal of congenital cholesteatoma in (**A**).

COMPLICATIONS

Complications include the following:

1. *Recurrence.* Routine reexploration is not necessary when the cholesteatoma is confined to the anterior superior quadrant of the middle ear. Any recurrence in this group will usually be limited and detected by routine otoscopy. An open cholesteatoma or a closed cholesteatoma that extends into the antrum and mastoid is associated with a significantly higher rate of recurrence. Thus routine reexploration is advised between 6 and 12 months postoperatively. Surgical indications for reexploration are primarily dictated by the surgeon's opinion that residual disease may have been left behind at the original operation or if there is an open type cholesteatoma with its increased potential for residual disease. Patients with congenital cholesteatoma are routinely followed for at least 36 months.

2. *Lateralization of the tympanic membrane.* There is a small risk of lateralization of the tympanic membrane from the malleus if it was released from the umbo for exposure. This can be prevented by placing a circular disc of Gelfoam 7 mm in diameter on the lateral surface of the tympanic membrane.

CONCLUSION

Congenital cholesteatoma is rare, occurring primarily between the ages of 1 and 3 years. It occurs classically as a white mass in the anterior superior segment of the middle ear behind an intact tympanic membrane. Surgical removal is mandatory, and residual or recurrent disease in those lesions confined to the anterior superior segment and removed by an extended posterior superior tympanotomy is unlikely. If the diagnosis is delayed until the lesion has extended beyond the middle ear and into the attic and antrum, or in the case of an open cholesteatoma, ossicular erosion and a higher recurrence rate can be expected.

REFERENCES

1. Derlacki EL, Clemis JD. Congenital cholesteatoma of the middle ear and mastoid. *Ann Otol Rhinol Laryngol* 1965;74:706–727.
2. Teele DW, Klein JO, Rosner BA. Epidemiology of otitis media in children. *Ann Otol Rhinol Laryngol* 1980;89[Suppl 68]:5–6.
3. Levenson MJ, Parisier SC, Chute P, et al. A review of twenty congenital cholesteatomas of the middle ear in children. *Otolaryngol Head Neck Surg* 1986;94:560–567.
4. McGill TJ, Merchant S, Healy GB, et al. Congenital cholesteatoma of the middle ear in children: a clinical and histopathological report. *Laryngoscope* 1991;101:606–613.
5. House JW, Sheehy JL. Cholesteatoma with intact tympanic membrane: a report of 41 cases. *Laryngoscope* 1980;90:70–76.

6. Aimi K. Role of the tympanic ring in pathogenesis of congenital cholesteatoma. *Laryngoscope* 1983;93:1140–1146.

7. Sobol SM, Reichert TJ, Faw KD, et al. Intramembranous and meso-tympanic cholesteatomas associated with an intact tympanic membrane in children. *Ann Otol Rhinol Laryngol* 1980;89:312–317.

8. Northrop C, Piza J, Eavey RD. Histological observations of amniotic fluid cellular content in the ear of neonates and infants. *Int J Pediatr Otorhinolaryngol* 1986;11:113–127.

9. Michaels L. Evolution of the epidermoid formation and its role in the development of the middle ear and tympanic membrane during the first trimester. *J Otolaryngol* 1988;17:22–28.

10. Lee TS, Liang JN, Michaels L, et al. The epidermoid formation and its affinity to congenital cholesteatoma. *Clin Otolaryngol* 1998;23:449–454.

11. Peron DL, Schuknecht HF. Congenital cholesteatoma with other anomalies. *Arch Otolaryngol* 1975;101:498–505.

PART VI

Surgery for Sensorineural Hearing Loss

CHAPTER 26

Surgery for Sensorineural Hearing Loss: Perilymph Fistula

Steven D. Rauch

Simply put, perilymphatic fistula is an abnormal communication between the perilymphatic space of the inner ear and the pneumatized space of the middle ear. There is abundant evidence that this condition can occur due to head trauma and barotraumas or as a complication of stapedectomy for otosclerosis. Furthermore, there is general consensus among otologists that a spontaneous fistula can be produced by a Valsalva maneuver or sudden increase in intracranial pressure, with symptoms identical to the traumatic or barotrauma cases. Such patients present with fluctuating, progressive sensorineural hearing loss (SNHL), episodic vertigo, dysequilibrium, tinnitus, and aural pressure or fullness, symptoms virtually indistinguishable from Meniere's syndrome. There is an unproven underlying assumption that sudden volume shift of perilymph from the inner ear into the middle ear via a disrupted stapediovestibular ligament or round window membrane causes some undefined inner ear injury that results in the symptoms. In recent years, controversy has arisen concerning the possibility of chronic perilymph leakage via microfissures in the otic capsule or occult intermittent leakage via the oval or round window. These present with "atypical" constellations of signs and symptoms, such as chronic imbalance without hearing loss or sudden hearing loss without vertigo. Proponents of this idea have offered no convincing explanation of the mechanism by which such occult leaks might produce symptoms.

A reliable way of diagnosing a perilymphatic fistula has yet to be developed. The standard of practice is to explore the ear surgically, place soft tissue patches in the oval and round window niches, and observe the patients for evidence of improvement in symptoms. Because there is no preoperative method to confirm the diagnosis and no objective method to measure the patients' symptoms of vertigo postoperatively, there is tremendous potential for abuse of this procedure by applying it to any patient with sudden hearing loss or imbalance of undetermined etiology. Hopefully, a thorough understanding of the physiology and biophysics of the inner ear will lead to rational management of patients with presumed perilymphatic fistula and to avoidance of unnecessary surgery.

This chapter covers the topics that bear directly on our understanding of perilymphatic fistula, including conceptual history, clinical presentation, diagnosis, and management.

CONCEPTUAL HISTORY OF PERILYMPHATIC FISTULA

Stapedectomy Experience

The concept of perilymphatic fistula (PLF) as a cause of hearing loss and imbalance has evolved slowly over the last 30 to 40 years. In 1962 Farrior (1) first described a postsurgical PLF as a complication of polyethylene tube stapedectomy, stating, "The polyethylene strut placed over the mobilized footplate may gradually work its way into the inner ear so that the perilabyrinthine fluid escapes submucosally up the polyethylene tube. The perilabyrinthine fluid may escape all the way to the incus, producing submucosal blebs and resultant separation of the incus and polyethylene strut." Subsequently, Steffen et al. (2) described "slipped strut syndrome" following stapedectomy. They found 24 of 52 cases (46%) explored for drop in hearing to have PLF, "usually in the nature of perilymph ascending through the lumen of the tube." In 1967 Harrison et al. (3) brought attention to the vestibular component of PLF in their report of 46 cases of PLF confirmed by surgical exploration for revision of stapes surgery. According to Harrison et al. (3), "The symptoms in the proven cases are so similar to those of labyrinthine hydrops that it makes the differential diagnosis very difficult, if not impossible." They observed vertigo in 35%, tinnitus in 28%, fluctuating progressive hearing loss in 87%, imbalance in 39%, and fullness or aural pressure in 35% of patients with surgically confirmed fistulas. Their surgical findings included:

a punched out funnel-shaped or round hole in a pliable membrane, to a crescent-shaped opening conforming to the semicircular shape of the beveled cut end of the polyethylene prosthesis. A slit-like opening was often observed after the stainless steel wire with Gelfoam or fat graft techniques. The perilymph escaped freely in a few cases with continued rapid refilling of the oval window niche, while in others the perilymph could be seen to pulsate and slowly seep through passages not clearly defined (3).

Their results state that "prognosis for hearing improvement after fistula repair is guarded at best. Only 11 patients (24%) achieved a practical level of 30 dB or better after fistula repair" (3). They conclude that "those patients with a definite sudden onset of symptoms of moderate severity explored early had the best prognosis. Those explored and repaired after symptoms had been present over a long period of time did not obtain good results" (3). In addition to post-surgical PLF, several groups noted congenital PLF in the region of the stapes (4–8). In all these cases the patients presented with recurrent meningitis or frank cerebrospinal fluid (CSF) otorrhea.

Membrane Breaks

A major conceptual advance in understanding the role of hydrodynamics in damage to the inner ear was the theory of membrane breaks in sudden hearing loss proposed by Simmons (9). In this landmark paper, he reviewed animal work by Lawrence and McCabe (10), in which intense sound caused disruption of Reissner's membrane, and his own demonstration in cats of intracranially applied endolymphatic duct pressure causing sudden loss in electrical activity of the ear without signs of dysequilibrium (11). He also reported 15 clinical cases meeting specific criteria:

1) Each could document exactly when the loss occurred. 2) Each had previously normal hearing in that ear and (with two exceptions) had a negative history for any auditory disorder other than childhood otitis. 3) None had vertigo associated with his sudden hearing loss or developed dizziness subsequently. 4) None had a history or physical examination positive for recent respiratory infection, cardiovascular disease, diabetes, or other serious systemic disease (11).

He noted that prognosis for recovery is strongly correlated with time of initial examination. Specifically, "If a patient was examined less than two days after hearing loss, likelihood of recovery (regardless of therapy) was about 50%. By three weeks, chance for recovery was about 5%. Almost no one seen later than two months recovered their hearing completely. No patient over 45 years of age recovered their hearing" (9).

Perilymphatic Fistula Following Head Trauma

Fee (12) gave the first report of PLF resulting from head trauma in patients with otherwise normal ears. Based on his three cases, Fee (12) stated that the "most common combination of presenting complaints resembles the syndrome of labyrinthine hydrops and tinnitus, fluctuating hearing loss, fullness, and vertigo. Less commonly, the patient will complain of sudden hearing loss, popping, gurgling, or a sensation of sudden linear movement." He stated that audiometric findings in traumatic PLF are consistent with hydrops, showing low-tone SNHL progressing to flat loss. Discrimination scores fluctuate initially and then drop disproportionately low. Reduced discrimination may be the only audiometric finding in a patient with primarily vestibular symptoms. He observed that the "most consistent labyrinthine finding, regardless of the presenting complaint, is a direction fixed positional nystagmus usually directed toward the affected ear when it is lowermost. A canal paresis in response to caloric stimuli is usually present early in the course of fistula" (12). He recommends exploration of any ear with persisting positional vertigo and hearing loss following trauma, regardless of whether the hearing loss was conductive or sensorineural.

Spontaneous Perilymphatic Fistula

Stroud and Calcaterra (13) were the first to propose spontaneous oval window PLF. A summary of clinical features in their four cases suggests significant similarity to Meniere's disease. However, age of onset was younger than typically seen in Meniere's; three fourths of cases began with an episode of increased intracranial or venous pressure such as bending over, laughing, or singing; and all cases showed predominantly high frequency hearing loss with disproportionate decrease in discrimination, in contrast to the low-tone loss often seen in early Meniere's. All cases showed progressive canal paresis on caloric testing, consistently negative fistula test with pneumatic otoscope, and no positional nystagmus above and beyond that already present spontaneously in some patients. They postulated that, unlike Simmon's presumption of inner ear membrane rupture, patients with increased intracranial pressure will transmit it equally to all membranous compartments of the inner ear, resulting in a pressure gradient across the stapediovestibular ligament or round window membrane leading to rupture and perilymph leakage. According to Stroud and Calcaterra (13), "If a congenital weakness of the mucoendosteal articulation of stapes footplate and vestibular fenestra were combined with a rapid equilibration system between the cerebrospinal fluid space and the perilymphatic space, it would be easy to explain how transient rises in intracranial pressure could occasionally produce perilymph fistulas." They go on to say,

Although the incidence of spontaneous perilymph fistula is completely unknown, we suspect that it occurs only rarely. If this were commonly to mimic Meniere's disease, it most certainly would have been discovered during the many thousands of destructive labyrinthine operations. It is possible that these leaks occur intermittently, and the fistulas heal over between attacks of symptoms (13).

Perilymphatic Fistula Following Exertion

Goodhill (14) presented three cases of oval and/or round window perilymphatic fistulas resulting from exertion. All presented with sudden hearing loss. Some had immediate or delayed vertigo, and some had no vestibular symptoms. Goodhill (14) advanced the now famous theory of implosive and explosive membrane rupture routes. The explosive route transmits increased intracranial pressure to the perilymphatic space via a patent cochlear aqueduct or internal auditory canal and cribrose area, resulting in rupture of the stapediovestibular ligament or round window membrane and perilymph volume shift into the middle ear. The implosive route transmits increased air pressure (e.g., Valsalva maneuver) from the nasopharynx via the eustachian tube and middle ear to the round and oval windows, with resultant membrane rupture driving air into the inner ear and displacing perilymph into the middle ear. Goodhill (14) concludes, "Where there is a distinct exertion history, and where spontaneous improvement is not observed at bed rest, exploratory tympanotomy and careful search for an oval window or round window rupture may be indicated." In this theory, as in explanations of PLF after trauma or stapedectomy, there is an assumption of perilymph volume shift from the inner ear to the middle ear (with or without pneumolabyrinth) to account for hearing loss or imbalance.

A variety of basic science studies have been undertaken that bear directly on the validity of Goodhill's theory of explosive rupture of the round window membrane or stapediovestibular ligament. Anatomic studies of human cochlear aqueduct patency have observed variable patency with a general trend to progressive soft tissue occlusion of the aqueduct lumen with increasing age (15–19). Jackler and Hwang (20) emphasized that previous reports identifying a dilated cochlear aqueduct as a possible explanation for PLF have only assessed configuration of the medial end of the aqueduct. Their more thorough evaluation of the radiographic anatomy looked at the diameter of the different segments in computed tomography (CT) scans of 100 ears. The medial end is highly variable in dimension. The portion that traverses the wall of the otic capsule was so small, however, that it was only radiographically identifiable in 56% of cases and never exceeded 2 mm in diameter. Others have studied the pressure relationships between intracranial and perilymphatic spaces (21–27). In cases of wide open disruption of stapediovestibular ligament or round window membrane, it is conceivable that there is a volume shift of perilymph from inner ear to middle ear associated with increased intracranial pressure. However, the pressure transfer function across the inner ear should be markedly mitigated by the narrowness of the vestibular and cochlear aqueducts in most patients.

Perilymphatic Fistula and Microfissures

Okano et al. (28) noted microfissures in the region of the oval window in 25% of temporal bones by age 10 years, with a sharp increase in the number of fissures up to age 40 years.

They consider these and round window microfissures to be normal developmental structures. Harada et al. (29) proposed nontraumatic mechanical stress fractures as the explanation for these microfissures. Not all authors believe that significant sudden perilymph volume shift is a requisite occurrence to produce clinical symptoms. Kamerer et al. (30) report four cases of sudden hearing loss with variable degrees of dysequilibrium or vertigo attributed to microfissure PLF. They described the representative intraoperative finding to be gradual accumulation of clear fluid in one of the windows despite repeated suctioning. Relative to the studies on patency of cochlear and vestibular aqueducts and pressure relationships between intracranial and inner ear compartments listed earlier, it is improbable that significant sudden volume shift of perilymph can occur via a microfissure. That being the case, there remains no convincing explanation of the mechanism of vertigo or hearing loss in these cases.

CLINICAL FEATURES OF PERILYMPHATIC FISTULA

As mentioned earlier, the clinical features of classical PLF occurring after head trauma, stapedectomy surgery, or barotrauma are virtually indistinguishable from those of Meniere's disease. Singleton et al. (31) tabulated clinical features of a large number of surgically confirmed PLF cases and used discriminant-analysis statistical methods to identify and rank the features most useful in differentiating PLF from other causes of dizziness and hearing loss. Trauma and sudden symptom onset were the two most important aspects of the history. Reduced speech discrimination was the most important audiometric variable. Salient findings on electronystagmography included positive fistula test, canal paresis on the affected side, and positional nystagmus different from the classic benign paroxysmal type. Specifically, the positional nystagmus, usually with the affected ear down, had little or no latency, was less violent than in benign paroxysmal positional vertigo, had long duration, fatigued slowly or not at all, rarely reversed direction on returning to upright position, had unpredictable direction relative to the affected ear, and was only occasionally rotatory. Singleton (32) described a new clinical test, the "eyes-closed turning test," that he observed to have a greater positive predictive value than any other clinical feature. In this test the patient was instructed to walk a straight line with eyes closed and, on command, to stop short, turn 180 degrees right or left, and stand still with feet together (Romberg position). The test was considered positive if the patient was unable to maintain stable posture after turning toward the affected ear, a finding in 23 of 26 patients tested. Singleton treated his patients with 5 days of strict bed rest. Surgery was reserved for those who failed conservative treatment and was accomplished with perichondrial graft and Gelfoam packing. Excepting infrequent graft failures, all patients had relief of vertigo but rarely had recovery of hearing.

Clinical Predictors of Perilymphatic Fistula

Shott and Pensak (33) have enumerated the clinical situations in which PLF should be considered:

1. Hearing loss preceded by trauma (head trauma, barotraumas, or penetrating ear trauma)
2. New onset SNHL in a child with craniofacial anomalies
3. Fluctuating or progressive hearing loss
4. New onset hearing loss in an only hearing ear
5. Progressive hearing loss in patients with CT-documented inner ear anomalies
6. History of recurrent meningitis or labyrinthitis
7. New onset SNHL in a child with other sensory impairments (e.g., blindness)
8. Unexplained vestibular or balance abnormalities with or without hearing loss

Several large series of clinical cases have been reported.

Surgical Series of Perilymphatic Fistula

Seltzer and McCabe (34) reported the University of Iowa experience with 214 exploratory tympanotomies in 177 patients with suspected PLF. Every possible combination of hearing loss, tinnitus, and vertigo was represented in the study group, and the authors do not define their indications for exploration of these particular patients. Including some surgeries for recurrent PLF, they report 132 surgically confirmed PLFs in 91 of 177 patients (51%) and 93 (49%) negative explorations. Twenty (22%) of the patients with negative explorations went on to have sac surgery for presumed endolymphatic hydrops. Slightly more than half of PLFs were at the oval window. Of those with PLF, 26% had a history of prior ear surgery (stapedectomy and other), 23% experienced trauma (barometric, acoustic, head injury, or blow to the ear), 12% had exertion, 10% had congenital anomalies, 4% had URI, 1% had congenital syphilis, and 24% were idiopathic. Of 61 PLF patients tested, 22 (36%) had a positive fistula test at initial presentation. Results of fistula testing in the PLF-negative ears was not reported. With regard to outcome of surgery, those patients with vestibular symptoms had complete resolution in 53%, improvement in 41%, and no change in 6%; overall a benefit in 94% was shown. Hearing outcome was at least a 10-dB improvement in 49%, but improvement to the serviceable range (SRT less than 35 dB, discrim greater than 80%) was shown in only 23%. Hearing was stabilized in 40% and worse in 11%.

Shelton and Simmons (35) reported the Stanford University experience with 78 exploratory tympanotomies in 65 patients suspected of PLF. Indications for exploration included Meniere's symptoms; fluctuating, sudden, or progressing SNHL; and various balance disturbances exacerbated by exertion or increased intracranial/intrathoracic pressure. Explorations were scored "positive" for PLF if two observers confirmed clear fluid accumulation despite repeated aspirations. All "maybe" and "possibility" cases

were excluded. These are by far the most stringent intraoperative diagnostic criteria in any published study. No intraoperative maneuvers to increase CSF pressure improved detection. PLF was identified in 51% of patients: two thirds at the oval window and one third at the round window. When audiometric configuration was analyzed, 56% of downward sloping, 50% of flat, 60% of upward sloping, and 50% of normal hearing patients had PLF. Analysis of vestibular symptoms revealed PLF in 58% of patients with spinning, nausea, and vomiting; 50% of those with spinning alone; and 50% of those with postural unsteadiness. In the 47 patients with vestibular dysfunction as the major symptom, 78% had episodic symptoms. Of PLF patients with spinning, nausea, and vomiting, 63% were improved by surgery, 39% of those with spinning only were improved, and 70% of those with postural unsteadiness were improved. Resolution of the major presenting symptom was achieved in 64% of PLF patients. The same success was observed in those who had no PLF noted at surgery. Hearing was stabilized in 50% of PLF patients. Only four patients (6%) had improvement in hearing of at least 20 dB.

Rizer and House (36) reported the House Ear Clinic experience with 86 patients explored for presumed PLF. The primary symptom was hearing loss in 52.3%, dizziness in 46.5%, and tinnitus in 1.2%. Of the 45 patients with hearing loss as the primary complaint, 29 (64%) reported dizziness as a secondary complaint. Thirty-five of 86 patients (40.7%) explored had PLF. All PLFs had fat, fascia, or perichondrium patching. Of 80 patients available for follow-up, 67.7% of PLF cases and 28.6% of non-PLF cases were improved by their own subjective judgment. If no PLF was seen, 26 were patched anyway and 24% reported improvement. In those who received no patch, 33.3% reported improvement. When analyzed by primary symptom, PLF was found in 42% of those with hearing loss and 40% of those with dizziness. Outcome judged by those patients showed 48% with primary hearing loss felt improved and 40% of those with primary dizziness felt improved. By objective measurement, only 18.7% of patients had hearing improvement and 12% had significant decline. However, the authors did not separate results for those with and without PLF. The authors concluded that it is difficult to justify exploration for PLF when the primary symptom is hearing loss, that prophylactic repair when no PLF is seen did not affect outcome, and that preoperative testing was of no help in predicting intraoperative findings.

In summary, the archetypical PLF patient presents with episodic vertigo and stepwise progressive SNHL accompanying each attack of vertigo. The attacks are precipitated by episodes of increased intrathoracic or intracranial pressure, such as heavy lifting, straining, or sneezing. However, patients with PLF can present with virtually any combination of SNHL and vertigo or imbalance. The best predictor of the presence of PLF is a history of prior stapedectomy, barotraumas, or head trauma. However, the absence of any of these historical features does not exclude the possibility of PLF. In those patients with vestibular symptoms, between 50% and 80% will have subjective improvement after surgical patching of the oval and round windows (compared with roughly the same benefit for those in whom no PLF is observed intraoperatively). Up to 20% of PLF patients may achieve improved hearing, and approximately 50% will get stabilization of a fluctuating or progressive loss following surgical intervention.

DIAGNOSIS OF PERILYMPHATIC FISTULA

Vestibular Testing

Many authors have lamented the lack of a reliable preoperative diagnostic workup for PLF. Patients are expected to have audiometric evidence of sensorineural hearing loss in the affected ear. Electronystagmography may show spontaneous or positional nystagmus or caloric asymmetry in perhaps 50% to 75% of cases. As noted earlier, the classic fistula test, in which eye movements are monitored while positive and negative pressure is administered to the ear canal, is neither sensitive nor specific.

Several lines of investigation have tried to improve diagnostic accuracy. Black et al. (37) described a variation of the traditional fistula test performed on a posturography platform. They found surgically confirmed PLF in 73 of 75 (97%) patients with abnormal platform fistula testing. This compares favorably with other vestibular tests showing PLF confirmation in 50% of patients with abnormal bithermal calorics, 30% with rotation abnormalities, 61% with abnormal Hallpike position tests, and 70% with abnormal posturography. However, others have not found this degree of sensitivity or specificity (38). It is possible that the rhythmic sinusoidal application of ear canal pressure for the fistula test results in a concomitant "phase-locked" sway that gives false-positive test results.

Bhansali et al. (39) created a cat model of PLF by inserting a ventilating tube into the round window membrane of three animals. In the early postoperative period all three animals showed evidence of acute unilateral vestibulopathy, with gait instability, head tilt, spontaneous nystagmus, and changes in vestibuloocular reflex on rotation testing. In two of the three cats, all vestibulospinal responses and caloric testing were normal within 1 week of surgery and rotation testing was normal by 2 weeks after surgery. One animal had markedly slower recovery and upon surgical reexploration of all three animals at 2 weeks after fistulization was noted to have brisk perilymphatic leakage, compared with intermittent and slight leakage in the two recovered animals. Histopathologic evaluation of the animals' temporal bones demonstrated a substantially larger cochlear aqueduct in the cat with persistent leakage. This work showed that intubation of the round window membrane in cats was an effective model of PLF. However, objective measures of vestibular function rapidly returned to normal despite persistent patency of the fistula.

Wall and Casselbrant (40) have used chinchillas to study the relationship between vestibuloocular reflex and inner ear fistulas. They compared electrooculographic tracings in animals with fistulas in the round window, oval window, or horizontal semicircular canal. The fistulized animals received a pseudorandom pattern of positive and negative pressure pulses to the ear canal as the test stimulus. The nature of the vestibuloocular reflex (nystagmus) response was highly correlated with the site of fistula. Clinical trials of this systems identification fistula test (SIFT) are currently in progress.

Endoscopy

Poe et al. (41,42) have used mini-endoscopes to perform tympanoscopy in patients with presumed PLF. The endoscopy is performed under iontophoretic anesthesia through a myringotomy. This eliminates any potential misidentification of serum or local anesthetic in the middle ear as perilymph. The prototype endoscopes used for the study have recently become commercially available. They promise to be extremely useful in evaluating potential PLF patients and avoiding unnecessary surgery.

β$_2$-Transferrin Assay

Bassiouny et al. (43) have advanced the work of others to develop a clinically applicable electrophoretic assay of middle ear fluid to try and identify β$_2$-transferrin. Electrophoretic comparison of 4-μl samples of cadaveric perilymph, serum, CSF, and middle ear secretions showed similar results: Both β$_1$- and β$_2$-transferrin bands were present in CSF and perilymph but only the β$_1$ band in serum (44). Weber et al. (45) reported electrophoretically detectable β$_2$-transferrin in fluid samples obtained from 67% of nine pediatric cases of PLF. In a follow-up study, Weber et al. (46) found β$_2$-transferrin in 26% of 23 pediatric PLF patients. This same study also found β$_2$-transferrin in 10% of 20 cases with anatomic middle ear anomalies but no observable PLF.

As greater experience has been gained with electrophoretic assay for β$_2$-transferrin, early successes have given way to less encouraging results. Skedros et al. (47) noted an assortment of technical factors that may introduce error into the β$_2$-transferrin assay. These include sample collection, delivery, and extraction factors; assay factors; physician-related factors; and patient-related factors. More recently, Levenson et al. (48) reported negative β$_2$-transferrin assay results in 85% of 13 perilymph samples obtained during cochlear implantation and stapedectomy. Likewise, Buchman et al. (49) found β$_2$-transferrin in only 5% of 20 inner ear fluid samples obtained during cochlear implantation or translabyrinthine removal of acoustic neuroma. Rauch (50), using a microelectrophoretic assay, found no β$_2$-transferrin in 20 inner ear fluid samples obtained during stapedectomy or cochlear implantation. Unequivocal confirmation of the presence of perilymph in the middle ear may enable correlation with other preoperative diagnostic studies to eventually develop a reliable noninvasive workup.

Electrocochleography

Electrocochleography (EcochG) to measure the ratio of summating and compound action potentials (SP/AP ratio) has been proposed as a diagnostic study for endolymphatic hydrops, as well as for PLF. Arenberg et al. (51) reported guinea pig experiments showing abnormal EcochG only if there was active PLF with volume shift of perilymph out of the inner ear or if hydrops developed. They also reported a finding of abnormal EcochG in 14 of 27 patients (51.9%) with surgically confirmed PLF.

Meyerhoff and Yellin (52) reported EcochG results in 39 ears explored for presumed PLF. Ten of 19 ears (52.6%) with normal preoperative SP/AP ratio had surgically confirmed PLF, whereas 16 of 20 ears (80%) with abnormal preoperative SP/AP ratio had PLF. Of these latter 20, 18 (90%) had normal postoperative SP/AP ratio after round and oval window patching. The authors conclude that EcochG is specific for inner ear fluid imbalance but not sensitive at differentiating PLF from other conditions.

Gulya et al. (53) reported results of guinea pig experiments comparing prefistula, postfistula, and postfistula repair EcochG. No EcochG differences were detected in any group. No animals developed hydrops. They conclude that in the guinea pig EcochG does not detect creation, healing, or repair of PLF.

Gibson (54) performed intraoperative EcochG in stapedectomy patients. Opening the oval window produced no changes in SP/AP ratio. However, if perilymph was removed from the oval window, marked changes occurred and could be reversed by raising intrathoracic pressure or otherwise replacing perilymph. He developed an office procedure to measure EcochG with and without increased intrathoracic pressure. He identified 206 patients strongly suspected of PLF based on clinical history and vestibular signs. Using his modified EcochG, 90 patients had an abnormality and 116 did not. Forty-six patients with abnormal EcochG were explored, and 38 (82%) had confirmed PLF. Thirty-two patients with normal EcochG were explored, and 10 (30%) had confirmed PLF. He concludes that the raised intrathoracic pressure modification of EcochG may be a useful adjunct to diagnosis. Likewise, Sass et al. (55) noted that transtympanic EcochG in PLF showed enhanced SP/AP ratio as seen in Meniere's disease, but PLF patients had EcochG responses that varied with intrathoracic pressure, whereas patients with Meniere's disease showed no such dependence.

In summary, there is no reliable gold standard for diagnosis of PLF. Currently, the best predictors are aspects of the history combined with corroborative evidence of hearing loss or vestibular system dysfunction. Perhaps future development of middle ear endoscopy, β_2-transferrin assay, and, ultimately, noninvasive vestibular testing paradigms will eventually define a sensitive, specific, reliable means of diagnosing this disorder.

MANAGEMENT OF PERILYMPHATIC FISTULA

Medical Management

Though controversy abounds in the area of PLF diagnosis, there is virtually none in the area of treatment. Treatment of suspected PLF in which diagnosis is doubtful or symptoms minimal consists of a trial of bed rest with head elevation and avoidance of any Valsalva maneuver (such as by bending, lifting, straining, or nose blowing). Stool softeners are indicated for patients prone to constipation. Duration of this treatment is empirical. Recommendations ranging from 48 hours to 12 weeks have been proposed (31,32,56–58). Because stapedectomy surgery creates an obvious large PLF and patients heal well with 18 to 24 hours of bed rest and 2 weeks of restricted bending, lifting, and straining, this seems a reasonable protocol for other causes of PLF as well.

Surgical Management

Patients with recurrent symptoms after conservative treatment by bed rest and reduced activity and those with severe or progressive symptoms require surgery. Transcanal exploratory tympanotomy with soft tissue patching of the oval and round window niches is the standard of care. Though a free fat graft is often adequate, many cases of failed fat grafts have been reported, leading most otologists to favor perichondrium or temporalis muscle fascia as more durable alternatives. Surgery can be performed under either general anesthesia or local anesthesia with intravenous sedation. If mini-endoscopes are available, transtympanic endoscopy should be performed prior to elevation of the eardrum to search for evidence of perilymph leakage before the field is contaminated with local anesthetic or serum. Patients can be placed in Trendelenburg position and large positive airway pressures delivered to try inducing perilymph flow into the middle ear. If perilymph leakage is identified, the mucosa surrounding the niche is stripped or lasered away and the perichondrial or fascial graft applied. Absorbable gelatin sponge (Gelfoam) is used to cover the grafts and hold them in place. The eardrum is then returned to its original position and the canal packed lightly. Postoperative care is the same as that described earlier for stapedectomy. In many cases, no perilymph leakage is observed intraoperatively. In such cases, some otologists forego patching. However, the majority will patch both oval and round windows in the case of a negative exploration based on the fact that the small risk of the patch is far outweighed by the potential risk of failing to repair an occult leak (56).

REFERENCES

1. Farrior JB. Abstrusse complications of stapes surgery. In: Schuknecht HF, ed. *International Symposium on Otosclerosis.* Boston: Little Brown, 1962;509–521.
2. Steffen TN, House HP, Sheehy JL. The slipped strut problem. A review of 52 cases. *Ann Otol Rhinol Laryngol* 1963;72:191–205.
3. Harrison WH, Shambaugh GE Jr, Derlacki EL, et al. Perilymph fistula in stapes surgery. *Laryngoscope* 1967;77:836–849.
4. Skolnick EM, Ferrer JL. Cerebrospinal otorrhea. *Arch Otolaryngol* 1959;70:795–799.
5. Barr B, Wersäll J. Cerebrospinal otorrhea with meningitis in congenital deafness. *Arch Otolaryngol* 1965;81:26–28.
6. Bennett RJ. On subarachnoid-tympanic fistulae. A report of two cases of the rare indirect type. *J Laryngol Otol* 1966;80:1242–1252.
7. Crook JP. Congenital fistula in the stapedial footplate. *South Med J* 1967;60:1168–1170.
8. Rice WJ, Waggoner LG. Congenital cerebrospinal fluid otorrhea via a defect in the stapes footplate. *Laryngoscope* 1967;77:341–349.
9. Simmons FB. Theory of membrane breaks in sudden hearing loss. *Arch Otolaryngol* 1968;88:41–48.
10. Lawrence M, McCabe B. Inner-ear mechanics and deafness: special consideration of Meniere's syndrome. *JAMA* 1959;171:1927–1932.
11. Simmons FB, Mongeon CJ. Endolymphatic duct pressure produces cochlear damage. *Arch Otolaryngol* 1967;85:143–150.
12. Fee GA. Traumatic perilymph fistulas. *Arch Otolaryngol* 1968;88:477–480.
13. Stroud MH, Calcaterra TC. Spontaneous perilymph fistulas. *Laryngoscope* 1970;80:479–487.
14. Goodhill V. Sudden deafness and round window rupture. *Laryngoscope* 1971;81:1462–1474.
15. Anson BJ, Donaldson JA, Warpeha RL, et al. The vestibular and cochlear aqueducts: their variational anatomy in the adult human ear. *Laryngoscope* 1965;75:1203–1223.
16. Palva T, Dammert K. Human cochlear aqueduct. *Acta Otolaryngol* 1969;[Suppl 246]:1–58.
17. Rask-Andersen H, Stahle J, Wilbrand H. Human cochlear aqueduct and its accessory canals. *Ann Otol Rhinol Laryngol* 1977;86[Suppl 42]:1–16.
18. Wlodyka J. Studies on cochlear aqueduct patency. *Ann Otol Rhinol Laryngol* 1978;87:22–28.
19. Carlborg B, Densert B, Densert O. Functional patency of the cochlear aqueduct. *Ann Otol Rhinol Laryngol* 1982;91:209–215.
20. Jackler RK, Hwang PH. Enlargement of the cochlear aqueduct: fact or fiction? *Otolaryngol Head Neck Surg* 1993;109:14–25.
21. Kerth JD, Allen GW. Comparison of the perilymphatic and cerebrospinal fluid pressures. *Arch Otolaryngol* 1963;77:581–585.
22. Beentjes BIJ. *On the pressure of the endolymphatic, the perilymphatic and the cerebrospinal fluid with data on the endolymphatic membranes.* Amsterdam: North-Holland Publishing, 1970.
23. Densert O, Carlborg B, Stagg J. Pressure-regulating mechanisms in the inner ear. *ORL J Otorhinolaryngol Relat Spec* 1979;40:319–324.
24. Carlborg BI, Farmer JC Jr. Transmission of cerebrospinal fluid pressure via the cochlear aqueduct and endolymphatic sac. *Am J Otolaryngol* 1983;4:273–282.
25. Densert B, Densert O, Erlandsson B, et al. Transmission of square wave pressure pulses through perilymphatic fluid in cats. *Acta Otolaryngol* 1986;102:186–193.
26. Allen GW. Fluid flow in the cochlear aqueduct and cochlea-hydrodynamic considerations in perilymph fistula, stapes gusher, and secondary endolymphatic hydrops. *Am J Otol* 1987;8:319–322.
27. Carlborg B, Farmer J Jr, Carlborg A. Effects of hypobaric pressure on the labyrinth. Cochlear aqueduct patent. *Acta Otolaryngol* 1990;110:386–393.
28. Okano Y, Myers EN, Dickson DR. Microfissure between the round window niche and posterior canal ampulla. *Ann Otol Rhinol Laryngol* 1977;86:49–57.
29. Harada T, Sando I, Myers EN. Microfissure in the oval window area. *Ann Otol Rhinol Laryngol* 1981;90:174–190.
30. Kamerer DB, Sando I, Hirsch B, et al. Perilymph fistula resulting from microfissures. *Am J Otol* 1987;8:489–494.
31. Singleton GT, Post KN, Karlan MS, et al. Perilymph fistulas. Diagnostic criteria and therapy. *Ann Otol Rhinol Laryngol* 1978; 87:797–803.
32. Singleton GT. Diagnosis and treatment of perilymph fistulas without hearing loss. *Otolaryngol Head Neck Surg* 1986;94:426–429.
33. Shott SR, Pensak ML. Perilymphatic fistula. *Ear Nose Throat J* 1992;71:568, 571–572.
34. Seltzer S, McCabe BF. Perilymph fistula: the Iowa experience. *Laryngoscope* 1986;96:37–49.
35. Shelton C, Simmons FB. Perilymph fistula: the Stanford experience. *Ann Otol Rhinol Laryngol* 1988;97:105–108.
36. Rizer FM, House JW. Perilymph fistulas: the House Ear Clinic experience. *Otolaryngol Head Neck Surg* 1991;104:239–243.
37. Black FO, Lilly DJ, Nashner LM, et al. Quantitative diagnostic test for perilymph fistulas. *Otolaryngol Head Neck Surg* 1987;96:125–134.
38. Shepard NT, Telian SA, Niparko JK, et al. Platform pressure test in identification of perilymphatic fistula. *Am J Otol* 1992;13:49–54.
39. Bhansali SA, Cass SP, Benitez JT, et al. Vestibular effects of chronic perilymph fistula in the cat. *Otolaryngol Head Neck Surg* 1990;102:701–708.
40. Wall C III, Casselbrant ML. System identification of perilymphatic fistula in an animal model. *Am J Otol* 1992;13:443–448.
41. Poe DS, Rebeiz EE, Pankratov MM. Evaluation of perilymphatic fistulas by middle ear endoscopy. *Am J Otol* 1992;13:529–533.
42. Poe DS, Rebeiz EE, Pankratov MM, et al. Transtympanic endoscopy of the middle ear. *Laryngoscope* 1992;102:993–996.
43. Bassiouny M, Hirsch BE, Kelly RH, et al. Beta 2 transferrin application in otology. *Am J Otol* 1992;13:552–555.
44. Naiberg JB, Flemming E, Patterson M, et al. Perilymphatic fistula: the end of an enigma? *J Otolaryngol* 1990;19:260–263.
45. Weber PC, Kelly RH, Bluestone CD, et al. Beta 2-transferrin confirms perilymphatic fistula in children. *Otolaryngol Head Neck Surg* 1994;110:381–386.
46. Weber PC, Bluestone CD, Kenna MA, et al. Correlation of beta-2 transferrin and middle ear abnormalities in congenital perilymphatic fistula. *Am J Otol* 1995;16:277–282.
47. Skedros DG, Cass SP, Hirsch BE, et al. Sources of error in use of beta-2 transferrin analysis for diagnosing perilymphatic and cerebral spinal fluid leaks. *Otolaryngol Head Neck Surg* 1993;109:861–864.
48. Levenson MJ, Desloge RB, Parisier SC. Beta-2 transferrin: limitations of use as a clinical marker for perilymph. *Laryngoscope* 1996;106:159–161.
49. Buchman CA, Luxford WM, Hirsch BE, et al. Beta-2 transferrin assay in the identification of perilymph. *Am J Otol* 1999;20:174–178.
50. Rauch SD. Transferrin microheterogeneity in human perilymph. *Laryngoscope* 2000;110:545–552.
51. Arenberg IK, Ackley RS, Ferraro J, et al. ECoG results in perilymphatic fistula: clinical and experimental studies. *Otolaryngol Head Neck Surg* 1988;99:435–443.
52. Meyerhoff WL, Yellin MW. Summating potential/action potential ratio in perilymph fistula. *Otolaryngol Head Neck Surg* 1990;102:678–682.
53. Gulya AJ, Boling LS, Mastroianni MA. ECoG and perilymphatic fistulae: an experimental study in the guinea pig. *Otolaryngol Head Neck Surg* 1990;102:132–139.
54. Gibson WP. Electrocochleography in diagnosis of perilymphatic fistula: intraoperative observations and assessment of a new diagnostic office procedure. *Am J Otol* 1992;13:146–151.
55. Sass K, Densert B, Magnusson M. Transtympanic electrocochleography in the assessment of perilymphatic fistulas. *Audiol Neurootol* 1997;2:391–402.
56. Hughes GB, Sismanis A, House JW. Is there consensus in perilymph fistula management? *Otolaryngol Head Neck Surg* 1990;102:111–117.
57. Davis RE. Diagnosis and management of perilymph fistula: the University of North Carolina approach. *Am J Otol* 1992;13:85–89.
58. Nomura Y. Perilymph fistula: concept, diagnosis and management. *Acta Otolaryngol* Suppl 1994;514:52–54.

CHAPTER 27

Cochlear Implantation and Implantable Hearing Aids

Joseph B. Nadol, Jr.

Since early attempts at experimental electrical stimulation of the auditory nerve in deaf patients (1–3), there have been rapid advances in electrode and processing technology, and three implant systems (Nucleus, Clarion, and Med-El) have been approved by the Food and Drug Administration (FDA) for rehabilitation of individuals with severe to profound sensorineural hearing loss in both ears.

Study of temporal bones from individuals profoundly deaf during life (4) has demonstrated that despite great variability, the mean number of remaining spiral ganglion cells ranges from 28% to 75% of normal, suggesting that an "adequate" number of ganglion cells is available for stimulation in most patients with profound deafness. The most significant determinant of the number of remaining spiral ganglion cells appears to be the cause of deafness. Thus individuals who are deafened by aminoglycoside toxicity generally have a higher individual cell count than those who became deafened from postnatal viral or bacterial labyrinthitis. However, the minimum requisite number of functioning spiral ganglion cells and their optimal distribution within the cochlea are as yet undetermined. Nevertheless, cochlear implantation is a rehabilitative option in the majority of both prelingually and postlingually deafened individuals. Because of the tonotopic arrangement of receptor units within the organ of Corti and the low electrical impedance encountered in the scala tympani, contemporary electrode arrays are designed to be placed into the scala tympani via the round window.

Despite a variety of electrode arrays and strategies for speech processing, all cochlear implants have several elements in common (Fig. 27.1). A microphone, usually at ear level, detects acoustic energy, which is then encoded into an electrical signal by the external sound processor. The electrical stimulus is then transmitted to the implanted electrode array either in the middle ear or inner ear through some form of signal coupler. This may take the form of a direct (percutaneous) or induction-coupled (transcutaneous) system. The most commonly used commercially available implants in the United States are those manufactured by Clarion (Advanced Bionics Corporation) with eight pairs of electrodes and by Nucleus (Cochlear Corporation) with 22 or 24 active electrodes. Both systems employ a transcutaneous signal coupler. The most important difference between sound processors is the use of single-channel versus multichannel strategies. A single-channel processor presents the same information to one or more electrodes, whereas in a multichannel processor each of the implanted electrodes receives a different stimulus based on its position within the cochlea. Both the Clarion and Nucleus devices are multichannel systems capable of a variety of processing strategies.

PREOPERATIVE EVALUATION AND PATIENT SELECTION

At present, cochlear implantation has clinical approval of the FDA for both prelingually and postlingually deafened children and adults.

Clinical Evaluation and Criteria

The first stage of evaluation includes an otologic and audiologic history and examination. Particularly for prelingually deafened individuals, the current preferred form of communication (oral or sign) will be important for evaluating candidacy for implantation. An evaluation of the daily social interaction of the candidate is important to assess the importance and motivation for oral communication. An audiologist, rehabilitation audiologist, and speech language pathologist will be valuable colleagues in this evaluation.

Clinical Auditory Testing and Criteria

All patients should receive a thorough behavioral audiometric examination including pure-tone thresholds and speech discrimination and, if necessary, confirmation by auditory

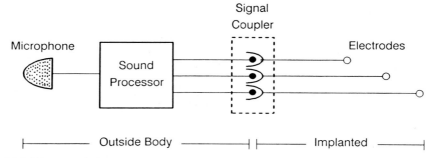

FIG. 27.1 Diagrammatic representation of common elements of a cochlear implant system.

evoked response techniques. In the last several years, the threshold for candidacy for implantation based on audiometric results has been somewhat liberalized to include some patients with severe, as well as profound, sensorineural hearing loss. Individuals with a pure-tone average of greater than 80 dB in the better hearing ear and less than 30% open set speech recognition using sentence materials with the best fitting hearing aids are considered candidates for implantation (5).

Radiologic Evaluation

Computed tomographic (CT) scanning of the temporal bone is useful for several purposes: (i) to determine the pneumatization of the mastoid; (ii) to evaluate the patency of the inner ear—that is, lack of labyrinthitis ossificans; and (iii) to evaluate the possibility of anomalies of the inner ear (6). Obliteration of part or all of the inner ear by new bone formation may occur in certain forms of deafness, particularly that due to bacterial meningitis (7) (Fig. 27.2), and may be detected by CT (8–10) (Fig. 27.3). CT may also be helpful in evaluating patients following cochlear implantation (8). Magnetic resonance imaging (MRI) may also be helpful in evaluating lesions of the inner ear (11).

Psychosocial and Educational Evaluation

Assessment of a patient's motivation for implantation and its subsequent use and the potential effects of surgical success or failure on the patient and his or her family is important. For children, educational plans that include the cochlear implant must be formulated by educators, rehabilitative audiologists, and parents before cochlear implantation.

Informed Consent

In addition to the risks inherent in a mastoidotomy, the patient should be informed of the risks related to the cochlear implant. These include immediate or delayed mechanical or electric failure, infection, or extrusion of the implanted device. Most importantly, the patient should understand that any residual hearing in the operated ear will be lost following insertion of a multielectrode implant and that the hearing

results achieved postoperatively are variable and may not include open set speech comprehension without lip reading. Postoperatively, there may be limitations on the ability to undergo an MRI because postoperative exposure to an MR scan may demagnetize the coupling magnet. Even with a removable magnet as available in the Nucleus device, the implanted electronics may be damaged if the power of the MRI exceeds 1.5 tesla. Hence, postoperative MR scanning is at least relatively contraindicated. Given the hearing status of the patient, a preprinted consent form is useful to ensure comprehension of these important issues.

SURGICAL PROCEDURE

The most commonly used surgical approach for cochlear implantation is the postauricular mastoidotomy and posterior tympanotomy for implantation of the scala tympani via the round window.

Incision and Soft Tissue Flaps

The two most commonly employed incisions are the anteriorly based flap, or Cincision, or a variant of an extended postauricular incision (Fig. 27.4). For the anteriorly based flap, it is essential that the superior limb be 5 cm above the root of the helix and that the inferior limb be 3 cm below the attachment of the lobule to preserve the blood supply from branches of the superficial temporal and the postauricular arteries. The incision should be extended approximately 8 cm posterior to the postauricular crease to be certain that no limb of the incision is in proximity to the eventual location of the signal coupler (percutaneous pedestal or transcutaneous coil). The signal coupler should be located well behind the auricle to prevent interference with eyeglass frames.

Another useful skin incision and skin flap is shown in Fig. 27.4B. The standard postauricular incision is carried 5 to 6 cm above the root of the helix and then extended posteriorly. This incision also results in no incision line over the eventual location of the implanted receiver coil.

The skin flap is then elevated in the plane of the temporalis fascia superiorly and the cervical fascia inferiorly (Fig. 27.5). The lateral mastoid cortex is then exposed. Incisions

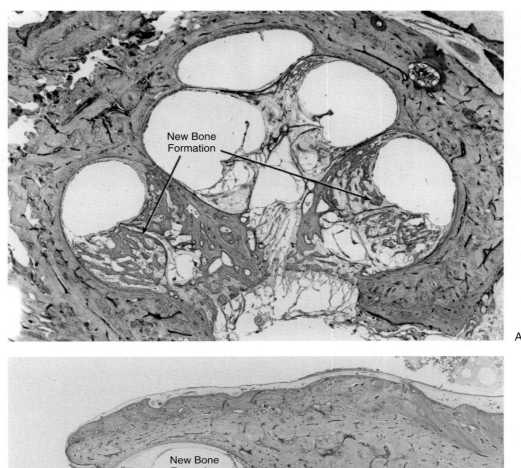

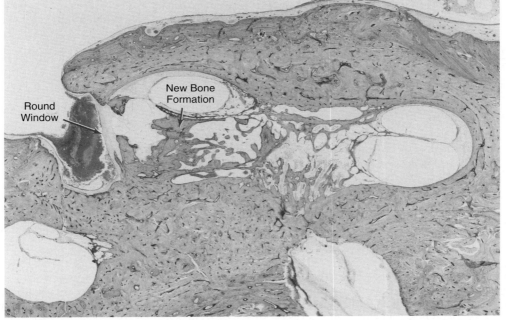

FIG. 27.2 A: Midmodiolar section of the right cochlea in an 84-year-old man who had been profoundly deaf since childhood secondary to bilateral bacterial labyrinthitis. New bone formation is visible, particularly in the scala tympani of the basal turn. **B:** Axial histologic section through the basal turn of the left cochlea from a 70-year-old woman who had been profoundly deaf since childhood secondary to bacterial meningogenic labyrinthitis. New bone formation obstructs the scala tympani at the level of the round window.

through the periosteum are designed in a way to allow a musculoperiosteal layer over the transcutaneous implant, thus helping it to minimize subsequent displacement or extrusion of the implant. The total thickness of the soft tissue coverage over the implanted transcutaneous induction coil should not exceed 6 mm to allow the magnetic coupling between the coil and the external device. Therefore defatting of the cutaneous flap or thinning of the musculoperiosteal fascial flap over the site of the receiver package may be necessary in some patients.

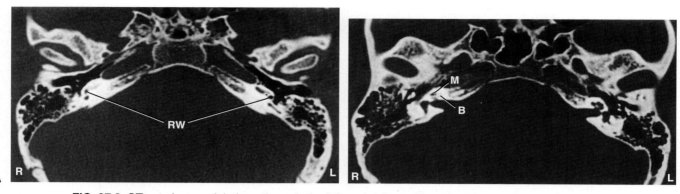

FIG. 27.3 CT cuts in an axial plane through the left and right cochlea of a 26-year-old cochlear implant candidate. **A:** At the level of the round window *(RW)*, the cochlear duct of the basal turn is patent on the left and obliterated by material of bone density on the right. **B:** On a midmodiolar plane, the cochlear duct is patent on the left side, whereas on the right only portions of the middle turn *(M)* appear patent and the basal turn *(B)* is obliterated by bone density.

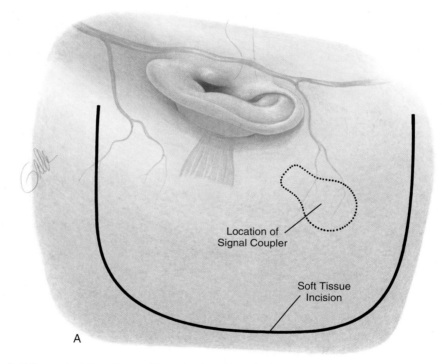

FIG. 27.4 Soft tissue incisions for cochlear implantation. **A:** For the Cincision, the superior limb should be created 5 cm above the attachment of the auricle to preserve branches of the superficial temporal artery. The inferior limb should lie 3 cm below the inferior attachment of the auricle to preserve the postauricular artery. The posterior limb of the Cincision should lie 8 cm posterior to the postauricular crease to be certain that no line of incision will lie across the location of the signal coupler.

Mastoidotomy and Approach to Round Window

A canal wall–up mastoidotomy and posterior tympanotomy are performed (Chapter 17) to provide exposure of the round window niche (Fig. 27.6). The site for the signal coupler is determined and prepared. An inset is created in the lateral mastoid cortex to accommodate the signal coupler. A groove is then developed from the coupler site to the mastoidotomy to accommodate the electrode bundle. The location of the signal coupler should be sufficiently distant from the postauricular crease as to not interfere with eyeglasses and to allow the option of a postauricular ear level signal processing unit. Tie-down holes are created on both sides of the bony inset to allow bony fixation of the signal coupler.

Working through the posterior tympanotomy, the bony overhang of the round window is removed with microdrills.

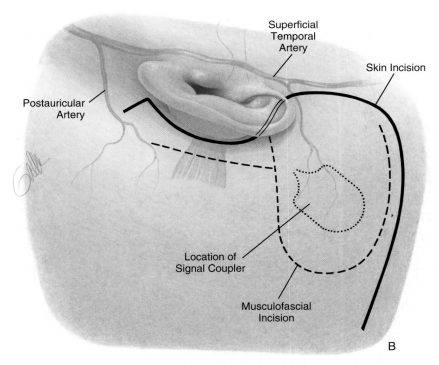

FIG. 27.4, cont'd. Soft tissue incisions for cochlear implantation. **B:** The inverted U incision extends the standard postauricular incision to create a wide inferiorly based pedicle.

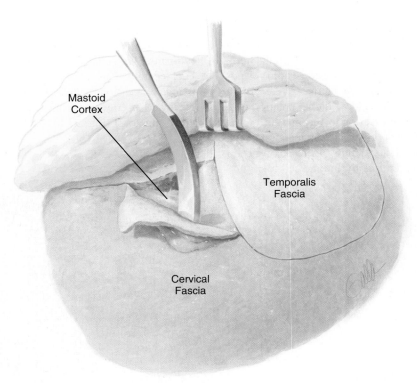

FIG. 27.5 The skin flap has been raised in the plane above the temporalis and cervical fascia. These fascial planes are incised to the level of lateral mastoid cortex to create musculofascial flaps that may be used to cover the signal coupler.

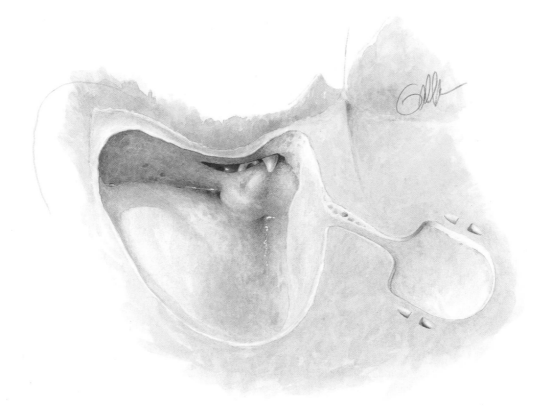

FIG. 27.6 A canal wall–up mastoidotomy and posterior tympanotomy have been performed to expose the round window. The site for the signal coupler is prepared using burs or an end-mill.

An anterior/inferior cochleostomy is created anterior to the round window or by drilling away the anterior bony margin of the round window niche (Fig. 27.7) to straighten the hook portion of the basal turn and provide adequate room for positioning of the electrode and insertional guide. In cases with bony obliteration of the round window niche, creation of a cochleostomy starting 2 mm inferior to the margin of the stapediovestibular joint will approximate the location of the round window and prevent accidental electrode insertion into the hypotympanum and infralabyrinthine cell tract.

The round window membrane and inner periosteum of the anteroinferior cochleostomy are reflected to enter the scala tympani. The electrode array is then inserted into the cochleostomy and gently advanced in an apical direction, using an insertional guide, a rubber-shod alligator, or a claw electrode inserter to prevent damage to the insulation of the electrode array (Fig. 27.8). Although full insertion is desir-

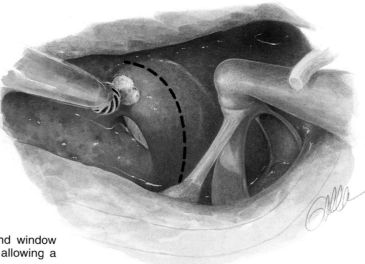

FIG. 27.7 Through the posterior tympanotomy, the round window niche is expanded, particularly anteriorly and inferiorly, allowing a wide cochleostomy.

Scala Tympani

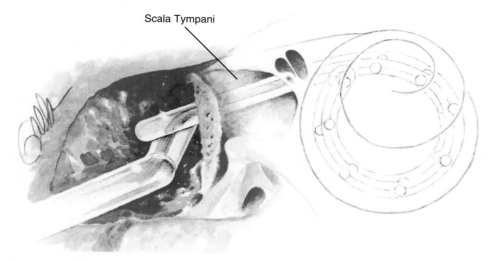

FIG. 27.8 The electrode array is inserted in the scala tympani through the cochleostomy of the basal turn.

able to access the more apical fibers, partial insertion should be accepted when resistance is encountered. The round window and cochleostomy are then sealed with a free fat periosteal or fascial graft placed around the electrode cable.

The signal coupler is then secured using a permanent suture between bony tunnels developed on both sides of the transcutaneous induction coil (Fig. 27.9). An impediment should be created to postoperative migration of the electrode array out of the cochlea. This may be accomplished first by creating some redundancy in the electrode near its exit point from the round window, by securing it to the bony bridge between the aditus ad antrum and posterior tympanotomy using suture material or alternatively by creating a pocket in the mastoid tip covered by the lateral mastoid cortex to take advantage of the natural spring effect of the electrode (see Fig. 27.9).

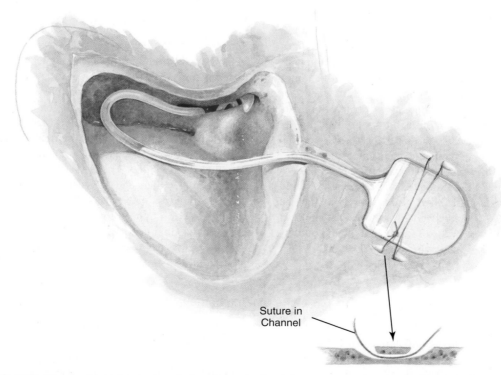

Suture in Channel

FIG. 27.9 The cochlear implant and signal coupler have been placed. The transcutaneous signal coupler is stabilized with two nonabsorbable ties fixed to bone tunnels on both sides of the coupling unit.

Closure

The musculofascial/periosteal flaps are returned to their anatomic position to close the mastoidotomy site in an effort to prevent migration of the electrode and also to provide additional fixation of the implanted signal coupler. The skin incisions are closed in two layers. A Penrose drain is placed at the inferior aspect of the wound, and a standard mastoid dressing is applied. After placement of the cochlear implant, electrocautery should be limited to bipolar technique to avoid an electrical damage to the implanted device. Following skin closure, telemetry is used to verify electrical integrity of the implanted device.

POSTOPERATIVE CARE

Antibiotic prophylaxis begun preoperatively is continued intraoperatively and postoperatively. Postoperative care is identical to that for mastoidotomy. Postoperative electrical testing in preparation for customizing the processor is begun 6 to 8 weeks following implantation.

COMPLICATIONS

The surgical complications are similar to those for mastoidotomy. In addition, meningitis in the perioperative period is a theoretical possibility, but it is rare. Postoperative dizziness may occur, but it is unusual.

Bony Obliteration of Round Window Niche and Scala Tympani

Labyrinthitis ossificans is a common sequela of many of the causes of profound sensorineural hearing loss and hence is a common finding in cochlear implant surgery. Modern algorithms for CT (8) will identify most cases of severe bony obstruction. The surgeon should be prepared to remove minor bony obstruction by use of a microdrill through the facial recess approach. For more severe degrees of obstruction, particularly beyond the first 8 mm of the basal turn, the surgeon should be prepared to modify the insertion technique. The posterior canal wall and tympanic membrane may be removed, converting the exposure to wide-field mastoidectomy. This will allow wide exposure of the promontory and basal and middle turns (12). An electrode array may then be laid into the opened recreated cochlear turns and held in place with overlying free grafts of fascia and fat and obliteration of the tympanomastoid cavity.

Injury to Facial Nerve

The posterior tympanotomy approach requires skeletonizing the fallopian canal. The use of intraoperative electrophysiologic monitoring of facial nerve, polishing or diamond burs, and suction irrigation will minimize this risk. In some patients with high cochlear electrical thresholds to stimulation, electrical stimulation of the facial nerve via the cochlear implant may result in twitching of the face. This may be minimized by placing a small fat graft between the electrode lead and the underlying fallopian canal or by discontinuing stimulation of the offending electrode.

False Insertion of Electrode Array into Hypotympanic Cells and Infralabyrinthine Cell Tract

Labyrinthitis ossificans may totally obliterate the round window niche, thus removing an important landmark for cochleostomy. There have been reports of false insertions of the electrode into the infralabyrinthine cell tract discovered postoperatively by radiography. If the round window is obliterated, beginning a cochleostomy 2 mm anteroinferior to the inferior margin of the oval window niche will result in fenestration of the basal turn. Where there is question about proper placement of the electrode array, intraoperative radiographic confirmation may be helpful.

Late Failure, Extrusion, Migration, or Infection of the Implanted Device

The implant or the system may fail after surgery due to a variety of causes, including electrical malfunction or mechanical injury to the hermetic seal. Migration of the implanted receiver package or electrodes may result in extrusion or infection of the implant, which may require removal of the device.

BONE-ANCHORED AND IMPLANTABLE HEARING AIDS

Bone-Anchored Hearing Aids

Patients with conductive hearing loss that is not otherwise rehabilitated by surgery or hearing aids are candidates for a bone-anchored hearing aid (BAHA) that bypasses the defective external and middle ear structures. Candidates for this device include individuals with congenital malformations of the middle and external ears such as aural atresia, those with chronic active otitis media, and individuals who cannot tolerate conventional air-conduction threshold because of a reaction to the ear mold. The BAHA is contraindicated in patients younger than age 18 years and in individuals with sensorineural loss in excess of 30 dB. Thus patients who are candidates for a conventional bone conduction hearing aid are also potential candidates for the bone-anchored device. Commercially available devices include the BAHA (Nobelpharma) (13).

Implantable Hearing Aids

Implantable hearing aids have recently been approved by the FDA. The theoretical advantages of replacing a conventional ear level hearing aid include elimination of acoustic distortion and feedback and the obvious cosmetic advantage of eliminating an externally visible device. In addition, some patients with chronic dermatologic disorders of the external ear canal cannot tolerate a conventional hearing aid. At present, devices use either an electromagnetic or piezo-ceramic transduction system. In the electromagnetic devices, a magnet is attached to the drum or ossicles and a coil is positioned in proximity to induce a magnetic flux thus moving the attached magnet. The piezo-ceramic devices depend on the fact that the volume of a piezo-ceramic crystal changes when exposed to an electric current. The crystal may be attached to an ossicle to allow in an induced motion. Both classes of devices suffer at least at the current time by limited amplification and the requirement for a surgical procedure to implant them. In addition, the electromagnetic device would theoretically preclude magnetic resonance imaging (14).

REFERENCES

1. Simmons FB, Mongeon CJ, Lewis WR, et al. Electrical stimulation of the acoustical nerve and inferior colliculus: results in man. *Arch Otolaryngol* 1964;79:559–567.
2. Michelson RP. Electrical stimulation of the human cochlea. A preliminary report. *Arch Otolaryngol* 1971;93:317–323.
3. House WF, ed. Cochlear implants. *Ann Otol Rhinol Laryngol* 1976; 85[Suppl 27]:1–93.
4. Nadol JB Jr, Young Y-S, Glynn RJ. Survival of spiral ganglion cells in profound sensorineural hearing loss: implications for cochlear implantation. *Ann Otol Rhinol Laryngol* 1989;98:411–416.
5. Cochlear implants in adults and children. NIH consensus development panel on cochlear implants in adults and children. *JAMA* 1995;274: 1955–1961.
6. Woolley AL, Oser AB, Lusk RP, et al. Preoperative temporal bone computed tomography scan and its use in evaluating the pediatric cochlear implant candidate. *Laryngoscope* 1997;107:1100–1106.
7. Balkany T, Gantz B, Nadol JB Jr. Multichannel cochlear implants in partially ossified cochleas. *Ann Otol Rhinol Laryngol* 1988;97[Suppl 135]:3–7.
8. Ketten DR, Skinner MW, Wang G, et al. In vivo measures of cochlear length and insertion depth of Nucleus cochlear implant electrode arrays. *Ann Otol Rhinol Laryngol* 1998;107[Suppl 175]:1–16.
9. Jackler RK, Luxford WM, Schindler RA, et al. Cochlear patency problems in cochlear implantation. *Laryngoscope* 1987;97:801–805.
10. Balkany TJ, Dreisbach JN, Seibert CE. Radiographic imaging of the cochlear implant candidate: preliminary results. *Otolaryngol Head Neck Surg* 1986;95:592–597.
11. Himi T, Akiba H, Yamaguchi T. Topographic analysis of inner ear lesions in profoundly deafened patients with tympanogenic and meningogenic labyrinthitis using three-dimensional magnetic resonance imaging. *Am J Otol* 1999;20:581–586.
12. Gantz BJ, McCabe BF, Tyler RS. Use of multichannel cochlear implants in obstructed and obliterated cochleas. *Otolaryngol Head Neck Surg* 1988;98:72–81.
13. Tjellström A, Håkansson B. The bone-anchored hearing aid. Design, principles, indications, and long-term clinical results. *Otolarynol Clin North Am* 1995;28:53–72.
14. Hüttenbrink K-B. Current status and critical reflections on implantable hearing aids. *Am J Otol* 1999;20:409–415.

PART VII

Surgery for Vertigo

CHAPTER 28

Labyrinthectomy

Joseph B. Nadol, Jr. and Michael J. McKenna

Unilateral surgical vestibular ablation is an effective treatment for unilateral peripheral vestibular dysfunction in the presence of ipsilateral severe profound sensorineural hearing loss in patients in whom medical management has failed to result in satisfactory control or compensation. Certainly the most common indication for this surgery includes unilateral Meniere's disease. However, the procedure may also be indicated in unilateral peripheral vestibular dysfunction in other disorders, such as posttraumatic or postinfectious labyrinthitis, in which there is no useful cochlear function. The physiologic rationale for peripheral vestibular ablation is based on the fact that compensation for peripheral vestibular dysfunction seems to be more rapid when (i) unilateral vestibular dysfunction is fixed rather than fluctuating and (ii) the absence of unilateral peripheral input to vestibular stimuli is more easily compensated, compared with disordered vestibular input (1).

Unilateral vestibular ablation can be accomplished in a variety of ways, including section of the vestibular or cochleovestibular nerve, transmastoid labyrinthectomy, and transcanal labyrinthectomy. Unilateral eighth nerve section or selective vestibular nerve section was introduced by Dandy (2) in 1928 for Meniere's disease, and transmastoid labyrinthectomy was described by Jansen (3) in 1895 for peripheral vestibulopathy caused by suppurative labyrinthitis. The transmastoid approach was applied to other peripheral vestibulopathies, including Meniere's disease by Milligan (4) and Lake (5) in 1904. Pulec (6) emphasized the importance of total ablation of the peripheral vestibular apparatus, a tenet that has been adopted in modern surgical procedures for unilateral vestibular ablation.

A transcanal approach for a labyrinthectomy was introduced by Lempert (7) using an endaural exposure of the middle ear. A transcanal approach was popularized by Schuknecht (8) and Cawthorne (9). A modification of transmeatal labyrinthectomy with and without cochleovestibular neurectomy was described by Silverstein (10) to be more certain of complete peripheral vestibular ablation. The importance of total surgical ablation was also emphasized by Armstrong (11) and Ariagno (12).

PATIENT SELECTION FOR PERIPHERAL VESTIBULAR ABLATION

The patient's vestibular episodes must be debilitating and ascribable to vestibular dysfunction in one ear, as indicated by preoperative evaluation. Reasonable attempts at medical management, including pharmacologic and rehabilitative measures, must have failed. Hearing loss in the affected ear should be in the severe to profound range, that is, with a pure-tone average of 75 dB or worse and speech discrimination of 20% or less. Particularly in Meniere's disease, in which bilateral involvement may occur in 10% to 40% of patients (13,14), surgical intervention, especially in the form of labyrinthectomy, which will destroy all residual hearing, should be reserved as a last resort. Documentation that the vestibulopathy is debilitating is not always straightforward and depends on a variety of clinical and patient variables that include not only frequency, duration, and severity of vertiginous episodes but also such issues as age and occupation.

Preoperative Evaluation

A thorough history of the vestibular complaint, including severity, duration, frequency of attacks, and contributing factors, should be documented. The nonotologic medical history should clearly document other disorders that may compound the vestibulopathy or interfere with compensation once a labyrinthectomy is performed. These include age, other debilitating disorders, peripheral neuropathies as may be seen in diabetes, cardiac disease, proprioceptive disorders, generalized arthritis, visual disturbances such as cataract, and evaluation of any potential secondary gain. A complete otolaryngologic and head and neck examination should be performed, including a neurotologic examination with evaluation of cranial nerves, cerebellar testing, and office vestibular testing such as Dix-Hallpike maneuver. Behavioral audiometry, including pure-tone thresholds for air and bone conduction and speech discrimination, is essential. A fistula and Hennebert's sign should be sought (15).

Formal vestibular testing should include, as a minimum, bilateral caloric function, preferably documented by electronystagmography. A complete vestibular evaluation using the rotating chair and posturography may give further clues and confirmation that the vestibulopathy may be ascribed to the suspect ear and that there is no evidence of significant bilateral vestibular dysfunction. Imaging may not be necessary in every case. However, given the fact that lesions in the posterior fossa may at times mimic the symptoms of Meniere's syndrome, magnetic resonance imaging (MRI) with gadolinium is useful to rule out the presence of a cerebellopontine angle or other posterior fossa tumor or the presence of demyelinating lesions. Other neurologic dysfunction elicited by history or physical examination should be evaluated by referral to a neurologist. In some patients with Meniere's disease, the caloric function in the affected ear will remain normal or minimally reduced. In such cases, labyrinthectomy may still be justified based on clearly localizing symptoms and signs such as fluctuating severe to profound sensorineural loss, ipsilateral tinnitus, coincidence of unilateral aural symptoms of fullness and tinnitus, and hearing loss concurrent with the vestibular attack. Preoperative vestibular testing is also useful for the purpose of counseling the patient. In general, the more active the caloric response in the affected ear, the more severe the postoperative reaction to labyrinthectomy may be.

In summary, the ideal candidate for a labyrinthectomy is an otherwise healthy patient with clear-cut unilateral vestibular dysfunction and ipsilateral severe to profound sensorineural hearing loss who has failed conventional medical management and has no secondary gain in remaining disabled (16). The entity of delayed endolymphatic hydrops in a previous deafened ear and the presence of Tumarkin drop attacks are generally excellent indications for labyrinthectomy if other patient selection criteria have been satisfied.

Preoperative Counseling of a Patient and Informed Consent

Preoperatively, the patient should be aware of the natural history of Meniere's disease, including spontaneous remission rate of approximately 70% over 8 years (17) and the fact that Meniere's disease may become bilateral in up to 40% of patients (13,14). The patient should be informed that all hearing in the operated ear will be lost, although the potential for cochlear implantation of the labyrinthectomized ear, if bilateral sensorineural loss occurred in the future, may be preserved. The patient should also be aware that tinnitus, which is almost universally present in unilateral Meniere's disease, is not likely to be ameliorated by this procedure. It should be explained that postoperatively the patient, particularly one with relatively intact vestibular function in the affected ear, will suffer a severe and protracted episode of vertigo with nausea and vomiting lasting several days. A prolonged period of disequilibrium, possibly requiring

vestibular physical therapy, may ensue, particularly in patients with contributing factors such as age, obesity, arthritis, visual disturbance, or proprioceptive disorders. A permanent disability in the form of imbalance without vertigo may occur. The patient should be made aware of alternate forms of therapy, both medical and surgical, including those surgical techniques that are designed to preserve residual hearing, such as selective vestibular nerve section or endolymphatic sac decompression, or those surgical procedures that may abate the vestibular symptoms without significant postoperative vestibular morbidity—for instance, round window labyrinthotomy or endolymphatic sac decompression.

Finally, the complications generic to ear surgery, including infection and facial nerve paresis and a failure of the procedure to totally ablate vestibular nerve function, should be discussed with the patient. Particularly for the transmastoid labyrinthectomy, the possible risk of spinal fluid leakage or meningitis and the possible need for free tissue graft, such as abdominal fat, should be outlined. Although less likely with a transmeatal labyrinthectomy, spinal fluid leakage may occur due to anomaly or injury to the cribrose area.

Surgical Technique

For both transcanal and transmastoid labyrinthectomy, general anesthesia is indicated because of the vestibular response that may be anticipated during removal of the vestibular end organs. One possible exception is a patient with poor compensation following labyrinthectomy with documented minimal residual vestibular function. In such cases, the patient's response under local anesthesia may provide intraoperative confidence that residual functional vestibular end organs have been identified.

TRANSCANAL LABYRINTHECTOMY

The patient is placed in the supine position as for stapedectomy or other transcanal procedure. The head is shaved approximately 2 cm around the auricle to allow placement of a fenestrated drape, and antiseptic solution is used to prep the ear. In general, facial nerve monitoring is not required for transcanal labyrinthectomy but is useful for translabyrinthine labyrinthectomy or in a revision labyrinthectomy in which scar tissue may obscure the surgical anatomy in the middle ear around the facial nerve. A standard anterior-based tympanomeatal flap is elevated. In unusual cases with a small external auditory canal or meatus, an endaural or postauricular approach will facilitate exposure. The posterior bony annulus is curetted widely to provide exposure of the horizontal segment of the facial nerve and the entire limits of the round window niche. The chorda tympani may usually be preserved. The incus is removed.

The tendon of the stapedius muscle is sectioned, and using a 1-mm hook, the stapes is removed intact (Fig. 28.1). The oval window is enlarged by drilling away its inferior margin (Fig. 28.2A). This may be extended inferiorly to the level of

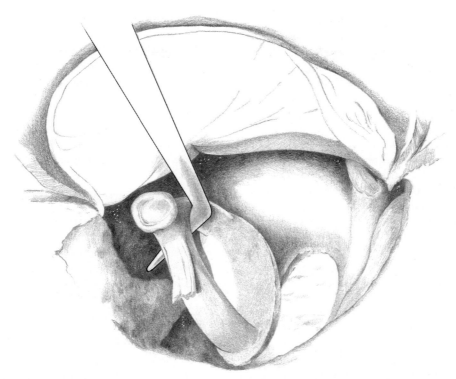

FIG. 28.1 Transcanal labyrinthectomy of the left ear. The tympanomeatal flap is reflected anteriorly, and sufficient tympanic bony annulus is removed to provide a full view of the posterior mesotympanum. The incus is disarticulated and removed. The stapedius tendon is cut, and the stapes is disarticulated from the oval window and removed.

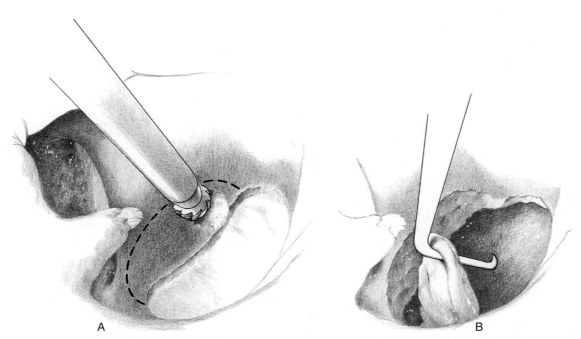

A

B

FIG. 28.2 Left ear. **A:** The oval window can be enlarged by removing bone at its inferior margin utilizing a small cutting or diamond-surfaced bur. **B:** A modified 3-mm right-angled pick is used to engage and remove the utricular macula. The pick shown here features a small hook at its distal tip and is known as a "utricle hook." The saccular macula is then removed by aspiration.

the round window. At a minimum, a 3- to 4- mm right-angled hook should easily be placed in the vestibule. As little of the vestibular perilymph should be aspirated as possible to avoid displacement of the macula utriculi. A suction tip no greater than 24 gauge should be used to avoid inadvertent and unrecognized removal of the utricle. A 3- to 4-mm right-angled hook, a "utricle hook," or a whirlybird may be used to locate and remove the utricle (Fig. 28.2B). The utricle will generally be located posterosuperiorly in the vestibule medial to the horizontal segment of the facial nerve. Care should be exercised with the right-angled instrument to avoid trauma to the medial surface of the facial nerve. It is essential that the utricle be identified and removed. Avulsion of the utricle generally results in simultaneous removal of the ampullae of the superior and lateral semicircular canals but not of the posterior semicircular canal.

Following identification and removal of the utricle, the ampullate ends of the three semicircular canals are probed to ensure destruction of vestibular neuroepithelium of the superior, lateral, and posterior semicircular canals. In addition, the posterior ampullary nerve may be separately identified and sectioned in the floor of the round window niche. In an experimental study of labyrinthectomy, Schuknecht (18) reported that incomplete ablation of the vestibular end organs occurred in 10 of 24 ears and that residual neuroepithelium of the posterior semicircular canal was the most common. Hence, section of the posterior ampullary nerve will enhance the probability of complete peripheral vestibular ablation. Usually the macula sacculi will be removed by aspiration.

Care should be taken to avoid trauma to the medial wall of the vestibule to prevent fracture and spinal fluid leak from the internal auditory canal. After removal and destruction of all five vestibular end organs, the vestibule is filled with absorbable gelatin sponge or a small fat graft taken from the postauricular area or the lobule. Filling the vestibule with an aminoglycoside antibiotic may also be done to ensure ablation of the vestibular end organs. A tissue graft within the vestibule is essential if even a small spinal fluid leak is suspected. The tympanic membrane is then returned to its anatomic location and held in place with rosebud packing.

Postoperative Care

Hospitalization for 1 to several days may be required to manage postoperative vestibular disturbance, nausea, and vomiting. Intravenous fluids may be necessary to maintain hydration. Control of vestibular symptomatology with promethhazine, droperidol, or other vestibular suppressants should be tapered as quickly as possible because prolonged vestibular suppression may interfere with central compensation for unilateral vestibular ablation. Rapid resumption of activity should be encouraged consistent with the safety of the patient. Ambulation with help is generally achieved within the first 2 postoperative days. The patient is discharged from the hospital when self-sufficient but generally before achieving complete vestibular compensation. Postop-

erative outpatient vestibular physical therapy may be necessary in some cases. Maximal vestibular compensation may take many months to achieve.

Packing in the external auditory canal is removed at 1 week, and the patient is seen at monthly postoperative intervals to evaluate progress. A postoperative ice water caloric of the operated ear is advisable after a resolution of any residual spontaneous nystagmus using 20 ml of ice water and Frenzel lenses or electronystagmography to document completion of unilateral vestibular ablation.

TRANSMASTOID LABYRINTHECTOMY

The transmastoid labyrinthectomy provides assurance of complete peripheral vestibular ablation by opening the vestibule and removing the neuroepithelium of the vestibular end organs under direct vision, as described by Graham and Colton (19) and Benecke et al. (20).

Surgical Procedure

The lateral mastoid cortex is exposed via a postauricular incision, and a canal wall–up mastoidectomy is performed. The incus is exposed and removed. The semicircular canals are skeletonized and then opened to identify the three ampullae (Fig. 28.3). The vestibule is opened by extending the drilling through the semicircular canals. The macula utriculi is identified under direct vision and removed, as are the cristae ampullares of the three semicircular canals (Fig. 28.4). The vestibule is aspirated with a 20-gauge French

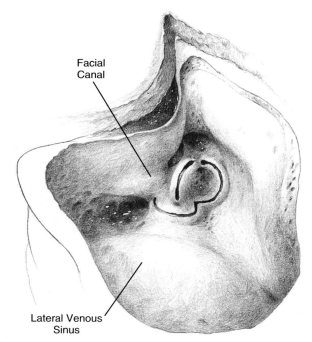

Facial Canal

Lateral Venous Sinus

FIG. 28.3 Transmastoid labyrinthectomy of left ear. A canal wall–up mastoidectomy has been performed and the semicircular canals opened and followed to the vestibule.

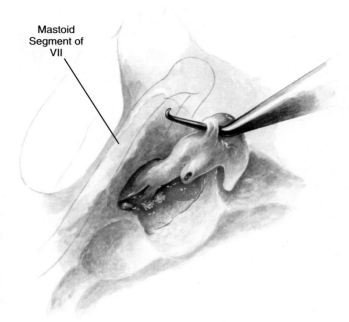

Mastoid
Segment of
VII

FIG. 28.4 Transmastoid labyrinthectomy of left ear. The vestibule has been opened posterior to the mastoid segment of the facial nerve and the utricle and ampullae removed.

suction to ensure that the macula sacculi has been destroyed. The opened vestibule is then packed with Gelfoam soaked in gentamicin or streptomycin solution followed by pledgets of fat to prevent any leakage of spinal fluid from the cribrose area of the vestibule. The postauricular incision is then closed.

TRANSLABYRINTHINE VESTIBULAR NERVE SECTION

The principal indication for this procedure is failure of previous labyrinthectomy either by the transcanal or by the transmastoid approach. The incidence of incomplete labyrinthectomy is less than 5%. Thus Hammerschlag and Schuknecht (21) reported a cure rate of episodic vertigo in 97% of patients operated on by transcanal labyrinthectomy. Likewise, Ariagno reported a success rate of 98% by the transcanal approach modified by joining the oval and round windows (12). However, some authors state that a labyrinthectomy alone is less reliable in completely ablating vestibular function. Thus Linthicum et al. (22) reported a 40% failure rate, which they ascribed to formation of a postoperative traumatic neuroma. The survival of vestibular nerve fibers has been documented in experimental labyrinthectomy in the cat (23). The usual clinical presentation of incomplete unilateral vestibular ablation is failure to compensate following labyrinthectomy, although the acute vestibular attacks of spinning vertigo may disappear completely. In some patients, residual vestibular function may be

documented by caloric testing. However, a vestibular nerve section should be considered in any patient in whom a labyrinthectomy has failed, even in the face of absent caloric responses postoperatively. Before proceeding with a translabyrinthine vestibular nerve section, particularly in the face of absent calorics, the patient's record and clinical finding should be reviewed to rule out other reasons for poor compensation, such as central nervous system disease, proprioceptive and visual defects, bilateral vestibular disease, or secondary gain. A trial of vestibular rehabilitation should be attempted before resorting to this procedure.

Surgical Procedure

The lateral mastoid cortex is exposed through a postauricular incision, and the semicircular canals are skeletonized. A transmastoid labyrinthectomy is performed, and the internal auditory canal is skeletonized. The medial aspect of the vestibule identifies the distal extent of the internal auditory canal. The axis of the internal auditory canal can be visualized by an imaginary line drawn through the external and internal auditory canals of both ears. The distal half of the internal auditory canal is opened (Fig. 28.5). The superior vestibular nerve is identified as distinct from the facial nerve and separated from it by the vertical crest (Bill's bar). The superior and inferior vestibular nerve trunks are resected distally and dissected from the underlying facial and cochlear nerves to be sure of a total vestibular nerve section (Fig. 28.6). Approximately 5 mm of the distal nerve trunk is resected. This will also result in removal of Scarpa's ganglion, preventing regeneration of vestibular nerve fibers.

Following transection and resection of a segment of the vestibular nerve, the internal auditory canal is covered with a free graft of temporalis fascia and the aditus ad antrum and mastoid defect filled with adipose tissue taken as a free graft from the abdominal wall to prevent development of a spinal fluid leak. The mastoid incisions are closed carefully in layers without drainage, and a standard mastoid dressing is applied.

Complications of Translabyrinthine Vestibular Nerve Section

The potential for complications is greater for translabyrinthine vestibular nerve section than for either transcanal or transmastoid labyrinthectomy, principally because of potential damage to the facial nerve and the greater potential for spinal fluid leakage because the subarachnoid space has been open. During the dissection of the vestibular nerve, monitoring and stimulation of the facial nerve will help confirm the location of that nerve. In addition, care should be taken to avoid damage to an intracanalicular loop of the anterior/inferior cerebellar artery. Although the cochlear nerve may be sectioned, there does not appear to be a specific indication to do so unless there is a concern about complete ablation of the inferior vestibular nerve.

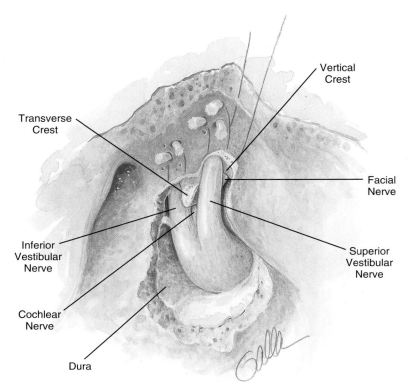

FIG. 28.5 Transmastoid-translabyrinthine vestibular nerve section of left ear. After a canal wall–up mastoidectomy and skeletonization of the semicircular canals has been completed (Fig. 28.3), the internal auditory canal is skeletonized and opened and the superior and inferior vestibular nerves sectioned. The vertical crest (Bill's bar) helps to distinguish the facial nerve from the superior vestibular nerve.

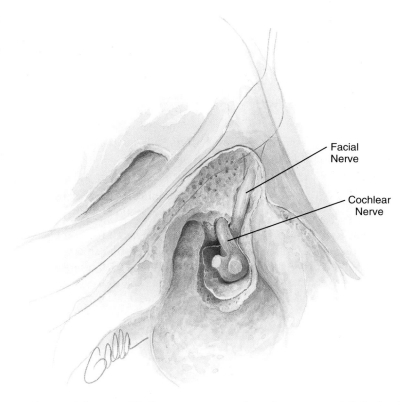

FIG. 28.6 The superior and inferior vestibular nerves are sectioned and 5 mm of their distal segments resected to ensure removal of Scarpa's ganglion.

REFERENCES

1. Stockwell CW, Graham MD. Vestibular compensation following labyrinthectomy and vestibular neurectomy. In: Nadol JB Jr, ed. Second International Symposium on Meniere's Disease. Amsterdam: Kugler & Ghedini Publications, 1989:489–498.
2. Dandy WE. Meniere's disease: its diagnosis and a method of treatment. *Arch Surg* 1928;16:1127–1152.
3. Jansen A. Referat ueber die Opertionsmethoden bei den verschiedenen otitischen Gehirskomplicationen. *Verh Dtsch Otol Ges Jena* 1895;96.
4. Milligan W. Meniere's disease: a clinical and experimental inquiry. *Br Med* 1904;2:1228.
5. Lake R. Removal of the semicircular canals in a case of unilateral aural vertigo. *Lancet* 1904;1:1567–1568.
6. Pulec JL. Labyrinthectomy: indications, technique and results. *Laryngoscope* 1974;84:1552–1573.
7. Lempert J. Lempert decompression operation for hydrops of the endolymphatic labyrinth in Meniere's disease. *Arch Otolaryngol* 1948; 47:551–570.
8. Schuknecht HF. Ablation therapy for the relief of Meniere's disease. *Laryngoscope* 1956;66:859–870.
9. Cawthorne TE. Membranous labyrinthectomy via the oval window for Meniere's disease. *J Laryngol Otol* 1957;71:524–527.
10. Silverstein H. Transmeatal labyrinthectomy with and without cochleovestibular neurectomy. *Laryngoscope* 1976;86:1777–1791.
11. Armstrong BW. Transtympanic vestibulotomy for Meniere's disease. *Laryngoscope* 1959;69:1071–1074.
12. Ariagno RP. Transtympanic labyrinthectomy. *Arch Otolaryngol* 1964; 80:282–286.
13. Greven AI, Oosterveld WJ. The contralateral ear in Meniere's disease. A surgery of 292 patients. *Arch Otolaryngol* 1978;101:608–612.
14. Paparella MM, Griebie MS. Bilaterality of Meniere's disease. *Acta Otolaryngol (Stockh)* 1984;97:233–237.
15. Nadol JB Jr. Positive "fistula sign" with an intact tympanic membrane. *Arch Otolaryngol* 1974;100:273–278.
16. Nadol JB Jr, Weiss AD, Parker SW. Vertigo of delayed onset after sudden deafness. *Ann Otol Rhinol Laryngol* 1975;84:841–846.
17. Silverstein H, Smouha E, Jones R. Natural history versus surgery for Meniere's disease. In: Nadol JB Jr, ed. Second International Symposium on Meniere's Disease. Amsterdam: Kugler & Ghedini Publications, 1989:543–544.
18. Schuknecht HF. Behavior of the vestibular nerve following labyrinthectomy. *Ann Otol Rhinol Laryngol* 1982; 9[Suppl 97]:16–32.
19. Graham MD, Colton JJ. Transmastoid labyrinthectomy indications. Technique and early postoperative results. *Laryngoscope* 1980;90: 1253–1262.
20. Benecke JE Jr, Tubergen LB, Miyamoto RT. Transmastoid labyrinthectomy. *Am J Otol* 1986;7:41–43.
21. Hammerschlag PE, Schuknecht HF. Transcanal labyrinthectomy for intractable vertigo. *Arch Otolaryngol* 1981;107:152–156.
22. Linthicum FH Jr, Alonso A, Denia A. Traumatic neuroma. A complication of transcanal labyrinthectomy. *Arch Otolaryngol* 1979;105: 654–655.
23. Cass SP, Davidson P, Goshgarian H. Survival of the vestibular nerve after labyrinthectomy in the cat. *Otolaryngol Head Neck Surg* 1989;101: 459–465.

CHAPTER 29

Shunt Procedures

Harold F. Schuknecht and Michael J. McKenna

EXTERNAL ENDOLYMPHATIC SHUNT

The external endolymphatic shunt operation purports to alleviate the vertiginous symptoms of Meniere's disease by preventing the accumulation of excess endolymph by shunting it from a presumably incompetent endolymphatic sac to either the subarachnoid space or the mastoid. Ever since Guild (1) presented the theory of longitudinal flow of endolymph toward the endolymphatic sac and Portmann (2) proposed the shunt operation, the procedure has been steeped in controversy. There are strong advocates for shunting, many of whom have devised modifications based on some conceived notion for improving drainage, and there are almost as many skeptics who point out the improbability of achieving drainage by any shunt operation.

Portmann's (2) original procedure consisted of removing part of the lateral wall of the sac, thus exposing the lumen to the mastoid. Yamakawa and Naito (3) modified the method by removing part of the medial wall of the sac to expose its lumen to the subarachnoid space, and House (4) devised a silicone tube that extended from the sac into the subarachnoid space. Subsequently, Shea (5), Paparella and Hanson (6), and many others (7–10), not being enamored of the idea of opening into the subarachnoid space, proposed draining the sac into the mastoid using a variety of tubes or sculptured sheets of plastic material. Arenberg et al. (11) have advocated the use of a unidirectional valve, which is a modification of the valve designed for filtering the anterior chamber of the eye. Brackmann and Nissen (12) could show no significant differences between subarachnoid and mastoid shunts in the control of vertigo, with both procedures reporting a 70% success rate.

The endolymphatic sacotomy procedures have suffered some loss of credibility from the reports of Shambaugh (13) and Larouere and Graham (14) that merely decompressing the sac achieves the same success rate as opening it and the report of Bretlau et al. (15) that sham surgery limited to merely entering the mastoid is as successful as sac drainage procedures.

There are also several histopathologic observations that challenge the rationale of sac drainage procedures: (i) Any device implanted in the sac is almost certain to become encapsulated in fibrous tissue (16), which certainly would compromise its presumed function in promoting drainage. (ii) In some cases the endolymphatic sac is too small to be identified and drained (17). (iii) In some cases the endolymphatic duct is blocked by bone or fibrous tissue, which prevents endolymph from reaching the sac (18). (iv) In many ears the membranous labyrinths are severely distorted by dilation and collapse, causing blockage of longitudinal flow at the ductus reuniens, saccular duct, utricular duct, and sinus of the endolymphatic duct (18).

This preface should alert the reader to some significant flaws in the therapeutic concept of endolymphatic sac shunt procedures. We have used the shunt at the Massachusetts Eye and Ear Infirmary on a limited basis for patients with Meniere's disease who were experiencing intractable and disabling vertigo in the presence of good hearing. The results are similar to the reports of others, that is, approximately 70% of patients are initially relieved of vertigo or are greatly improved. Our enthusiasm has been dampened, however, by the previously mentioned temporal bone findings and the high incidence of delayed postoperative failures.

From perusing reports in the literature, it seems quite clear that shunting into the subarachnoid space does not give better results than shunting into the mastoid and therefore does not warrant the increase in potential morbidity that comes with opening the subarachnoid space. If hearing is useless, it is generally preferable to ablate vestibular function by labyrinthectomy unless the patient is elderly, in which case a cochleosacculotomy may be preferable.

Indications for Endolymphatic Shunt Surgery

Surgical intervention for Meniere's disease should be considered only for patients with disabling episodic vertigo that has failed to respond to medical management. Because endolymphatic shunt surgery is not an ablative procedure, it offers the advantage for potential alleviation of episodic vertigo without the loss of residual vestibular function in the operated ear. For this reason and because of a relatively low incidence of surgically induced sensorineural hearing loss, it is often considered among the best first options for the management of recalcitrant Meniere's disease. These advantages must be weighed against the relatively high failure rate of approximately 30%. Endolymphatic shunt surgery does not preclude other forms of surgical intervention, including labyrinthectomy and selective vestibular neurectomy, if the symptoms of episodic vertigo are not relieved. It is our practice to present patients with a thorough discussion of both endolymphatic shunt surgery and intratympanic gentamycin therapy as the first best options for the management of Meniere's disease that has failed medical management and when the affected ear has serviceable hearing. For intratympanic gentamycin therapy, the advantages are that it can be performed in an outpatient setting without the need for a general anesthetic and that the success rate for the control of vertigo is superior to endolymphatic shunt surgery, in the range of 85% to 90%. The disadvantages of intratympanic gentamycin therapy are that it is an ablative procedure that results in loss of vestibular function in the treated ear and that it has a higher incidence of sensorineural hearing loss, in the range of 10% to 15%. Because endolymphatic shunt surgery is not ablative and has a relatively low incidence of associated sensorineural hearing loss, it may be considered as a viable treatment option for some patients with bilateral Meniere's disease. In rare cases, endolymphatic shunt surgery may be considered in patients with Meniere's disease in an only hearing ear. The indication for surgery in such cases is a progressive disease process with declining sensorineural hearing that has failed all forms of medical management, including immunosuppressive therapy, when it is clear that the active disease process poses a greater risk to hearing than the surgical intervention. Endolymphatic shunt surgery is contraindicated in cases of enlarged vestibular aqueducts or in ears with concurrent active chronic otitis media.

Some patients who have undergone successful endolymphatic shunt surgery may develop a recurrence of symptoms in the operated ear years following surgery. If it is clear that the initial surgery resulted in a significant benefit, many of these patients will benefit from a revision endolymphatic shunt surgery.

Surgical Technique

Prior to endolymphatic saccotomy, an axial computed tomographic (CT) scan of the temporal bone is done to determine if there is sufficient space between the sigmoid sinus and the posterior semicircular canal to permit access to the area of the dura mater in which the sac is located. A separation of at least 3 mm is necessary to identify and enter the sac. Also, the CT scan will show the relationship of the posteromedial cell tract to the endolymphatic sac. This cell tract may lie between the endolymphatic sac and the dura, in which case the sac is surrounded by air cells and does not enter the dura until it reaches the sigmoid sinus. In such cases an unsus-

pecting surgeon may drill through the endolymphatic sac without ever having identified it.

The operation is performed under general anesthesia and normally requires 1 to 1.5 hours operating time. The mastoid is entered via a postauricular approach, and the lateral semicircular canal and incudal fossa are identified. Once exposed, the mastoid antrum is temporarily occluded with a piece of compressed Gelfoam to prevent spillage of bone dust into the middle ear and a resultant conductive hearing loss. The mastoid air cell system is sufficiently exenterated to identify and skeletonize the bony prominence of the sigmoid sinus. Bone is removed anterior to the sigmoid sinus and posterior to the posterior semicircular canal to expose the dura mater (Fig. 29.1). The endolymphatic sac can be identified as a thickened whitish-appearing area of the dura. A no. 11 Bard-Parker knife blade is used to incise the lateral wall of the sac (Fig. 29.2A). A dental excavator is introduced into the sac, and its anatomic configuration and size are explored. An implant of the surgeon's choosing (e.g., Silastic or Teflon sheeting or tube) is introduced into the sac, and Gelfoam or tissue graft is placed over the implant. The author fashions a dumbbell-shaped implant from Silastic sheeting,[1] one lobe of the dumbbell to fit the sac and the other extending into the mastoid cavity (Fig. 29.2B). The expectation is that fibrous tissue will grip the narrow middle part of the implant and thereby prevent extrusion of the implant from the sac. The postauricular incision is closed in layers.

Surgical Complications

Among the possible surgical complications are (i) inadvertent fistulization of the posterior semicircular canal, (ii) cerebrospinal fluid leak, (iii) laceration of the sigmoid sinus, and (iv) postoperative fixation of ossicles by bone dust entering the middle ear. Each can be avoided by attention to surgical detail.

Fistulization of the Posterior Canal

Fistulization of the posterior canal usually causes temporary postoperative vertigo and may cause permanent profound hearing loss. The posterior canal lies within a 10-mm arc of the incudal fossa and can be avoided by limiting the exposure of dura mater to an area beyond this arc (19,20). Most surgeons avoid extensive thinning of bone overlying the canal (blue-lining) simply because of the increased risk of fistulization.

Cerebrospinal Fluid Leak

Cerebrospinal fluid leak is rare with the mastoid shunt method; however, one or more small leaks may occur as the surgeon penetrates the dura with a knife in search of a small

---

[1]Medium Silastic sheeting, 500-5 nonreinforced all silicone, 0.02 inch (0.5 mm) in thickness (Dow Corning, 1 Wells Ave., Newton, MA 02159).

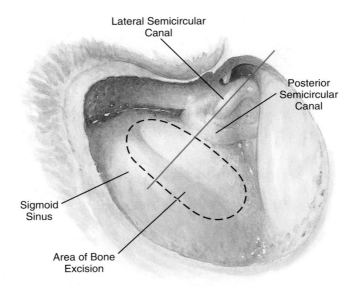

FIG. 29.1 Endolymphatic shunt. Via a transmastoid approach, the dura is exposed along a broad front between the sigmoid sinus and the posterior semicircular canal. The endolymphatic sac lies within the presigmoid dura inferior to the imaginary line that runs through the lateral semicircular canal (Donaldson's line).

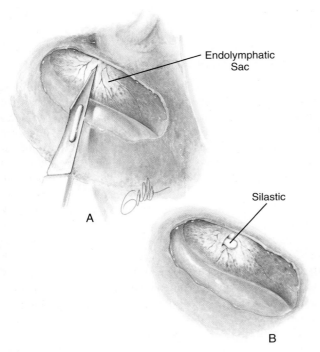

FIG. 29.2 A: An incision is made into the outer layer of the endolymphatic sac. **B:** A Silastic sheet that has been fashioned into a dumbbell shape is placed within the sac.

or hidden endolymphatic sac. Usually the leaks repair themselves within a week, but during this time the risk of meningitis is present and prophylactic antibiotics should be given. Adipose tissue or temporalis fascia can be placed over these small dural fistulas to promote healing.

Laceration of the Sigmoid Sinus

In the normal mastoid the sigmoid sinus can be readily identified by its prominent bony bulge into the mastoid and by its bluish color. In cases with an anteriorly positioned sigmoid, it may be necessary to remove the overlying bone and decompress the sinus to achieve optimal exposure of the presigmoid dura. The wall of the sinus is quite tough, and only by a grossly errant maneuver with drill or curette can it be lacerated. Oxycel or similar hemostatic substance should suffice to stop the bleeding and allow the operation to continue.

Postoperative Fixation of Ossicles

Postoperative fixation of ossicles occurs when bone dust generated by mastoid drilling is allowed to pass through the aditus into the middle ear. After 3 or 4 months, this bone dust forms a fibroosseous mass that can fix the stapes, and less commonly the malleus and incus, causing a conductive hearing loss. This complication is reduced by temporarily blocking the aditus with Gelfoam and by the judicious use of suction irrigation.

INTERNAL ENDOLYMPHATIC SHUNT

Among the internal shunt procedures are the sacculotomy of Fick (21,22), the tack operation of Cody and others (23,24), the otic-perotic shunt of House and Pulec (25), and the cochleosacculotomy of Schuknecht (26).

In the sacculotomy and tack operations, picks are introduced through the footplate of the stapes to puncture the saccule, with the objective of producing a permanent fistula in the saccular wall by which endolymph can drain into the perilymphatic space. Unfortunately, this approach fails to take into consideration the histologic observation that in Meniere's disease the dilated saccular wall is usually adherent to the footplate (27).

The otic-perotic shunt as conceived by House and Pulec is done under local anesthesia through the ear canal and involves the placement of a platinum tube through the basilar membrane to connect the scala media and scala tympani. Pulec subsequently reported that the procedure had been discontinued because 25% of patients having the operation experienced severe hearing losses (28). The operation as originally described, however, is simply not feasible because of the small size of the cochlear duct.

It has been observed that spontaneous fistulization may occur in any part of the membranous labyrinth in Meniere's disease. These ruptures are presumed to be the result of distention, thinning, and rupture of the membranes. In the vestibular labyrinth it is common to find the inner layer of the wall to be ruptured and the outer layer to be herniated outward, a condition that Altmann and Kornfeld (29) have termed outpouching. It has been speculated that spontaneous ruptures, including outpouchings, might act as sites for the escape of excessive endolymph and therefore explain the long remissions that are common in Meniere's disease.

It is known that the membranous labyrinth has a strong propensity for self-repair. Animal studies have shown that permanent fistulization is impossible to achieve by planned surgical disruption of Reissner's membrane (30), utricle, saccule, or semicircular canals (31). However, it has been demonstrated in experimental studies on cats (32–34) and guinea pigs (35) that fracture-disruption of the cochlear duct can sometimes result in permanent fistulization.

The concept of producing an internal shunt between endolymph and perilymph has a logical basis. Theoretically, it should arrest the progression of hydrops and ruptures of the endolymphatic system and therefore alleviate the attacks of vertigo. To be effective, it would seem logical that the shunt should be done early in the course of the disease before the membranous labyrinth becomes so distended and deformed that it blocks the longitudinal flow of endolymph toward the fistula.

The cochleosacculotomy is such an internal shunt procedure and is based on the following clinical, pathologic, and experimental observations: (i) Both human temporal bone studies and animal experiments show that fistulas of the membranous labyrinth are compatible with normal or near-normal sensory function in areas remote to the site of the fistula (36). (ii) Human temporal bone studies have shown that permanent spontaneous fistulas occur in the membranous labyrinth in Meniere's disease. (iii) Prolonged and even permanent remission of symptoms is occasionally observed in Meniere's disease and may be related to the occurrence of these spontaneously occurring fistulas. (iv) Animal studies have demonstrated that the only method of consistently producing permanent fistulization of the endolymphatic system is by creating a fracture-disruption of the cochlear duct.

It is clear, however, that many cochleosacculotomies could not be successful because the membranes of the dilated membranous labyrinth block access routes to the surgically created fistula (18).

Indications for Cochleosacculotomy

The cochleosacculotomy operation, like other surgical procedures for unilateral Meniere's disease, has the objective of arresting disabling episodic vertigo. It has the advantage of being technically simple to perform, is almost totally free of morbidity, and carries little or no risk of mortality. It is preferable to vestibular ablative procedures for patients who for health reasons are at risk for general anesthesia and the stress of postoperative vertigo. The procedure should be considered for elderly patients who often poorly compensate for vestibular ablation.

Experience with 142 cochleosacculotomies performed since April 1979 has shown that (i) prolonged relief of vertigo occurred in 70% of cases, (ii) hearing loss was aggravated in 35% of cases (15-dB worse pure-tone hearing loss or 15% worse discrimination), and (iii) an additional 11% of cases experienced profound hearing loss as a result of the operation.

Technique of Cochleosacculotomy

Under local anesthesia, a tympanomeatal flap is elevated and the round window niche is exposed. In rare cases the round window niche is partly hidden behind the posteroinferior margin of the tympanic bony annulus. In this situation a 3-mm sharp cutting bur can be used to remove bony annulus sufficient to gain access to the round window niche. Rarely a high jugular bulb can block access to the niche, in which case it may be prudent to abort the operation. A prominent subiculum may interfere with the introduction of the pick and require removal with a bur.

Usually the niche will accommodate a 3-mm right-angled pick without removal of bone. The pick is advanced through the round window membrane in the direction of the oval window. Care is taken to hug the lateral wall of the inner ear to ensure that the cochlear duct is traversed. When the pick is introduced to its full 3-mm length, the end of the pick is located beneath the footplate of the stapes (Fig. 29.3).

In the event that the round window niche will not accommodate a 3-mm right-angled pick, the bony lip of the niche is removed with a 2-mm bur. If this is done, a 2-mm (rather than a 3-mm) right-angled pick should be used to avoid excessive deep penetration into the vestibule with the possibility of injury to the utricular macula.

Occasionally a slight loss of resistance is felt as the pick passes through the osseous spiral lamina. Usually the patient experiences no sensation, but a few have noted momentary vertigo and some have reported hearing a "click" as the pick

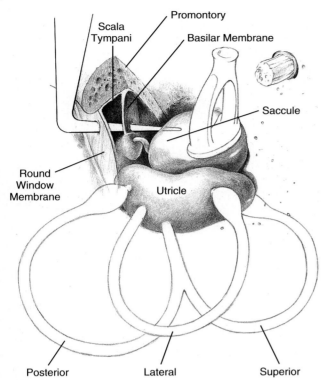

FIG. 29.3 Cochleosacculotomy. Sketch showing position of a 3 mm right-angled pick at full depth traversing the dilated cochlear duct and entering the dilated saccule. The pick, which measures approximately 300 μm in diameter, passes through the cochlear duct approximately 1.5 mm from its basal end. In this region the basilar membrane is approximately 115 μm wide.

Labels: Promontory, Scala Tympani, Basilar Membrane, Saccule, Round Window Membrane, Utricle, Posterior, Lateral, Superior

fractures the osseous spiral lamina. The maneuver does not produce vertigo, presumably because (i) the vestibular sense organs (maculae and cristae) are not mechanically disturbed and (ii) the endolymph drainage is into the surgical wound (scala tympani of the basal turn and round window niche) rather than into the perilymphatic spaces of the vestibule.

The pick is withdrawn and the perforation of the round window membrane is covered by a tissue graft of perichondrium, earlobe fat, or temporalis fascia. The operation is terminated by returning the tympanomeatal flap to its original position and packing it in place.

Most patients experience no postoperative vertigo. A few note slight unsteadiness for a day or two; however, all feel well enough to be discharged from the hospital on the following day.

REFERENCES

1. Guild SR. The circulation of endolymph. *Am J Anat* 1927;39:57–81.
2. Portmann G. Vertigo. Surgical treatment by opening the saccus endolymphaticus. *Arch Otolaryngol* 1927;6:309–315.
3. Yamakawa K, Naito T. The modification of Portmann's operation for Meniere's disease (Yamakawa-Naito's operation). *Med J Osaka Univ* 1954;5:167–175.
4. House WF. Subarachnoid shunt for drainage of endolymphatic hydrops. A preliminary report. *Laryngoscope* 1962;72:713–729.
5. Shea JJ. Teflon film drainage of the endolymphatic sac. *Arch Otolaryngol* 1966;83:316–319.
6. Paparella MM, Hanson DG. Endolymphatic sac drainage for intractable vertigo (method and experiences). *Laryngoscope* 1976;86:697–703.
7. Gardner G. Endolymphatic sac shunt operation in Meniere's disease. *Trans Am Acad Ophthalmol Otolaryngol* 1975;80:306–313.
8. Palva T, Ylikoski J, Paavolainen M, et al. Vestibular neurectomy and saccus decompression surgery in Meniere's disease. *Acta Otolaryngol* 1979;88:74–78.
9. Miller GW, Welsh RL. Surgical management of vestibular Meniere's disease with endolymphatic mastoid shunt. *Laryngoscope* 1983;93:1430–1440.
10. Spector GJ, Smith PG. Endolymphatic sac surgery for Meniere's disease. *Ann Otol Rhinol Laryngol* 1983;92:113–118.
11. Arenberg IK, Stahle J, Wilbrand H, et al. Unidirectional inner ear valve implant for endolymphatic sac surgery in Meniere's disease. *Arch Otolaryngol* 1978;104:694–704.
12. Brackmann DE, Nissen RL. Meniere's disease: results of treatment with the endolymphatic subarachnoid shunt compared with the endolymphatic mastoid shunt. *Am J Otol* 1987;8:275–282.
13. Shambaugh GE Jr. Surgery of the endolymphatic sac. *Arch Otolaryngol* 1966;83:305–315.
14. Larouere MJ, Graham MD. Wide bony decompression of the endolymphatic sac in the surgical management of Meniere's disease. *Op Tech Otolaryngol Head Neck Surg* 1991;2:7–8.
15. Bretlau P, Thomsen J, Tos M, et al. Placebo effect in surgery for Meniere's disease: nine-year follow-up. *Am J Otol* 1989;10:259–261.
16. Belal A Jr, House WF. Histopathology of endolymphatic subarachnoid shunt surgery for Meniere's disease. *Am J Otol* 1979;1:37–44.
17. Khetarpal U, Schuknecht HF. Temporal bone findings in a case of bilateral Meniere's disease treated by parenteral streptomycin and endolymphatic shunt. *Laryngoscope* 1990;100:407–414.
18. Schuknecht HF, Ruther A. Blockage of longitudinal flow in endolymphatic hydrops. *Eur Arch Otorhinolaryngol* 1991;248:209–217.
19. Shea JJ, Emmett JR, Moore RE. The surgical treatment of Meniere's disease. *Laryngoscope* 1979;89:1244–1257.
20. Paparella MM, Goycoolea M. Panel on Meniere's disease. Endolymphatic sac enhancement surgery for Meniere's disease: an extension of conservative therapy. *Ann Otol Rhinol Laryngol* 1981;90:610–615.
21. Fick IA, Van N. Decompression of the labyrinth. A new surgical procedure for Meniere's disease. *Arch Otolaryngol* 1964;79:447–458.
22. Fick IA, Van N. Meniere's disease: aetiology and a new surgical approach: sacculotomy. (Decompression of the labyrinth.) *J Laryngol Otol* 1966;80:288–306.
23. Cody DTR. The tack operation for endolymphatic hydrops. *Laryngoscope* 1969;79:1737–1744.
24. Cody DTR, Simonton KM, Hallberg OE. Automatic repetitive decompression of the saccule in endolymphatic hydrops (tack operation). Preliminary report. *Laryngoscope* 1967;77:1480–1501.
25. Pulec JL. The otic-perotic shunt. *Otolaryngol Clin North Am* 1968;1:643–648.
26. Schuknecht HF. Cochleosacculotomy for Meniere's disease: theory, technique and results. *Laryngoscope* 1982;92:853–858.
27. Schuknecht HF. Pathology of Meniere's disease as it relates to the sac and tack procedures. *Ann Otol Rhinol Laryngol* 1977;86:677–682.
28. Pulec JL. The surgical treatment of vertigo. *Laryngoscope* 1969;79:1783–1822.
29. Altmann F, Kornfeld M. Histological studies of Meniere's disease. *Ann Otol Rhinol Laryngol* 1965;74:915–943.
30. Duvall AJ III, Rhodes VT. Ultrastructure of the organ of Corti following intermixing of cochlear fluids. *Ann Otol Rhinol Laryngol* 1967;76:688–708.
31. Kimura RS, Schuknecht HF. Effect of fistulae on endolymphatic hydrops. *Ann Otol Rhinol Laryngol* 1975;84:271–286.
32. Schuknecht HF, Neff WD. Hearing losses after apical lesions in the cochlea. *Acta Otolaryngol (Stockh)* 1952;42:263–274.
33. Schuknecht HF, Sutton S. Hearing losses after experimental lesions in basal coil of cochlea. *Arch Otolaryngol* 1953;57:129–142.
34. Schuknecht HF, Seifi AE. Experimental observations on the fluid physiology of the inner ear. *Ann Otol Rhinol Laryngol* 1963;72:687–712.
35. Kimura RS, Schuknecht HF, Ota CY, et al. Experimental study of sacculotomy in endolymphatic hydrops. *Arch Otorhinolaryngol* 1977;217:123–137.
36. Schuknecht HF. Cochlear endolymphatic shunt. *Am J Otol* 1984;5:546–548.

CHAPTER 30

Neurectomy Procedures for Vertigo

Herbert Silverstein

When medical management of patients with Meniere's disease fails, vestibular neurectomy is among the procedures of choice if hearing is to be preserved. The operation is effective in relieving vertigo attacks caused by Meniere's disease while preserving hearing in 90% of patients. Although the most common inner ear disorder treated by vestibular neurectomy is classic Meniere's disease, vestibular neurectomy is useful in selected cases of recurrent vestibular neuronitis, traumatic labyrinthitis, and vestibular Meniere's disease. In deciding when to operate, the patient's preference is a strong consideration. Some patients may have one or two severe episodes per month that do not affect their lifestyle sufficiently to warrant a major surgical procedure. Other patients, even those with only a few attacks per year, may be so severely affected that they live in constant dread of the next recurrence. There should be objective evidence of unilateral inner ear disease. Unless patients are experiencing an acute Meniere's attack, they should be able to perform a tandem gait test reasonably well.

Contraindications to vestibular neurectomy include bilateral vestibular disease; poor general health, particularly when associated with physiologic old age; disequilibrium; an only hearing ear; or indications of other central nervous system disease. Vertigo from an ear with very poor hearing (80-dB speech reception threshold [SRT] with less than 20% discrimination) is usually more appropriately treated with transtympanic cochleovestibular neurectomy or labyrinthectomy. Previous transmastoid surgery of the endolymphatic sac is not a contraindication, nor is old age when the patient is healthy and has good balance function. Elderly people usually require more time to regain good balance function than do younger individuals. Vestibular neurectomy has been performed successfully in patients in their 70s, with no additional morbidity.

Although the middle fossa approach for selective vestibular neurectomy provides control of vertigo, the procedure is formidable and anatomic landmarks are difficult to determine. In general, patients more than age 60 years are not candidates for this approach because of the difficulty in elevating thin dura from the floor of the middle fossa and decreased tolerance for retraction of the temporal lobe.

ANATOMY: VESTIBULAR, COCHLEAR, AND FACIAL NERVES

At the fundus of the internal auditory canal, six separate branches of the seventh and eighth cranial nerves enter the internal auditory canal. They are the facial nerve, nervus intermedius, superior vestibular, saccular, posterior ampullary, and cochlear nerve. The transverse (falciform) crest divides the fundus into superior and inferior compartments. The vertical crest separates the superior half of the fundus into an anterosuperior quadrant for the facial nerve and nervus intermedius and a posterosuperior quadrant for the superior vestibular nerve. Anterior and inferior to the falciform crest lies the cochlear nerve, hidden from the surgeon by the inferior vestibular nerve. The posterior ampullary nerve lies in a separate canal (the singular canal) that enters the internal auditory canal in the posteroinferior quadrant, approximately 2 mm medial to the falciform crest. This reliable landmark is the point at which drilling stops when the posterior wall of the internal auditory canal is being surgically removed. A thin section computed tomograph (CT) of the labyrinth is routinely obtained to visualize the location of the singular canal. The inferior vestibular nerve is formed by the junction of the saccular nerve and joins the posterior ampullary nerve at the level of the singular canal in the posteroinferior quadrant.

The superior vestibular nerve innervates the superior and lateral cristae, the utricular macula, and sends a small twig to the anterosuperior part of the saccular macula. The inferior vestibular nerve innervates most of the saccular macula and the posterior crista.

Whereas the superior and inferior vestibular nerves are separated in the lateral part of the internal auditory canal, they fuse as they travel toward the porus acusticus. In the lateral part of the internal auditory canal, the cochlear nerve lies anteroinferior and the vestibular nerves lie posterior, but they fuse into a single trunk, known as the eighth cranial nerve, near the porus or medial to it. As the combined nerve trunk passes toward the porus, the cochlear and vestibular segments rotate 90 degrees (1). As viewed by the surgeon, the rotation is clockwise on the left and counterclockwise on the right, so that the cochlear nerve shifts from an anteroinferior to a posteroinferior position relative to the vestibular nerve as it travels toward the porus (2). Most of the rotation occurs within the internal auditory canal; only a slight rotation occurs in the cerebellopontine angle (Fig. 30.1). The 90-degree rotation of the cochlear and vestibular nerves is not recognized in modern neurologic publications (3). The cochlear nerve enters the brainstem caudal and slightly dorsal to the vestibular nerve. The flocculus of the cerebellum covers 5 mm of the eighth cranial nerve at the brainstem.

The cochleovestibular cleavage plane can usually be identified grossly. The surgical view will show the vestibular fibers to be cephalad or superior and the cochlear fibers to be caudal or inferior. Occasionally, inferior vestibular fibers will course with the cochlear nerve (Fig. 30.2). In the cerebellopontine angle, the cochleovestibular cleavage plane appears grossly as a fine septum along the eighth cranial nerve in 75% of patients.

The facial nerve remains ventrally positioned and hidden by the eighth cranial nerve along much of its course and assumes a ventral-caudal position as it enters the brainstem. In the internal auditory canal, the facial nerve is connected to the superior vestibular nerve by the Rasmussen facial-vestibular anastomosing fibers, and in the cerebellopontine angle the facial nerve lies adjacent but distinct from the eighth nerve. Although it remains hidden from the surgeon's view by the eighth cranial nerve in the retrosigmoid approach, the facial nerve can easily be seen by gentle retraction of the superior vestibular nerve in the internal auditory canal or the eighth nerve in the cerebellopontine angle. The facial nerve enters the brainstem 3 mm ventral and usually caudal to the eighth nerve route entry zone. In the internal auditory canal, the facial nerve appears whiter than the eighth nerve, and in the cerebellopontine angle it appears grayer.

The nervus intermedius, which may consist of a single nerve or multiple bundles, travels between the facial and eighth nerves through their entire course. The nervus intermedius enters the brainstem closest to the eighth nerve and usually delineates the cochleovestibular cleavage plane on the anterior surface of the eighth nerve.

OPERATIVE APPROACHES FOR VESTIBULAR NEURECTOMY

Retrolabyrinthine Vestibular Neurectomy

The retrolabyrinthine approach had been previously described for use in patients with trigeminal neuralgia, and it is also a convenient approach for selective vestibular nerve section (4).

In this procedure, a simple mastoidectomy is performed. Both the lateral venous sinus and posterior fossa dura anterior and posterior to it are exposed. The endolymphatic sac is widely exposed, and the bony contour of the posterior semicircular canal is identified. The lateral venous sinus is retracted posteriorly, and the dura is incised anterior to the sinus to create an anteriorly based dural flap. Intravenous mannitol (1.5 g/kg) is administered when the drilling begins. This causes contraction of the cerebellum and allows a wider exposure of the cerebellopontine angle (Fig. 30.3). Cochlear nerve action potentials may be monitored during the course of surgery if desired.

In 75% of cases an identifiable cleavage plane exists between the cochlear and vestibular fibers of the eighth cranial nerve in the cerebellopontine angle. From the surgeon's view, the cochlear fibers compose the inferior portion of the nerve and the vestibular fibers compose the superior portion. The fifth cranial nerve is identified superiorly and the ninth, tenth, and eleventh nerves inferiorly. After the cleavage plane is visualized under high magnification, an incision is made in the cleavage plane, the cochlear and vestibular

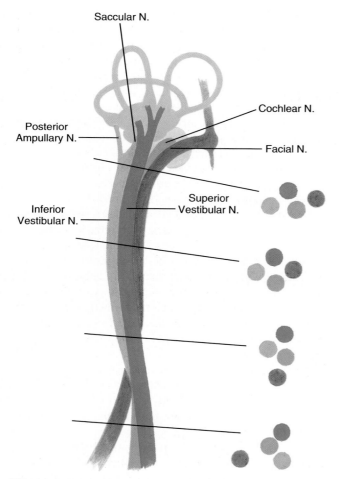

Saccular N.

Posterior Ampullary N.

Cochlear N.

Facial N.

Inferior Vestibular N.

Superior Vestibular N.

FIG. 30.1 Anatomy of the seventh and eighth cranial nerves as seen from the surgical position during the left retrosigmoid-internal auditory canal approach. Note the 90-degree rotation of the cochlear and vestibular nerves.

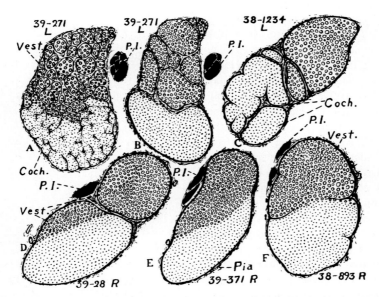

FIG. 30.2 Diagrams showing the funicular pattern of the eighth nerve from human adults. The cochlear and vestibular regions are distinguished from each other by different types of stippling. The *solid black areas (P.I.)* represent pars intermedia (nerve of Wrisburg) of the seventh cranial nerve. **A:** Cross-section slightly central to the vestibular ganglia. Both cochlear and vestibular portions consist of many small bundles, the cochlear having commenced to fuse. **B:** A section of the same nerve as **A** taken 2 mm farther centrally, showing not only complete fusion of the cochlear but several vestibular fasciculi. The vestibular bundles ultimately fuse with each other and with the cochlear component until a single trunk is formed (similar to **E**). **C:** A case where neither cochlear nor vestibular nerves are completely fused through most of their course in the internal auditory meatus and subarachnoid space. **D:** Example of the condition where the eighth nerve is represented by two distinct trunks, one of which was apparently purely vestibular, whereas the other was mostly cochlear, but with a prominent vestibular region amounting to about one-fifth of the cross-sectional area of the cochlear trunk. **E:** Example of a common condition where there is a single trunk, a little more than half of which (upon microscopic examination) is found to be vestibular and the rest cochlear. **F:** A case where incomplete glial septa roughly indicate the division between cochlear and vestibular trunks. There are generally at least a few vestibular fibers on the cochlear side of such septa. (From Rasmussen GL. Studies of the VIIIth cranial nerve of man. *Laryngoscope* 1940;50:67–83.)

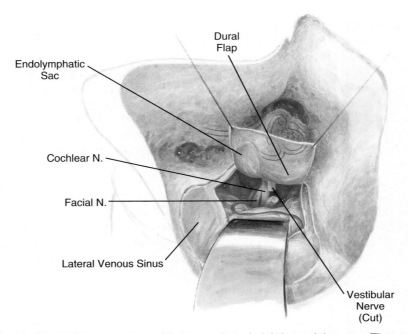

FIG. 30.3 The retrolabyrinthine exposure of the seventh and eighth cranial nerves. The vestibular nerve has been transected.

fibers are separated, and the vestibular nerve is transected with microscissors. Helpful landmarks to find the cochleovestibular cleavage plane are as follows: (i) The cochlear nerve appears whiter because its fibers are more numerous and closely packed. (ii) A fine blood vessel may be seen passing on the surface between the cochlear and vestibular fibers. (iii) The cochleovestibular cleavage plane is sometimes more visible from the anterior surface of the eighth cranial nerve (a mirror can be used to view this). (iv) The nervus intermedius, if identified, usually lies in the cleavage plane. When a cleavage plane cannot be readily identified, the superior half of the eighth cranial nerve is transected. When this technique is used, most vestibular fibers will be cut and most cochlear fibers will be spared.

In reviewing 67 patients, 82% were free of vertigo, 10% were improved, and 8% noted no change postoperatively. Sensorineural hearing has been maintained within 20 dB of the preoperative level in 71% (5). Some patients experienced a mild conductive loss in the low frequencies, presumably from bone dust entering the middle ear causing fixation of ossicles.

Retrosigmoid Vestibular Neurectomy

Because the cleavage plane between cochlear and vestibular fibers is more completely developed within the internal auditory canal, a more complete and selective vestibular neurectomy can be performed by cutting those nerves within the internal auditory canal. During this procedure, a posterior fossa craniotomy is made posterior to the lateral venous sinus, and the cerebellum is gently retracted to give exposure to the seventh and eighth cranial nerves and the internal auditory canal (6). The posterior wall of the internal auditory canal is removed with a diamond bur as far as the singular canal, thereby exposing the branches of the eighth cranial nerve (Fig. 30.4). The superior vestibular nerve is sectioned, and the singular nerve is divided. The inferior vestibular fibers that innervate the saccule are not divided because of their close association with cochlear fibers. The saccule has no known vestibular function in humans, and it appears that sparing these fibers does not compromise the success of surgery.

This procedure has resulted in freedom from vertigo in 87% of patients, with hearing results similar to those of the retrolabyrinthine vestibular neurectomy (5). Advantages over the latter are that (i) it can be performed on patients who have had chronic ear disease or poorly pneumatized mastoids because the mastoid is not entered, and (ii) it can be done on ears that have an anteriorly located lateral venous sinus.

Severe postoperative headaches uncontrolled by nonnarcotic analgesics may persist for many months. Because this approach has been used successfully for vascular decompression or section of the fifth cranial nerve apparently without significant postoperative headache, bone dust created by

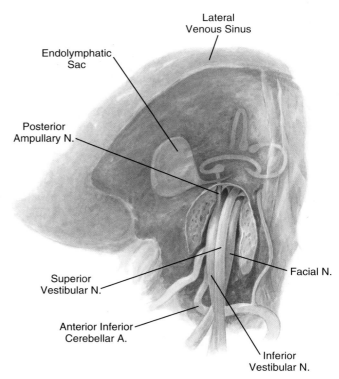

FIG. 30.4 The retrosigmoid-internal auditory canal (suboccipital) approach for vestibular neurectomy (left ear). Note the 90-degree rotation of the eighth nerve from the ear to the brain. Most of the rotation occurs in the internal auditory canal.

entering the internal auditory canal may be the cause of an arachnoiditis and resultant headache.

Combined Retrolabyrinthine-Retrosigmoid Vestibular Neurectomy

Vestibular neurectomy may also be done by the combined retrolabyrinthine-retrosigmoid approach (7). This procedure incorporates the advantages of both the retrolabyrinthine and retrosigmoid-internal auditory canal approaches. The combined retrolabyrinthine-retrosigmoid neurectomy allows the surgeon to assess the cochleovestibular cleavage plane in the posterior fossa and to decide where the neurectomy should be performed. If a satisfactory cleavage plane exists in the cerebellopontine angle, the section can be performed at that location. If not, the internal auditory canal can be opened, and the superior vestibular and posterior ampullary nerves can be sectioned within the internal auditory canal, as in the retrosigmoid-internal auditory canal procedure.

In the combined retrolabyrinthine-retrosigmoid vestibular neurectomy, a limited mastoidectomy is performed to expose 3 cm of the lateral venous sinus extending inferiorly from the transverse sinus. The lateral venous sinus is skele-

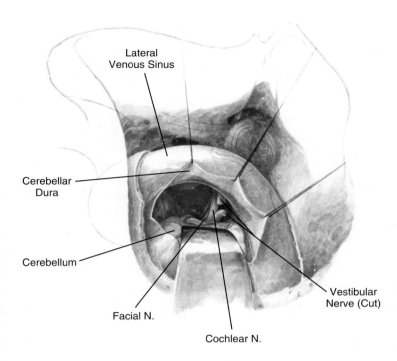

FIG. 30.5 Combined retrolabyrinthine-retrosigmoid vestibular neurectomy in the cerebellopontine angle. There is a good cochleovestibular cleavage in the cerebellopontine angle, and neurectomy is done in the posterior fossa (left ear).

tonized. The posterior fossa dura is exposed for 1 cm posterior to the lateral sinus. A dural incision is made 3 mm behind and parallel to the lateral venous sinus, and the lateral sinus is retracted anteriorly using stay sutures placed in the dural cuff (Fig. 30.5). A Penrose drain is placed against the cerebellum, and using a Penfield elevator the cerebellum is gently retracted until the arachnoid layer is identified at the cerebellopontine angle. After the arachnoid layer is opened and cerebrospinal fluid is released, the cerebellum falls away from the temporal bone, providing a wide exposure of the cerebellopontine angle. The eighth cranial nerve is examined and a cleavage plane is sought between the cochlear and vestibular fibers. If the cochleovestibular cleavage plane is present, the vestibular nerve section is performed as in the retrolabyrinthine approach. If no cleavage plane is identified, then the dura is reflected off the temporal bone, the internal auditory canal is opened with a diamond bur, and the superior vestibular and posterior ampullary nerves are divided, as in the retrosigmoid-internal auditory canal approach (Fig. 30.6). The dura is closed in a watertight manner, the air cells are filled with bone wax, and the defect is filled with abdominal adipose tissue.

The combined retrolabyrinthine-retrosigmoid procedure offers certain advantages compared with the retrolabyrinthine or retrosigmoid approaches. The surgical time is shortened because much less bone removal is needed than in the retrolabyrinthine approach. In addition, the surgeon has the option of opening the internal auditory canal and cutting the vestibular nerve more laterally where the cochleovestibular cleavage plane is better defined. The advantage that this procedure has over the retrosigmoid approach is that less cere-

bellar retraction is necessary and the bony defect is smaller. In a recent review (5), vertigo was relieved in 93% of patients, hearing was preserved within 20 dB of preoperative levels in 89%, and speech discrimination was maintained within 20% of the preoperative level in 84%. It appears that drilling the posterior lip of the internal auditory canal for vestibular neurectomy will result in headache in 50% of

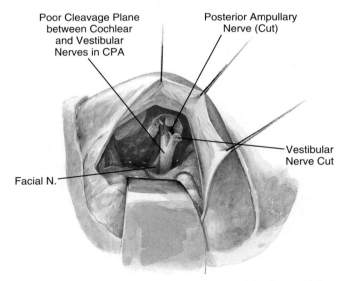

FIG. 30.6 Exposure during a left combined retrolabyrinthine/retrosigmoid approach in a patient with a poor cochleovestibular cleavage plane in the cerebellopontine angle (CPA). Vestibular neurectomy was performed after removing bone from the posterior aspect of the internal auditory canal.

patients (5). Opening of the internal auditory canal for better exposure of the vestibular nerve is necessary in approximately 20% of patients.

Complications of Selective Vestibular Neurectomy

Intraoperative

In retrolabyrinthine vestibular neurectomy, bleeding from injury to the lateral venous sinus or jugular bulb is usually managed by placing Avitene microfibrillar collagen over the bleeding site and holding it in place with a cottonoid sponge. Bleeding from a large emissary vein is controlled with Avitine pack. However, this problem can be prevented if a stump of vein is left on the lateral venous sinus that can be cauterized. If the emissary vein can be seen before bleeding occurs, dissection should proceed with a diamond bur. Bleeding from small vessels of the dura is controlled with microbipolar cautery. Lifting the dura and cutting with scissors helps avoid cutting these vessels.

After opening the dura, there is a slight chance that brain swelling may occur. This is prevented by lowering the Pco_2 during surgery by hyperventilating the patient, and by giving the patient mannitol (1.5 g/kg) intravenously when bone work is begun. Damage to the cerebellum is prevented by using a Penrose drain placed against the cortex while retracting the cerebellum to gain exposure of the cerebellopontine angle and release cerebrospinal fluid. In younger patients, the cerebellum may be tense and protrude slightly through the dural incision. The Penrose drain is slid along the cerebellum at the inferior margin of the wound toward the ninth cranial nerve. After cerebrospinal fluid is released from the cerebellopontine angle by opening the arachnoid layer with a blunt instrument over the ninth cranial nerve, the cerebellum will fall away from the temporal bone, allowing satisfactory exposure of the cerebellopontine angle without cerebellar retraction. If brain swelling occurs from trauma to the cerebellum and the posterior fossa cannot be easily exposed, it may be prudent to retreat from further surgery. Care must be taken not to traumatize the petrosal veins located above the fifth cranial nerve and near the tentorium. Because of the brain shrinkage from mannitol, these veins are stretched and can easily rupture. Bleeding is controlled with Avitine or microbipolar electrocautery.

When the thin arachnoid layer is dissected away from the seventh and eighth cranial nerves, bleeding from capillaries may occur. This is controlled by first cauterizing the vessels with microbipolar cautery and then transecting them with microscissors. Sometimes the flocculus of the cerebellum is attached to the structures of the cerebellopontine angle and must be dissected away from it. Locating cranial nerves V, IX, and X helps orient the surgeon to the vestibular portion of the eighth cranial nerve (the superior half is closest to the fifth cranial nerve). To prevent injury to the facial nerve, a small mirror is used to view the anterior aspect of the eighth cranial nerve. In 4% of cases the facial nerve is attached to the vestibular nerve and must be separated from it with a round knife. The cleavage between the cochlear and vestibular nerves is first made with a sharp sickle knife and then completed with a blunt nerve separator. The electrophysiologic monitoring of facial nerve function is essential for these procedures.

If the facial nerve lies close to the anterior aspect of the eighth cranial nerve, the vestibular nerve should be sectioned piecemeal with scissors and sickle knife to avoid injury to the facial nerve and labyrinthine artery. If the facial nerve is inadvertently transected, it should be repaired at the time of surgery with a great auricular nerve graft. Because this procedure is done in the posterior fossa, a neurosurgeon must be available if an unusual complication occurs with which the otologist is unfamiliar.

Postoperative

Early postoperative bleeding in the posterior fossa requires assessment by a neurosurgeon. The wound may have to be opened immediately. Meningismus with mild temperature elevation occurring soon after surgery usually represents chemical meningitis due to small amounts of blood in the cerebrospinal fluid and requires no treatment. Wound infection secondary to serum collected beneath the flap in the postauricular crease is treated by incision and drainage, culture of pus, and appropriate treatment, usually with cephalosporin antibiotics given intravenously or by mouth. This complication is prevented by keeping the skin flap and muscle layer together when elevating the skin flap and by using perioperative antibiotics. If there is spiking temperature elevation with nuchal rigidity and headache, a spinal tap for culture and sensitivity should be done and the patient should be treated for meningitis. Following retrolabyrinthine vestibular neurectomy, the most common early complication is cerebrospinal fluid leak (10%) from the wound edge or through the eustachian tube. A cerebrospinal fluid leak is best treated with continuous lumbar drainage for 3 or 4 days. Because the dura cannot be closed in a watertight fashion using the retrolabyrinthine exposure, there is no apparent way to prevent the high incidence of cerebrospinal fluid leak. When the dural incision can be closed in a watertight fashion, as in the combined retrolabyrinthine-retrosigmoid procedure, the incidence of cerebrospinal fluid leakage is reduced.

Transmeatal Cochleovestibular Neurectomy

For patients suffering incapacitating vertigo of Meniere's disease or iatrogenic vestibular symptoms following otologic surgery, and whose hearing loss is greater than 80 dB and discrimination score is 20% or less, ablation of auditory and vestibular function may be considered. A relative contraindication to ablative surgery may be advanced physiologic age in a patient with active vestibular function as determined by caloric tests, because central compensation for the loss of one labyrinth may be incomplete. Other contraindications include poor hearing in the opposite ear, bilateral Meniere's disease, disorders of the central nervous system, low vision, and a young individual who may later be a candidate for a cochlear implant. The transmeatal approach to the internal auditory canal for cochleovestibular neurectomy was independently described by Alvarez de Cozar and Antoli-Candela (8) and Silverstein (9). The results compare favorably with any ablative procedure. Experience has been gained in 140 such procedures (10). The most common indication for cochleovestibular neurectomy surgery is Meniere's disease in a patient with persistent vertigo, tinnitus, and no serviceable hearing.

The tympanic cochleovestibular neurectomy ensures complete ablation of the labyrinth and possible relief of tinnitus. Abdominal adipose tissue is not necessary because a transmastoid exposure is not needed.

The patient is placed in a supine otologic position, and general endotracheal anesthesia is administered. Perioperative antibiotics are not used. A postauricular incision is made 1 cm behind the postauricular crease, and the skin of the posterior wall of the external auditory canal is incised below the spine of Henle. Exposure of the external canal is maintained with a self-retaining mastoid retractor. A large tympanomeatal flap is elevated and reflected anteriorly to expose the middle ear structures. Cutting and diamond burs are used to create a large bony canalplasty until the horizontal and vertical portions of the facial nerve are identified. This allows wide exposure of the middle ear and an excellent view of the round window niche. To improve exposure of the middle ear, the chorda tympani nerve, pyramidal process, and bone anterior to the vertical segment of the facial nerve are removed. The superior lip of the round window niche is removed with a fine diamond bur to expose the entire round window membrane. Movement of the stapes will produce an obvious round window reflex.

After removing bone from the floor of the round window niche, the posterior ampullary nerve is identified (Fig. 30.7). This nerve can be found traversing a 45-degree angle, 1 mm deep to the round window membrane, just anterior to the

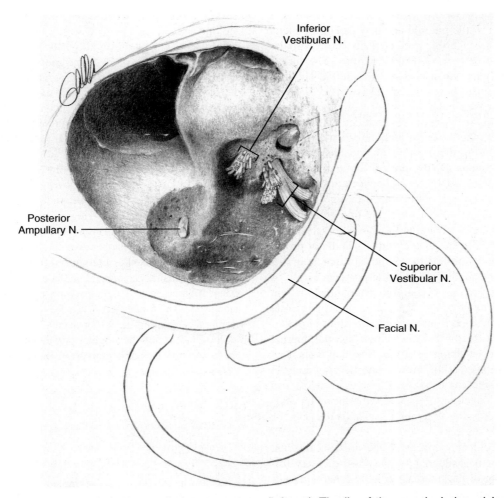

Inferior Vestibular N.

Posterior Ampullary N.

Superior Vestibular N.

Facial N.

FIG. 30.7 Transcanal cochleovestibular neurectomy (left ear). The lip of the round window niche has been removed, exposing the basal turn of the cochlea. The posterior ampullary nerve is identified. The incus and stapes have been removed, and promontory bone connecting oval and round windows has been drilled away. The posterior ampullary nerve is followed toward the internal auditory canal.

ampulla of the posterior semicircular canal. The posterior ampullary nerve will appear as a white structure, and palpation with a pick will identify the nerve and the singular canal. If the posterior ampullary nerve cannot be found in the round window niche, it can be found entering the ampulla.

The incus and stapes are now removed, and the horizontal portion of the facial nerve is palpated to determine if any portion of the nerve is dehiscent. An exposed horizontal portion of the facial nerve makes it susceptible to injury either by the drill shaft or suction tip during exposure of the internal auditory canal. The promontory bone connecting the round and oval windows is removed, and, using a 3-mm right-angled pick, the utricle is removed from the elliptical recess. The posterior ampullary nerve and singular canal (usually 4.5 mm long) are followed toward the internal auditory canal. The posteroinferior aspect of the internal auditory canal is skeletonized, and the transverse crest is removed. To orient the surgeon to the cochlear nerve's direction, the basal turn of the cochlea is opened anteriorly. When the modiolus is opened, free flow of cerebrospinal fluid occurs, which provides irrigation during the drilling.

In this approach to the internal auditory canal, the facial nerve lies anterior, superior, and beneath the vestibular nerves and is therefore less vulnerable to injury. The dura is opened along the posterior aspect of the internal auditory canal over the superior vestibular nerve. The superior vestibular, inferior vestibular, posterior ampullary nerve, cochlear nerve, and facial nerve are identified. The inferior vestibular nerve and the posterior ampullary nerve are routinely transected during the drilling. The cochlear nerve is transected at the fundus of the internal auditory canal. A good cleavage plane is usually found between the facial and superior vestibular nerves. Once the cleavage plane is clearly identified, the vestibular fibers are transected, a few fibers at a time, to avoid stretching the facial nerve. The facial nerve is electrically stimulated with a stimulator probe. Stimulation thresholds of 0.05 to 0.2 mm are typical in this area and indicate normal facial function postoperatively. A free temporalis muscle and fascia graft is obtained and cut into three pieces. The first piece is inserted into the internal auditory canal, the second is inserted into the anterior part of the middle ear, and the third is placed between the internal auditory canal and tympanomeatal flap. The flap is then returned to its position over the muscle and held securely in place by packing the ear canal with polyester strips and round cottonoid pledgets impregnated with antibiotic ointment. A mastoid dressing is applied for 24 hours and the packing removed in 2 weeks.

Cerebrospinal fluid may appear on the dressing the first day. If the leak persists, reoperation may be necessary followed by repacking of the internal auditory canal and middle ear. If a cerebrospinal fluid leak occurs, continuous lumbar drainage can be used for several days, which may allow the patient to avoid repeat surgery. Postoperative facial paralysis should be immediately investigated surgically and the facial nerve decompressed or repaired. A slight facial weakness may be treated expectantly.

Delayed facial paralysis is treated expectantly or with prednisone (20 mg three times a day) for 1 week. Delayed cerebrospinal fluid leak is treated with reexploration. The surgeon must be especially careful, because the exposed facial nerve may become adherent to the muscle graft.

Cawthorne (11) reported total relief of tinnitus in 8% and Simonton and Sciarra (12) in 16% of patients undergoing labyrinthectomy. In the current series of 82 patients having cochleovestibular neurectomy, there were 24 (29%) who had complete relief of tinnitus and 24 (29%) who had substantial improvement. The patients with persistent tinnitus after cochleovestibular neurectomy probably have a central etiology of their tinnitus.

Denervating a labyrinth, especially in elderly patients, will produce certain immediate postoperative side effects. The patients are usually vertiginous with severe nystagmus for the first 24 to 48 hours. Patients with prolonged, severe Meniere's disease and a reduced caloric response as demonstrated by electronystagmography usually will not have as severe a vestibular reaction. The period of central compensation varies in each patient; steady improvement in balance occurs over a 3- to 6-month period. In general, young patients recover more quickly and more completely. Seven of 10 patients who described postoperative unsteadiness as severe were still satisfied with their results because their vertigo had been relieved. It was noted that 90% of patients who complained of severe unsteadiness had experienced unsteadiness preoperatively and that half of these had undergone previous labyrinthectomy.

The transmeatal approach to the internal auditory canal has the following advantages over the transmastoid-translabyrinthine approach to the internal auditory canal: (i) It is the most direct approach and requires much less bone removal than the translabyrinthine approach, which shortens the operating time. (ii) The postoperative cerebrospinal fluid leak rate is low (1%) because the internal auditory canal is grafted with muscle tissue that can be held in place for 2 weeks by the tympanic membrane and tight packing in the external auditory canal. (iii) The facial nerve may be less vulnerable. (iv) Abdominal adipose tissue is not needed. (v) The surgeon gains skill in transecting the singular nerve, a procedure that is useful in certain cases of benign positional vertigo.

REFERENCES

1. Silverstein H. Cochlear and vestibular gross and histologic anatomy (as seen from postauricular approach). *Otolaryngol Head Neck Surg* 1984;92:207–211.
2. Silverstein H, McDaniel A, Wazen J, et al. Retrolabyrinthine vestibular neurectomy with simultaneous monitoring of the 8th nerve and brain stem auditory evoked potentials. *Otolaryngol Head Neck Surg* 1985; 93:736–742.
3. Silverstein H, Norrell H, Haberkamp T, et al. The unrecognized rotation of the vestibular and cochlear nerves from the labyrinth to the brain tem: its implications to surgery of the eighth cranial nerve. *Otolaryngol Head Neck Surg* 1986;95:543–549.

4. Silverstein H, Norrell H. Retrolabyrinthine surgery: a direct approach to the cerebellopontine angle. *Otolaryngol Head Neck Surg* 1980;88: 462–469.
5. Silverstein H, Norrell H, Smouha E, et al. An evaluation of approach in vestibular neurectomy. *Otolaryngol Head Neck Surg* 1990;102: 374–381.
6. Silverstein H, Norrell H, Haberkamp T. A comparison of retrosigmoid IAC, retrolabyrinthine, and middle fossa vestibular neurectomy for treatment of vertigo. *Laryngoscope* 1987;97:165–173.
7. Silverstein H, Norrell H, Smouha E, et al. Combined retrolab-retrosigmoid vestibular neurectomy. An evolution in approach. *Am J Otol* 1989;10:166–169.
8. Alvarez de Cozar F, Antoli-Candela F. Transvestibular surgery. *Rev Laryngol Otol Rhinol (Bord)* 1970;91:927–935.
9. Silverstein H. Transmeatal labyrinthectomy with and without cochleovestibular neurectomy. *Laryngoscope* 1976;86:1777–1791.
10. Jones R, Silverstein H, Smouha E. Long-term results of transmeatal cochleovestibular neurectomy: an analysis of 100 cases. *Otolaryngol Head Neck Surg* 1989;100:22–29.
11. Cawthorne T. Membranous labyrinthectomy via the oval window for Meniere's disease. *J Laryngol Otol* 1957;71:524–527.
12. Simonton KM, Sciarra PA. Destructive labyrinthotomy: study of prognosis of postoperative disability. *Ann Otol Rhinol Laryngol* 1958;67: 775–788.
13. Rasmussen GL. Studies of the VIIIth cranial nerve of man. *Laryngoscope* 1940;50:67-83.

CHAPTER 31

Surgical Treatment for Benign Paroxysmal Positional Vertigo

Richard R. Gacek, Mark R. Gacek, and Michael J. McKenna

Benign paroxysmal positional vertigo (BPPV) is a disorder of the peripheral vestibular end organ that results in brief but severe bouts of vertigo that are precipitated by change in head position. Although in most cases this is a self-limiting condition lasting from weeks to months, in a small percentage of patients the clinical course may be protracted and not resolve with time or physical therapy. Under such circumstances and when the disorder becomes psychologically or physically incapacitating, surgical intervention may be considered. Until recently, the best and most discriminating surgical approach has been selective posterior ampullary nerve section by a transcanal approach. However, over the past decade another surgical option for the management of BPPV has emerged, the transmastoid occlusion of the posterior semicircular canal. These two techniques have different physiologic effects on the peripheral vestibular system and result in similar rates of success.

When first described by Barany (1), benign paroxysmal positional vertigo was thought to be a disorder of the otolithic system, specifically the utricular macula. However, the brisk transient rotatory nystagmus produced by the provocative positioning maneuver (Hallpike) cast doubt on a purely otolithic mechanism (2). A reasonable hypothesis supported by human temporal bone histopathology is that the cupula of the posterior semicircular canal is transformed into a gravity-sensitive receptor by the deposition of high specific gravity deposits onto the cupula or floating in the endolymph of the canal (3) (Fig. 31.1). The canal sense organ is then excited by gravitational forces when the characteristic ear-down or head-back position is assumed (Fig. 31.2). Selective surgical denervation or ablation of the posterior canal function has been shown to relieve the subjective symptoms and objective nystagmus of the disorder (4,5), thus affirming that the posterior semicircular canal sense organ is responsible for BPPV. Similarly, disruption of endolymph flow by mechanical occlusion of the posterior semicircular canal results in similar findings, adding further evidence that the symptoms associated with BPPV

originate from the posterior canal ampulla. What is not clear at present is the exact pathophysiologic mechanism that results in the symptoms of BPPV. Features of this disorder that are not explained on a purely mechanical basis are the limited duration of the ocular response despite maintaining the provocative position and its fatigability on repeat provocation (3). Recent observations in temporal bone specimens of patients with BPPV reveal focal degeneration of axons in the inferior vestibular division (6,7). This suggests that there may be a neural component to the pathophysiology of BPPV that may account for these features that provoke the vestibuloocular response. Evidence of a primary mechanical etiology includes the observation of pathologic deposits within the cupula of the ampulla of the posterior canal in temporal bone specimens from patients with BPPV (3), evidence of free-floating particles within the endolymph of the posterior semicircular canal that are gravity sensitive and have been observed at the time of posterior canal occlusion (8,9), and the clinical observation that a high percentage of patients with acute BPPV can be cured of their symptoms by a particle repositioning maneuver designed to redistribute free-floating particles within the posterior canal.

The fact that some cases of BPPV have evidence of axonal degeneration on postmortem examination and the clinical observation that the majority of cases result from a stressful precipitating event such as trauma, upper respiratory tract infection, and surgery on other parts of the body are highly suggestive of a viral etiology as is suspected in Bell's palsy and vestibular neuritis.

SIGNS AND SYMPTOMS OF BENIGN PAROXYSMAL POSITIONAL VERTIGO

Patients with BPPV complain of a rotatory experience accompanied by nausea when the head is placed in the head-back or ear-down position (10). The vertigo and nystagmus typically have a 1- to 4-second latency and duration of 20 to

391

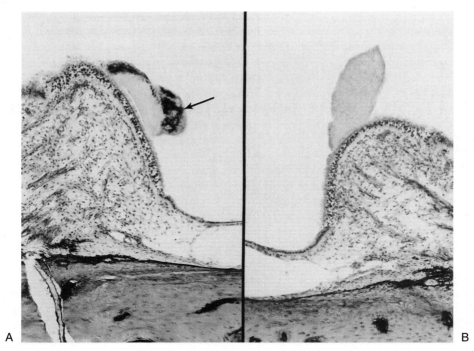

FIG. 31.1 A: Basophilic deposit (*arrow*) embedded in the posterior canal cupula of the symptomatic ear of a patient with BPPV. **B:** Contralateral posterior canal crista of patient in **A.**

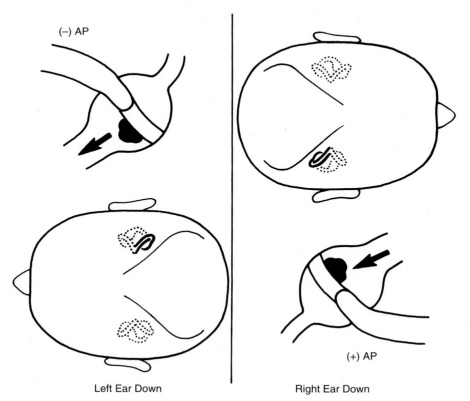

Left Ear Down   Right Ear Down

FIG. 31.2 Schematic representation of the mechanism of cupulolithiasis. *AP,* nerve action potential.

25 seconds. Repeat positioning results in decreased signs and symptoms.

The Hallpike maneuver on the patient fitted with Frenzel's glasses is used to reproduce nystagmus and symptoms of BPPV (2). In severe cases of BPPV, the nystagmus can be observed without suppression of visual fixation. The direction of nystagmus is usually rotatory in a counterclockwise direction with the right ear down and clockwise with the left ear down. This type of nystagmus is the result of the vestibuloocular projections from the posterior semicircular canal (Fig. 31.3). Occasionally, a horizontal nystagmus may be observed with the same latency, duration, and fatigability as is seen with the rotatory nystagmus (11). The responsible sense organ in this instance is thought to be the lateral semicircular canal crista. Another group of patients experience balance symptoms, not typically paroxysmal positional vertigo, resulting from incomplete ablation of labyrinthine function attempted either by transcanal labyrinthectomy or vestibular nerve transection. Because the posterior canal sense organ and its nerve supply are anatomically inaccessible in these procedures, they may escape ablation. This residual function of the posterior canal sense organ may be responsible for persistent symptoms following vestibular ablation procedures. In these patients, transection of the singular nerve can be performed to provide relief of their symptoms.

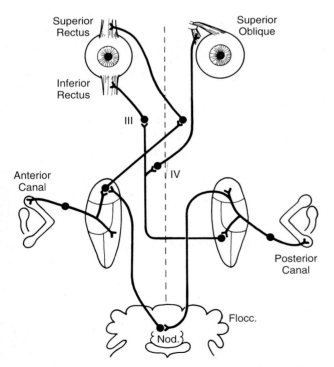

FIG. 31.3 Diagram of neural pathways activated in BPPV. *III*, oculomotor nucleus; *IV*, trochlear nucleus; *Nod*, nodulus of cerebellum; *Flocc*, flocculus of cerebellum.

PATIENT SELECTION

Because most patients with BPPV undergo spontaneous resolution within a 6- to 12-month period or may be only mildly disabled by their symptoms, surgical treatment is not often employed (6). Exercise programs that use the head and neck and upper trunk muscles may be helpful to reduce the severity of symptomatology and promoting spontaneous resolution (12). Repositioning maneuvers intended to redistribute high density particles in the endolymph of the posterior canal are also effective to relieve symptoms, particularly in acute BPPV (13,14). However, for a small group of patients who demonstrate chronic positional vertigo for more than 1 year despite conservative measures and are sufficiently disabled from their normal activities, singular neurectomy or transmastoid posterior canal occlusion provide an effective means of relief from the disabling symptoms (4,5,7,15–17). Some patients with chronic BPPV continue to live with their symptoms by avoiding the provocative position and changing their lifestyle. Surgical relief is offered only to those who request it and are willing to accept the low risk of hearing loss.

PREOPERATIVE EXAMINATION

The evaluation and diagnosis of BPPV consist of an accurately obtained history documenting labyrinthine trauma, such as head injury; viral labyrinthitis; inner ear or general surgery; or aging. Tests of auditory and vestibular function are essential. Most patients with this syndrome are middle age (mean age in the sixth decade). There is a 2:1 female predominance. Most patients have a normal ear examination, although occasionally a patient with chronic middle ear inflammatory disease experiences BPPV. Patients with chronic inflammatory disease should undergo attempted surgical eradication of the disease in an effort to control the vestibular symptoms. The functional evaluation consists of pure-tone and speech audiometry, as well as electronystagmographic assessment of the vestibular sensitivity by the caloric method. Auditory brainstem response and electrocochleographic examinations are not necessary in the evaluation of patients with this disorder. The most important diagnostic test is the Hallpike maneuver, properly performed with or without Frenzel's glasses with the patient on an examining table (Fig. 31.4). The test has been well described in the literature (2) and consists of the examiner taking the patient to a head-handing position, first right and then left, from the sitting position and observing the patient's ocular response, along with his or her subjective vestibular experience. Posterior canal BPPV typically produces a rotatory nystagmus either clockwise or counterclockwise after a latency of a few seconds. The nystagmus builds to a crescendo and then disappears over 25 to 30 seconds but reappears in reverse direction when the sitting position is again assumed. Repeat testing produces less nystagmus and fewer subjec-

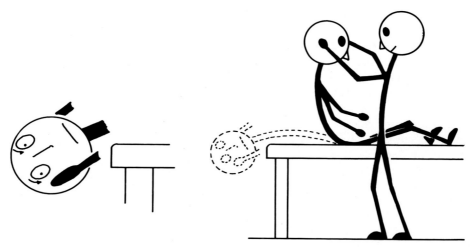

FIG. 31.4 The positioning (Hallpike) maneuver used to elicit BPPV.

tive symptoms, supporting the peripheral location of the pathology (fatigability). It is important to test both right and left head-down positions because approximately 15% to 18% of patients with BPPV have bilateral disease that is usually worse in one ear (18). In patients with BPPV, nystagmus response is not seen when the contralateral (noninvolved) ear is placed geotropically because the gravity-sensitive cupula is deflected utriculopetally (opposite to hair cell polarization). When the involved ear is geotropic, cupula deflection is utriculofugal and in the direction of hair cell polarization, thereby causing depolarization (Fig. 31.2). Occasionally, the Hallpike test may reveal a horizontal nystagmus with the same time characteristics and fatigability observed with the rotatory nystagmus (11). These patients are not candidates for singular neurectomy or posterior canal occlusion because their symptoms may be caused by pathology in other labyrinthine sense organs, such as the lateral canal crista.

Because a central nervous system lesion may rarely cause similar findings (19,20), an imaging study such as enhanced magnetic resonance imaging (MRI) of the posterior fossa is recommended to rule out the small chance of a central lesion being responsible for the positional vertigo.

Once a patient has been identified as having BPPV of the peripheral type, the degree of disability from the positional vertigo must be determined from an evaluation of the patient's work and lifestyle. If the patient is willing to risk sensorineural hearing loss for relief of the positional vertigo, it is considered sufficiently disabling to warrant surgical intervention.

SURGICAL TECHNIQUE OF POSTERIOR AMPULLARY NERVE SECTION

Preoperative preparation is similar to that for any transcanal middle ear surgery. Preoperative or intraoperative antibiotics are not used; however, postoperative antibiotics are rou-

tinely used to prevent ascending infection through the singular canal. Such infection has not occurred in our series of more than 203 patients. The surgical site is prepared with a sterilized solution, such as povidone-iodine (Betadine), and draped for transcanal surgery. A bifenestrated drape with an opening over the patient's face and one that fits around the auricle is available commercially. The patient is in prone position with the head turned so that the operated ear is facing up toward the surgeon and the head is in somewhat of a dependent position, placing the ear canal on a straight line with the surgeon's view. A small amount of hair is shaved around the postauricular area so that the drape can adhere to the skin's surface. The surgical procedure is carried out with the patient under local anesthesia with 1% lidocaine (Xylocaine with 1:100,000 dilution of adrenaline) injected into the external auditory meatus and the posterior and inferior canal wall skin. A 27-gauge needle is helpful to successfully place local anesthetic in the subperiosteal layer of the ear canal and dissect down to the level of the tympanic annulus. Medically assisted anesthesia with intravenous medication from an anesthesiologist helps allow local anesthesia to be effective.

Instruments

The instruments for this procedure are the same as those used for routine middle ear surgery, including various size specula, speculum holder, angled canal wall elevators, and hooks and picks used in oval window surgery. The most essential instrument for this procedure is an electric powered microdrill for use through an ear speculum with diamond burs of 1-mm and 0.5-mm diameters. The drill is preferably angled so that the visualization around the drill and the transcanal speculum approach is permitted to remove the round window niche overhang and to approach the singular canal in the floor of the round window niche. Monitoring of hearing or facial nerve function is not included in our experi-

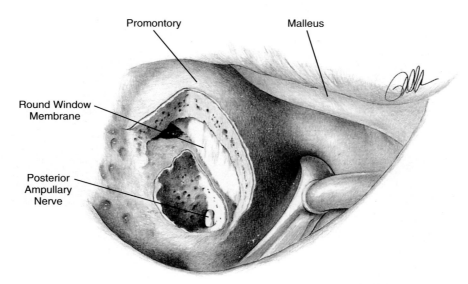

FIG. 31.5 Pertinent anatomic landmarks in transcanal transection of the posterior ampullary nerve (singular neurectomy).

ence. With the patient under local anesthesia, the surgeon can monitor the patient's subjective symptoms of vertigo and pain when the singular nerve is transected and can observe a vertical or rotatory nystagmus at this transection.

Surgery

After elevation of the tympanomeatal flap, the drill is used to remove the overhang of the round window niche so that the entire round window membrane can be visualized from anterior to posterior (Figs. 31.5 and 31.6). Often, a mucous

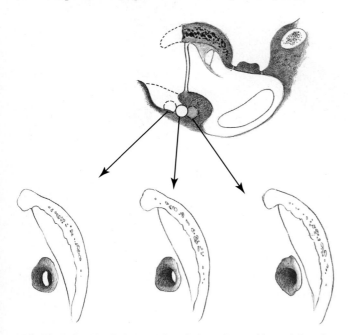

FIG. 31.6 Surgical view and variations in position of the singular canal are shown in this drawing of a left ear and a section through the labyrinth.

membrane fold will cover the aperture of the round window niche and should not be confused with the round window membrane (Fig. 31.7). This membrane fold is dissected free with small hooks and picks so that the round window membrane can be clearly identified by its dark gray appearance and its displacement when the ossicular chain is depressed. After the round window membrane has been satisfactorily exposed, the drill is used to create a depression in the floor of the round window niche just inferior to the bony attachment of the posterior segment of the round window membrane. This bony depression is deepened to a level of 2 to 3 mm, at which point the singular canal is usually encountered and is recognized by the white myelinated nerve bundle that runs at an angle to the alignment of the round window membrane (Fig. 31.5). The preferred segments of the singular nerve for transection are the intermediate and cribrose portions (Figs. 31.8 and 31.9). If the singular canal is not identified at the level of 2 mm or more, the singular canal may be superiorly located under the attachment of the round window membrane (Fig. 31.6). The drill can be used to enlarge the base of the bony depression in the floor of the niche to reach the singular canal from the inferior direction by undercutting the attachment of the round window membrane. In these cases, identification of the nerve in the singular canal is highlighted by the patient's abrupt response of vertigo or pain. The canal is then entered with a small right-angled hook probing only the proximal end of the singular canal. Probing the distal end of the canal is not advised because of proximity to the posterior canal ampulla. After repeat probing of the canal, with destruction of nerve tissue, the bony defect is drilled lightly to place bone dust into the canal lumen. This dust should form a bony barrier to regeneration of nerve fibers. Adipose tissue harvested from the earlobe is then used to fill the bony defect. Because the segment of singular canal exposed is either the intermediate or cribrose

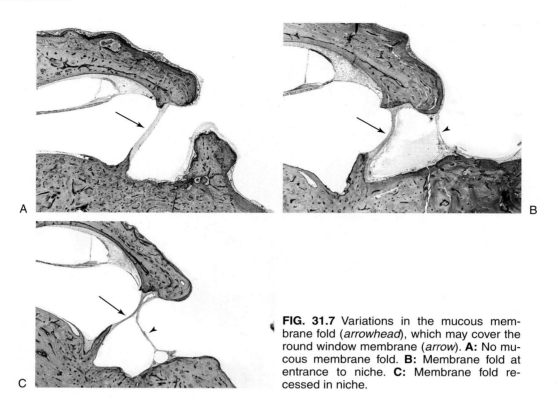

FIG. 31.7 Variations in the mucous membrane fold (*arrowhead*), which may cover the round window membrane (*arrow*). **A:** No mucous membrane fold. **B:** Membrane fold at entrance to niche. **C:** Membrane fold recessed in niche.

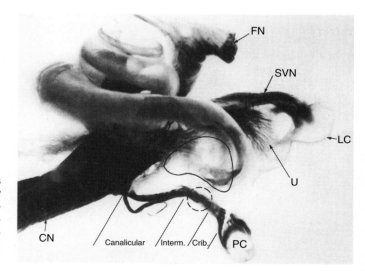

FIG. 31.8 Specimen of the inner ear innervation illustrates the relationship of the singular nerve to the round window membrane (*solid line*). *Dashed line* denotes the preferred location for transection of the intermediate segment of the singular nerve. *FN,* facial nerve; *CN,* cochlear nerve; *SVN,* superior vestibular nerve; *LC,* lateral canal ampulla; *PC,* posterior canal ampulla; *U,* utricular nerve.

segment, cerebrospinal fluid leak is not usually encountered. The nerve is surrounded by cerebrospinal fluid in the proximal canalicular segment, which lies inferior to the floor of the vestibule. Rarely, a leak of spinal fluid may be seen if the singular canal is probed too far proximally. In these cases, a small piece of adipose tissue will satisfactorily control the leak. On a few occasions, the singular nerve was exposed at its entrance into the recess of the posterior canal ampulla (Fig. 31.10). After the tympanic membrane and flap are returned to their original position, a small pack is used to hold them in position for approximately 1 week while healing oc-

curs. A small cotton ball in the external auditory meatus and a small outer ear dressing are applied for the first 24 hours. Beyond that, a sterile cotton ball is placed in the external auditory meatus and the pack is removed 1 week later in an outpatient visit.

Postoperative Care

Oral antibiotics are used routinely for 1 week. Postoperatively, patients have varying degrees of ataxia and dizziness; most patients are able to leave the hospital 1 day after sur-

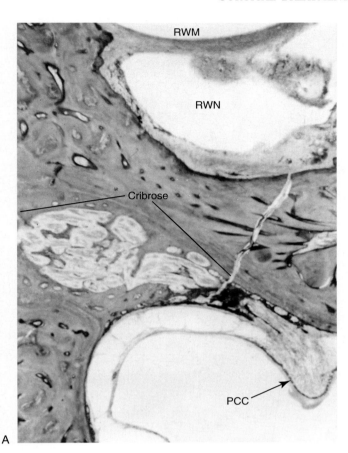

A

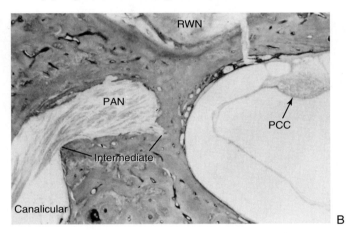

FIG. 31.9 Photomicrographs of the cribrose (**A**) and intermediate (**B**) segments of the singular canal.

B

gery; others require 2 to 3 days. The Hallpike maneuver, when carried out on the first postoperative day, fails to demonstrate a rotatory nystagmus as in the preoperative positional test but instead will provoke a persistent down-beating vertical nystagmus reflecting the imbalance between eye muscles supplied by complimentary vertical canals. An unopposed pull of the superior rectus from the contralateral anterior canal follows the innervation of its coplaner posterior canal (Fig. 31.3). This nonfatiguing positional down-beating nystagmus will be observed for 1 to 3 days and usually parallels the patient's ability to leave the hospital. Vestibular exercises are not necessary but may help to allow some patients to complete the compensatory process necessary to overcome the vestibular deficit created by singular neurectomy.

Nonselective Singular Neurectomy

Nonselective singular neurectomy implies that the procedure is performed in association with transtympanic labyrinthectomy (Fig. 31.10). This is accomplished by first removing the promontory to expose the vestibule and basal turn of cochlea. The saccular and utricular maculae and the cristae are removed. The singular canal is found by drilling in the medial wall of the vestibule between the spherical recess and the scala vestibuli of the basal turn. The canal lumen with its nerve component is encountered at a depth of 1 to 2 mm at this point. Although a small amount of cerebrospinal fluid leakage usually occurs from the singular canal, it is readily controlled by packing the vestibule with Gelfoam.

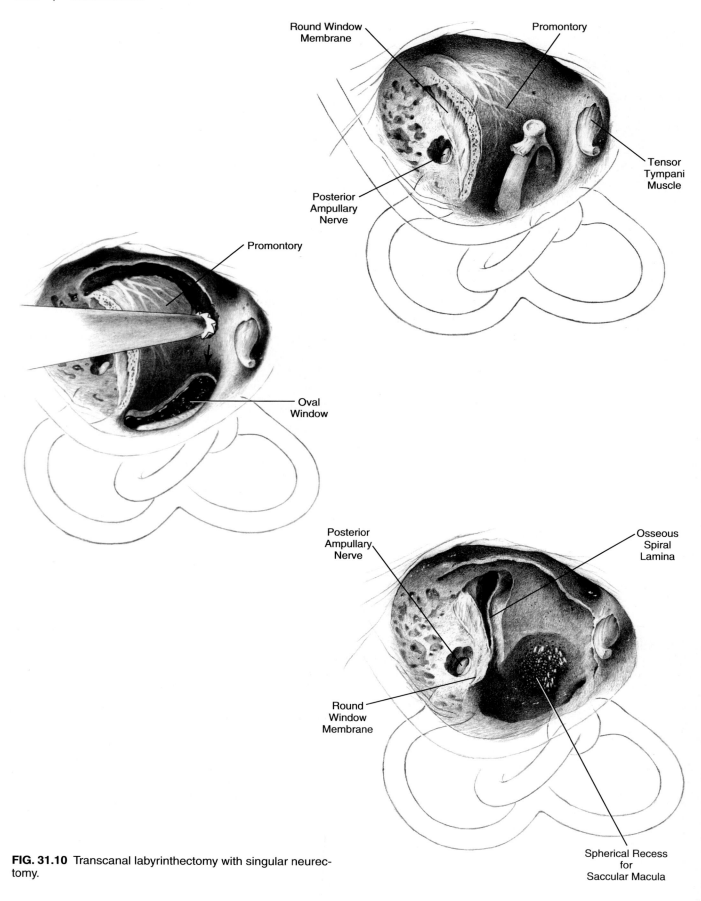

FIG. 31.10 Transcanal labyrinthectomy with singular neurectomy.

Pitfalls of Surgery

The primary risk of this surgery is injury to the cochlea through the round window membrane. This injury can be avoided by carefully identifying the round window membrane and avoiding injury to it with instrumentation, particularly the drill. Maintaining a ridge of bone between the attachment of round window membrane and the site created for exposing the singular canal is helpful to avoid this undesirable result. Another significant complication of the procedure is not finding the singular canal and the nerve. Because of variability in the anatomic position of the canal, this may occur when the singular canal is located superiorly under the round window membrane attachment. The use of local anesthesia to permit the patient's response when the canal is exposed and probed is crucial to avoid this pitfall of surgery.

Results

From 1972 through 1999, 203 patients have undergone singular neurectomy for disabling, chronic (greater than 1 year) positional vertigo. One hundred ninety-three patients had a unilateral singular neurectomy and 10 patients underwent bilateral sequential singular neurectomies at intervals of 6 months to 1 year for bilateral BPPV. The incidence of bilateral BPPV in this group of patients was 18%. There were 144 females and 59 males age 21 to 93 years. The peak incidence was in the sixth decade. The etiology for the BPPV was idiopathic in 144, head trauma in 39, surgery (other than otologic) under general anesthesia in 18, endolymphatic sac surgery in 1, and cerebrovascular accident in 1.

Complete relief from the positional vertigo was obtained in 205 patients (96.2%) and partial relief from vertigo in 3 patients (1.4%). No relief was experienced in 5 patients (2.4%). In this group of failures, clear exposure of the singular canal was lacking. Sensorineural hearing loss of various levels and severity was encountered in 5 patients (2.4%).

Complications

Infection and delayed healing of the tympanic membrane should not occur in the hands of a trained otologic surgeon. The primary problems following this surgery are a recurrence of symptoms and sensorineural hearing loss. Recurrence of vertigo following singular neurectomy may be caused by incomplete transection of the singular nerve or BPPV involving the contralateral ear. Incomplete transection may occur if there is compartmentalization of the singular canal by bony partitions (Fig. 31.11), though probing of the canal should minimize this event. Carefully performing Hallpike maneuvers with documentation of the nystagmus response is necessary to determine the presence of positional vertigo in either ear. Approximately 15% to 18% of patients may exhibit bilateral BPPV. Other forms of disequilibrium may be experienced by patients following singular neurectomy and are related to inadequate vestibular compensation for the ablation procedure.

Sensorineural hearing loss in the operated ear is the most serious complication of singular neurectomy. It is the reason for reluctance to use this form of surgical relief for chronic BPPV. However, precise knowledge of the anatomic landmarks and variations in the location of the singular canal are responsible for the low incidence of sensorineural hearing loss (2.4%) in this series of 203 singular neurectomies. The severity of sensorineural hearing loss in five patients ranged from moderate to severe and most occurred in the first half of the experience with singular neurectomy. Therefore this complication is similar in incidence to other routine otologic procedure (e.g., stapedectomy, tympanoplasty) and less than is associated with selective vestibular denervation techniques (e.g., vestibular neurectomy, intratympanic gentamicin).

POSTERIOR CANAL OCCLUSION

Unlike singular neurectomy, the principal goal of posterior canal occlusion is to disrupt the flow of endolymph within the posterior semicircular canal and thereby prevent or retard the defection of the posterior canal crista that occurs in response to geotropic stimuli from high density particles that are either attached to the crista or located within the endolymphatic space of the posterior canal and move freely in response to positional change, which in turn incites the flow of endolymph within the posterior canal. Yakushin et al. (21) compared canal afferents after nerve section and canal plugging in the monkey. They found that after nerve section, the canal afferents were inactivated, whereas after canal plugging, the afferent neurons were still activated by rotation. Their data indicated that with the plugging technique the canals are not inactivated but have an altered dominant time constant and corresponding frequency response.

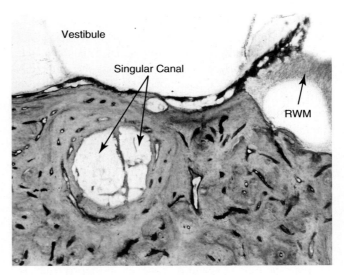

FIG. 31.11 Photomicrograph illustrates compartmentalization of the singular canal.

Surgical Technique

Although it is possible to perform a posterior canal ablation under local anesthesia, unless medically contraindicated, this procedure is best accomplished under general anesthesia. We have routinely employed the use of perioperative antibiotics as a preventative measure to avoid problems with bacterial labyrinthitis. The surgical site is prepped and draped in a manner similar to that for any transmastoid procedure. Facial nerve monitoring and the monitoring of auditory function are not necessary. Four to 5 ml of 1% Xylocaine with 1:100,000 epinephrine is routinely injected into the postauricular area to help reduce bleeding from the skin edges. A curved incision is made in the postauricular area approximately 2 cm posterior to the postauricular crease. Inferiorly, the incision is carried down to the level of the mastoid cortex using either a no. 15 blade or the electric cautery on a cutting mode. Superiorly, the incision is carried down to the level of the temporalis fascia. A transverse incision is made in the temporalis muscle at the level of the temporal line that extends anteriorly to just above the external auditory canal. A large periosteal elevator is then used to elevate the periosteum off the mastoid cortex up to and including the periosteum of the lateral aspect of the posterior bony external auditory canal. Once the mastoid cortex has been exposed, a single self-retaining retractor is positioned. Using suction irrigation and a combination of cutting and diamond burs, a canal wall–up mastoidectomy is performed. It is important to try to avoid the spilling of bone dust liberated from drilling through the aditus ad antrum and into the middle ear. This can result in a postoperative conductive hearing loss similar to that which can occur following endolymphatic saccotomy or retrolabyrinthine vestibular neurectomy. Once the antrum is identified, a piece of Gelfoam soaked in sterile saline should be packed into the antrum in an effort to reduce the flow of bone dust through this region. To achieve adequate exposure of the posterior semicircular canal, it is often necessary to skeletonize the sigmoid sinus and the posterior fossa dura anterior to the sigmoid. The facial nerve from the second genu to the stylomastoid foramen and the lateral and posterior semicircular canals are skeletonized. If necessary, bone is removed over the sigmoid sinus and the presigmoid posterior fossa plate so that this can be gently compressed to achieve adequate working room and visualization of the posterior semicircular canal. With a 2-mm diamond bur, the posterior semicircular canal is blue lined for an arc of at least 120 degrees. Using a 1-mm diamond bur, the bone overlying the endosteum of the posterior semicircular canal is slowly thinned until a 3- to 4-mm eliptoid island of bone overlying the canal becomes freely mobile (Fig. 31.12). At this point the cavity should be thoroughly irrigated with sterile saline and punctate areas of hemorrhage controlled with bipolar cautery. Under high magnification, a 0.6-mm hook is used to carefully lift and separate the mobile island of bone and posterior canal endosteum. Effort should be made not to disrupt the membranous labyrinth within the posterior semicircular canal. Once removed, it is essential not to use suction within the open posterior canal (Fig. 31.13). Once the cap of bone overlying the posterior canal is removed, a small ball of bone wax on the tip of a cotton-tipped applicator is gently pressed into the opening of the posterior canal. Once the bony opening has been sealed with bone wax, the posterior canal is covered with a small piece of temporalis fascia. Any Gelfoam that had been previously placed in the mastoid antrum is removed, and a layered closure of the wound is accomplished. A mastoid dressing is used for the first 24 hours.

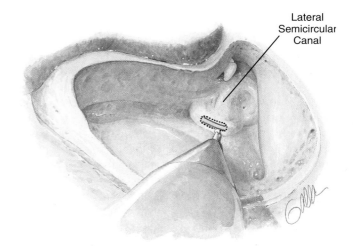

FIG. 31.12 The posterior semicircular canal has been blue lined. Using a 1-mm diamond bur, an eliptoid island of bone over the posterior canal is created.

Postoperative Care

As is the case with singular neurectomy, most patients have some disequilibrium and ataxia in the immediate postoperative period. The average hospital stay is 2 days following surgery. The symptoms of dizziness and mild vertigo are exacerbated by positional change. However, the Hallpike maneuver, when performed in the immediate postoperative period, fails to demonstrate the rotatory nystagmus that was present preoperatively. Although most patients report a dramatic improvement in their symptoms of positional vertigo, some patients continue to complain of mild disequilibrium that is exacerbated by movement for up to 6 weeks following surgery. Rarely is this incapacitating, and most patients are able to resume normal activity.

Pitfalls of Surgery

As is the case with singular neurectomy, the primary risk of posterior canal occlusion is hearing loss, which may be either conductive or sensorineural. The conductive hearing loss occurs as a result of bone dust that spills through the aditus ad antrum into the middle ear and ultimately inter-

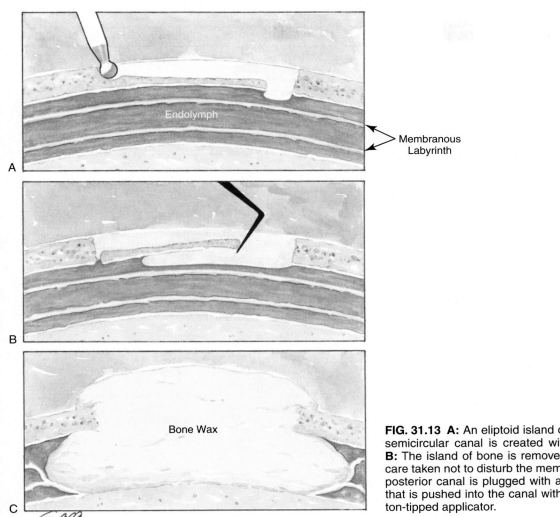

FIG. 31.13 A: An eliptoid island of bone over the posterior semicircular canal is created with a 1-mm diamond bur. B: The island of bone is removed with a small hook, with care taken not to disturb the membranous labyrinth. C: The posterior canal is plugged with a small patty of bone wax that is pushed into the canal with a small cottonoid or cotton-tipped applicator.

feres with ossicular motion. As is the case with endolymphatic saccotomy and retrolabyrinthine vestibular neurectomy, this may occur in 20% to 30% of cases. It can be avoided by judicious use of irrigation and by blocking the mastoid antrum with Gelfoam during the drilling process. Sensorineural hearing loss can also occur following posterior canal occlusion, although this is a rare complication, with profound sensorineural hearing loss occurring in only 1% to 2% of cases. A transient mild high-tone sensorineural hearing loss has been reported to occur in approximately 50% of cases. Although the cause of sensorineural hearing loss in posterior canal ablation is difficult to attribute to any specific factor, intuitively this would be most likely related to trauma incurred during removal of bone overlying the posterior canal. Every effort should be made to accomplish this is an atraumatic fashion. If interruption of the membra-

nous labyrinth occurs during removal of bone overlying the posterior canal, the bony defects should be immediately sealed with bone wax to prevent decompression and collapse of the endolymphatic space.

Results

The hallmark of a good surgical procedure is one that results in a predictable outcome with a high success rate, low complication rate, and results that are reproducible among different surgeons. Such is the case with posterior canal ablation (Table 31.1). Since its inception approximately 10 years ago, the results reported are practically identical from center to center, with a cure rate of approximately 98% and a 1% to 2% incidence of significant sensorineural hearing loss.

TABLE 31.1 *Combined results of posterior semicircular canal occlusion surgery*

Study (ref)	Total patients	Patients relieved of vertigo	Number with SNHL
Parnes & McClure, 1991 (15)	8	8	0
Pace-Balzan & Rutka, 1991 (22)	5	5	0
Anthony, 1993 (23)	14	13	1
Hawthorne & el-Naggar, 1994 (24)	15	15	1
Kartush & Sargent, 1995 (25)	4	4	0
Zappia, 1996 (16)	8	8	0
MEEI	7	7	0
TOTALS	61	60 (98%)	1 (1.6%)

SNHL, sensorineural hearing loss.

REFERENCES

1. Barany R. Diagnose von Krankheitserscheinungen im Bereiche des Otolithenapparates. *Acta Otolaryngol (Stockh)* 1921;2:434–437.
2. Carmichal EA, Dix MR, Hallpike CS. Pathology, symptomatology and diagnosis of the organic affectations of the eight nerve system. *Br Med Bull* 1956;12:146–152.
3. Schuknecht HF. Cupulolithiasis. *Arch Otolaryngol* 1969;90:765–778.
4. Gacek RR. Pathophysiology and management of cupulolithiasis. *Am J Otolaryngol* 1985;6:66–74.
5. Gacek RR. Singular neurectomy update. II. Review of 102 cases. *Laryngoscope* 1991;101:855–862.
6. Gacek RR. The pathology of facial and vestibular neuronitis. *Am J Otolaryngol* 1999;20:202–210.
7. Gacek RR, Gacek MR. Update on the pathophysiology and management of benign paroxysmal positional vertigo. *Otorhinolaryngol Nova,* in press.
8. Parnes LS, McClure JA. Free-floating endolymph particles: a new operative finding during posterior semicircular canal occlusion. *Laryngoscope* 1992;102:988–992.
9. Welling DB, Parnes LS, O'Brien B, et al. Particulate matter in the posterior semicircular canal. *Laryngoscope* 1997;107:90–94.
10. Barber HO. Positional nystagmus, especially after injury. *Laryngoscope* 1964;74:891–944.
11. McClure JA. Horizntal canal BPV. *J Otolaryngol* 1985;14:30–35.
12. Brandt T, Daroff RB. Physical therapy for benign paroxysmal positional vertigo. *Arch Otolaryngol* 1980;106:484–485.
13. Wolf JS, Boyev KP, Manokey BJ, et al. Success of the modified Epley maneuver in treating benign paroxysmal positional vertigo. *Laryngoscope* 1999;109:900–903.
14. Coppo GF, Singarelli S, Fracchia P. Benign paroxysmal positional vertigo: follow-up of 165 cases treated by Sermont's liberating maneuver. *Acta Otorhinolaryngol Ital* 1996;16:508–512.
15. Parnes LS, McClure JA. Posterior semicircular canal occlusion in the normal hearing ear. *Otolaryngol Head Neck Surg* 1991;104:52–57.
16. Zappia JJ. Posterior semicircular canal occlusion for benign paroxysmal positional vertigo. *Am J Otol* 1996;17:749–754.
17. Walsh RM, Bath AP, Cullen JR, et al. Long-term results of posterior semicircular canal occlusion for intractable benign paroxysmal positional vertigo. *Clin Otolaryngol* 1999;24:316–323.
18. Longridge NS. Barber HO. Bilateral paroxysmal positional nystagmus. *J Otolaryngol* 1978;7:395–400.
19. Dunniway HM, Welling DB. Intracranial tumor mimicking benign paroxysmal positional vertigo. *Otolaryngol Head Neck Surg* 1998;118:429–436.
20. Sakata E, Ohtsu K, Shimura H, et al. Positional nystagmus of benign paroxysmal type (BPPN) due to cerebellar vermis lesions. Pseudo-BPPN. *Auris Nasus Larynx (Tokyo)* 1987;14:17–21.
21. Yakushin SB, Bukharina SE, Dai M, et al. Differential effects of canal nerve-section and canal plugging on a VOR spatial gain and phases. *Abstracts of the Twenty-Second Midwinter Research Meeting,* Association for Research in Otolaryngology. Abstract 419. St. Petersburg Beach, FL, Feb 13–18, 1999:106.
22. Pace-Balzan A, Rutka JA. Non-ampullary plugging of the posterior semicircular canal for benign paroxysmal positional vertigo. *J Laryngol Otol* 1991;105:901–906.
23. Anthony PF. Partitioning the labyrinth for benign paroxysmal positional vertigo: clinical and histologic findings. *Am J Otol* 1993;14:334–342.
24. Hawthorne M, el-Naggar M. Fenestration and occlusion of posterior semicircular canal for patients with intractable benign paroxysmal positional vertigo. *J Laryngol Otol* 1994;108:935–939.
25. Kartush JM, Sargent EW. Posterior semicircular canal occlusion for benign paroxysmal positional vertigo-CO_2 laser-assisted technique: preliminary results. *Laryngoscope* 1995;105:268–274.

CHAPTER 32

Surgery for Vertigo: Chemical Labyrinthectomy

Steven D. Rauch

The vertigo of unilateral Meniere's disease is controllable by conservative, medical means in 90% to 95% of patients. The remaining 5% to 10% are considered intractable cases, manifesting frequent, severe, or otherwise incapacitating symptoms. These patients are candidates for invasive therapy. Invasive therapies have traditionally been surgical procedures classified as either drainage operations (cochleosacculotomy and endolymphatic sac decompression or shunt) or destructive operations (labyrinthectomy and vestibular neurectomy). Early attempts to capitalize on the ototoxicity of streptomycin to achieve "chemical labyrinthectomy" ablated vestibular function but also caused total hearing loss in the treated ear (1). Newer aminoglycosides, such as gentamicin, offer a fair margin of safety between vestibulotoxicity and cochleotoxicity, and low-dose titration protocols for administration further enhance this margin. Over the last 15 years, a number of investigators have revisited chemical labyrinthectomy using intratympanic gentamicin (2–20). In these reported protocols, administration of gentamicin until onset of labyrinthine symptoms often results in hearing loss. However, gradual administration of very low doses over weeks or months can reliably achieve reduction or elimination of vertigo attacks while preserving hearing. The protocols for treatment vary widely, but there is consensus that the procedure achieves a high degree of successful control of vertigo with acceptably small risk to hearing. Intratympanic gentamicin (ITG) therapy has thus achieved status as a minimally invasive technique in the destructive category. It offers the advantages of high success and low risk plus the added benefit that it is performed in the outpatient setting and has a far more benign course of recovery than that often seen in surgical labyrinthectomy.

TREATMENT RATIONALE

At the outset, intratympanic aminoglycoside therapy was seen as a chemical labyrinthectomy, with every effort made to achieve complete vestibular ablation. When this was performed with streptomycin by Schuknecht, the drug was administered repeatedly until patients developed gait ataxia and oscillopsia (1). Labyrinthine destruction was assured, but it came at the price of total hearing loss in the treated ear; no clear advantage over surgical labyrinthectomy was demonstrated. Treatment with alternative drugs and less aggressive dosing was undertaken in an effort to maintain a high degree of labyrinthine destruction but spare hearing. Gentamicin dosing schemes with two or more injections weekly achieved vertigo control rates of 80% to 97%, but hearing loss rates approached 20% to 40% in some series (3,7–9,11,18). Some small proportion of aminoglycoside ototoxicity represents an idiosyncratic hypersensitivity to the drug, possibly on a genetic basis. However, the majority of hearing loss cases arise because treating physicians emphasize vestibular ablation as the therapeutic end point, administering gentamicin doses that can fall into a cochleotoxic range. However, it may be feasible to obtain good vertigo control without dosing that achieves a high degree of vestibular ablation (21). This more gentle approach to therapy aims to downregulate vestibular symptoms while preserving hearing. It is unclear whether the efficacy of this very low dose therapy is truly due to ototoxic destruction of hair cells: There are reports that aminoglycosides can have actions as ion channel blockers (22) and can exert an effect on the vestibular dark cells (23) that might alter endolymph homeostasis in a beneficial way. If, as some suggest (11), incomplete vestibular ablation leads to higher relapse rate, it is an easy matter to retreat with more gentamicin when symptoms reactivate to an unacceptable level. Over the long term, giving a single intratympanic injection of gentamicin once or twice yearly appears to give good control of vestibular symptoms with minimal risk to hearing. This philosophy is gaining acceptance because it appears to offer the best balance of symptomatic relief and minimum morbidity.

ADMINISTRATION PROTOCOL

Gentamicin sulfate is supplied in a 40 mg/ml injectable solution. Some authors have recommended diluting or buffering the mixture to reduce chemical irritation of the middle ear and tympanic membrane. However, if administered no more than once every 2 to 4 weeks, this measure is unnecessary. Only a single injection is given, and then 2 or more weeks are allowed to pass to see if symptoms abate. If not, supplemental doses are given at 2- to 4-week intervals until symptoms are adequately controlled or hearing is adversely affected. It is rare to require more than two doses to achieve noticeable benefit.

AUDIOMETRY

Hearing is tested by pure-tone audiometry and speech discrimination before initiation of ITG treatment, immediately before each new cycle of therapy, and at 1 month after treatment.

VESTIBULAR TESTING

Vestibular function tests are performed in all patients before initial ITG treatment. The test battery includes electronystagmography, sinusoidal vertical axis rotation, visual-vestibular interactions, and computerized dynamic posturography. The objectives of vestibular testing are to confirm which ear is affected, to quantify the magnitude of hypofunction, and to confirm that the contralateral ear is normal. Intratympanic gentamicin therapy, presumably a destructive treatment, is relatively contraindicated in bilateral Meniere's disease because of the risk of inadequate vestibular compensation after treatment. Indicators of binaural disease include binaural hearing fluctuation, vestibular test findings of bilateral caloric paresis on electronystagmogram, and sinusoidal vertical axis rotation test showing reduced vestibuloocular reflex gain at all frequencies or markedly shortened time constant.

ADMINISTRATION TECHNIQUE

The patient is positioned supine under an operating microscope with the affected ear up. The tympanic membrane is anesthetized with topical phenol at two sites, anteroinferiorly and posteroinferiorly. A tuberculin syringe filled with injectable gentamicin sulfate, 40 mg/ml, is fitted with a 1.5-inch 27-gauge needle and quickly warmed to body temperature in the surgeon's hands to prevent a caloric effect. The needle is used to create a puncture at the anteroinferior anesthetized site as a vent hole to let air escape as the drug is instilled. Gentamicin is injected through the posterior anesthetized site until the fluid level reaches the umbo and the patient tastes the drug as it flows down the eustachian tube (0.3 to 0.7 ml). The patient remains supine with the head turned 30 degrees toward the normal ear for 1 hour and is then released. Patients are instructed to observe strict water precautions until the injection perforations are well healed, a few weeks after the treatment is complete. The sites painted with topical phenol will remain anesthetic for several weeks and need not be retreated.

LOCAL EFFECTS

Gentamicin is mildly irritating. Approximately one third of patients experienced 5 to 20 seconds of burning at the time of each administration. The likelihood of burning increases with each injection as a local inflammatory response develops in the tympanic membrane and middle ear, but longer intervals between doses lessens this side effect. Tympanic inflammation subsides within a few days. Perforation of the tympanic membrane at the injection site persists for at least 2 weeks after treatment in all patients. Permanent perforation occurs in approximately 2% of cases.

ACUTE LABYRINTHINE EFFECTS

The degree of symptoms experienced in the days following the ITG injection is highly variable. Patients with significantly intact vestibular function, and those very sensitive to the ototoxic effects of the drug, tend to be more symptomatic, whereas patients with substantial vestibular hypofunction before treatment have little noticeable discomfort from the treatment. If it occurs, onset of labyrinthine upset typically begins 3 to 5 days after injection. Patients notice a continuous mild dysequilibrium characterized by a swimming sensation in the head. They often describe the feeling that, if they turn their head quickly, the world keeps swirling after the head stops, a sensation likened to water swirled in a glass. A number of patients state that when they bend over they feel as though their head will roll off their shoulders. Unanimously, patients easily distinguish this ototoxic drug effect from their Meniere's attacks. Once it begins, the labyrinthine reaction becomes progressively worse, peaking in approximately 1 week. Patients typically stay in bed or miss work for 1 or 2 days at the peak of symptoms. Gradual resolution takes an additional 2 to 4 weeks. Patients are encouraged to be as active as they can tolerate to facilitate central vestibular compensation. Rarely a patient with persistent dysequilibrium beyond 6 weeks is referred for vestibular rehabilitation physical therapy. Because baseline vestibular function declines over time in Meniere's disease and each treatment with ITG presumably causes some decrement in vestibular function, patients requiring retreatment for relapsed Meniere's attacks have less post-ITG vestibulopathy than patients having their first cycle of treatment.

VESTIBULAR OUTCOME

By the time any acute labyrinthine reaction subsides, approximately 95% of patients have elimination of their acute attacks of vertigo. Over the next 12 months, approximately 30% of patients develop return of some attacks. However, most patients find the relapsed symptoms to be far less severe than the pre-ITG attacks. Some patients with relapse can tolerate the symptoms at the new, lower intensity, electing to continue sodium-restricted diet and diuretics. Other patients want more complete control of vertigo and elect to retreat with ITG or proceed to alternative invasive therapies.

Two special situations are worthy of comment: patients with Tumarkin drop attacks and patients who have failed previous endolymphatic sac surgery. This author's anecdotal and unpublished experience with ITG for Tumarkin drop attacks has been successful in 5 of 5 cases. Obviously, Tumarkin drop attacks are a relative emergency, and thorough discussion with patients regarding the potential risks of delaying definitive surgical therapy are necessary prior to embarking on a trial of ITG. Most patients at the Massachusetts Eye and Ear Infirmary who have failed to achieve benefit from ITG were patients who had failed previous endolymphatic sac-to-mastoid shunt surgery. This phenomenon has been observed by others. There are several plausible explanations: Patients who have failed sac surgery may have worse disease and therefore fail other treatments as well. Patients who have had sac surgery may have bone dust and fibrosis occluding the round window niche, preventing access of gentamicin solution to the inner ear. Endolymphatic sac surgery may alter inner ear function to change endolymphatic fluid flow patterns or change endolabyrinthine electrical potential, altering distribution of the gentamicin molecules so they do not reach their targets effectively.

HEARING OUTCOME

Although a few reports of ITG treatment note no adverse hearing effects, most reports observe a range of outcomes. Across studies, the trend is for hearing to be unaffected in approximately 50% of cases, worse in 20% to 30% of cases, and improved in 20% to 30% of cases. As noted earlier, excluding idiosyncratic hypersensitivity to gentamicin, which can cause profound deafness within 24 hours of a single injection, risk of hearing loss tends to go up with increasing dosage. Therefore newer approaches utilizing infrequent single injections will likely result in lower hearing loss rates than the 20% to 30% seen to date.

CONCLUSIONS AND FUTURE DIRECTIONS

The many reports of ITG treatment all claim good results and low risk despite a variation in the dosing scheme. This puzzling observation has led to questions about the actual amount of gentamicin reaching the round window and a search for better ways to administer the drug. Recently some investigators have advocated use of surgically implanted delivery devices to carry gentamicin directly to the round window (24,25). They claim a theoretical advantage of delivering a more consistent drug dose directly to the round window membrane, eliminating the variability produced by soft tissue or bony obstructions in the round window niche, and rapid evacuation of gentamicin solution down the eustachian tube. To date, these theoretical advantages do not justify the time and expense of converting a 2-minute office procedure into a surgical undertaking in the operating room.

Intratympanic gentamicin therapy is a widely accepted, minimally invasive option for treatment of intractable, unilateral Meniere's disease. It is an outpatient office treatment with an initial success in approximately 95% of cases and a long-term success in approximately 70% of cases. Anecdotally, ITG is also effective for management of Tumarkin drop attacks. Its role in management of bilateral Meniere's disease is not clear, but this use seems ill advised because of the likelihood of incomplete central compensation after destructive procedures in bilateral disease. On the other hand, if all medical options have been exhausted, a small dose of ITG in an active ear may reduce attacks without producing so much peripheral vestibular ablation that central compensation is taxed. Hearing loss has occurred in 20% to 30% of patients, but newer once-a-month dosing schemes may lower that risk.

When risk and benefit statistics are considered, ITG appears to be equivalent in efficacy and risk to endolymphatic sac surgery. Sac surgery requires hospitalization and general anesthesia, whereas ITG is done with local anesthesia on an outpatient basis. Post treatment morbidity is also equivalent: Both therapies produce mild dysequilibrium for 2 to 4 weeks; ITG avoids the low facial nerve risk of sac surgery; sac surgery avoids the low risk of persistent ear drum perforation seen with ITG. Conventional wisdom holds that sac surgery, a drainage procedure, should be tried before a destructive procedure such as ITG. However, there remains considerable uncertainty whether sac surgery truly acts by altering endolymphatic drainage and whether ITG acts by destroying hair cells. A strong argument can be made for letting patients choose between both treatments as first line invasive procedures, on the basis of both risk/benefit and cost/benefit analyses.

REFERENCES

1. Schuknecht HF. Ablation therapy in the management of Meniere's disease. *Acta Otolaryngol Suppl* 1957;132:1–42.
2. Sala T. Transtympanic administration of aminoglycosides in patients with Meniere's disease. *Arch Otorhinolaryngol* 1988;245:293–296.
3. Ödkvist LM. Middle ear ototoxic treatment for inner ear disease. *Acta Otolaryngol Suppl* 1989;457:83–86.
4. Magnusson M, Padoan S, Karlberg M, et al. Delayed onset of ototoxic effects of gentamicin in treatment of Meniere's disease. *Acta Otolaryngol Suppl* 1991;481:610–612.
5. Magnusson M, Padoan S. Delayed onset of ototoxic effects of gentamicin in treatment of Meniere's disease. Rationale for extremely low dose therapy. *Acta Otolaryngol* 1991;111:671–676.
6. Magnusson M, Padoan S, Karlberg M, et al. Delayed onset of ototoxic effects of gentamicin in patients with Meniere's disease. *Acta Otolaryngol Suppl* 1991;485:120–122.
7. Nedzelski JM, Schessel DA, Bryce GE, et al. Chemical labyrinthectomy: local application of gentamicin for the treatment of unilateral Meniere's disease. *Am J Otol* 1992;13:18–22.
8. Nedzelski JM, Bryce GE, Pfleiderer AG. Treatment of Meniere's disease with topical gentamicin: a preliminary report. *J Otolaryngol* 1992;21:95–101.
9. Nedzelski JM, Chiong CM, Fradet G, et al. Intratympanic gentamicin instillation as treatment of unilateral Meniere's disease: update of an ongoing study. *Am J Otol* 1993;14:278–282.
10. Pyykkö I, Ishizaki H, Kaasinen S, et al. Intratympanic gentamicin in bilateral Meniere's disease. *Otolaryngol Head Neck Surg* 1994;110:162–167.

11. Rauch SD, Oas JG. Intratympanic gentamicin for treatment of intractable Meniere's disease: a preliminary report. *Laryngoscope* 1997; 107:49–55.

12. Harner SG, Kasperbauer JL, Facer GW, et al. Transtympanic gentamicin for Meniere's syndrome. *Laryngoscope* 1998;108:1446–1449.

13. Kaasinen S, Pyykkö I, Ishizaki H, et al. Intratympanic gentamicin in Meniere's disease. *Acta Otolaryngol* 1998;118:294–298.

14. McFeely WJ, Singleton GT, Rodriguez FJ, et al. Intratympanic gentamicin treatment for Meniere's disease. *Otolaryngol Head Neck Surg* 1998;118:589–596.

15. Pfleiderer AG. The current role of local intratympanic gentamicin therapy in the management of unilateral Meniere's disease. *Clin Otolaryngol* 1998;23:34–41.

16. Youssef TF, Poe DS. Intratympanic gentamicin injection for the treatment of Meniere's disease. *Am J Otol* 1998;19:435–442.

17. Atlas JT, Parnes LS. Intratympanic gentamicin titration therapy for intractable Meniere's disease. *Am J Otol* 1999;20:357–363.

18. Minor LB. Intratympanic gentamicin for control of vertigo in Meniere's disease: vestibular signs that specify completion of therapy. *Am J Otol* 1999;20:209–219.

19. Kaplan DM, Nedzelski JM, Chen JM, et al. Intratympanic gentamicin for the treatment of unilateral Meniere's disease. *Laryngoscope* 2000; 110:1298–1305.

20. Longridge NS, Mallinson AI. Low-dose intratympanic gentamicin treatment for dizziness in Meniere's disease. *J Otolaryngol* 2000; 29:35–39.

21. Driscoll CL, Kasperbauer JL, Facer GW, et al. Low-dose intratympanic gentamicin and the treatment of Meniere's disease: preliminary results. *Laryngoscope* 1997;107:83–89.

22. Schacht J. Biochemical basis of aminoglycoside ototoxicity. *Otolaryngol Clin North Am* 1993;26:845–856.

23. Pender DJ. Gentamicin tympanoclysis: effects on the vestibular secretory cells. *Am J Otolaryngol* 1985;6:358–367.

24. Hoffer ME, Balough B, Henderson J, et al. Use of sustained release vehicles in the treatment of Meniere's disease. *Otolaryngol Clin North Am* 1997;30:1159–1166.

25. Silverstein H. Use of a new device, the MicroWick, to deliver medication to the inner ear. *Ear Nose Throat J* 1999;78:595–598, 600.

CHAPTER 33

Superior Semicircular Canal Dehiscence Syndrome

Michael J. McKenna and Mitchell J. Ramsey

Only a fraction of patients who present with vestibular complaints will ultimately be diagnosed with a clear pathologic condition amenable to surgical intervention. To this short list of disorders a recent addition has been made, superior semicircular canal dehiscence (SSCD) syndrome. The astute recognition that bony dehiscence of the superior semicircular canal in humans can give rise to auditory- and pressure-evoked vestibular disturbances was made by Lloyd Minor (1). Minor's work was in part based on the experimental findings of Tullio (2) and Huizinga (3) many years earlier. Recent advances in computed tomography (CT) technology have made possible the definitive radiologic demonstration of SSCD along the floor of the middle cranial fossa. Patients affected by SSCD typically present with auditory- or pressure-induced vestibular symptoms. Although these acute symptoms are very distinctive, it is more common that patients with SSCD complain of chronic disequilibrium and unsteadiness. The unremitting nature of the chronic disequilibrium is the most significant complaint in most patients and in many cases is debilitating enough to justify surgical intervention.

PATHOPHYSIOLOGY

Nager (4) in 1947 first described a bony dehiscence of the superior semicircular canal in the middle cranial fossa from an individual with no accompanying clinical history. He attributed the defect to "senile osteoporosis" of the temporal bone. A recent systematic survey of temporal bones by Carey et al. (5) found dehiscence of the bone overlying the superior semicircular canal in approximately 0.5% of temporal bones. Bilateral dehiscence was found in approximately half of the cases identified (5). Their findings also revealed that a thin covering of bone (0.1 ml or less) was present in 1.4% of all cases studied (5). The clinical histories of these patients did not reflect the typical symptoms associated with SSCD. It is likely that many if not most individuals who have bony dehiscence of the superior semicircular

canal remain asymptomatic. This is further supported by incidental observation of superior canal dehiscence in temporal bone CT studies of nonvertiginous patients (H. Curtin, personal communication).

Factors that lead to the development of symptomatic bony dehiscence of the superior canal have yet to be determined. Our experience, and that of others, has been the occurrence of superior canal dehiscence in extremely well-pneumatized temporal bones with thin or defective tegmental plates, suggesting abnormal temporal bone development as one contributing factor. Some patients associate the onset of symptoms with minor head trauma, which has been suggested as a contributing factor in predisposed individuals. The third potential process leading to dehiscence is pressure-induced resorption of the tegmen tympani.

The mechanism of the evoked eye movements and vertigo can be explained by the presence of a third inner ear mobile window at the site of the superior semicircular canal dehiscence. Pressure changes transmitted through the third mobile window create motion of the endolymph and deflection of the superior canal cupula. Stimuli that produce inward displacement of the dehiscent membranous labyrinth result in ampullopetal deflection of the cupula. These inhibitory stimuli produce a decrease in the basal firing rate and include Valsalva maneuver, jugular venous compression, and negative middle ear pressure. Stimuli that cause outward deflection of the dehiscent membranous labyrinth produce ampullofugal deflection. These excitatory stimuli include increased middle ear pressure from Valsalva maneuver against closed nostrils, positive pressure on pneumotoscopy, and tragal compression.

SYMPTOMS AND SIGNS

Patients with SSCD syndrome may present with a variety of complaints, including hyperacusis, oscillopsia, auditory sensation with eye movement, and auditory- or pressure-evoked visual field shifts, vertigo, and disequilibrium. The auditory-

and pressure-evoked symptoms are most characteristic of SSCD, but chronic disequilibrium is also common and often the most debilitating symptom. A combined review of the clinical data from the Massachusetts Eye and Ear Infirmary and the one published series indicates 75% of patients complained of chronic disequilibrium; furthermore, this was the most common reason patients sought medical evaluation (6). Other common complaints included sound-evoked symptoms in 95%, pressure-evoked symptoms in 55%, and gaze-evoked symptoms in 20% of patients.

In most patients, careful examination reveals a vertical torsional nystagmus elicited in response to high level auditory stimuli, changes in middle ear pressure, or increased intracranial pressure. The torsional nystagmus is distinguishable from the horizontal nystagmus present in patients with a positive Hennebert's sign or positive fistula test. The direction of the nystagmus corresponds to a change in the basal rate of firing from the superior canal cupula. Excitatory stimulation of the right superior canal will produce a vertical-torsional nystagmus with a slow phase that is upward and counterclockwise to the patient. The resulting nystagmus can be appreciated using Frenzel lenses or infrared video-oculography or by placement of specialized ocular coils that are capable of measuring torsional eye movements. It is important to note that standard vestibular testing with electronystagmography (ENG) or rotatory chair is unlikely to reveal an abnormality in these patients. Standard ENG ocular leads may be inadequate because they are incapable of sensing purely rotational eye movement. In the combined series of patients, nystagmus could be elicited by auditory stimuli in 84%, Valsalva maneuver in 53%, and tragal pressure in 47% of patients.

A small subset of patients with SSCD will experience vestibular symptoms without changes in eye movement in response to appropriate stimuli. When this occurs in the presence of a CT-confirmed unequivocal bony dehiscence, the diagnosis may be highly suspect but not absolute. Ultimately, it is the constellation of symptoms, the physical and radiographic findings, and the determination of an incapacitating disability that makes a particular individual a surgical candidate.

Patients with SSCD may also present with purely auditory complaints, including hearing loss, pulsatile tinnitus, and autophony. Conductive hearing loss may be present and in some cases may mimic the clinical features of otosclerosis. In recent years, at least four patients at the Massachusetts Eye and Ear Infirmary underwent surgical exploration and stapedectomy without improvement in hearing and ultimately were discovered to have SSCD as the cause of the conductive hearing loss. In all cases, the conductive loss was greatest in the low frequencies, and low frequency bone conduction scores were elevated above 0 dB. Most cases of SSCD are accompanied by a mild conductive loss 5 to 10 dB, and some cases have no conductive loss. At present the cause of the conductive loss is unknown and under investigation. Patients with conductive hearing loss from SSCD have intact stapedial reflexes and lower stimulus thresholds for vestibular evoked myogenic responses (VEMP), two distinguishing features that can be used to differentiate them from true conductive hearing loss. Because of the incumbent risks of middle fossa plugging of the superior canal, including sensorineural hearing loss, we have not repaired the SSCD for patients with purely auditory symptoms.

PATIENT EVALUATION

As is the case for all patients who present for vestibular evaluation, a complete neurotologic and neurologic history and examination provide the basis for establishing an accurate diagnosis. Because the symptoms associated with SSCD are often atypical and variable, the patient's complaints may at first seem vague. It is unfortunately clear that many patients whom we have evaluated over the years for symptoms consistent with the diagnosis of SSCD have escaped accurate diagnosis. Details regarding the onset, frequency, and fluctuation of symptoms, as well as eliciting factors, such as auditory stimuli, tragal pressure, Valsalva maneuver, straining, and eye movements, must all be specifically probed. A complete review of auditory and vestibular symptoms, including hearing loss, tinnitus, aural fullness, oscillopsia, vertigo, and disequilibrium, must be conducted. Patients should be questioned about an individual and family history of migraine and other neurologic disorders.

Essential to the diagnosis of SSCD syndrome is the demonstration of a torsional vertical nystagmus in response to auditory stimuli or changes in middle ear or intracranial pressure. No patient should be considered a good surgical candidate unless vestibular symptoms can be provoked by auditory or pressure stimuli regardless of demonstrable changes in eye movement. Eye movements can be demonstrated in the office with the patient wearing Frenzel lenses. Nystagmus can often be evoked by one or more of the following: auditory stimuli from a Barany noisemaker placed directly in the suspected ear, positive or negative insufflation of the ear canal, and a Valsalva maneuver against a closed glottis or with plugged nose. If an immediate vertical torsional movement of the eyes cannot be readily demonstrated, efforts should be made to document the response with infrared video-oculography or with the use of specialized electromagnetic ocular coils capable of measuring rotatory nystagmus. As mentioned earlier, this is often not possible with conventional ENG leads and requires placement of a specialized coil directly on the surface of the cornea. If nystagmus is detected with conventional ENG leads, it may be horizontal and reflective of other inner ear pathology. This methodology, which is most often employed as a research tool, carries a low risk of minor corneal irritation and trauma, necessitating appropriate institutional approval and informed consent. A general neurologic examination, including cerebellar and cranial nerve evaluation, should be completed.

The patient's evaluation requires complete audiometric testing, including measurement of pure-tone air and bone thresholds, and speech discrimination. Sensorineural asymmetry should be appropriately evaluated with either auditory evoked response testing or magnetic resonance imaging (MRI). Standard vestibular testing, including ENG and rotational testing, should also be performed in all cases. The purpose of this testing is to rule out other vestibulopathies, both peripheral and central, which may be contributing to the patient's symptoms.

Of the auditory and vestibular testing available, the most useful is the VEMP. The VEMP responses are short latency relaxation potentials measured from tonically contracting sternocleidomastoid muscles that relax in response to ipsilateral presentation of loud clicks (7). Patients with SSCD have lowered VEMP thresholds compared with healthy persons. The VEMP responses are typically absent in patients with conductive hearing loss; however, as mentioned previously, some patients with SSCD have mild to moderate conductive hearing loss, but in these patients VEMP thresholds have been demonstrated to be present despite the conductive hearing loss (8). This may serve as a very useful tool in distinguishing between conductive hearing loss associated with SSCD and conductive hearing loss from other etiologies.

Ultimately, the clinical features suggesting a diagnosis of SSCD syndrome will be confirmed by the demonstration of a bony dehiscence of the superior canal along the floor of the middle cranial fossa by specifically requested high resolution CT scanning. The diagnosis cannot be made, and in fact is often missed, by standard temporal bone CT protocols. The essential component of an accurate CT protocol is the ability to produce sections parallel and perpendicular to the plane of the superior semicircular canal. Ultrahigh resolution CT of the temporal bones using fine cuts (0.5 mm) in an axial plane is performed. Coronal and sagittal reconstructions are performed to obtain images parallel and perpendicular to the plane of the superior semicircular canal; these are often referred to as the Poschl and Stenvers views, respectively (Fig. 33.1).

Patient Selection

Once a diagnosis of SSCD syndrome has been established, the treatment recommendations must be based on an assessment of an individual's symptoms, comorbidities, and preferences. In considering the patient's symptoms, one must assess the level of disability, both physical and psychologic; estimate their capability for recovery, including central compensation for a new unilateral vestibular loss; and determine their ability to compensate for unilateral hearing loss if it were to occur. Conservative treatment options include observation; behavioral modifications, such as avoidance of inciting stimuli; and pressure-equalization tubes.

Patients who are surgical candidates must consider themselves incapacitated to the point where they are willing to risk permanent sensorineural hearing loss, symptoms of persistent disequilibrium, and risks intrinsic to intracranial surgery. Furthermore, no patient should be considered a good surgical candidate without auditory- or pressure-evoked vestibular symptoms, regardless of associated eye movements. These clinical features are absolutely necessary to establish the diagnosis of superior canal dehiscence. Most surgical candidates suffer from the symptoms of chronic disequilibrium and oscillopsia. Surgery for patients who are solely bothered by auditory-induced vestibular symptoms is rarely justified unless these symptoms are preventing them from engaging in a chosen occupational pursuit. Surgery should not be done on a better or only hearing ear. In such cases, the diagnosis should be carefully reconsidered because sensorineural asymmetry may herald the presence of an associated vestibulopathy unrelated to SSCD dehiscence.

Patients with bilateral SSCD may have bilateral symptoms. At present, it is not clear how these patients will fair following bilateral superior canal occlusion. Clearly, the occurrence of a complication, including sensorineural hearing loss or increased disequilibrium, would represent a relative contraindication for contralateral ablation. The choice of which side to operate first should be based on the patient's perception of the more symptomatic ear. If this is not absolutely clear based on the patient's perception and CT scanning reveals a significant difference in the degree of dehiscence between the two sides, the side with the greater dehiscence should be considered first.

INFORMED CONSENT

At the time of this writing, our own experience and that reported in the literature with plugging or resurfacing of the superior semicircular canal in symptomatic patients is limited to fewer than 10 individuals with no follow-up longer than 3 years. This relatively small series forms the basis on which a major surgical procedure is being considered. It is of fundamental importance that patients be made aware of this relative lack of data when considering surgical intervention. This alone will discourage some patients from proceeding. The following are the most significant complications patients must consider in electing surgical therapy:

1. *Failure to achieve the surgical objective.* In the case of SSCD syndrome, the primary objective of surgery is to alleviate the associated vestibular symptoms while preserving vestibular and auditory function. Our experience, as well as others', suggests that more than 90% of patients experience improvement or complete resolution of their vestibular symptoms with treatment. However, recovery in most cases is not immediate and may require weeks to months. In many ways, the recovery is similar to that which follows posterior semicircular canal ablation for benign paroxysmal positional vertigo. Most patients experience a sense of disequilibrium in the immediate postoperative period, which differs subjectively from their preoperative symptoms and gradually improves over time. The auditory-evoked vestibular symptoms should be immediately improved. The per-

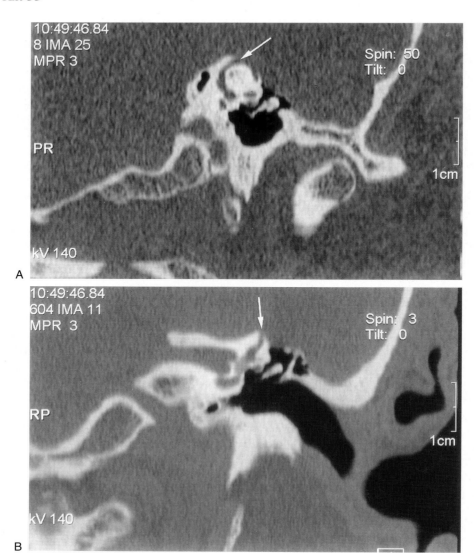

FIG. 33.1 CT imaging of SSCD requires the planes of imaging to include sections parallel and perpendicular to the superior canal. These planes are known as Poschl and Stenvers views, respectively. **A:** A CT coronal reformation in a plane parallel to the superior semicircular canal reveals absence of bone along the superior aspect of the canal approximately 4 mm long *(arrow)*. **B:** A CT coronal reformation in a plane perpendicular to the superior semicircular canal transects the canal and reveals a small bony dehiscence at the superiormost aspect of the canal *(arrow)*.

sistence of the auditory-evoked symptoms should cast doubt on the success of canal plugging. Another cause of persistent disequilibrium may be damage to the vestibular labyrinth from canal plugging. This may be revealed by a reduced ipsilateral peripheral vestibular response on postoperative vestibular testing. Patients with persistent incapacitating vestibular symptoms may require revision canal plugging if improvement does not occur over time and with vestibular physical therapy. Selective vestibular neurectomy or labyrinthectomy may be considered, depending on the status of the hearing in the operated ear.

2. *Hearing loss.* Of the five cases reported in the literature and the eight treated at the Massachusetts Eye and Ear Infirmary, a moderate sensorineural hearing loss has occurred in one patient, or 7%. Thus far the incidence of hearing loss is notably higher with SSCD treatment than that which occurs with posterior canal ablation for benign paroxysmal positional vertigo, where sensorineural hearing loss occurs in approximately 1% to 3% (9,10). Intuitively, this difference is likely related to surgical trauma from elevation of the middle fossa dura off a widely dehiscent superior canal. Under these conditions, preservation of the en-

dosteum is difficult and disruption of the membranous canal is likely.

Some surgeons have begun to approach the dehiscent superior canal through the mastoid, thus avoiding a middle fossa craniotomy with its intrinsic risks. The results of this approach have yet to be reported. One intrinsic risk of transmastoid superior canal occlusion is a conductive hearing loss from bone dust, which spills through the antrum into the attic and middle ear, resulting in bony fixation of the ossicular chain. Extrapolating from experience with posterior canal ablation, endolymphatic saccotomy, and retrolabyrinthine vestibular neurectomy, it can be estimated that conductive hearing loss will occur in 10% to 15% of cases when operated by a mastoid approach.

3. *Complications associated with middle fossa craniotomy.* Exposure and plugging of the superior canal by the middle fossa approach introduces potential risks intrinsic to all middle fossa procedures: cerebrospinal fluid (CSF) leak, meningitis, epidural hematoma, trismus, headache, temporal lobe swelling, and contusion from retraction.

Because the approach is extradural, the incidence of CSF leak should be low. However, because most cases occur in temporal bones with extremely thin tegmental plates, often containing multiple small bony defects, it may be difficult to achieve a watertight seal between the middle fossa and tympanomastoid cavity if a CSF leak were to occur. If the temporal dura is violated during the procedure, a large piece of temporalis fascia should be placed along the floor of the middle fossa to cover potential avenues for egress of spinal fluid into the middle ear and mastoid. Lumbar drainage for 3 to 5 days may be considered in cases with profuse intraoperative CSF leakage. Broad-spectrum antibiotics are started at the time of surgery and continued for 72 hours or for as long as a lumbar drain is in place.

SURGICAL APPROACHES

Reports on surgical repair of SSCD have described canal plugging, as well as resurfacing of the bony defect, as effective alternatives. At present it is not clear which method is superior. Thus far the patients operated on at our institution have undergone a plugging procedure using bone wax through a middle fossa approach. This method seems more advantageous because it is likely to achieve an immediate and lasting physical barrier.

Although some surgeons are beginning to approach the SSCD through the mastoid, reports of their results have not yet emerged.

Middle Fossa Superior Canal Occlusion

The patient is positioned supine with the head turned in a soft headrest. Facial nerve monitoring is not necessary ex-

cept as a precaution to prevent injury of an exposed geniculate ganglion, which may be dehiscent in approximately 5% of cases. The incision, soft tissue approach, and craniotomy are the same as for middle fossa resection of an acoustic neuroma except that the craniotomy has an epicenter directly over the external auditory canal rather than the anterior bias used for acoustic neuroma removal (see Chapter 12 on transtemporal approaches). Once the craniotomy has been accomplished and the bone of the inferior margin is lowered to the level of the middle cranial fossa floor, the dura over the floor of the middle fossa is elevated along a broad front. In patients with SSCD, the white labyrinthine bone in the region of the arcuate eminence usually stands in stark contrast to the thin, translucent bone of the tegmental plate. Before uncovering the dehiscent superior canal, the middle fossa retractor should be positioned and homeostasis maximized. Extreme care is necessary during dural elevation to avoid injury to the exposed membranous labyrinth. Once the dura is removed from the top of the dehiscent superior canal, care must be taken to avoid suctioning within the open canal. The dura over the canal is elevated under direct visualization through the operating microscope and continued medially to the point where the retractor blade can be positioned without obstructing access to the canal dehiscence (Fig. 33.2A). A small, flat piece of bone wax is then placed atop the opening in the canal and pressed into the canal with a quarter-inch cottonoid and bipolar forceps (Fig. 33.2B,C). Excess bone wax is removed with a small drum elevator or straight dissector, and the sealed fistula covered by a layer of temporalis fascia followed by an overlapping layer of Surgicel which serves to hold it in position as the middle fossa retractor blade is removed. Closure of the craniotomy wound is accomplished in a manner similar to other middle fossa procedures.

POSTOPERATIVE CARE

As with other intracranial procedures, patients are monitored overnight in the intensive care unit with observation of their neurologic status and tight blood pressure control. Once transferred from the unit, recovery and discharge from the hospital is most dependent on the severity of vestibular symptoms and the ability to safely ambulate, eat, and drink. Most patients can be discharged within 3 days of surgery. A minority of patients who suffer more severe vestibular symptoms may benefit from vestibular physical therapy prior to discharge.

Patients are seen for follow-up 10 days after surgery for suture removal and evaluation of progress. Outpatient vestibular physical therapy may be helpful for those patients who are continuing to experience disequilibrium and difficulty ambulating. A postoperative audiogram is performed 6 weeks following surgery. Some patients may complain of dryness of the ipsilateral eye, which results from stretching the greater superficial petrosal nerve at the time of surgery. Artificial tears may help to alleviate these symptoms while lacrimal function recovers.

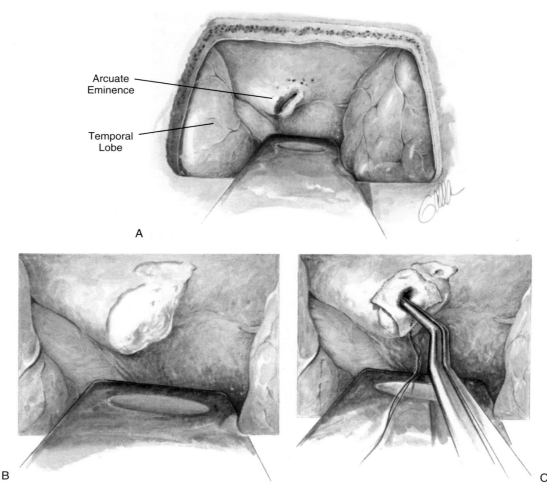

FIG. 33.2 The subtemporal craniotomy approach to the repair of the superior semicircular canal dehiscence. **A:** A middle cranial fossa exposure has been performed, and the temporal lobe is retracted exposing the canal dehiscence. During this portion of the surgery, extreme care must be taken to prevent injury to the membranous labyrinth during elevation of the dura. This exposure often reveals multiple areas of thin bone and dehiscent bone in the tegmen. The SSCD is identified as a dark, linear osseous defect in the otic capsule bone in the region of the arcuate eminence. **B:** Once adequate exposure is obtained, wax is applied over the dehiscent region. **C:** A small cotton pledget is used to contour the wax into the osseous defect, and the excess is removed. Temporalis fascia is often used to cover the repaired defect.

SURGICAL RESULTS

The surgical results from the one published series have been combined with the surgical series from the Massachusetts Eye and Ear Infirmary for a total of eight patients (6). Follow-up times range from 6 months to 36 months. Overall the success rate in resolving the evoked and chronic symptoms has been 75% (six of eight). One patient with initial failure to control symptoms underwent a successful revision surgery. One patient of ours was within 3 months of surgery and still moderately symptomatic; he noted only mild improvement postoperatively. In the one published report, two patients had vestibular hypofunction postoperatively. None of the patients from the Massachusetts Eye and Ear Infirmary have undergone postoperative vestibular testing thus far. Hearing was preserved at preoperative levels in 6 patients. Two patients developed a mild sensorineural hearing loss that has remained stable. A third patient developed mild to moderate loss that fully recovered with steroid treatment. No complications of meningitis, CSF leak, or seizures have been reported with the middle cranial fossa repair of SSCD.

COMMENT

The signs and symptoms of SSCD are similar to those that occur in patients with perilymphatic fistulas. The diagnosis of SSCD should be considered in all patients with presumed spontaneous perilymphatic fistula. The torsional quality of the nystagmus and the failure to elicit nystagmus with positional testing may be helpful in differentiating the two disorders.

REFERENCES

1. Minor LB, Solomon D, Zinreich JS, et al. Sound- and/or pressure-induced vertigo due to bone dehiscence of the superior semicircular canal. *Arch Otolaryngol Head Neck Surg* 1998;124:249–258.
2. Tullio P. *Das Ohr und die Entstehung der Sprache und Schrift.* Berlin: Urban and Schwarzenberg, 1929.
3. Huizinga E. On the sound reaction of Tullio in the pigeon and the fenestration operation in man. *Acta Otolaryngol Suppl* 1951;100: 174–180.
4. Nager FR. *Pathology of the labyrinthine capsule, and its clinical significance.* New York: Thomas Nelson & Sons, 1947.
5. Carey JP, Minor LB, Nager GT. Dehiscence or thinning of bone overlying the superior semicircular canal in a temporal bone survey. *Arch Otolaryngol Head Neck Surg* 2000;126:137–147.
6. Minor LB. Superior canal dehiscence syndrome. *Am J Otol* 2000; 21(1):9–19.
7. Colebatch JG, Halmagyi GM, Skuse NF. Myogenic potentials generated by a click-evoked vestibulocollic reflex. *J Neurol Neurosurg Psychiatry* 1994;57:190–197.
8. Streubel SO, Cremer PD, Carey JP, et al. Vestibular-evoked myogenic potentials in the diagnosis of superior canal dehiscence syndrome. *Acta Otolaryngol Suppl* 2001;545:41–49.
9. Zappia JJ. Posterior semicircular canal occlusion for benign paroxysmal positional vertigo. *Am J Otol* 1996;17:749–754.
10. Parnes LS. Update on posterior canal occlusion for benign paroxysmal positional vertigo. *Otolaryngol Clin North Am* 1996;29:333–342.

PART VIII

Surgery for Trauma to the Temporal Bone and Dysfunction of the Facial Nerve

CHAPTER 34

Trauma of the Tympanic Membrane and Ossicles

Herbert Silverstein

Injury to the tympanic membrane and ossicles may occur in many ways, including a blast injury, slap to the auricle, slag-burn, waterskiing accident, and introduction into the ear canal of objects that penetrate the tympanic membrane. It may also occur in association with temporal bone fractures. A secondary infection is a common sequela of these injuries. Management depends on determining the probable extent of injury by careful history. Important questions to ask include the following: How and when did the injury occur? Has there been bleeding or drainage of clear fluid from the ear? Is there a hearing loss and, if so, how severe? Was dizziness experienced at the time of injury or later? It is essential to examine the ear with magnification, preferably the operating microscope, to determine the extent of injury and formulate a plan of treatment. A workup should include audiometric tests, including air, bone, and speech discrimination testing.

Nonpenetrating injuries, such as a slap to the auricle, a blast injury, or a waterskiing accident, usually heal without surgery; however, the area of injury should be cleared of wax, keratin, and loose hair that may have been imploded and that retard or prevent spontaneous healing. After cleaning the ear, torn segments of the tympanic membrane can be repositioned on a bed of Gelfoam and splinted with silk strips and cotton packing. Earlobe adipose tissue can be introduced as a medial onlay graft if the perforation is large.

Experience with 27 penetrating injuries reported in 1973 is representative of the continued experience with these cases (1). The most common cause of self-inflicted injury is the cotton-tipped applicator being used to clean the ear. The second most common occurs in children who introduce objects into their ears. About one-third of the lacerations of the tympanic membrane are associated with ossicular dislocations or fractures and most commonly involve the incus or stapes (Figs. 34.1 to 34.4). Fracture of the manubrium or neck of the malleus is less common (Fig. 34.5).

The acute symptoms include some or all of the following: pain, conductive hearing loss, bleeding from the ear, laceration of the skin of the concha and canal, vertigo, unsteadi-

ness, facial palsy, and drainage of clear fluid (perilymph, cerebrospinal fluid). The decision regarding the need for emergent surgery is dictated by the symptoms and the findings on microscopic otoscopy. For children, this preliminary examination may require general anesthesia, and the surgeon should be prepared to complete the repair, if indicated, while the child is anesthetized. For adults, the preliminary examination, done with or without local anesthesia, will determine whether a surgical procedure is indicated. If the symptoms and findings suggest a complicated problem, such as a large perforation, dislocated or fractured ossicles, or a perilymph fistula, the repair can be done immediately or scheduled to be done within 24 hours.

About 20% of penetrating injuries result in fistulization of the perilymphatic space by either a subluxated stapes or a fractured footplate. The occurrence of immediate or subsequent vertigo is an important symptomatic clue for the presence of such an injury. The repair may take the form of a graft of adipose or other tissue on the footplate, return of a dislocated stapes to its normal position, or removal of a fractured or dislocated stapes followed by oval window grafting. If the stapes footplate is subluxated into the vestibule and cannot be elevated into the oval window, a control hole can be drilled at the inferior edge of the promontory so that a small instrument can be used to elevate the footplate. The Argon or KTP laser may be helpful if a stapedotomy opening is needed in a mobile or floating footplate. Correction of a dislocated incus or fractured long process may take the form of replacement to its normal position or removal followed by sculpting and replacement as a strut. After all surgery has been completed, the tympanic graft can be momentarily elevated for a final inspection of the integrity of the ossicular reconstruction.

If facial nerve injury has occurred, the fallopian canal is examined for a depressed fracture and the bony fragments are elevated or removed. The nerve trunk should be exposed for several millimeters on each side of the injury.

The torn fragments of tympanic membrane are placed on a bed of Gelfoam, and a tissue graft of earlobe adipose tissue

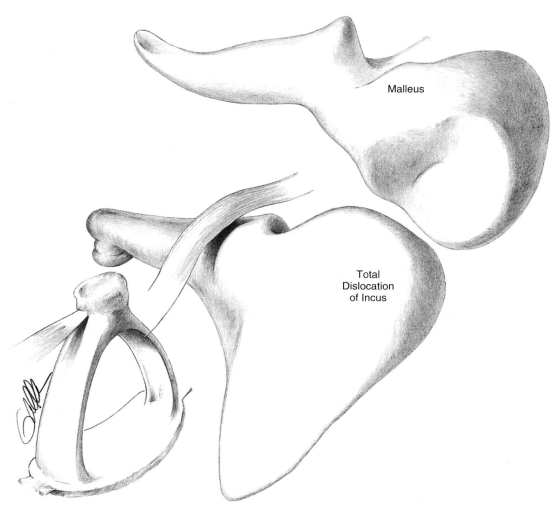

FIG. 34.1 Dislocated incus *(left ear).* This sketch shows a traumatic dislocation of the incus at both the incudostapedial and incudomalleal articulations. Reconstruction will require removal of the incus and introduction of a minor columella strut.

Malleus

Total
Dislocation
of Incus

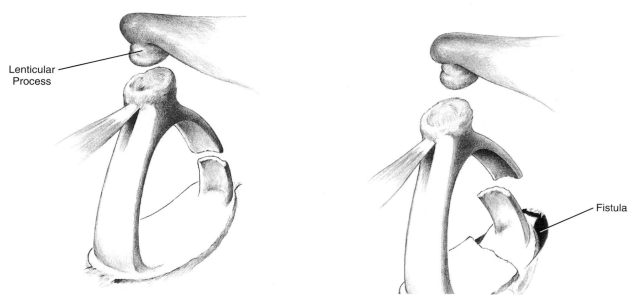

Lenticular
Process

Fistula

FIG. 34.2 Incus subluxation and crural fracture. The sketch shows a fracture of the anterior crus and lateral dislocation of the lenticular process causing discontinuity at the incudostapedial articulation. If the incudomalleal articulation seems stable, the reconstruction can consist of interposing a bone chip between the lenticular process of the incus and the head of the stapes.

FIG. 34.3 Stapes fracture-dislocation and oval window fistula. This sketch demonstrates a fracture of the footplate and anterior crus with an inward displacement of the footplate fragment resulting in an oval window fistula. The incudostapedial articulation is also separated. If the other ossicles are intact, the reconstruction can consist of a total stapedectomy and implantation of a fat-wire prosthesis.

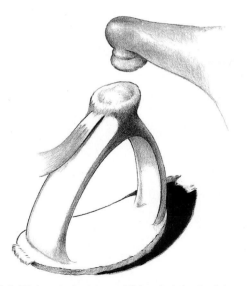

FIG. 34.4 Dislocated stapes. This sketch depicts a dislocated stapes at both the incudostapedial and stapediovestibular articulations without fracture. In this situation it is usually possible to return the stapes to its normal position and, with the aid of Gelfoam pledgets or autogenous tissue graft, to stabilize the stapes and acquire a satisfactory functional result.

or other tissue is used as a medial underlay graft to assist the healing process.

Early postoperative complications are unusual after middle ear surgery. If a perilymph fistula was repaired, there may be vertigo and nausea. These symptoms are treated with fentanyl/droperidol combination (Innovar), 1 ml every 6 hours, and prochlorperazine (Compazine) (25 mg) suppositories. Postoperative infection can occur. If there is drainage and pain from the ear, the packing is removed, a culture is obtained, and appropriate antibiotics are given. A delayed facial weakness is treated expectantly. Late complications include graft failure and conductive hearing loss, both of which will require revision surgery.

Chronic symptoms of the neglected or untreated cases include some or all of the following: suppurative otorrhea, continuing conductive hearing loss, sensorineural hearing loss, persisting vertigo or unsteadiness, persisting facial palsy, and cholesteatoma of the middle ear. These cases are managed as planned tympanoplasty procedures.

REFERENCES

1. Silverstein H, Fabian RL, Stool SE, et al. Penetrating wounds of the tympanic membrane and ossicular chain. *Trans Am Acad Ophthalmol Otolaryngol* 1973;77:125–135.

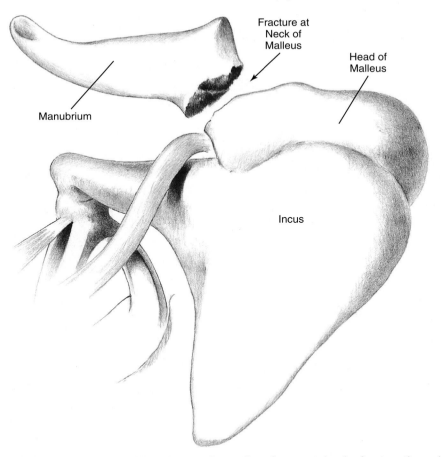

FIG. 34.5 Malleus fracture *(left ear).* In this case the malleus has sustained a fracture through its neck. A fracture in this location rarely heals, and hearing loss may be severe. Reconstruction will require removal of the incus and a columella strut, preferably bone, to bridge the gap from the head of the stapes to either the manubrium or tympanic membrane.

CHAPTER 35

Management of Dural Defects of the Temporal Bone

Jamie M. Rappaport, Michael J. McKenna, and William W. Montgomery

Cerebrospinal fluid (CSF) leak remains a potentially serious complication of temporal bone trauma or surgery, particularly with respect to meningitic infection. Embryologic pneumatization of the temporal bone occurs by extension of air cell tracts from the middle ear into the mastoid, petrous, and accessory areas. As such, the air cells of the temporal bone are all interconnected in a honeycomb fashion with the middle ear space (1). The eustachian tube represents the final common pathway for leakage of CSF from the pneumatized temporal bone.

Cerebrospinal fluid otorrhea or otorhinorrhea from the temporal bone is the end result of rupture of the arachnoid membrane or herniation of the brain through a defect in the protective dura mater and calvarium. The rupture may be small, admitting only a herniation of arachnoid (meningocele), or may be large enough to accommodate brain tissue (encephalocele). Flow of CSF through either type of fistula may be a trickle or profuse, chronic or intermittent, and usually ceases temporarily for a few weeks following an attack of meningitis. Cerebrospinal fluid otorrhea indicates a leakage of spinal fluid from the posterior or middle cranial fossa by way of the mastoid or middle ear through a defect in the tympanic membrane or the external auditory canal. Cerebrospinal fluid otorhinorrhea has a similar origin to otorrhea. If the tympanic membrane is intact, the spinal fluid flows through the middle ear and eustachian tube and exits by way of the nasal cavity.

ANATOMY OF CEREBROSPINAL FLUID LEAK

Cerebrospinal fluid is produced by the choroid plexus at a rate of 0.3 ml per minute, or a total of approximately 500 ml per day. Cerebrospinal fluid may enter the interior of the temporal bone by a number of routes (Fig. 35.1). There may be a defect in the middle ear or mastoid tegmen that most commonly follows mastoid or intracranial surgery. A defect in the posterior fossa may enter the mastoid air cell system by way of Trautmann's triangle or cells anterior and poste-

rior to the sigmoid portion of the lateral sinus. This occurs most commonly following posterior fossa surgery and occasionally with mastoid surgery (2). Occasionally there is a defect directly through the medial aspect of the internal auditory canal. A defective, fractured, or diseased oval window may be the site of the exit of CSF into the middle ear. A widely patent cochlear aqueduct or defect of the modiolus may result in CSF leakage into the middle ear through the oval or round window either spontaneously or following surgical or external trauma. Rarely, the CSF finds its way to the mastoid antrum by way of a defect in the petromastoid canal or into the middle ear space by way of Hyrtl's fissure (3).

PATHOGENESIS

Otorrhea or otorhinorrhea arises from disorders of the temporal bone that may be divided into (i) trauma, (ii) congenital defects, (iii) infection of the middle ear and mastoid, and (iv) tumors of the skull base (most commonly as a complication of their surgical removal).

Trauma

Trauma of the temporal bone may result in a longitudinal or transverse fracture or a combination of both. *Longitudinal* fractures follow a blow to the front or side of the head. They extend along the longitudinal axis of the petrous bone, passing through the external auditory canal, tegmen tympani, and anterior surface of the petrous pyramid, usually sparing the inner ear structures of the otic capsule. Longitudinal fractures account for 80% of temporal bone fractures. If hearing is affected, it is usually a conductive loss due to middle ear fluid (CSF or blood). Occasionally, the ossicular chain may be disrupted. Injury to the facial nerve occurs in about 15% of cases and is usually at the level of the geniculate ganglion. Cerebrospinal fluid leakage, when it occurs, is by way of a laceration of the dura at the tegmen tympani. Most often this type of leakage is self-limiting and does not

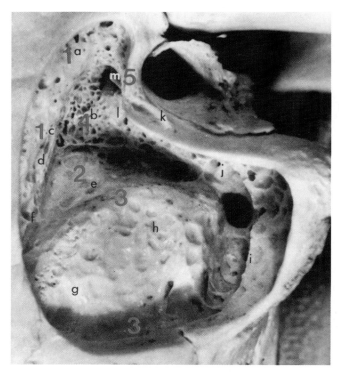

FIG. 35.1 Anatomy of CSF leak—temporal bone. *a:* anterior superior cells; *b:* perilabyrinthine cells; *c:* tegmen middle fossa; *d:* Citelli's angle (superior petrosal sinus); *e:* bony plate anterior to posterior fossa dura; *f:* posterior superior cells; *g:* sigmoid sinus plate; *h:* posteromedial cells; *i:* digastric crest; *j:* anterior inferior cells; *k:* Macewen's triangle (Henle's spine); *l:* horizontal semicircular canal; *m:* short process of incus. Routes of CSF leakage: *1:* by way of the middle ear and mastoid tegmen from the middle fossa dura; *2:* into the mastoid air cell system by way of Trautmann's triangle and the posterior fossa dura; *3:* cells anterior and posterior to the sigmoid portion of the lateral sinus from the posterior fossa dura; *4:* petrous pyramid: petrous cells to mastoid antrum through the lateral aspect of the internal auditory canal into the perilymph; *5:* through the oval window (not shown).

require surgical repair. Cerebrospinal fluid otorrhea occurs when the tympanic membrane or external ear canal is breached; otherwise the CSF flows down the eustachian tube and is evident as rhinorrhea. Vertigo is not common.

Transverse fractures of the temporal bone follow a blow to the occiput, which produces a line of fracture perpendicular to the long axis of the petrous pyramid; they account for 15% of temporal bone fractures. Often this fracture crosses the vestibule and internal auditory canal and results in a complete sensorineural hearing loss and loss of vestibular function. The site of injury to the facial nerve is medial to the geniculate ganglion and occurs in approximately 45% of transverse fractures. Ecchymosis may develop within hours over the mastoid (Battle's sign). Examination of the tympanic membrane may reveal blood or CSF in the middle ear. Injury to the ossicles and tympanic membrane are rare. Spinal fluid leakage and vertigo are quite common. A *com-*

bined longitudinal and transverse fracture of the temporal bone follows severe trauma and represents 5% of temporal bone fractures.

Penetrating wounds, either directly through the skin into the temporal bone or indirectly through the external auditory canal and tympanic membrane, can result in CSF otorrhea or otorhinorrhea. Barotrauma, such as descending rapidly in an airplane or a rapid change in pressure while scuba diving, can occasionally result in CSF leakage. A congenital defect is most likely a predisposing factor in these cases.

Congenital Defects

Congenital defects resulting from malformation and incomplete closure of fissures can result in communications between the middle ear space and the middle and posterior cranial fossae. These defects can occur both in the mastoid portion of the temporal bone and the bony labyrinth. Congenital absence of bone and dural barriers between the subarachnoid space and the mastoid air cells are common causes of CSF leak in infants and children who have experienced recurrent bacterial meningitis. Congenital malformations resulting in CSF leakage occur most commonly in the cochlear aqueduct and internal auditory canal and permit direct communication between the subarachnoid space and the perilymph. These defects usually remain asymptomatic until a defect in either the round or oval window occurs as a result of an external trauma or surgery.

Spontaneous CSF fistulas in adults most commonly occur through defects in the floor of the middle cranial fossa (4). It is theorized that constant, physiologic intracranial pressure and CSF pulsations cause focal ischemia, which weakens the dura to the point of rupture (5). More recent theories propose the formation of arachnoid granulations, macroscopic enlargements, or distensions of minute projections of arachnoid villi. These project into the intradural venous sinuses, allowing for resorption of CSF into the bloodstream (6–8).

The necessity for dural injury in the pathogenesis of CSF leakage by way of the temporal bone appears to be evident in the work by Åhrén and Thulin (9). They reviewed the autopsy findings in 94 skulls in patients more than age 40 years. Defects in the tegmen were found in 21% of these skulls. There were multiple defects in 6% of the skulls. Another 16% had thin transparent bone in the tegmen tympani. There were no meningeal or cerebral herniations in these cases. A small to large area of exposed dura during mastoid surgery, whether primary or secondary, does not necessarily preclude a cerebral herniation. One must be particularly careful to avoid full-thickness cauterization of dura using monopolar cautery and avoid tearing the dura with a cutting bur or curette. Herniations usually occur through the central portion of normal exposed dura. Encephaloceles can herniate through a defect as small as 2 mm. Herniation of dura may occur in the area where brain abscesses were drained through the tegmen in the past.

Infection

Cerebrospinal fluid leakage as a complication of both acute and chronic infection occurs because the mastoid air cells are in close contact with the posterior fossa and the roof of the middle ear (tegmen tympani), which is the floor of the middle cranial fossa. Consequently, infection can destroy this thin, bony communication and erode dura to establish a communication between the subarachnoid space and the tympanomastoid compartment. Chronic middle ear and mastoid infection can result in spontaneous CSF leakage by formation of an erosive granulation tissue or cholesteatoma. Cerebrospinal fluid leakage occurs much more commonly following the surgical treatment of this disease.

The bacterial flora of chronic otitis media and mastoiditis are distinct from the usual respiratory pathogens. Gramnegative organisms, both aerobes (*Proteus, Klebsiella,* and *Pseudomonas*) and anaerobes (*Bacteroides* species) predominate. Mixed infections are common. Chronic infections rarely produce meningitis, presumably because the chronicity permits adhesions of the meninges to the infected bone. Ipsilateral brain abscesses of the temporal lobe or cerebellar hemisphere with mixed organisms are the more common intracranial complications of chronic otitis media and mastoiditis. Other complications include subdural abscesses, sigmoid sinus thrombophlebitis, and otitic hydrocephalus.

Skull Base Tumors and Surgery

Tumors of the temporal bone are a rare cause of spontaneous CSF leakage. However, CSF leak remains a fairly common postoperative complication following skull base surgery. Subsequent meningitis adds a significant source of morbidity and mortality to these patients, many of whom are already handicapped by neurologic dysfunction, including cranial nerve deficits. Factors that contribute to the formation of CSF fistulas include suboptimal wound closure, formation of granulation tissue, and elevated intracranial pressure. The dura of the posterior fossa is tightly adherent to the temporal and occipital bones. A partial or total excision of the temporal bone almost invariably results in a dural defect.

Early surgeries for large acoustic neuromas were reported to be complicated by CSF leak in up to one third of cases. Subsequent advances in neurotologic technique, including waxing of air cells at the internal auditory canal petrosotomy site and fat obliteration of the mastoid defect, have reduced this incidence to less than 20% in more current series, with some reporting rates lower than 10% (10–13). Hoffman reviewed several previous series and calculated an overall incidence of 12% for both translabyrinthine and suboccipital approaches (14). In a multicenter review of the Acoustic Neuroma Registry, 175 of 1579 patients (11.1%) developed CSF leak. Meningitis was seen in 39 patients (2.5%) (15). Some studies have shown even higher rates of meningitis (1,16).

Cerebrospinal fluid leaks are more likely to occur following the removal of larger tumors (1,16,17). The onset of CSF leaks following skull base surgery is often delayed, with more than one third diagnosed more than a week postoperatively (1,18,19).

We reviewed our own experience in 504 skull base cases managed between 1988 and 1996 (20). There were 63 cases of CSF leakage in this series, for an overall incidence of 12.5%, as shown in Table 35.1. Rates for meningitis are depicted as well. The mean postoperative interval of diagnosis of CSF leak was 5.7 days, with a range of presentation from immediately postoperatively to 33 days. An additional three cases of late postoperative presentation of CSF leak were seen. Seven of the 63 patients with CSF leak were noted postoperatively to have hydrocephalus, two of whom required placement of ventriculoperitoneal shunts. Noninvasive expectant management was associated with cessation of CSF leakage in only two of eight cases (25%), suggesting that observation alone is not a reasonable option. Lumbar drainage was successful in 30 of 41 patients (73%). Standard mastoid obliteration, with or without obliteration of the eustachian tube orifice via a posterior tympanotomy, was successful in 7 of 10 cases (70%). Extended tympanomastoid obliteration was used in 24 cases, including those patients who failed the aforementioned techniques. All 24 of these patients (100%) had no recurrent or persistent leak.

DIAGNOSIS

Signs and Symptoms

The signs and symptoms that can be associated with a CSF leak are shown in Table 35.2. Unless leakage of CSF is profuse and persistent, its source can be difficult to ascertain. Thus the investigation must be systematic and thorough. Leakage should be considered in patients who have had severe trauma to the head, especially if there is evidence of skull base fracture (e.g., Battle's sign, raccoon eyes). A patient who has had repeated episodes of meningitis should be thoroughly investigated for CSF otorrhea or otorhinorrhea.

TABLE 35.1 *CSF leaks in 504 skull base cases (1988 to 1996)*

Pathology/ approach	Incidence of CSF leak	Incidence of meningitis
Acoustic neuroma/ suboccipital	53/426 = 12.4%	8/426 = 1.9%
Acoustic neuroma/ translabyrinthine	3/35 = 8.6%	3/35 = 8.6%
Glomus jugulare/ infratemporal fossa	0/12 = 0.0%	0/12 = 0.0%
Meningioma/ subtemporal- suboccipital	2/8 = 25.0%	0/8 = 0.0%
Others/various	5/23 = 21.7%	2/23 = 8.7%
TOTAL	63/504 = 12.5%	13/504 = 2.6%

TABLE 35.2 *Signs and symptoms of CSF leak*

- Repeated episodes of meningitis
- History of otorrhea or rhinorrhea
- Salty taste and frequent swallowing
- Rhinorrhea from dependent side of nose when recumbent and on side
- Hearing loss (usually conductive)
- Sensation of fluid in ear
- Visualization of bubbles or liquid behind the tympanic membrane
- Mass behind tympanic membrane
- Mass encountered at the time of mastoidectomy; the mass may pulsate, and a tegmental bony defect may be palpable behind the mass
- Seizure activity

The CSF otorrhea or otorhinorrhea may be intermittent. It is most often unilateral. An acceleration in the flow rate with change in position is rather characteristic. Flow is usually increased with a Valsalva maneuver or compression of the jugular veins. If the rate of flow is profuse, the patient will swallow frequently when in a recumbent position. The fluid is clear unless there is an associated acute trauma, when it may be serosanguineous. It is odorless, salty, and nonsticky. Leakage through the mastoid or middle ear may be attended with a conductive hearing loss and the appearance of fluid or air bubbles behind the tympanic membrane.

The diagnosis and localization of a dural defect may often be made by acquiring from the patient an accurate and detailed history and a description of the present illness. The interrogation should include the following questions:

1. Has there been a leakage of clear fluid?
2. Is the leakage from the ear or the nose?
3. Which side is leaking?
4. Is the leakage constant or intermittent?
5. Is there a salty taste associated with the leakage?
6. Is there frequent swallowing when in the recumbent position?
7. Is there excessive liquid entering the throat from above?
8. Has there been a sensation of fluid in the ear?
9. When in the recumbent position, does the leakage occur only from the dependent side of the nose? An affirmative answer would be consistent with spinal fluid passing from the middle ear by way of the eustachian tube into the nasopharynx and out by way of the dependent nasal cavity.
10. Does the leakage occur in gushes? This happens when a paranasal sinus becomes filled with spinal fluid and suddenly evacuates with a change of position.
11. Is there a history of trauma to the head?
12. Is there a history of ear or intracranial surgery?

Cerebrospinal Fluid Tests

Unless contaminated by blood from trauma or infection, CSF is a clear, colorless liquid with a low specific gravity (1.006) containing no mucus, low protein (less than 50 mg/dl), and a modest glucose content (50 to 70 mg/dl). Cerebrospinal fluid will not stiffen a handkerchief when dried, as do nasal secretions and those of serous otitis media. A halo test may be positive.

Testing of rhinorrhea fluid for glucose and protein content can be confusing. Normally, CSF contains more glucose and less protein than nasal secretions; however, nasal secretions may contain glucose as a result of lacrimation and may be watery and contain little protein. We have abandoned the use of the testing of rhinorrhea fluid with laboratory paper test strips. After standing in a test tube, sediment will be found in nasal secretion or the secretions of middle ear effusion, whereas spinal fluid will remain clear without sediment (Fig. 35.2). At this same time, one should consider culturing the fluid.

More recently, immunologic identification of ß$_2$-transferrin (tau band) serum protein electrophoresis has been recommended (21–23). ß$_2$-transferrin is present in CSF and not in serous otitis, serous effusion, or nasal secretions. Staining the sample with silver nitrate adds a 40-fold higher sensitivity to this test, so that samples less than 1 ml are usually sufficient.

At the Massachusetts Eye and Ear Infirmary sodium fluorescein in a concentration of 0.5% is the preferred method of identifying CSF leaks. A stronger concentration of fluorescein has been reported to cause transient neurologic symptoms. It is thus very important that this concentration be exact. The fluorescein test should not be performed for at least 1 month after meningitis has been successfully treated or until CSF leak recurs. An accurate method of identifying and localizing the source of CSF rhinorrhea or otorhinorrhea is a test consisting of intrathecal injection of fluorescein dye solution and subsequent detection of its presence intranasally or by otoscopy. The patient is placed in the sitting position for the first portion of this examination. After examination of the nasal cavities, nasopharynx, pharynx, and ears

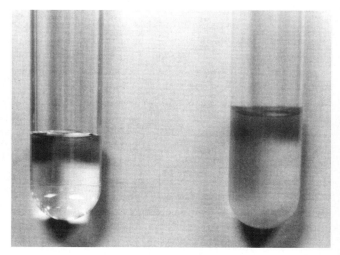

FIG. 35.2 The left test tube contains clear spinal fluid, the right cloudy nasal precipitate. Both have been standing for longer than 24 hours.

for the presence of fluid, both nasal cavities are packed with 4% cocaine-impregnated cottonoid strips to produce topical anesthesia and shrink the nasal mucous membrane. The cocaine packing is removed after 10 minutes. Next, a separate moist cottonoid strip is inserted into (i) the sphenoethmoidal recess, (ii) the region of the olfactory slit and middle meatus, and (iii) the anterosuperior nasal cavity (Fig. 35.3). A lumbar puncture is done and the CSF pressure recorded. In patients with a large dural defect, the CSF pressure is often quite low, making a spinal tap in the recumbent position difficult. In these cases the tap is carried out with the patient in the sitting position. (If increased intracranial pressure is present, the patient may be in need of a ventriculoperitoneal shunt. Taking the pressure is thus an important part of the CSF leakage workup.)

Fluorescein (0.5 to 1 ml of a 10% solution) diluted with at least 10 ml of CSF is slowly injected intrathecally (Fig. 35.4). During this injection, CSF is repeatedly withdrawn as the injection progresses to make certain that the fluid is being injected intrathecally. In cases in which 10 ml of CSF cannot be obtained because of low spinal fluid pressure, Hartmann's solution or normal saline solution may be used to dilute the fluorescein dye.

Following the lumbar puncture, the patient is placed in the horizontal supine position. If the leakage has been profuse, the head is elevated on one or two pillows. After a period of 10 minutes to 1 hour, depending on the rate of the CSF leakage, the cotton pledgets are carefully removed and labeled according to their intranasal location. The room is darkened, and the pledgets are inspected for the presence of fluorescein dye using an ultraviolet light source (Wood's lamp). The presence of fluorescein dye on the pledget that was placed in the sphenoethmoidal recess most likely indicates leakage by way of a posterior ethmoidal cell, sphenoidal sinus, or eustachian tube or as a result of otorhinorrhea. Fluorescein on the pledget placed in the olfactory region and middle meatus indicates a leakage by way of the cribriform plate or anterior ethmoidal cells. Fluorescein on the pledget placed in the anterosuperior nasal cavity indicates that the dural defect is probably behind the posterior wall of the frontal sinus.

In addition to the foregoing technique, the posterior pharyngeal wall is examined for the presence of fluorescein. Both tympanic membranes are also examined. If fluorescein dye is present in the middle ear, the yellow-green color of the tympanic membrane will be readily apparent by standard otoscopy. If equipment and facilities for nasal packing are not available, a fiber-optic scope can be used to identify fluorescein in the nasopharynx and ear. When relying on direct inspection, however, one must consider that CSF rhinorrhea coming from the middle or posterior fossa and draining into the mastoid antrum and down the eustachian tube may be intermittent.

Imaging

Routine radiographs of the skull and temporal bones may demonstrate an intracranial abnormality such as air or a tumor, fluid in the middle ear or mastoid, or fractures of the temporal bone. Nuclear medicine scans may provide additional information. As with fluorescein, pledgets are placed in the nasal cavity and technetium-99–labeled serum albumin or indium 111-DPTA is injected intrathecally. These pledgets are subsequently removed and examined for their radioisotope content. High-resolution computed tomography (HRCT) and magnetic resonance imaging (MRI) are a more exacting technique for pinpointing the sight of a dural defect. One of the various pneumatized cavities may show

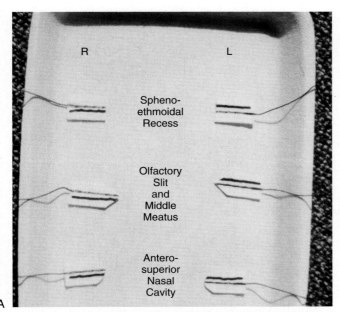

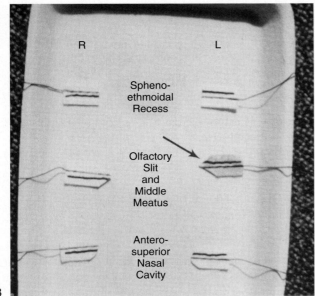

FIG. 35.3 A: The technique used to organize the cottonoid strips in localizing the site of CSF leakage. **B.** A positive test in the left cribriform ethmoid region.

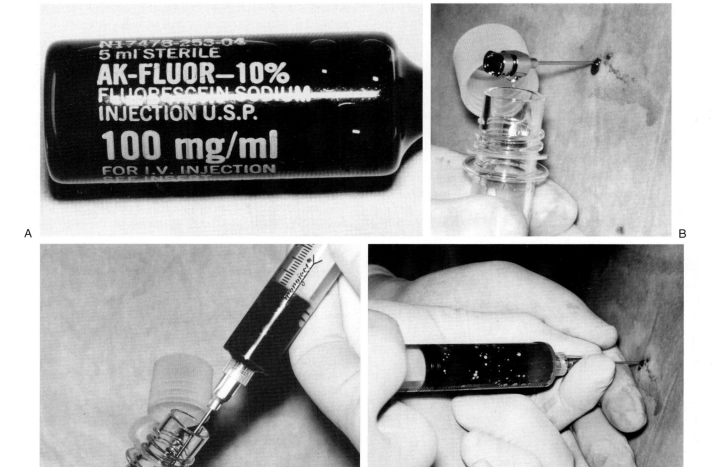

FIG. 35.4 A: Vial of 10% fluorescein (100 mg/ml). **B:** Collection of 10 ml spinal fluid in a test tube. **C:** 0.5 ml of 10% solution of fluorescein is diluted with 10 ml of spinal fluid. **D:** During injection of the diluted fluorescein, the clinician must be certain that the spinal fluid is being injected intrathecally, using frequent aspiration of spinal fluid during the injection.

increased density owing to the presence of CSF. A small fracture may be demonstrated. Pneumocephalus is diagnostic of a dural defect, and its location may indicate the sight of leakage.

If there is active drainage, contrast-enhanced (pantopaque, metrizamide) cysternography can both identify and localize a dural defect (24). Although computed tomographic (CT) scanning offers the best information regarding bony structures, an MRI scan is more useful for assessing the status of the dural and brain tissue.

The diagnosis of CSF leak in many cases remains a challenge. Clinical acumen and an index of suspicion are essential to the management of these patients. This workup may be lengthy, and, if a delay is expected while the patient is being investigated, one should give consideration to vaccinat-

ing the patient against the more common organisms causing meningitis, namely *Haemophilus influenzae* and *Streptococcus pneumoniae*.

MANAGEMENT OF CEREBROSPINAL FLUID LEAKS

Conservative Treatment

In most cases of CSF leak, especially following trauma or surgery, a short period of observation is warranted (25). The patient is placed on bed rest with head-of-bed elevation. Pressure dressings are reinforced, and the patient is instructed to avoid sniffing, sneezing, or straining pressure. Stool softeners are prescribed to minimize straining. Medication may be used to decrease CSF production, including acetazolamide (Diamox) or furosemide (Lasix). The use of prophylactic antibiotics is controversial (26).

A lumbar drain is placed and left in situ for 3 to 5 days. Alternatively, serial lumbar punctures may be performed daily. One should carefully observe the patient for signs of meningitis or increased intracranial pressure. These may include fever, headache, nausea, neck stiffness, or change in mental status. If intracranial pressure remains elevated or if hydrocephalus is present, a shunt procedure may be indicated.

The majority of CSF leaks can be successfully managed with such conservative treatment. Early CSF leaks are more likely to respond to conservative management than those of later onset (11).

Surgical Treatment

On occasion, an erroneous diagnosis of serous effusion is made when in fact the middle ear contains CSF. This becomes obvious when a myringotomy is performed (with or without a ventilating tube). Immediate intervention is warranted because of the potential for meningitis and its complications.

Middle Ear Approach

On rare occasions, one may encounter an obvious CSF leakage from the oval window during middle ear surgery such as a stapedectomy (perilymph gusher). If possible, the operation should be completed, using either a vein graft or perichondrium to form an oval window seal. Alternatively, a fat-wire prosthesis may be used (Chapter 22). If there is no hearing in the involved ear, the vestibule can be obliterated with adipose or fibrous tissue by way of the oval window. Some surgeons prefer not to enlarge the oval window, citing advantages in maintaining the grafts in place, whereas others preface the obliteration by connecting the oval and round windows.

Mastoid Approach

Most small leaks that are encountered during mastoid surgery will cease spontaneously but are best covered with a layer of fascia and Surgicel. It is best to repair a dural injury intraoperatively when it is recognized. Paparella et al. (27) recommend removal of surrounding tegmental bone to expose normal middle fossa dura 5 mm circumferentially. (For posterior fossa dura, 1 cm is recommended because less arachnoid tissue is available for spontaneous repair in that region [27].) A temporalis fascia graft can then be tucked between the dura and bone and further secured with Surgicel, fibrin glue, or Tisseel. Slits in the dura can sometimes be repaired with sutures. If the leakage is profuse and the defect in the dura is large, then it is first covered with Surgicel or Gelfoam, followed by repeated packing and waiting. After

the leakage is controlled, the mastoid is obliterated with local pedicled flaps or adipose tissue (Chapter 17). The pedicled flaps are preferable to the adipose tissue when a radical mastoidectomy has been performed.

When repairing a CSF leak in the mastoid, a postauricular incision is used to expose the mastoid after fluorescein has been injected intrathecally using the technique outlined earlier. A complete mastoidectomy is carried out so as to expose the anterosuperior cells, the perilabyrinthine cells, the tegmen, the mastoid, Citelli's angle, the bony plate anterior to the sigmoid sinus, the posterior fossa dura posterior to the sigmoid sinus, and the digastric crest. In so doing, and having injected fluorescein intrathecally, a leakage into the mastoid from either the middle or posterior cranial fossa can be easily identified. If the leakage is by way of the perilabyrinthine cells from the petrous pyramid, these cells must be carefully dissected.

If prolapsed brain tissue is encountered in the mastoid, it is nonfunctional and thus can usually be excised (28,29). As a general rule, posterior and lateral defects in the dura can be repaired by way of the mastoid approach, whereas anterior and medial defects are best repaired using the middle cranial fossa approach alone or combined with the mastoid approach. If no hearing is present, the translabyrinthine approach may be used if the CSF leakage is by way of the petrous apex cells. A defect in the tegmen over the middle ear is repaired using dried temporalis fascia. The fascia is inserted and tucked in on the intracranial side of the defect external to the dura.

Middle Fossa Approach

Exposure for the middle fossa approach is accomplished by using a postauricular incision along with an extension superiorly over the squamous portion of the temporal bone (Figs. 35.5 to 35.9). The temporalis fascia is carefully preserved, or a large piece can be taken for grafting at this time. The squamous portion of the temporal bone is exposed using self-retaining retractors. A portion of squamosal bone is resected using first cutting, then diamond burs. If there is herniation of brain tissue into the mastoid, a mastoidectomy is performed. Small amounts of healthy brain tissue can be returned to the middle cranial fossa, but larger herniations should be amputated, especially if necrotic.

The temporal lobe dura is carefully elevated and exposure is accomplished using a House-Urban middle cranial fossa retractor. An appropriately sized piece of temporalis fascia is used to line the defect. For bony defects greater than 5 mm, many surgeons will split the calvarium of the craniotomy flap and use this to further reenforce the tegmen defect. The temporal lobe is then allowed to return to its anatomic position, sandwiching the graft reconstruction. Adkins and Osguthorpe (30) described a "mini-craniotomy" approach for repairing smaller brain hernias.

If the posterior canal wall has been surgically removed, a skin graft is applied over the defect in the mastoid cavity, the

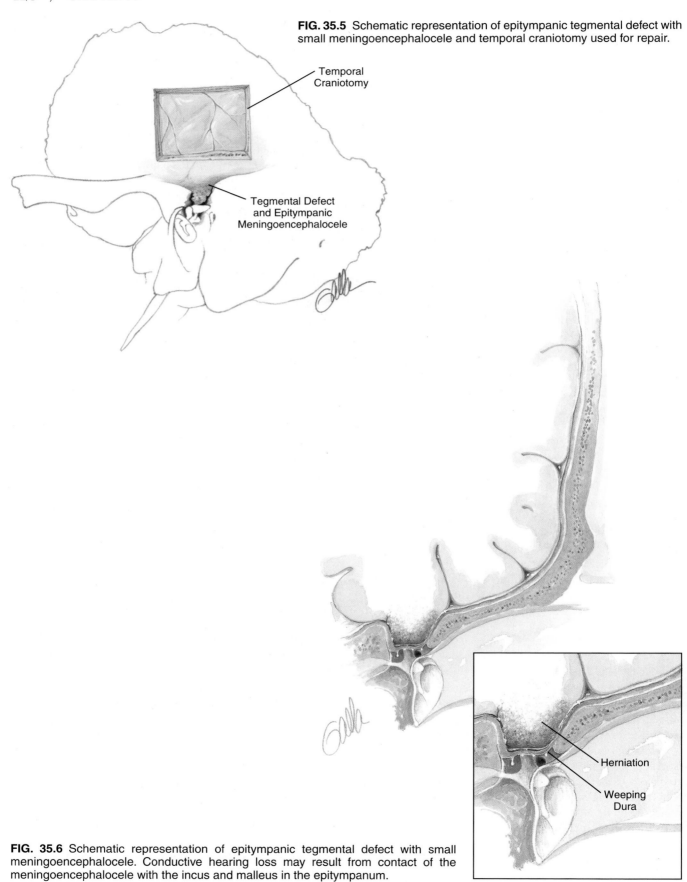

FIG. 35.5 Schematic representation of epitympanic tegmental defect with small meningoencephalocele and temporal craniotomy used for repair.

Temporal Craniotomy

Tegmental Defect and Epitympanic Meningoencephalocele

Herniation

Weeping Dura

FIG. 35.6 Schematic representation of epitympanic tegmental defect with small meningoencephalocele. Conductive hearing loss may result from contact of the meningoencephalocele with the incus and malleus in the epitympanum.

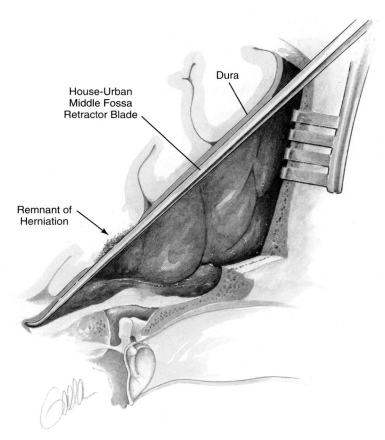

Dura

House-Urban
Middle Fossa
Retractor Blade

Remnant of
Herniation

FIG. 35.7 Middle fossa repair of epitympanic meningoencephalocele. The temporal lobe dura is elevated beyond the defect in the floor of the middle cranial fossa followed by placement of the middle fossa retractor.

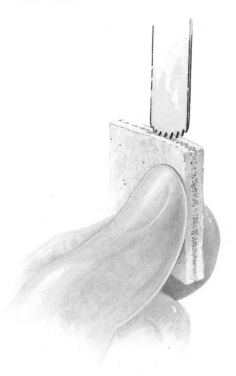

FIG. 35.8 A portion of the bone flap is split with a sagittal saw for use in the repair of the tegmental defect.

cavity is packed with half-inch iodoform gauze impregnated with bacitracin, and the gauze is removed 2 to 3 weeks later. If the posterior wall is intact, the mastoid cavity is obliterated with adipose tissue.

Cerebrospinal Fluid Leakage Following Skull Base Surgery

Management of CSF leakage in skull base surgery involves both primary prevention and secondary treatment of leaks once they develop. Several maneuvers can be performed at the initial procedure to minimize leaks. In suboccipital approaches, these include bone wax, fat, and muscle to close the mastoid air cells exposed during the craniotomy and to obliterate the petrosotomy defect created by removal of the posterior wall of the internal auditory canal. It is our practice in nonhearing preservation cases to drill this region widely to maximize exposure of the tumor limits, including extension toward the anterior face of the petrous ridge and lateral exposure to the fundus of the internal auditory canal. This ensures complete removal of tumor with less inherent risk of persistence or recurrence (31). This technique does, however, expose a greater proportion of air cells. The suboccipital approach does not afford any direct access to the middle ear or eustachian tube.

FIG. 35.9 A portion of the split bone flap is used to cover the bony defect in the floor of the middle fossa, sandwiched between two layers of temporalis fascia.

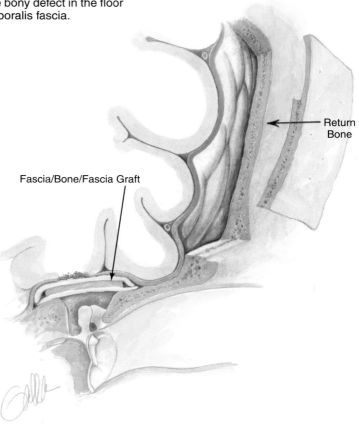

Return Bone

Fascia/Bone/Fascia Graft

In translabyrinthine approaches, primary prevention of CSF leakage can be accomplished with a wider range of obliteration options. Packing of the eustachian tube can be attempted in a limited fashion via a posterior tympanotomy approach following removal of the incus and head of the malleus or severing of the tensor tympani tendon. Dissection of the peritubal air cell tracts can only be accomplished by lowering the posterior canal wall, removing the tympanic membrane, and dissecting the protympanum to exenterate and plug the peritubal air cell region. There are some select reports of endoscopic closure of the eustachian tube via the nasopharynx (1,32,33).

The closure of a translabyrinthine defect must be done meticulously. The dural flaps are reapproximated, and a large piece of temporalis fascia or fascia lata is used to cover the defect. Montgomery introduced the use of abdominal fat in acoustic neuroma surgery (Fig. 35.10) (34). This adipose tissue becomes revascularized within days of implantation, assuming that it is not injured with instrumentation (35). House et al. (10) refined this technique by advocating the use of strips (0.5 by 3.0 cm) of fat as opposed to a single large piece. They noted that the free fat grafts tended to swell slightly after transplantation, thus forming a seal. This is in contrast to free muscle, which tends to atrophy. Tissue seal may be improved with the use of fibrin glue (36) or Tisseel (37). Other authors have proposed the utility of bacitracin irrigation (38),

factor XIII (39), and maintainance of a postoperative compression dressing for as long as possible (40).

Despite these preventive strategies, a CSF leak still may occur following a skull base procedure. The type of repair of such leaks will depend on the nature of the original procedure and the status of the patient's residual hearing. If hearing has been preserved, a mastoidectomy is performed, the bony labyrinth is skeletonized, and bone wax and paté are used to obliterate the air cell tracts. The antrum is sealed, and the mastoid is obliterated with fat. When hearing has not been preserved or if leakage persists despite a mastoid obliteration, a more definitive obliteration should be performed.

As mentioned, the ability of the surgeon to definitively obliterate the eustachian tube via a posterior tympanotomy route alone is limited. A review of the Massachusetts Eye and Ear Infirmary's temporal bone collection examined the prevalence and extent of peritubal aeration in normal specimens (41). In this study, histologic sections from 120 adult human temporal bones were examined by light microscopy. Peritubal pneumatization was present in 78 (65%) of the specimens. Of the 57 specimens in which the openings of the peritubal cells could be identified, in 52 (91%) the cells opened into the eustachian tube anterior to its tympanic orifice. In 13 temporal bones (21%), the tubal openings were at a distance of more than 5 mm anterior to the tympanic orifice of the eustachian tube. Therefore a CSF leak may persist

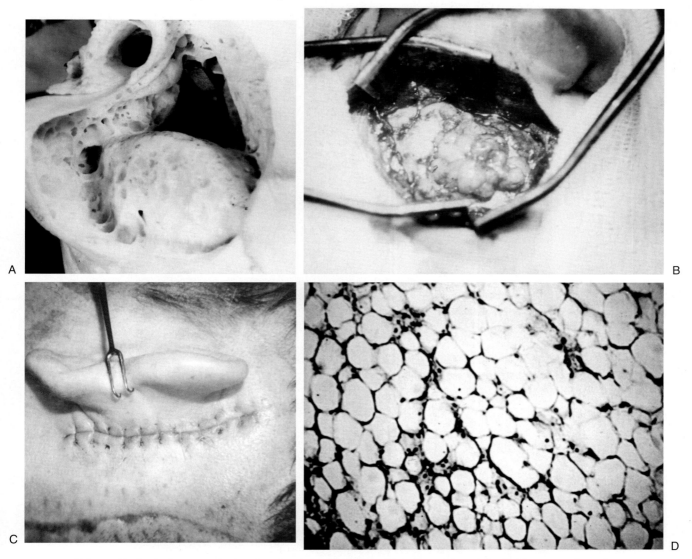

FIG. 35.10 A: A photograph showing the dural defect resulting from a translabyrinthine resection of a small acoustic neurinoma. **B:** The labyrinthine-mastoidectomy defect has been obliterated with abdominal subcutaneous adipose tissue. **C:** The skin incision is closed without drainage. **D:** A tissue section from an adipose autograft 1 month after being implanted into the mastoid cavity. There was no loss of adipose tissue and very little fibrous tissue.

through these tubal openings despite obliteration of the mastoid, middle ear, and tympanic orifice of the eustachian tube (Figs. 35.11 and 35.12). Other studies have supported this high incidence of peritubal cell aeration (42,43).

In consideration of these temporal bone findings, it is our approach to perform an extended typanomastoid obliteration technique. This is an extension of the modified Rambo procedure (44), which has been described by previous authors for skull base defects (42,43,45,46).

The extended tympanomastoid obliteration technique (Chapter 17) is accomplished via a postauricular incision (separate from any previous suboccipital craniotomy wound), followed by transection and two-layered closure of

the external auditory meatus. After meticulous removal of the tympanic membrane and epithelial remnants, a limited canal wall–down mastoidectomy is performed. The peritubal air cell tracts are exenterated by removing the anterior tympanic ring medial to the temporomandibular joint, exposing the anterior mesotympanum. The petrous carotid artery is skeletonized at its anterior turn within the protympanum, and the porus of the eustachian tube is widened and drilled distally toward its bony-cartilaginous junction. This region is then obliterated with bone wax on the ends of cotton-tipped applicators. Care must be taken to avoid overpacking in a situation of carotid dehiscence to prevent compression of the petrous carotid vessel within its bony canal.

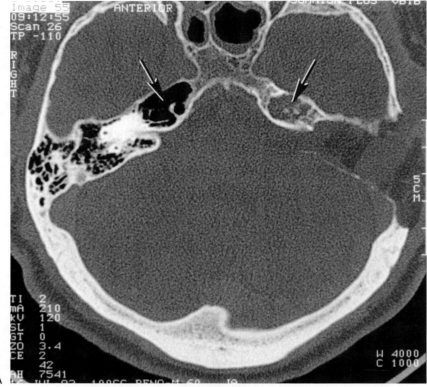

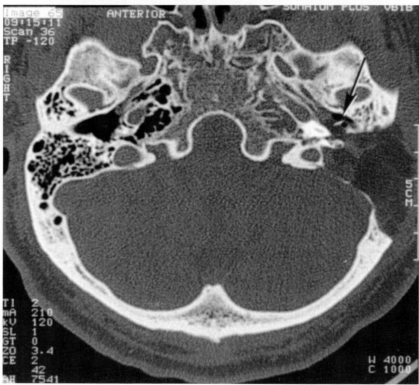

FIG. 35.11 A: Axial computed tomographic (CT) scan after translabyrinthine resection of a left acoustic neuroma with fat obliteration of the middle ear and mastoid. The petrous apex on both sides is well pneumatized (*arrows*). On the left, the petrous apex is filled with material of fluid density. **B:** An axial CT scan at the level of the eustachian tube shows extensive pneumatization of the petrous apex, including peritubal cells bilaterally. Although most of the petrous apex on the left is filled with material of fluid density, air is present in the peritubal cells near the tympanic orifice of the eustachian tube (*arrow*), suggesting passage of air via the eustachian tube, despite previous surgical obliteration of the tympanomastoid compartment. (From Saim L, McKenna MJ, Nadol JB Jr. Tubal and tympanic openings of the peritubal cells: implications for CSF otorhinorrhea. *Am J Otol* 1996;17:335–339. Reprinted with permission from Lippincott Williams & Wilkins.)

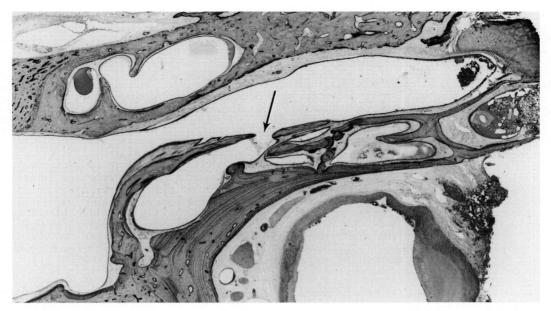

FIG. 35.12 Photomicrograph showing peritubal cells opening into the eustachian tube (*arrow*). The epithelial lining of peritubal air cells was in continuity with that of the eustachian tube and middle ear. (Hematoxylin and eosin, 13.8X.) (From Saim L, McKenna MJ, Nadol JB Jr. Tubal and tympanic openings of the peritubal cells: implications for CSF otorhinorrhea. *Am J Otol* 1996;17:335–339. Reprinted with permission from Lippincott Williams & Wilkins.)

Fat is then harvested from the abdominal wall, cut into strips, and used to fill the middle ear and mastoid cavities. The postauricular incision is then closed in a watertight manner with reapproximation of the mastoid periosteum, a deep layer of interrupted 3-0 vicryl sutures, and a skin layer of continuous, locking 3-0 nylon suture.

We recently reviewed a series of 54 patients managed with extended tympanomastoid obliteration (20). These patients were followed for a mean of 16.7 months postoperatively. Five of the 54 cases (9%) had minor complications, which included abdominal wound hematoma and granulation tissue at the meatal closure site. There were no major complications, that is, no patient developed recurrent or persistent CSF leak, meningitis, cholesteatoma formation, new facial nerve paralysis, or vascular injury.

Therefore we recommend that any hearing-sacrificing skull base procedures involving a lateral approach, including translabyrinthine removal of acoustic neuromas, should have primary closure accomplished with an extended tympanomastoid obliteration procedure. By directly addressing the peritubal air cells, this procedure has enabled us to decrease our CSF leak rate to zero since implementing this treatment philosophy. The added morbidity is minimal, and definitive packing of the eustachian tube can be accomplished in less than 1 hour of additional surgical time. In light of the significant morbidity and mortality of meningitis in patients undergoing skull base procedures, we recommend extended tympanomastoid obliteration for any patients who develop meningitis following skull base proce-

dures, regardless of hearing status or the presence of overt otorhinnorrhea.

REFERENCES

1. Bryce GE, Nedzelski JM, Rowed DW, et al. CSF leaks and meningitis in acoustic neuroma surgery. *Otolaryngol Head Neck Surg* 1991;104: 81–87.
2. Harner SG, Laws ER Jr. Translabyrinthine repair for CSF otorhinorrhea. *J Neurosurg* 1982;57:258–261.
3. Gacek RR, Leipzig B. Congenital cerebrospinal otorrhea. *Ann Otol Rhinol Laryngol* 1979;88:358–365.
4. Lundy LB, Graham MD, Kartush JM, et al. Temporal bone encephalocele and CSF leaks. *Am J Otol* 1996;17:461–469.
5. Ommaya AK. Cerebrospinal fluid rhinorrhea. *Neurology* 1964;14: 106–113.
6. Schuknecht HF, Gulya AJ. *Anatomy of the temporal bone with surgical implications.* Philadelphia: Lea & Febiger, 1986:125–126.
7. Gacek RR. Arachnoid granulation cerebrospinal otorrhea. *Ann Otol Rhinol Laryngol* 1990;99:854–862.
8. Gacek RR. Evaluation and management of temporal bone arachnoid granulations. *Arch Otolaryngol Head Neck Surg* 1992;118:327–332.
9. Åhrén C, Thulin C-A. Lethal intracranial complications following inflation in the external auditory canal in treatment of serous otitis media and due to defects in the petrous bone. *Acta Otolaryngol (Stockh)* 1965;60:407–421.
10. House JL, Hitselberger WE, House WF. Wound closure and CSF leak after translabyrinthine surgery. *Am J Otol* 1982;4:126–128.
11. Wiet RJ, Teixido M, Liang JG. Complications in acoustic neuroma surgery. *Otolaryngol Clin North Am* 1992;25:389–412.
12. Nadol JB Jr, Chiong CM, Ojemann RG, et al. Preservation of hearing and facial nerve function in resection of acoustic neuroma. *Laryngoscope* 1992;102:1153–1158.
13. Montgomery WW. Dural defects of the temporal bone. *Am J Otol* 1993;14:548–551.
14. Hoffman RA. CSF leak following acoustic neuroma removal. *Laryngoscope* 1994;104:40–58.

15. Wiegand DA, Ojemann RG, Fickel V. Surgical treatment of acoustic neuroma (vestibular schwannoma) in the United States: report from the Acoustic Neuroma Registry. *Laryngoscope* 1996;106:58–66.

16. Glasscock ME III, Kveton JF, Jackson CG, et al. A systematic approach to the surgical management of acoustic neuroma. *Laryngoscope* 1986;96:1088–1094.

17. Rodgers GK, Luxford WM. Factors affecting the development of CSF leak and meningitis after translabyrinthine acoustic tumor surgery. *Laryngoscope* 1993;103:959–962.

18. Gardner G, Robertson JH, Clark CW. 105 patients operated on for cerebellopontine angle tumours—experience using combined approach and CO₂ laser. *Laryngoscope* 1983;93:1049–1055.

19. Robson AK, Clarke PM, Dilkes M, et al. Transmastoid extracranial repair of CSF leaks following acoustic neuroma resection. *J Laryngol Otol* 1989;103:842–844.

20. McKenna MJ, Rappaport JM, Nadol JB Jr, et al. Extended tympanomastoid obliteration for the prevention and management of CSF leakage in skull base surgery. *Abstracts of the Second International Skull Base Congress,* San Diego, CA, June 29–July 4, 1996:8.

21. Oberascher G. CSF otorrhea—new trends in diagnosis. *Am J Otol* 1988;9:102–108.

22. Keir G, Zeman A, Brookes G, et al. Immunoblotting of transferrin in the identification of CSF otorrhoea and rhinorrhoea. *Ann Clin Biochem* 1992;29:210–213.

23. Bateman N, Jones NS. Rhinorrhoea feigning CSF leak: nine illustrative cases. *J Laryngol Otol* 2000;114:462–464.

24. Stone JA, Castillo M, Neelon B, et al. Evaluation of CSF leaks: high-resolution CT compared with contrast-enhanced CT and radionuclide cisternography. *Am J Neuroradiol* 1999;20:706–712.

25. Myers DL, Sataloff RT. Spinal fluid leakage after skull base surgical procedures. *Otolaryngol Clin North Am* 1984;17:601–612.

26. Brodie HA. Prophylactic antibiotics for posttraumatic CSF fistulae. A meta-analysis. *Arch Otolaryngol Head Neck Surg* 1997;123:749–752.

27. Paparella MM, Meyerhoff WL, Morris MS, et al. Mastoidectomy and tympanoplasty. In: Paparella MM, Shumrick DA, eds. *Otolaryngology,* 3rd ed. Philadelphia: WB Saunders, 1991:1405–1439.

28. Glasscock ME III, Dickins JR, Jackson CG, et al. Surgical management of brain tissue herniation into the middle ear and mastoid. *Laryngoscope* 1979;89:1743–1754.

29. Feenstra L, Sanna M, Zini C, et al. Surgical treatment of brain herniation into the middle ear and mastoid. *Am J Otol* 1985;6:311–315.

30. Adkins WY, Osguthorpe JD. Mini-craniotomy for management of CSF otorrhea from tegmen defects. *Laryngoscope* 1983;93:1038–1040.

31. Poe DS, Tarlov EC, Gadre AK. Translabyrinthine drillout from suboccipital approach to acoustic neuroma. *Am J Otol* 1993;14:215–219.

32. Kwartler JA, Schulder M, Baredes S, et al. Endoscopic closure of the eustachian tube for repair of CSF leak. *Am J Otol* 1996;17:470–472.

33. Sataloff RT, Zavod MB, Myers DL. Otogenic CSF rhinorrhea: a new technique for closure of CSF leak. *Am J Otol* 2000;21:240–243.

34. Montgomery WW, Ojemann RG, Weiss AD. Suboccipital-translabyrinthine approach for acoustic neuroma. Arch Otolaryngol 1966; 83:566–569.

35. Montgomery WW. The fate of adipose implants in a bony cavity. *Laryngoscope* 1964;74:816–827.

36. Nishihira S, McCaffrey TV. The use of fibrin glue for the repair of experimental CSF rhinorrhea. *Laryngoscope* 1988;98:625–627.

37. Symon L, Pell MF. CSF rhinorrhea following acoustic neurinoma surgery. Technical note. *J Neurosurg* 1991;74:152–153.

38. Kartush JM, Cannon SC, Bojrab DI, et al. Use of bacitracin for neurotologic surgery. *Laryngoscope* 1988;98:1050–1054.

39. Kawamura A, Tamaki N, Yonezawa K, et al. Effect of factor XIII on intractable CSF leakage after a transpetrosal-approach operation: a case report. *No Shinkei Geka* 1997;25:53–56.

40. Tos M, Thomsen J. CSF leak after translabyrinthine surgery for acoustic neuroma. *Laryngoscope* 1985;95:351–354.

41. Saim L, McKenna MJ, Nadol JB Jr. Tubal and tympanic openings of the peritubal cells: implications for CSF otorhinorrhea. *Am J Otol* 1996;17:335–339.

42. Grant IL, Welling DB, Oehler MC, et al. Transcochlear repair of persistent CSF leaks. *Laryngoscope* 1999;109:1392–1396.

43. Meyerson LR, Monsell EM, Rock JP. Preventive management of CSF leakage in translabyrinthine surgery. *Laryngoscope* 1996;106:610–613.

44. Rambo JHT. Primary closure of the radical mastoidectomy wound; a technique to eliminate postoperative care. *Laryngoscope* 1958;68: 1216–1227.

45. Coker NJ, Jenkins HA, Fisch U. Obliteration of the middle ear and mastoid cleft in subtotal petrosectomy: indications, technique, and results. *Ann Otol Rhinol Laryngol* 1986;95:5–11.

46. Meyerhoff WL, Stringer SP, Roland PS. Rambo procedure: modification and application. *Laryngoscope* 1988;98:795–796.

CHAPTER 36

Facial Nerve Injury and Decompression

Robert A. Sofferman

ANATOMY OF THE FACIAL NERVE

Temporal bone fractures following blunt trauma are the most common cause of facial nerve injury, with more than half caused by vehicular accidents (1). Other injuries related to sporting activities and assaults can similarly affect the temporal bone, especially falls that directly injure the occiput and transmit tremendous force to the skull base. Penetrating injury from weapons or missiles produce high-frequency fragmentation of the fallopian canal, mastoid air cells, and medial temporal bone, resulting in facial nerve injury and often transection of nerve integrity. Habercamp (2) has demonstrated that 75% of patients with gunshot wounds to the temporal bone have immediate-onset facial paralysis. Iatrogenic injury to the facial nerve by routine otologic surgery or during the process of neurosurgical procedures involving instrumentation along the floor of the middle cranial fossa may become apparent to the surgeon for the first time only in the recovery room as an unexpected complication. Each of these conditions has its own special anatomic, pathophysiologic, and management considerations. Understanding the comprehensive anatomy and topognostic information, electrophysiologic assessments, and basic science and clinical correlates allows a management schema that is somewhat predictable for each of these broad areas.

The facial nerve has the longest intraosseous course of any motor nerve in the body. Injury to the neurovascular supply of the facial nerve and intra- or extra-sheath hematoma within confined spaces may explain the special anatomic reasons for the development of facial paralysis in nontransection injury. Although the geniculate ganglion and proximal segments are amply supplied by branches of the labyrinthine artery and superficial petrosal branch of the middle meningeal artery, the vascular supply is essentially end-arterial with limited collateralization (3). The narrowest osseous path of the facial nerve is the labyrinthine segment, also the site of the most common physiologic impairment of facial nerve function in temporal bone trauma. These anatomic details might be among the most important factors responsible for the evolution of facial paralysis in the trauma condition under discussion (4).

The facial nerve originates at the facial nucleus within the medulla, courses medially around the abducens nucleus in the pons, and exits the brainstem at the cerebellopontine angle (Fig. 36.1). For the purpose of surgical discussion, five anatomic segments of the facial nerve can be identified (3) (Fig. 36.2):

1. The *pontine segment,* between the brainstem and porus, measures 23 to 24 mm in length. At this point the facial nerve is anterior to the cochleovestibular nerve. The special sensory and visceral efferent components of the facial nerve pass in a separate bundle adjacent to the main motor trunk as the nervus intermedius.
2. The *meatal segment,* within the internal auditory canal, is 7 to 8 mm in length. The facial nerve passes superior to the falciform crest in the lateral aspect of the canal and is separated from the superior vestibular nerve by a vertical crest of bone (Bill's bar).
3. The *labyrinthine segment,* between the meatal segment and geniculate ganglion, is 4 mm in length. The osseous canal surrounding the facial nerve is narrowest at the most proximal portion of the labyrinthine segment. This segment passes anterolaterally, paralleling the axis of the arcuate eminence of the superior semicircular canal, and passes superior and in proximity to the basal turn of the cochlea. The geniculate ganglion is triangular and averages 1.09 mm in length.
4. The *tympanic* or *horizontal segment,* between the geniculate ganglion and second genu, is 12 to 13 mm in length. The proximal edge of the geniculate ganglion is 5 mm anterosuperior to the posterior edge of the processus cochleariformis. The facial nerve passes superior to the oval window niche, a region where in approximately 55% of cases it is dehiscent (6).
5. The *mastoid* or *vertical segment,* between the second genu and stylomastoid foramen, measures 15 to 20 mm in length. At the second genu, the semicircular canal lies 0.5 mm posterosuperior to the facial nerve. The digastric ridge is a useful landmark just posterior to the stylomastoid foramen.

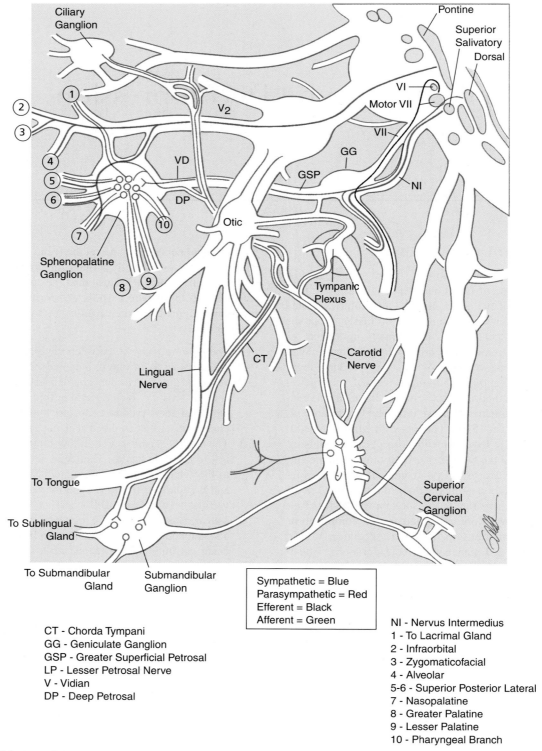

CT - Chorda Tympani
GG - Geniculate Ganglion
GSP - Greater Superficial Petrosal
LP - Lesser Petrosal Nerve
V - Vidian
DP - Deep Petrosal

Sympathetic = Blue
Parasympathetic = Red
Efferent = Black
Afferent = Green

NI - Nervus Intermedius
1 - To Lacrimal Gland
2 - Infraorbital
3 - Zygomaticofacial
4 - Alveolar
5-6 - Superior Posterior Lateral
7 - Nasopalatine
8 - Greater Palatine
9 - Lesser Palatine
10 - Pharyngeal Branch

FIG. 36.1 Schematic diagram of the facial nerve (5). The motor division is shown in *blue,* the sensory division in *black,* and the parasympathetic pathway in *red.* (Reprinted with permission from Janfaza P, Nadol JB Jr, Galla RJ, et al. *Surgical anatomy of the head and neck.* Philadelphia: Lippincott Williams & Wilkins, 2001.)

represent more than 50% of the cross-sectional area of the fallopian canal. These veins can bleed substantially during incision of the sheath.

MICROANATOMY OF THE FACIAL NERVE

The microanatomy of the facial nerve is important to an understanding of facial nerve dysfunction and recovery (8,9). The motor division of the facial nerve consists of approximately 7,000 motor axons with cell bodies located in the medullary brainstem (10). The connective tissue component of the nerve consists of endoneurium, perineurium, epineurium, and nerve sheath (Fig. 36.3). The endoneurium consists of longitudinally oriented fibrous tissue around and between individual axons. The perineurium consists of parallel, circumferential, tightly arranged fibrous tissue around individual fascicles of the nerve. The epineurium

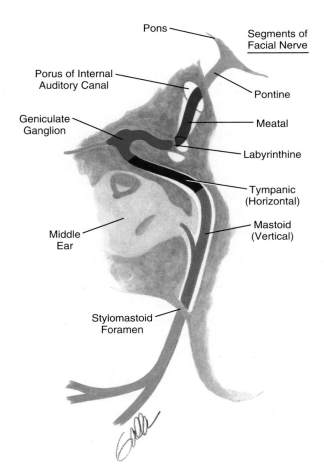

FIG. 36.2 The extramedullary segments of the facial nerve.

BLOOD SUPPLY OF THE FACIAL NERVE

The principal blood supply of the facial nerve originates from two opposite ends of the fallopian canal (2). The superficial petrosal artery, arising from the middle meningeal artery, enters the facial hiatus to supply the geniculate ganglion and horizontal and vertical segments of the facial nerve. The vessel anastomoses with the stylomastoid artery at the level of the oval window. The stylomastoid artery arises from the posterior auricular artery and passes through the stylomastoid foramen to supply portions of the mastoid cavity, tympanic membrane, and middle ear in addition to the facial nerve. There are anastomoses between the stylomastoid artery and posterior meningeal artery in the region of intersection of Arnold's and facial nerves. Despite the anastomotic blood supply, the principal arterial supply enters from each end of the facial canal, with resultant potential for ischemia in the intervening segments. Ogawa and Sando (7) have described significant variations in blood supply at the various segments of the facial nerve. Based on cross-sectional histology, the labyrinthine segment seems to have a much poorer blood supply than either the horizontal or vertical segments. Single or multiple large veins accompany the facial nerve within the epineural sheath and often

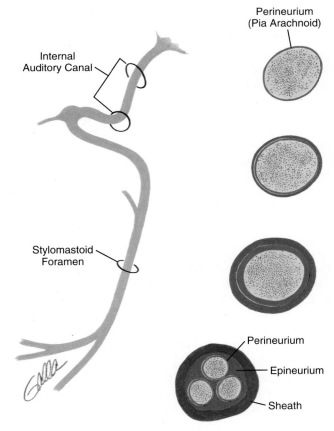

FIG. 36.3 Connective tissue components of the facial nerve. The endoneurium consists of longitudinally oriented fibrous tissue around and between individual axons. The perineurium *(green)* consists of parallel circumferential fibrous tissue around individual fascicles. The epineurium *(orange)* consists of loose connective tissue between and around fascicles and is continuous with the more dense nerve sheath *(purple)*. The facial nerve is monofascicular within its intratemporal course and develops a fascicular pattern as it emerges from the stylomastoid foramen. The perineurium is extremely thin in the proximal intratemporal course and becomes thicker distally.

consists of loose connective tissue between and around fascicles and is continuous with the more dense sheath. The arteries, veins, and lymphatics lie just within the epineural layer. Arteries and venules lie between fascicles, whereas capillaries are found within the nerve sheath. This nomenclature is confusing, particularly for the facial nerve, which varies considerably in microarchitecture from segment to segment. For example, the facial nerve is monofascicular within its intratemporal course and develops a typical fascicular pattern as it emerges from the stylomastoid foramen (Fig. 36.3). The perineurium is extremely thin in the proximal intratemporal course and becomes thicker more distally.

PATHOPHYSIOLOGY OF INJURY

In part, mechanisms of facial nerve injury may be ascribed to special anatomic considerations. Closed head trauma produces a deceleration injury, and some authorities have suggested that tethered neural structures are the most likely to be impaired during sudden deceleration (11). Two sites of consideration are the perigenicular region at the greater superficial petrosal nerve and the region of the facial nerve distal to the pyramidal eminence. The shearing forces produce intraneural contusion, edema, hemorrhage, and resultant ischemia.

In a cat experimental model, facial nerve transection at the stylomastoid foramen did not produce complete loss of distal electrical excitability until 72 hours had elapsed (12). The histopathology of facial nerve injury has been examined in a series of 12 patients with immediate traumatic facial palsy and eventual surgery for failed recovery 4 to 25 months after injury (13). Facial nerve biopsies revealed substantial axonal regeneration coexisting with other degenerating neurons. Axonal regeneration distal to the site of injury was blocked by fibrosis in the distal labyrinthine or proximal tympanic segments of the facial nerve in all cases. Others have theorized that intraneural fibrosis is a result of intraneural hematoma (14). Failed cases of nerve repair may be a result of suture line tension and subsequent fibrosis when primary anastomosis is attempted, arguing perhaps in favor of cable grafts for intralabyrinthine injury (15).

It is instructive to examine just what happens to patients with untreated traumatic facial paralysis and spontaneous complete or partial recovery. Adegbite et al. (16) reviewed 26 such patients who showed varying degrees of paralysis. Of patients with partial paralysis, 92.5% showed some evident recovery by 5 months, but only 10% of those with complete paralysis showed any recovery at this early time. Thus the course for recovery is more rapid for those with incomplete paralysis. Fisch (11) proposed that electroneurographic (ENoG) data in severe facial nerve injury in temporal bone trauma would be similar to that shown in his study on facial nerves with tumor and planned resection of the nerve. His analysis and that of Lieberherr et al. (17) suggest that the following ENoG results predict a favorable functional outcome: less than 90% degeneration for 6 days or no

progression to greater than 95% degeneration within 14 days of injury. Thus previous concern for nerve compromise greater than 90% also requires examination of time relationships. Similarly, Gantz et al. (18) have examined the natural history of facial nerve injury in the viral insult of Bell's palsy. Subjects who did not reach 90% degeneration on ENoG within 14 days of onset of complete paralysis all returned to House-Brackmann grade I (N = 48) or II (N = 6) by 7 months. Patients with greater than 90% degeneration on ENoG and no motor unit potentials on evoked electromyography (EMG) who elected to pursue conservative therapy had a 58% chance of poor outcome at 7 months (House-Brackmann grade III or IV [N = 19]). A similar group of patients who elected comprehensive middle fossa facial nerve decompression developed favorable recovery in 91% of cases (House-Brackmann grade I [N = 14] or II [N = 17]). However, the timing of decompression was critical: Patients having surgery within 2 weeks of onset of facial paralysis did well, but those submitted to surgery after 2 weeks had poorer results, similar to that of controls.

There may be some experimental validation for these clinical observations. Binns (12) produced a stretch injury at the second genu in cats and observed the expected facial paralysis and recovery at 6 to 8 weeks without treatment. Most animals subjected to facial nerve decompression of the second genu and vertical segment did not develop neural degeneration as long as surgery was performed within 48 hours. Decompression at 72 hours did not prevent neural degeneration. A separate study of compression injury in cats demonstrated clinical recovery if surgical decompression was performed within 12 days (19). Decompression between 14 and 21 days did not prevent synkinesis and reduction of electrical potentials.

ETIOLOGY OF TRAUMATIC FACIAL NERVE INJURY

Temporal Bone Fractures

Longitudinal Fracture

Seventy percent to 90% of temporal bone fractures are longitudinal as a result of a blow to the temporal or parietal skull, producing a fracture line that follows the long axis of the petrous pyramid (Figs. 36.4 and 36.5). The fracture crosses the floor of the middle cranial fossa near the foramen spinosum and courses anterior to the osseous labyrinth, injuring the facial nerve in 10% to 20% of cases at or near its labyrinthine segment. Fisch (11) has shown that 64% of longitudinal fractures involve the labyrinthine segment. The ossicular chain can be disrupted by fracture through the epitympanum, producing a conductive hearing loss. High-frequency sensorineural hearing loss occurs in approximately 20% of cases (20), presumably due to labyrinthine concussion. The fracture may pass through the external auditory canal, causing laceration of the skin and tympanic membrane. Bleeding and associated cerebrospinal fluid ot-

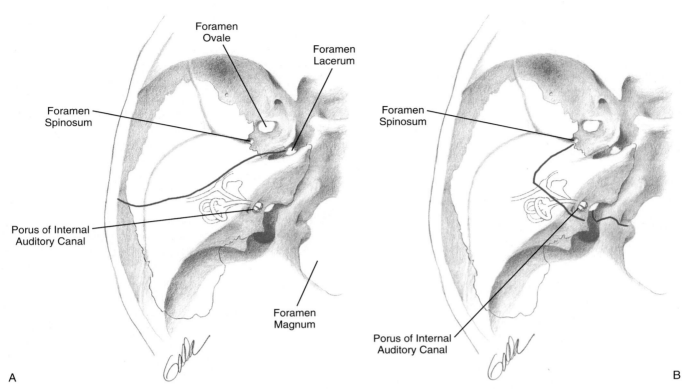

FIG. 36.4 A: Longitudinal fracture of the temporal bone follows the long axis of the petrous apex and crosses the floor of the middle cranial fossa near the foramen spinosum. The usual site of facial nerve injury is its labyrinthine segment. **B:** Transverse fracture of the temporal bone. The fracture line passes between the foramen magnum posteromedially and the foramen spinosum area anterolaterally and traverses the long axis of the petrous pyramid.

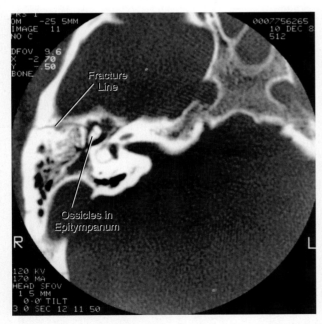

FIG. 36.5 High-resolution CT scan of a longitudinal skull fracture passing approximately parallel to the petrous ridge across the middle fossa floor and squamous portion of the temporal bone.

orrhea are common. Hasso and Ledington (21) have separated longitudinal fractures into anterior and posterior variants based on coronal computed tomographic (CT) scans. Posterior longitudinal fractures pass through the parietal skull and extend into the mastoid air cells, whereas anterior longitudinal fractures pass through the posterior and superior external auditory canal and tegmen. Both types may involve the eustachian tube, foramen lacerum, jugular canal, or carotid canal. Although facial paralysis develops in only 10% to 20% of longitudinal fractures, it is more common in well-pneumatized temporal bones, perhaps due to penetration of the nerve trunk by splinters of bone. Alternately, fixation of the facial nerve as it emerges from the internal auditory canal by the greater superficial petrosal nerve may predispose to traction injury. This may be associated with intraneural hematoma, leading to cicatricial obstruction of the fallopian canal. In a histologic study of a longitudinal fracture of the temporal bone occurring $1\frac{1}{2}$ years prior to death, Eby et al. (22) found reactive osteitis, exophytic new bone formation, and narrowing of the labyrinthine segment of the fallopian canal. Longitudinal fractures are more often associated with delayed onset of facial paralysis, which carries a good prognosis and often does not require surgical intervention.

Transverse Fractures

Transverse fractures pass in a plane perpendicular to the long axis of the temporal bone (21) between the foramen magnum and middle fossa floor, traversing the osseous labyrinth or internal auditory canal (23) (Figs. 36.4 and 36.6). As a result, profound sensorineural hearing loss and vertigo are common, and in 50% of cases there is an immediate onset of facial paralysis. The site of facial nerve injury is the labyrinthine segment in 90% and meatal segment in 10% of cases (11). Occasionally, the fracture may extend to the jugular fossa or carotid canal, the latter resulting in a unilateral hemispheric infarction. Axial CT scans best demonstrate transverse fractures with associated injury of the temporomandibular joint, mandibular condyle, and skull base.

Complex Fractures

Severe trauma to the head may produce a combination of longitudinal and transverse fractures that are often severely comminuted and dislocated. In addition to the clinical sequelae described, cerebrospinal fluid otorrhea, rhinorrhea, and brain herniation may be additional complications. Gunshot wounds usually produce complex fractures with unpredictable injuries to neurovascular structures. Carotid arteriography is usually indicated in complex penetrating temporal bone injuries.

Facial Nerve Injuries in Children

Birth Trauma

The earliest recognizable facial nerve injury occurs with birth trauma (24). The deficit may be difficult to recognize except with facial asymmetry during crying. Facial paralysis may not be identified early due to the excellent facial tone present in children. The most common cause of facial nerve injury in the newborn is traumatic forceps delivery. In the infantile mastoid, the facial nerve is vulnerable at the stylomastoid foramen, lying just beneath the soft tissues of the upper neck and unprotected by overlying bone. Other causes of injury include neural compression by the maternal sacral promontory or by the fetal shoulder. The risk of facial paralysis increases in large primiparous infants and multiple fetuses. Neuropraxia can be distinguished from complete avulsion by electrophysiologic studies. Agenesis of the facial nerve can be excluded if electrical stimulation can be elicited at birth. If electrical excitability is lost after 72 hours, severe injury or avulsion at the stylomastoid foramen should be assumed, warranting surgical exploration (25).

Facial nerve injury secondary to temporal bone fracture is less common in children than in adults. In two series of temporal bone fractures, facial paralysis occurred in 10% to 20% of children, well below the incidence in adults (24) (Table 36.1). In a series of 26 children with traumatic facial nerve injuries, 61% of those requiring operative intervention recovered satisfactory facial function. Unsatisfactory results in this series were attributed to a delay of 4 or more weeks in therapeutic intervention.

TABLE 36.1 *Incidence of facial paralysis in fractures of temporal bone*

	Incidence of fracture type	Incidence of facial paralysis
Adults		
Longitudinal type	70%–90%	10%–20%
Transverse type	10%–30%	50%
Children	Multidirectional	10%–20%

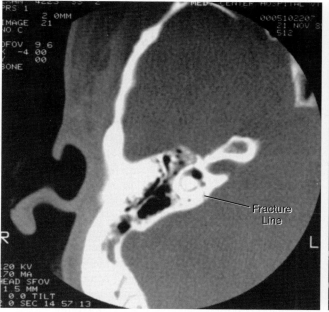
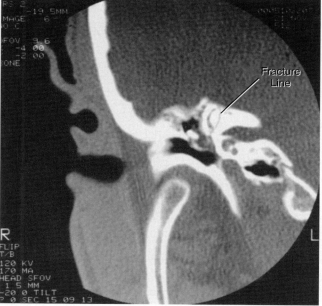

FIG. 36.6 Transverse fracture of the right temporal bone in the axial (**A**) and coronal (**B**) planes.

Iatrogenic Injuries

McCabe (25) stated that "mastoidectomy is of such complexity and so demanding of the surgeon today that virtually no temporal bone surgeon will fulfill his career without having a complication of the facial nerve." He defined the skill of the surgeon, not so much in frequency of facial nerve complications, but in his or her recognition of the injury at surgery. The incidence of injury to the facial nerve can be minimized by a thorough understanding of the anatomic locations where the facial nerve is most vulnerable and surgical practices designed to minimize trauma.

In at least 50% of cases, the facial nerve is dehiscent just craniad to the oval window. During stapedectomy, the use of angled otologic hooks may be required to remove mucosa around the stapes prior to techniques that require complete footplate removal and vein grafting. Instrumentation in the direction of the facial nerve with sharp instruments can injure the dehiscent nerve and produce edema with progressive functional loss. The facial nerve can be aberrant in the region of the second genu, even to the point of overlying the stapes. Occasionally, the nerve can be bifurcated (6), leading to misinterpretation of the anatomy and injury to the facial nerve. In surgery for congenital aural atresia, anomalies are expected and a heightened awareness will protect the nerve from injury.

During mastoidectomy, the best landmark to the facial nerve is the lateral semicircular canal. The nerve is then identified by thinning of the bone along its predicted pathway both proximally and distally. The facial nerve is particularly vulnerable in cases in which abundant granulation tissue and osteitis obscure surgical landmarks. Similarly, the facial nerve is more vulnerable to injury during revision surgery. Electrophysiologic monitoring of the facial nerve is particularly helpful when surgical landmarks are obscured.

In the facial recess approach for cochlear implantation, the nerve is the medial boundary of the dissection. Visualization of the round window niche and electrode insertion often require maximal lowering of the facial ridge. A thin layer of bone should be preserved over the vertical segment of the nerve in the facial recess to protect the nerve from injury during subsequent drilling in the middle ear.

In cases of facial paralysis following surgery for glomus jugulare or acoustic neuroma, much useful information can be gleaned from electrophysiologic testing over the first 4 to 7 days after surgery, despite that no immediate surgical intervention is contemplated. For example, ENoG is prognostic of early recovery and suggests the need for only nonsurgical protection of the eye. On the other hand, neurophysiologic evidence of axonotmesis or neurotmesis suggests the need for tarsorrhaphy or gold weight implants and early facial reanimation procedures.

IMAGING STUDIES

The most important imaging study in determining the location and extent of temporal bone fracture is the CT scan, because it provides both bone and soft tissue detail, including intracranial contents. Clinical findings that should raise the suspicion of temporal bone fracture include air fluid levels in the middle ear, opacification of the mastoid, intracranial air within the subarachnoid space of the cerebellopontine angle, and, occasionally, diffuse extracranial air over the posterior skull base (21). Epidural hematoma may follow fractures of the squamosa of the temporal bone with associated injury of the posterior branch of the middle meningeal artery or transverse sinus. Details of a temporal bone fracture are best visualized when the plane of tomographic sectioning is at 90 degrees to the plane of the fracture (21). Thus axial CT scans are most useful in delineating longitudinal fractures and coronal scans in evaluating transverse fractures (Figs. 36.5 and 36.6). When the facial nerve is injured, both axial and coronal planes may be helpful. High-resolution imaging of the facial nerve also requires frequent thin slices, preferably 1 to 2 mm in thickness. Coronal CT scans may be difficult to obtain in traumatized patients (23) due to the requirement for a supine-hanging head or the prone-extended head position. Although reconstructed images from the axial CT are helpful, the detail is less precise.

Shindo et al. (26) compared CT with magnetic resonance imaging (MRI) in seven patients with temporal bone fractures. Axial, coronal, and sagittal T1- and T2-weighted images were examined with a 1.5-Tesla magnet. The MRI scan identified important detail in six of eight fractures but underestimated the extent of the fractures compared with CT. However, several important concomitant intracranial injuries were discovered (five subdural and two epidural hematomas, two hemorrhagic brain contusions). Magnetic resonance imaging is less useful in determining localization of injury to the facial nerve due to the increased signal intensity of blood in the mastoid.

CLASSIFICATION OF FACIAL NERVE INJURY: ELECTRICAL AND TOPOGNOSTIC TESTS

A five-stage classification of injury of the facial nerve formulated by Sunderland (27), the details of topognostic and electrical stimulation tests, and a grading system for recovery of facial nerve function (House-Brackmann) are described in Chapter 6.

Long-standing facial paralysis may be best evaluated by EMG. Fibrillation potentials indicate denervation of an otherwise healthy muscle and the potential for reinnervation. Electrical silence suggests severe degeneration of facial muscles and hence suggests a poor prognosis for successful reinnervation. Following denervation, muscles can survive for 1 to 1½ years and, rarely, up to 3 years without innervation. Fibrillation potentials first occur 10 to 14 days after the onset of paralysis and thus are not useful in early prediction of denervation. However, polyphasic reinnervation potentials may develop as early as 4 to 6 weeks after palsy and predict satisfactory recovery (28).

Electroneurography is particularly helpful early in the course of traumatic facial paralysis. Neuropraxia, indicated by maintenance of the amplitude of summating potential 5 or more days after injury, predicts complete spontaneous recovery of facial nerve function.

One other curiosity exists regarding the utility of ENoG in deciding whether early surgical intervention will be required. Clinically, some patients with compression block from Bell's palsy may develop a delayed paralysis at day 14 to 21 and demonstrate 100% wallerian degeneration on ENoG. Despite these ENoG results, surgery would be deferred because spontaneous reasonable recovery of function is likely. In circumstances where nerve fibers are discharging at different rates due to degenerating and regenerating or remyelinating axons, ENoG recordings may not be accurate and register nearly 100% degeneration. Evoked EMG is performed by placing a concentric EMG electrode in both the orbicularis oculi and oris muscles and asking the patient to attempt a maximal facial contracture. Evoked EMG may demonstrate motor unit potentials, indicating early deblocking of neural conduction. These nerves have a good prognosis for recovery. Thus every patient considered a surgical candidate due to complete nondelayed facial paralysis should undergo evoked EMG in addition to ENoG. Those demonstrating voluntary motor unit potentials should be observed and are likely to demonstrate good facial nerve recovery.

Fisch (29) has examined the results of serial ENoGs in patients with delayed facial paralysis in internal auditory canal surgery. Three patients had facial palsies that developed 3 to 7 days after vestibular neurectomy. Although complete denervation occurred 14 to 21 days after the onset of palsy, all had nearly complete recovery. This suggests that the time relationships of degeneration may be as important a predictor of recovery as the degree of degeneration.

INDICATIONS FOR SURGICAL INTERVENTION

Iatrogenic Injury

Unanticipated postoperative facial palsy presents the surgeon with a therapeutic dilemma. When immediate facial palsy occurs after mastoid surgery, urgent reexploration of the facial nerve with decompression several millimeters on either side of the injured segment is indicated unless there is absolute confidence that the nerve is anatomically intact. Weit et al. (30) have suggested exploration within 24 hours, possibly by another otologic surgeon if the original surgeon is inexperienced in decompressive surgery. Neurolysis (slitting the epineural sheath) after decompression is performed if there is decrement of nerve excitability across the site of injury (25). When the operating surgeon is confident that the epineurium has not been violated, alternatives to immediate surgical intervention may be considered. If no cutting bur had been used along the course of the nerve or there is no suspicion of an injury that may have caused a disruption of the nerve, the surgeon may elect to observe the patient for a time. In this setting, it may be acceptable to place the patient on a high dosage of corticosteroids and follow the course of

degeneration by daily ENoG testing. If denervation reaches the 90% level within 6 days of injury, then a significant nerve injury has occurred demanding surgical decompression and neurolysis. In patients with a lesser degree or a slower rate of denervation, recovery can be expected without the need for revision surgery (Fig. 36.7).

Green et al. (31) have reviewed a retrospective series of 22 patients experiencing iatrogenic facial paralysis subsequent to ear surgery. Direct anastomosis or nerve grafts were performed only if greater than 50% of the nerves cross-sectional area was injured. Of the patients undergoing decompression alone, 38% experienced a result of House-Brackmann I or II and only 24% developed a poor result, House-Brackmann IV. If according to their criteria cable grafting was required, no patients accomplished a House-Brackmann I or II and 78% were House-Brackmann IV. Younger patients and those with lesser areas of injury had better outcomes. In addition, the longer time interval from injury to surgery did not seem to adversely affect the end result.

Temporal Bone Fracture

In traumatic facial nerve injury, slow degeneration of the nerve as indicated by loss of greater than 90% of the amplitude of the summating potential 2 to 3 weeks after the onset of paralysis is predictive of good recovery without surgical decompression. However, regardless of the immediacy of paralysis, degeneration of 90% or more of the facial nerve within 6 days of the onset of complete paralysis is predictive of poor recovery unless decompression is performed.

The timing of surgical intervention has received considerable attention in the literature. Attempts to rely on numerical parameters as adjunctive aids in surgical decision making are most attractive and can be summarized as follows:

1. Electroneurography demonstrating greater than 90% neural degeneration within the first 6 days suggests the need for surgical exploration.
2. Complete absence of stimulation on nerve excitability testing after the first 72 hours after onset of complete paralysis suggests a poor prognosis without surgery.
3. Maintenance of nerve excitability, but with reduced amplitude, suggests the potential for good recovery without surgery.

Adour et al. (32) have discussed a series of 13 patients with severe versus partial degeneration on electrical testing. The surgical results of decompression were uniform in both groups, raising questions about the predictability of testing. Indeed, the precision of ENoG is open to question. Hughes et al. (33) demonstrated significant test-retest variability in ENoG tests of 22 normal subjects. Additionally, most series of patients are too limited in size to allow adequate statistical evaluation. Finally, the futility of delayed surgical decompression for long-standing facial paralysis has been challenged by a small clinical series of patients operated on

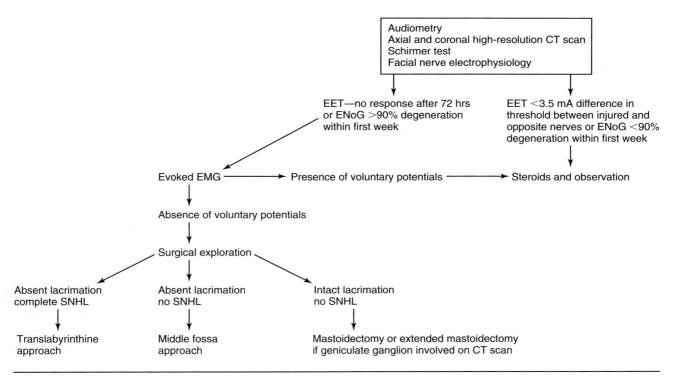

CT, computed tomography; EET, electrical excitability test; ENoG, electroneurography; EMG, electromyography; SNHL, sensorineural hearing loss.

FIG. 36.7 Management paradigm 1: temporal bone fracture.

well past the optimal time for decompression (34). Nerve decompression and sheath incision accomplished at 2½, 3, and 14 months after injury produced good results despite a poor prognosis suggested by neuromuscular tests. These and other anecdotal cases might argue in favor of exploration,

decompression, and primary nerve grafting if required in any patient with a posttraumatic complete paralysis regardless of the time delay. In equivocal situations beyond 1½ years, facial muscle biopsy may be helpful for prognosis of success (Fig. 36.8).

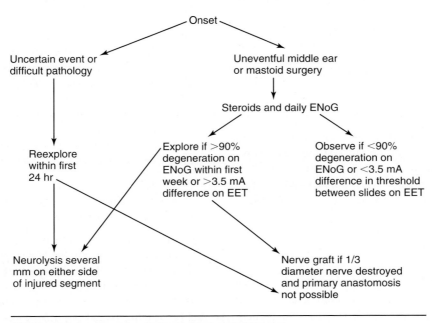

ENoG, electroneurography; EET, electrical excitability test.

FIG. 36.8 Management paradigm 2: immediate onset of complete iatrogenic facial palsy.

SURGICAL TECHNIQUE

Successful intervention in cases of surgical traumatic facial paralysis requires a thorough knowledge of the anatomy of the facial nerve, the availability of intraoperative electrical monitoring, and appropriate instrumentation. In cases of iatrogenic injury to the nerve during mastoid surgery, it is clear that a transmastoid approach will suffice. However, in cases of temporal bone fracture or penetrating injuries from gunshot wounds, the operating surgeon must be prepared to perform either a middle fossa or translabyrinthine approach and to transpose or graft the facial nerve in the labyrinthine segment. Electrical stimulation and monitoring of the facial nerve is essential. The ipsilateral face is exposed through transparent plastic drapes to allow direct inspection as an adjunct to electrophysiologic monitoring. A fine-tipped stimulating probe is essential. Monopolar stimulation with variable amperage provides less precise localization and stimulation of the facial nerve than "flush-tip" insulated electrodes and bipolar stimulation probes, particularly within the internal auditory canal (32). In more distal segments of the facial nerve, monopolar stimulation is adequate. Monitoring of facial muscle function is accomplished with a strain gauge (Silverstein nerve monitor) or electromyographic recording. Visual monitoring of facial muscle contraction is less precise than electrophysiologic or mechanical techniques but provides useful information if a reproducible threshold stimulus can be applied.

A protocol for localization of facial nerve injury has been advocated by Fisch and Esslen (35). Sequential stimulation of the facial nerve is accomplished in a distal-to-proximal direction. The site of conduction block is determined by identifying that segment of the nerve in which the amplitude of the neural response is abruptly diminished (36). Avoidance of muscle relaxants during facial nerve surgery is essential. The required instrumentation is found in the standard mastoidectomy set. Suction irrigation and diamond burs are important to avoid thermal injury to the nerve. A reversible drill can be a helpful adjunct when the nerve is widely exposed. Bipolar cautery at low settings and topical thrombin and Avitine (microfibrillar collagen hemostat) are useful for control of bleeding from the nerve sheath. Finally, curettes should be very sharp and never employed in such a manner that the convexity of the instrument compresses the nerve. Incision of the nerve sheath is accomplished when necessary with a sharp sickle knife, disposable Beaver keratotomy blade, or no. 11 scalpel blade to allow exposure and inspection of the perineural covering of individual fascicles.

Transmastoid Approach

Several authors have advocated a postauricular extended mastoidectomy to expose the facial nerve from the geniculate ganglion to the stylomastoid foramen (35,37) when (i) trauma is clearly localized to the vertical or horizontal segments of the nerve or (ii) there is blunt injury to the skull with preservation of lacrimation as demonstrated by Schirmer testing.

The lateral semicircular canal and fossa incudis are exposed with care to avoid contact of the drill with the short process of the incus. The digastric ridge is exposed to identify the stylomastoid foramen. The facial recess is opened after exposure of the facial nerve at the second genu (Fig. 36.9). The facial nerve is located approximately 0.5 mm anterior to the ampulla of the lateral semicircular canal. The horizontal portion of the facial nerve can be visualized through the facial recess, but opening of the fallopian canal in this segment is difficult without removal or disarticulation of the incus. The incus can be removed and then remodeled for reinsertion as an incus interposition with predictable excellent hearing results. May (38) and Goin (39) prefer to preserve the posterior incudal ligaments but disarticulate the incudomalleal and incudostapedial joints to eliminate the risk of high-frequency sensorineural hearing loss from acoustic trauma. Following facial nerve decompression, the incus can then be repositioned. The facial nerve can be traced forward to the geniculate ganglion, which has a mean distance of 2.36 mm from the anterior aspect of the cochleariform process to the beginning of the ganglion (39) (Fig. 36.10). The ganglion is superior and slightly medial to the horizontal facial segment. The geniculate ganglion can be exposed through the extended mastoidectomy, but the labyrinthine segment cannot be adequately exposed by this route without entering the ampulla of the lateral semicircular canal in two thirds of cases (37,39).

Troublesome bleeding from the area of the geniculate ganglion can be avoided by skeletonizing the labyrinthine segment before "turning the corner" at the geniculate ganglion. Drilling should be confined to the superior aspect of the labyrinthine segment to avoid injury to the superior vestibular nerve. The dura is easily torn near the geniculate ganglion (39). The nerve must be decompressed in 180 degrees of its circumference. The most common reported complication (38) of the extended transmastoid decompression of the facial nerve is hearing loss. A conductive loss of greater than 15 dB occurred in 14% of cases and a sensorineural hearing loss in the 4,000 to 8,000 cycle range in 51% of cases. A conductive hearing loss may be caused by stapes fixation from bone dust, dural herniation impinging upon the head of the malleus, or disarticulation of the incudomalleal joint.

Combined Middle Fossa–Extended Mastoidectomy Approach

The middle fossa approach provides the best exposure for management of injury in the labyrinthine segment of the facial nerve and allows nerve grafting while preserving cochleovestibular function. The procedure can be combined with transmastoid decompression to provide exposure of the nerve from the meatal segment to the stylomastoid foramen. Goin (39) has provided useful anatomic data supplementing the surgical principles of facial nerve decompression as de-

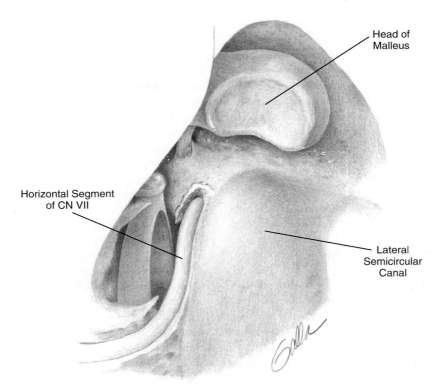

FIG. 36.9 Transmastoid facial nerve decompression of the left ear. The horizontal (tympanic) portion of the facial nerve can be visualized through the facial recess, but opening of the fallopian canal in this segment is difficult with removal or disarticulation of the incus.

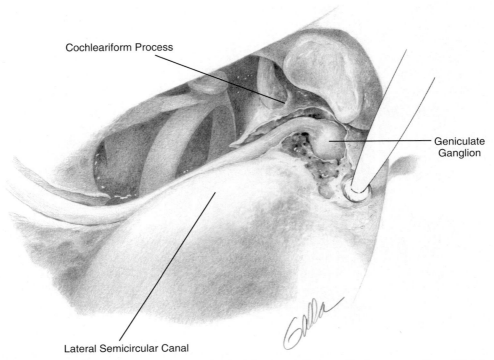

FIG. 36.10 Transmastoid decompression of the facial nerve, left ear, with decompression of the geniculate ganglion.

scribed by House (40) in 1961. The labyrinthine segment is 4 mm in length and subtends an angle of 120 degrees with the meatal segment. The nerve therefore passes around the basal turn of the cochlea en route to the geniculate ganglion (Fig. 36.11). The labyrinthine segment is parallel to the arch of the superior semicircular canal. The cochlea is located anteromedial and the vestibule and superior semicircular canal posterolateral to the geniculate ganglion. The distance between the ampulla of the superior semicircular canal and the cochlea is 3.89 mm. The distance between the cochlea and vestibular labyrinth is approximately 2.57 mm. A vertical segment of bone, triangular in shape, separates the vestibular and facial nerves just proximal to the geniculate ganglion. This vertical crest, also known as "Bill's bar," is a critical landmark to avoid surgical injury to the vestibular nerve during facial nerve decompression. At the geniculate ganglion, the nerve turns abruptly posteriorly at a 75-degree angle (Fig. 36.12). The greater superficial petrosal nerve lying in the hiatus of the facial canal courses anteriorly from the geniculate ganglion and lies just medial to the middle meningeal artery.

The skin incisions and craniotomy for the middle fossa approach (34,41) are discussed in Chapters 9 and 12. The tip of the House-Urban retractor is placed along the petrous ridge anteromedial to the arcuate eminence. The superior semicircular canal is exposed with the use of suction irrigation and diamond burs (Fig. 36.13). Some otologists prefer to "blue-line" the superior canal (36,42,43), whereas others do not feel this is necessary in facial nerve decompression (37). The geniculate ganglion can usually be identified by

following the greater superficial petrosal nerve. From this point, the dissection continues posteriorly for approximately 2 mm, roughly parallel to the superior semicircular canal, before proceeding in a more medial direction toward the meatal segment. At this point the nerve will have been followed into the internal auditory canal, where more proximal traumatic injury is uncommon.

Fisch and Esslen (35) prefer to enter the internal auditory canal early after identification of the superior semicircular canal and using an anterior 60-degree vector as a guide to the position of the internal auditory canal. After drilling in the area medial to the labyrinthine segment, the meatal dura is incised, providing access to the meatal segment of the facial nerve. Beginning at the meatal fundus, they then expose the labyrinthine segment and proceed in a lateral direction toward the geniculate ganglion.

When fractures, dural lacerations, and hematoma distort the middle fossa anatomy or when the arcuate eminence is ill defined, precluding precise localization of relationships, alternative methods of identifying the geniculate ganglion may be required. The greater superficial petrosal nerve is helpful in this regard. Occasionally, the location of the ganglion can only be ascertained by identification via an extended mastoidectomy. A small window in the tegmen is made to mark the location of the geniculate ganglion, which is then further exposed with diamond burs through the middle fossa.

After the labyrinthine segment and geniculate ganglion have been completely exposed, the tegmen tympani can be removed to expose the tympanic segment of the facial canal.

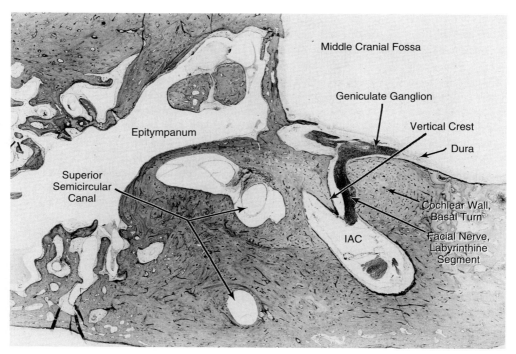

FIG. 36.11 Horizontal section through the left temporal bone at the level of the middle fossa floor. The labyrinthine segment of the facial nerve courses approximately parallel to the axis of the superior semicircular canal. IAC, internal auditory canal.

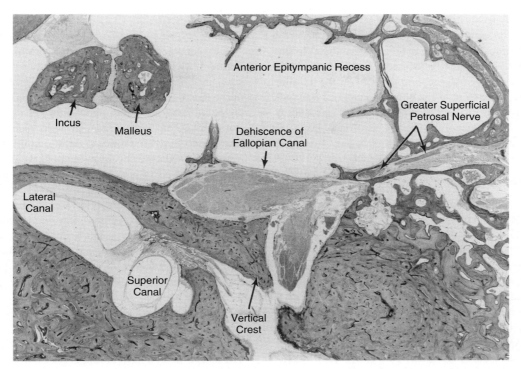

FIG. 36.12 Horizontal section through the left temporal bone at the level of the epitympanum.

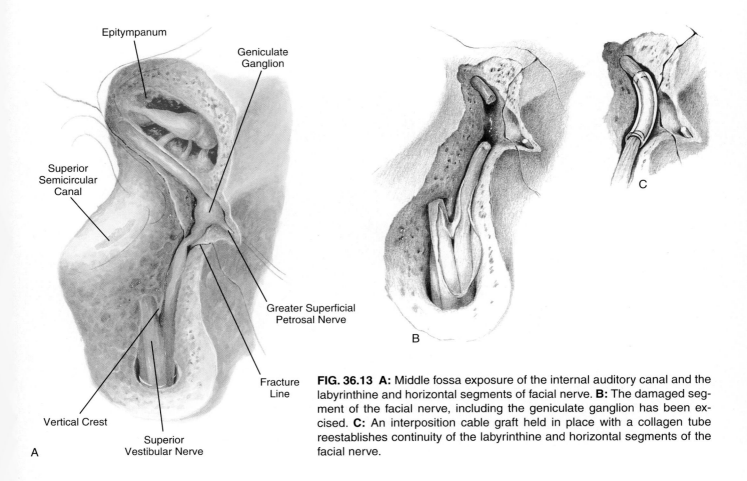

FIG. 36.13 A: Middle fossa exposure of the internal auditory canal and the labyrinthine and horizontal segments of facial nerve. **B:** The damaged segment of the facial nerve, including the geniculate ganglion has been excised. **C:** An interposition cable graft held in place with a collagen tube reestablishes continuity of the labyrinthine and horizontal segments of the facial nerve.

It is not necessary to disarticulate the ossicular chain unless there is need for decompressive drilling or nerve repair. Any definitive procedures involving the facial nerve distal to the geniculate ganglion should be accomplished through extended mastoidectomy. At the completion of the middle fossa procedure, a segment of the bone flap can be removed, thinned, and fashioned to reconstruct the roof of the attic. A temporalis fascia graft may be used to reinforce the dural floor or repair dural tears.

Translabyrinthine Approach

If cochlear and vestibular function have been destroyed by the initial trauma, the translabyrinthine approach provides excellent exposure of the entire intratemporal course of the facial nerve, including the labyrinthine segment (43). This technique is identical to that employed for translabyrinthine resection of acoustic neurinoma except that the dissection is extended laterally to the geniculate ganglion (Fig. 36.14). The procedure offers the distinct advantage of providing access to the entire facial nerve through one surgical field without the requirement for middle fossa dural dissection and retraction of the temporal lobe. Wide exposure of the facial nerve can be accomplished, facilitating rerouting or grafting techniques. Because the translabyrinthine pro-

cedure is described in Chapter 12, only a few special considerations germane to the facial nerve will be described here.

The facial nerve will have been skeletonized in its vertical segment, including the region of the horizontal canal. The keys to optimal facial nerve exposure are the wide opening of the vestibule after a labyrinthectomy and identification of the lateral end of the internal auditory canal (42). The superior division of the vestibular nerve is identified and traced laterally to the vertical crest. At this point the facial nerve lies anteromedial to the vertical crest, which is removed by drilling assisted by suction irrigation. The geniculate ganglion can be best exposed by removing the bone between the middle fossa dura and superior aspect of the internal auditory canal. In 90% of cases requiring repair of the facial nerve (11), reanastomosis can be accomplished by creating a new osseous channel between the stylomastoid foramen and internal auditory canal. Up to 10 to 14 mm of nerve can be resected without the need for cable grafting.

General Management of the Facial Nerve After Exposure

The safest method of avoiding surgical injury to the nerve is to drill to the point of seeing the vasa nervorum through translucent bone. Final removal of bone is accomplished

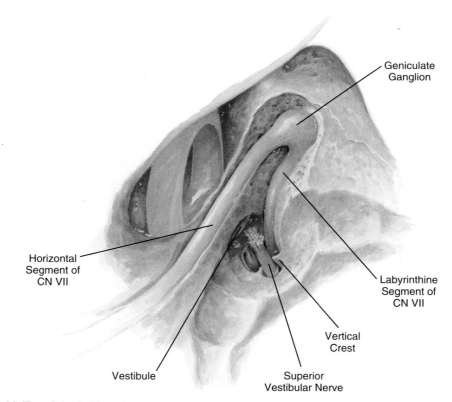

FIG. 36.14 Translabyrinthine decompression of the facial nerve, left ear. After a canal wall–up mastoidectomy has been completed, the semicircular canals are skeletonized and removed exposing the vestibule and internal auditory canal. The facial nerve is shown in its labyrinthine and horizontal segments. The vertical crest is an important landmark to distinguish the facial from superior vestibular nerves.

with sharp curettes, avoiding decompression of the nerve. The site of injury may be determined by recognition of obvious disruption of the nerve sheath, intraneural hematoma, or simply ecchymosis of the nerve as compared with the more normal appearing adjacent segments. It may also be possible to detect with some general degree of precision the site of injury by the use of a nerve stimulator, stimulating in a distal to proximal direction until the point of nerve block is detected by loss of stimulus response.

Studies by Greer et al. (44) have addressed the benefit or potential deficits in incising the nerve sheath in facial nerve decompression. In uninjured nerves, animals that underwent osseous decompression alone demonstrated better electrophysiologic parameters, but permanent histology was similarly favorable to animals whose nerve sheaths had been incised. However, when facial nerve crush injuries were produced in a separate set of animals, those that underwent sheath incision in addition to osseous decompression did poorer in every circumstance compared with osseous decompression alone. The authors suggested that sheath incision produces an additional devascularization injury. Whether these data can be transposed to the human circumstance is as yet unclear.

Those surgeons who subscribe to epineural sheath incision should incise several millimeters on either side of the point of injury utilizing a sharp sickle knife, disposable keratotomy blade, or no. 11 scalpel blade (45).

Incision of the nerve sheath should extend to the point where normal nerve is clearly identified. The most difficult decision after exposure of the initial perineurium and individual fascicles is whether to proceed with segmental resection and nerve graft. McCabe (25) has suggested that when one third or more of the cross-section of the nerve diameter has been destroyed, an interposition graft will be required. Nerve grafts are most easily obtained from the greater auricular nerve or sural nerve (Chapter 42). Fisch (11) has analyzed the findings in 30 patients with longitudinal fractures causing facial nerve paralysis. In 17% of cases the nerve was not interrupted and decompression with incision of the sheath was performed. In 26% of cases the facial nerve was interrupted within the labyrinthine segment, requiring resection of the geniculate ganglion and end-to-end anastomosis (Fig. 36.13). In 50% of cases an intraneural hematoma was identified after sheath incision. In these cases a silver clip was applied to the greater superficial petrosal nerve to avoid faulty regeneration of motor neurons. Intraneural hematoma in the region of the geniculate ganglion in the absence of fracture suggests a traction injury.

Because the osseous canal of the labyrinthine segment is a ready-made channel of appropriate dimension, interposition grafts are simply laid in place via the middle fossa approach. Exposure in this area is difficult, and the lack of epineurium in the meatal segment usually precludes approximation by sutures. Collagen tubes (11) or fibrin glue may facilitate neural approximation and alignment. In the mastoid segment, epineural or fascicular perineural sutures are possible. The ends of the nerve are sharply divided at a 45-degree angle to increase the surface area of contact (46). The epineurium is removed an additional 1 mm from the freshened ends of the graft and a four-quadrant epineural repair with 10.0 nylon accomplished. In the extended mastoidectomy approach where there is little room for manipulation or suture near the geniculate ganglion, microclips may be helpful to achieve apposition (47). Finally, in cases of late exploration of the facial nerve where degeneration and faulty regeneration may have occurred, histologic examination of a segment of the proximal stump may reveal absence of viable neurons, suggesting retrograde degeneration and a poor prognosis for regeneration. Alternate forms of reinnervation such as hypoglossal-facial anastomosis may then be considered.

In circumstances where the facial nerve is completely disrupted or severely traumatized, cable graft or complete end-to-end anastomosis is required. In these circumstances, no patients ever recover to House-Brackmann I or II, although 82% achieve House-Brackmann III or IV and only 18% stage V or VI (28,31,41,48–50). In addition, performing a repair of this magnitude produces the same result regardless of whether the surgery is performed at 1 month or 10 months from the point of injury. Thus the goal of early surgical intervention (before 14 days) is to identify patients with injuries amenable to facial nerve decompression, usually proximal to the labyrinthine segment and distally as far as required to encounter normal nerve. If there is uncertainty about the extent of damage in the early repair, cable grafting can be avoided and considered at a later date, such as in 6 to 8 months, to allow spontaneous recovery to at least House-Brackmann III or IV. Finally, if facial nerve surgery is inadvertently delayed beyond 14 days, either because of the patient's general condition or some other variable, there is no disadvantage to simple observation over the next several months. In summary, early facial nerve exploration is only considered when there is confidence that the nerve integrity is preserved and timing issues are favorable; otherwise, observation and watchful waiting may produce results identical or better than cable grafting.

REFERENCES

1. Adour KK, Wingerd J. Nonepidemic incidence of idiopathic facial paralysis. Seasonal distribution of 419 cases in three years. *JAMA* 1974;227:653–654.
2. Haberkamp TJ, McFadden E, Khafagy Y, et al. Gunshot injuries of the temporal bone. *Laryngoscope* 1995;105:1053–1057.
3. Schuknecht HF, Gulya AJ. *Anatomy of the temporal bone with surgical implications.* Philadelphia: Lea & Febiger, 1986.
4. Kumagami H, Nakao Y. Fluorescence findings of the facial nerve at decompression operation. *Acta Otolaryngol (Stockh) Suppl* 1988;446:126–131.
5. Janfaza P, Nadol JB Jr, Galla RJ, et al. *Surgical anatomy of the head and neck.* Philadelphia: Lippincott Williams & Wilkins, 2001.
6. Nager GT, Proctor B. Anatomical variations and anomalies involving the facial canal. *Ann Otol Rhinol Laryngol* 1982;91[Suppl 97]:45–61.
7. Ogawa A, Sando I. Spatial occupancy of vessels and facial nerve in the facial canal. *Ann Otol Rhinol Laryngol* 1982;91:14–19.
8. Horn KL, Crumley RL. The physiology of nerve injury and repair. *Otolaryngol Clin North Am* 1984;17:321–333.

9. Hughes GB. *Textbook of clinical otology.* New York: Thieme-Stratton, 1985.
10. Crumley RL. Mechanisms of synkinesis. *Laryngoscope* 1979;89: 1847–1854.
11. Fisch U. Facial paralysis in fractures of the petrous bone. *Laryngoscope* 1974;84:2141–2154.
12. Binns PM. Experimental studies of the facial nerve. *Trans Am Acad Ophthalmol Otolaryngol* 1967;71:665–676.
13. Felix H, Eby TL, Fisch U. New aspects of facial nerve pathology and temporal bone fractures. *Acta Otolaryngol (Stockh)* 1991;111: 332–336.
14. Ylikoski J. Facial palsy after temporal bone fracture: light and electron microscopic findings in two cases. *J Laryngol Otol* 1988:102:298–303.
15. Eby TL, Pollak A, Fisch U. Intratemporal facial nerve anastomosis: a temporal bone study. *Laryngoscope* 1990;100:623–626.
16. Adegbite AB, Khan MI, Tan L. Predicting recovery of facial nerve function following injury from a basilar skull fracture. *J Neurosurg* 1991;75:759–762.
17. Lieberherr U, Schwarzenbach D, Fisch U. Management of severe facial nerve paralysis in the temporal bone—a review of 82 cases. In: Castro D, ed. *Facial nerve: proceedings of the Sixth International Symposium on the Facial Nerve.* Amsterdam: Kugler and Ghedini Publications, 1990:285–289.
18. Gantz BJ, Rubinstein JT, Gidley P, et al. Surgical management of Bell's palsy. *Laryngoscope* 1999;109:1177–1188.
19. Yamamoto E, Fisch U. Experimentally induced facial nerve compression in cats. *Acta Otolaryngol (Stockh)* 1975;79:390–395.
20. Lambert PR, Brackmann DE. Facial paralysis in longitudinal temporal bone fractures: a review of 26 cases. *Laryngoscope* 1984;94:1022–1026.
21. Hasso AN, Ledington JA. Traumatic injuries of the temporal bone. *Otolaryngol Clin North Am* 1988;21:295–316.
22. Eby TL, Pollak A, Fisch U. Histopathology of the facial nerve after longitudinal temporal bone fracture. *Laryngoscope* 1988;98:717–720.
23. Cannon CR, Jahrsdoerfer RA. Temporal bone fractures. Review of 90 cases. *Arch Otolaryngol* 1983;109:285–288.
24. Kornblut AD. Facial nerve injuries in children. *Ear Nose Throat J* 1977;56:369–376.
25. McCabe BF. Injuries to the facial nerve. *Laryngoscope* 1972;82: 1891–1896.
26. Shindo ML, Fetterman BL, Shih L, et al. Gunshot wounds of the temporal bone: a rational approach to evaluation and management. *Otolaryngol Head Neck Surg* 1995;112:533–539.
27. Sunderland S. Some anatomical and pathophysiologic data relevant to facial nerve injury and repair. In: *Facial nerve surgery.* Birmingham, AL: Aesculapius, 1977.
28. Dobie RA. Electrical and topognostic tests of the facial nerve. In: Cummings CW, Fredrickson JM, Harker LA, et al, eds. *Otolaryngology—head and neck surgery,* vol 4. St. Louis: Mosby, 1986:2821–2827.
29. Fisch U. Prognostic value of electrical tests in acute facial paralysis. *Am J Otol* 1984;5:494–498.
30. Weit RJ, Davis WE, Shambaugh GE Jr. Iatrogenic facial paralysis: prevention and management. In: Graham MD, House WF. *Disorders of the facial nerve.* New York: Raven Press, 1982;351–356.
31. Green JD Jr, Shelton C, Brackmann DE. Surgical management of iatrogenic facial nerve injuries. *Otolaryngol Head Neck Surg* 1994;111: 606–610.
32. Adour KK, Boyajian JA, Kahn ZM, et al. Surgical and nonsurgical management of facial paralysis following closed head injury. *Laryngoscope* 1977;87:380–390.
33. Hughes GB, Josey AF, Glasscock ME III, et al. Clinical electroneurography: statistical analysis of controlled measurements in twenty-two normal subjects. *Laryngoscope* 1981;91:1834–1846.
34. Brodsky L, Eviatar A, Daniller A. Post-traumatic facial nerve paralysis: three cases of delayed temporal bone exploration with recovery. *Laryngoscope* 1983;93:1560–1565.
35. Fisch U, Esslen E. Total intratemporal exposure of the facial nerve. Pathologic findings in Bell's palsy. *Arch Otolaryngol* 1972;95:335–341.
36. Niparko JK, Kileny PR, Kemink JL, et al. Neurophysiologic intraoperative monitoring. II. Facial nerve function. *Am J Otol* 1989;10:55–61.
37. Farrior JB. Anterior facial nerve decompression. *Otolaryngol Head Neck Surg* 1985;93:765–768.
38 May M, Klein SR. Facial nerve decompression complications. *Laryngoscope* 1983;93:299–305.
39. Goin DW. Proximal intratemporal facial nerve in Bell's palsy surgery. A study correlating anatomical and surgical findings. *Laryngoscope* 1982;92:263–272.
40. House WF. Surgical exposure of the internal auditory canal and its contents through the middle cranial fossa. *Laryngoscope* 1961;71: 1363–1385.
41. Coker NJ, Kendall KA, Jenkins HA, et al. Traumatic intratemporal facial nerve injury: management rationale for preservation of function. *Otolaryngol Head Neck Surg* 1987;97:262–269.
42. House WF, Luetje CM, eds. *Acoustic tumors,* vol 2. *Management.* Baltimore: University Park Press, 1979.
43. Pulec JL. Total facial nerve exposure. *Arch Otolaryngol* 1969;89: 179–183.
44. Greer JA, Cody DTR, Lambert EH, et al. Experimental facial nerve paralysis: influence of decompression. *Am Otol Rhinol Laryngol* 1974;83:582–595.
45. Gacek R. Dissection of the facial nerve in chronic otitis media surgery. *Laryngoscope* 1982;92:108–109.
46. Gantz BJ. Intratemporal facial nerve surgery. In: Cummings CW, Fredrickson JM, Harker LA, et al, eds. *Otolaryngology—head and neck surgery,* vol 4. St. Louis: Mosby, 1986:3353–3366.
47. Williams JD. Microclip application in tympanoplasty. *Ann Otol Rhinol Laryngol* 1977;86:223–226.
48. McKennan KX, Chole RA. Facial paralysis in temporal bone trauma. *Am J Otol* 1992;13:167–172.
49. Kamerer DB. Intratemporal facial nerve injuries. *Otolaryngol Head Neck Surg* 1982;90:612–615.
50. Telischi FF, Patete ML. Blast injuries to the facial nerve. *Otolaryngol Head Neck Surg* 1994;111:446–449.

CHAPTER 37

Management of Bell's Palsy and Herpes Zoster

Bruce J. Gantz and Brian P. Perry

New information concerning the etiology of the most common causes of facial paresis or paralysis is altering our management of these disorders. It is now known that neurotropic viruses are important etiologic factors in both Bell's palsy and Ramsay Hunt syndrome. Herpes simplex virus type 1 has been identified in idiopathic facial paralysis or Bell's palsy, and herpes zoster virus has been isolated in Ramsay Hunt syndrome. The identification of a viral etiology in these two disorders allows the clinician to more effectively tailor management strategies and improve outcome as new antiviral medications are developed. This chapter will review the pathophysiology, diagnosis, and newer management algorithms for Bell's palsy and Ramsay Hunt syndrome.

PATHOPHYSIOLOGY

Bell's Palsy

As first proposed by McCormick in 1972 (1), the herpes simplex virus has recently been shown to be the etiologic agent of Bell's palsy (2–4). Using the polymerase chain reaction, herpes simplex virus type 1 (HSV-1) DNA has been identified in the saliva of patients with Bell's palsy (3), as well as in the geniculate ganglion of a patient who died shortly after the onset of Bell's palsy (2). The HSV-1 DNA has also been isolated in endoneurial fluid of patients undergoing facial nerve decompression for Bell's palsy, whereas it was not isolated in control patients undergoing facial nerve decompression procedures for other indications (4). Sugita et al. (5) and Carreno et al. (6) have designed animal models for Bell's palsy. Sugita et al. inoculated the ear (or tongue) of mice with HSV-1, demonstrating ipsilateral facial paralysis 6 days later. HSV-1 antigens were identified in both the facial nerve and nucleus following animal sacrifice. Using a rabbit model, Carreno found similar pathologic changes within the facial nerve and geniculate ganglion (edema, inflammatory cell infiltrates, vacuolar degeneration) without the associated facial paralysis.

It has been suggested that Bell's palsy begins with viral involvement of the sensory fibers followed by the motor fibers of the facial nerve, consistent with the idea that the disease is a herpes viral geniculate ganglionitis (7). The neural injury is thought to be secondary to edema within the nerve induced by the viral infection. Three factors determine the extent of injury: the size of the fallopian canal, the anatomy of the meatal foramen, and the degree of edema. The meatal foramen is the narrowest portion of the fallopian canal (0.68 mm) (8), with varying degrees of inclination from the labyrinthine segment to the geniculate ganglion. Contributing to the constriction at the meatal foramen is a tight band of arachnoid tissue that is adherent to the nerve at this location. Based on these findings, Fisch and Felix (9) first proposed that the facial nerve was entrapped at the meatal foramen as a result of edema leading to ischemia and subsequent wallerian degeneration. Intraoperative conduction studies have confirmed this theory (10).

A range of injuries occurs within the facial nerve fibers, from simple conduction block (neuropraxia) to axoplasmic disruption (axonotmesis) and neural tubule disruption (neurotmesis). The different degrees of nerve injury are helpful in differentiating the severity of the neural injury. Neuropraxia results in blockage of propagation of neural impulses, but the injury is not severe enough to induce neural degeneration (wallerian degeneration) distal to the injury. If a nerve that is in a stage of neuropraxia is stimulated distal to the injury, propagation of an electrically applied stimulus distal to the lesion can occur. In axonotmesis and neurotmesis, wallerian degeneration occurs distal to the injury, preventing electrically applied conduction. Electrodiagnostic testing is able to differentiate between neuropraxia and axonotmesis/neurotmesis but cannot distinguish between axonotmesis and neurotmesis. Nerves that have an axonotmesis type injury alone may achieve a complete return of facial function because the neural tubule remains intact. Neurotmesis, on the other hand, is a more severe injury, including disruption of neural tubules resulting in misdirection of healing fibers, leading to synkinesis and incomplete return of function. The rate of progression of wallerian degeneration, and therefore the rapidity of degeneration on electrical testing, provides useful information about the percentage of fibers undergoing neurotmesis (11). Nerves that degenerate slowly over 10 to 14 days are less likely to exhibit neurotmesis, whereas nerves that degenerate within 3 to 7 days most likely have undergone neurotmesis (11).

Ramsay Hunt Syndrome

In 1907 Ramsay Hunt suggested that the combination of facial paralysis and vesicular eruption of the ear was due to a geniculate ganglionitis. Since that time it has been shown that herpes zoster oticus is a polycranial neuronitis, induced by the reactivation of the virus. The varicella zoster virus remains latent within the cerebrospinal ganglion cells after primary infection with chicken pox during childhood (12). Deterioration of specific cellular immunity to the varicella virus is thought to be the trigger for reactivation (13). Wackym (14) demonstrated the presence of the varicella zoster virus (VZV) within the geniculate, spiral, and Scarpa's ganglia, as well as within the organ of Corti and macula of the saccule, in a patient with Ramsay Hunt syndrome and sudden hearing loss. Others, using the polymerase chain reaction, have shown the presence of the VZV in the oropharynx of patients with herpes zoster oticus and zoster sine herpete (15). Unlike Bell's palsy, in which the neural injury is secondary to edema and subsequent ischemia, the VZV invades the neuronal soma, leading to cell death (16,17) and a much more guarded prognosis.

DIAGNOSIS

Bell's Palsy

The acute onset of facial weakness or paralysis, occasionally associated with otalgia, hyperacusis, and dysgeusia without any additional findings, is classic for Bell's palsy. There is no side or gender predilection, and the annual incidence is 17 to 19 per 100,000 population (18). The occurrence of Bell's palsy during pregnancy is 3.3 times that for age-matched nonpregnant women (18). Peitersen (19) identified a 70% rate of complete paralysis and 30% rate of incomplete paralysis; usually the facial paresis progresses rapidly to facial paralysis in less than 48 hours.

The history and physical examination should be dedicated to making the diagnosis of Bell's palsy one of exclusion. A history of facial twitching or a slowly evolving paresis should be considered presumptive evidence of a tumor. Although both recurrent and bilateral facial paralyses can be due to Bell's palsy (HSV-1), their existence places the burden of proof upon the clinician, and imaging should be performed. Most patients begin to demonstrate the first signs of recovery within 3 weeks of onset, and nearly all patients have some return of function by 6 months (19). If some recovery of facial function has not occurred by 6 months, imaging is necessary to exclude a neoplasm. With the exception of the facial paralysis, the head and neck examination should be normal; occasionally one will identify loss of papillae on the ipsilateral tongue due to chorda tympani involvement. Audiologic evaluation often demonstrates a loss of the ipsilateral stapedial reflex with normal pure tones and speech discrimination.

Perhaps the most important aspect of the evaluation of a suspected case of Bell's palsy is electrodiagnostic testing. The combined use of electroneurography (ENoG) and voluntary contraction electromyography (EMG) can determine the extent of neural injury and provide prognostic information necessary for management decisions. ENoG, as originally described by Esslen (20), can differentiate between a conduction block (neuropraxia) and wallerian degeneration (axonotmesis/neurotmesis). Due to the delay in wallerian degeneration reaching the stylomastoid foramen (the site of electrodiagnostic stimulation), ENoG is not performed until 3 days after the onset of complete facial paralysis. It has been shown that degeneration of 90% or more of the nerve fibers within 14 days of the onset of the paralysis is associated with an incomplete recovery in more than 50% of cases (21). If this level of degeneration is not achieved within 3 weeks after onset of paralysis, the patient has an excellent prognosis for complete return of function. The rapidity of degeneration also has prognostic value; the more quickly one reaches complete electrical degeneration, the more severe the injury (11). The frequency of electrodiagnostic testing is therefore based on the percent degeneration given the duration of paralysis (Fig. 37.1).

Those patients who exhibit complete degeneration on ENoG should also undergo a voluntary evoked EMG to identify a false-positive ENoG result or deblocking phenomenon. Voluntary evoked EMG involves asking the patient to make a forceful facial contraction with EMG electrodes in place. Deblocking is the phenomenon in which asynchronous neural firing due to regeneration of axoplasmic flow fails to generate a surface, compound muscle action potential (CMAP). Any motor activity on voluntary evoked EMG testing indicates "deblocking" of the conduction block and subsequently a favorable prognosis. Poor prognosticators include electrical silence and fibrillation potentials.

Ramsay Hunt Syndrome

Herpes zoster oticus usually presents with severe otalgia, a vesicular eruption, and facial paralysis. The vesicles typically occur on the tympanic membrane, external auditory canal, conchal bowl, and the postauricular region; however, they may also present on the palate and pharyngeal mucosa. Unlike Bell's palsy, multiple cranial neuropathies are commonplace with the varicella zoster virus. The eighth cranial nerve is most commonly involved with associated sensorineural hearing loss and vertigo. Involvement of the cornea may also occur, necessitating prompt ophthalmologic consultation.

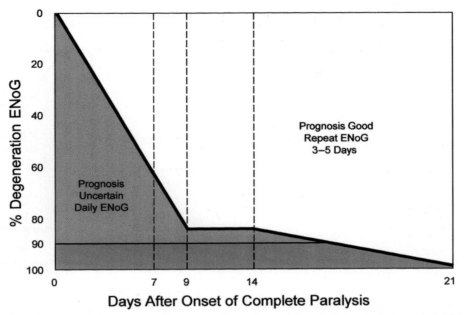

FIG. 37.1 ENoG retest protocol. The *pink area* represents an uncertain prognosis, and daily ENoG testing is recommended. The *blue area* indicates 90% degeneration, suggesting severe degeneration.

Ancillary testing, with the exclusion of an audiogram, is unnecessary. Electronystagmography (ENG) performed in the acute setting will be dominated by the underlying spontaneous nystagmus, which occurs with eighth nerve involvement. Persistent dysequilibrium months later may necessitate an ENG to document caloric weakness prior to initiation of vestibular rehabilitation. Electrical testing has demonstrated variable results in herpes zoster oticus, which may be due to the multiple regions of neural injury in this disorder, in contrast to the single site of injury in Bell's palsy.

MANAGEMENT

Bell's Palsy

Until recently, considerable controversy existed regarding the management of Bell's palsy. The treatment algorithm followed at our institution for the past 20 years is shown in Fig. 37.2. Those patients who present with facial paresis within 7 days of onset are treated with a combination of prednisone (1mg/kg/day for 7 days, without taper) and valacyclovir (500 mg t.i.d. for 10 days). Follow-up evaluation is arranged for 1 week to determine if neural degeneration has occurred, as evidenced by progression to a complete paralysis. If the patient progresses to a complete paralysis, electrodiagnostic testing is performed 3 days after the onset and the patient follows the algorithm for a total paralysis (Fig. 37.1). So long as any facial motion is present, electrodiagnostic evaluation is unnecessary. If a patient is seen later than 1 week after the onset of a facial paresis, and function is either stable or improving, medical treatment is unnecessary. Although the use of steroids and antivirals has not definitively

been shown to be superior to either one alone (22–26) or to the natural history of the disease (19,25), we continue to use this combination in an attempt to reduce the number of degenerating axons.

Those patients who present within 3 to 14 days of the onset of total paralysis undergo electrodiagnostic testing. If patients are seen before 3 days of a complete paralysis, they are started on prednisone and valacyclovir as per the aforementioned schedule and seen 2 to 3 days later for ENoG and EMG evaluation. If seen at least 3 days after the onset of a complete paralysis, electrodiagnostic studies are performed the same day. The degree of degeneration on ENoG will determine the timing of follow-up examinations (Fig. 37.1). Patients who exhibit 70% to 80% degeneration on ENoG or are degenerating rapidly should be evaluated every 1 to 2 days. If at least 90% degeneration is reached within 14 days of the onset of facial paralysis, an evoked EMG is also performed to eliminate the possibility of deblocking. Demonstration of CMAPs and polyphasic potentials on EMG portends a good prognosis despite complete degeneration on ENoG. Electrical silence or fibrillation potentials are indicative of denervation of the motor end plate, suggestive of a poor prognosis. (For a complete review of electrodiagnostic testing, see Perry and Gantz [27].) For those patients who demonstrate greater than 90% degeneration on ENoG and electrical silence or fibrillation potentials on evoked EMG within 14 days of their paralysis, a recommendation is made for middle cranial fossa facial nerve decompression. The option of continued medical management is always offered.

Decompression of the facial nerve for Bell's palsy has been performed for more than 50 years (28); however, until recently it was quite controversial. For those patients who

Bell's Palsy Management Algorithm

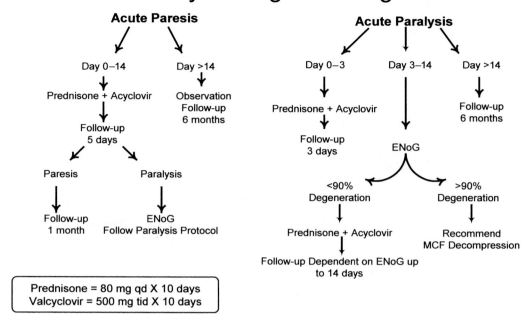

FIG. 37.2 Bell's palsy management algorithm.

have met electrodiagnostic criteria, it has been shown that prompt facial nerve decompression from the internal auditory canal to the tympanic segment offers a significant improvement in outcome when compared with medical management alone (29). When performed within 2 weeks of onset of paralysis, 91% of patients who underwent decompression achieved a House-Brackmann grade I or II (29). Only 42% of those patients who declined surgical therapy, after having met electrodiagnostic criteria, achieved a House-Brackmann grade I or II (29). It should be noted that all patients recovered to some degree with or without decompression.

Those patients who do not demonstrate greater than 90% neural degeneration on ENoG testing (the overwhelming majority of those affected) have an excellent prognosis with medical management alone. Most, if not all, will regain normal or nearly normal function with minimal synkinesis. The single most important aspect of their management may be eye care. As with all patients with facial paralysis, proper eye care is mandatory in Bell's palsy. The liberal use of lubricating drops during the day, ophthalmologic ointment at night, and a moisture chamber for sleep will usually suffice. If patients complain about irritation, or demonstrate erythema of the cornea or sclera, then they should be referred to an ophthalmologist.

Ramsay Hunt Syndrome

The management of facial paralysis secondary to the varicella zoster virus has evolved with the development of antiviral agents. Devriese and Moesker (30) evaluated the nat-

ural history of Ramsay Hunt syndrome, identifying only a 10% rate of complete facial nerve recovery during medical therapy. Subsequent studies have demonstrated an improvement in facial nerve recovery using a combination of steroids and antiviral agents (31–34). Complete return of facial function can be anticipated in as many as 75% of patients if both prednisone and antiviral agents are employed within 3 days of onset (32). The dosing schedule is the same as for Bell's palsy. Patients report a rapid reduction in pain and will occasionally notice facial nerve recovery while on therapy. Because the overall return of facial movement is better using this combination of drugs than with surgical decompression, the latter is no longer recommended. Of interest, patients who initially present with vertigo and facial paralysis will often notice a recurrence of the vertiginous episodes after initiating therapy with antiviral agents. Presumably this is caused by vestibular nerve recovery after the drug eliminates the viral source, whereas in years past the patient simply lost unilateral function with the illness and underwent spontaneous compensation.

Because of the possibility of corneal involvement by the varicella zoster virus, ophthalmologic consultation at the onset of the disease is not unreasonable. Similar to the management of Bell's palsy, proper eye care with drops, ointment, and a moisture chamber will suffice for most patients.

Facial Nerve Decompression

The risks of middle cranial fossa decompression are explained to the patient (Table 37.1) after the decision to proceed with decompression is made. Auditory brainstem re-

TABLE 37.1 *Risks of middle cranial fossa decompression*

Facial nerve injury	0
Hearing loss	1%
Conductive	1%
Sensorineural	<1%
CSF leak	4%
Meningitis	<1%
Intracranial hemorrhage	<1%
Stroke	<1%
Seizure	<1%
Aphasia	<1%
Death	0

Gantz BJ, Rubinstein JT, Gidley P, et al. Surgical management of Bell's palsy. *Laryngoscope* 1999;109:1177–1188.

sponse (ABR) audiometry is performed preoperatively for auditory monitoring during surgery. A Stenver's-view plain radiograph is obtained to evaluate the landmarks along the floor of the middle cranial fossa, including identification of the superior semicircular canal. Coagulation studies, a blood count, a baseline electrocardiogram, and a chest X-ray examination are also obtained if the history dictates further investigation.

The patient is placed on an operating room table that rotates from side to side, with a narrow headrest, allowing the surgeon access to the entire cranium. Support (thromboembolic deterrent [TED]) hose and pneumatic compression stockings are placed prior to the patient's undergoing general anesthesia without the use of muscle relaxants. After the endotracheal tube is secured to the contralateral side, the bed is rotated 180 degrees from the anesthesia personnel. At this point, several maneuvers are performed simultaneously. The surgical team inserts a Foley catheter and a temperature probe, after which the patient is securely padded with foam and strapped to the bed. The anesthesia team obtains any additional intravenous or arterial lines necessary and administers 1 g of cefazolin (repeated every 8 hours) and 6 mg of dexamethasone (Decadron) (repeated every 6 hours). For brain dehydration, 250 ml of mannitol (20% solution) is administered at the beginning of the craniotomy.

The ipsilateral cranium is then shaved 10 cm around the ear, and a posteriorly based skin flap is drawn on the skin (Fig. 37.3) and infiltrated with 10 ml 1% lidocaine with 1:100,000 epinephrine. The ABR recording electrodes are then placed into both mastoid tips, the vertex, and the superior brow. Insert earphones are secured within the external auditory canals bilaterally, for ABR stimulation and direct auditory nerve whole nerve action potential recording. The entire ipsilateral face, neck, and scalp are then scrubbed with povidone-iodine (Betadine) solo prep and covered with

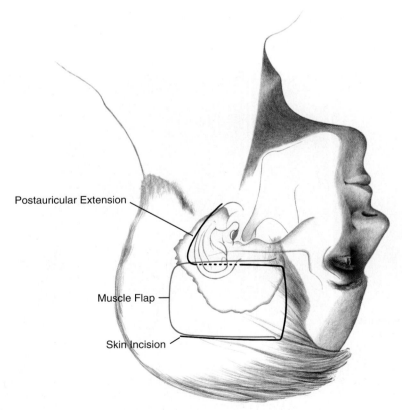

Postauricular Extension

Muscle Flap

Skin Incision

FIG. 37.3 The skin flap incision is posteriorly based to allow posterior elevation. The inferior limb can be extended postauricularly to expose the mastoid if necessary. The temporalis muscle flap is reflected anteriorly and offset to ensure temporalis muscle and skin incisions do not overlap. The craniotomy is centered on the zygomatic root and measures approximately 4 by 5 cm.

a clear plastic drape for facial nerve monitoring by the scrub nurse (Fig. 37.4). The NIMS recording electrodes are inserted for electrical monitoring of the facial nerve.

The incision is carried through the scalp down to the level of the temporalis fascia and retracted posteriorly. A 4-cm by 4-cm piece of fascia is harvested and set aside. An anteriorly based muscle flap, which is staggered inferiorly in relation to the skin flap, is raised. Two large Adson cerebellar retractors are inserted to separate the skin and muscle flaps, exposing the zygomatic root and cranium. A 4-cm wide by 5-cm high craniotomy is created using an otologic drill, centered inferiorly upon the zygomatic root (Fig. 37.5). The bone flap is elevated off the dura and set aside. Branches of the middle meningeal artery are encountered, both within the bone and on the dura, which are easily controlled with either bone wax or bipolar cautery. A 2-cm elevation of the dura is performed superiorly, anteriorly, and posteriorly to facilitate retractor placement.

The dura along the floor of the middle cranial fossa is elevated from posterior to anterior to avoid disruption of the greater superficial petrosal nerve and geniculate ganglion. Dural elevation can be quite difficult, especially in those older than age 65 years. After identifying the arcuate eminence, the greater superficial petrosal nerve, and the petrous ridge, the House-Urban middle fossa retractor is placed un-

der the lip of the ridge, overlying the suspected site of the internal auditory canal (Fig. 37.6). Drilling is thus begun over the arcuate eminence until the blue-line of the superior semicircular canal is identified. The anatomy of the middle fossa floor is quite variable, and, although the Stenver's radiograph is helpful, it is not a substitute for experience. The most consistent anatomic feature of the middle fossa anatomy is the position of the superior semicircular canal, which is almost always 90 degrees perpendicular to the petrous ridge (Fig. 37.7).

Drilling over the arcuate eminence should *always* be in a direction perpendicular to the petrous ridge until the blue-line of the canal is identified. Color differences of the bone are also extremely important in this type of surgery. The whitish-yellow color of the dense otic capsule bone helps to differentiate the superior semicircular canal from surrounding whiter membranous temporal bone. The internal auditory canal is located 60 degrees anterior to the blue-lined canal. The internal auditory canal should then be skeletonized up to the transverse crest. Anterior lateral exposure of the internal auditory canal should not extend more caudal than the labyrinthine segment of the facial nerve to avoid entrance into the cochlea. The labyrinthine segment of the facial nerve is identified at the transverse crest, where the nerve will angle both anterior and superior toward the genic-

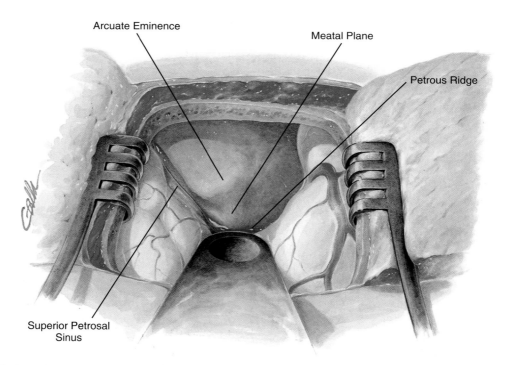

FIG. 37.4 Placement of the self-retaining House-Urban middle cranial fossa retractor at the petrous ridge. The meatal plane is the flattened area anterior and medial to the arcuate eminence. It is helpful to hook the edge of the retractor blade under the petrous ridge, but care must be taken to prevent injury to the superior petrosal vein. The first step in exposure of the facial nerve is identification of the superior semicircular canal by blue-lining. This is accomplished by carefully removing bone over the superior semicircular canal in the direction parallel to the canal with a diamond bur. Next, removal of bone over the internal auditory canal begins anterior and medial to the superior canal at the medial extent of the meatal plane.

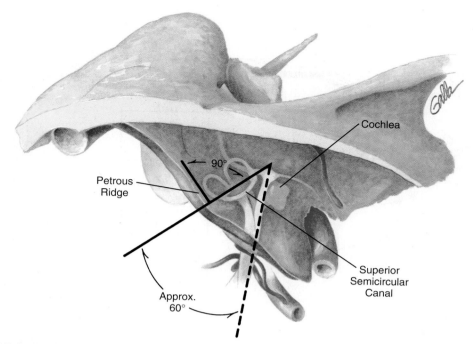

FIG. 37.5 Important anatomy of the otic capsule contents and internal auditory canal. The superior semicircular canal is almost always perpendicular to the petrous ridge. It does not always correspond to the longitudinal direction of the arcuate eminence. Finding the superior canal landmark is critical for providing orientation to the internal auditory canal, which is not more than 60 degrees anterior to the longitudinal line of the superior canal. The labyrinthine segment of the facial nerve lies a fraction of a millimeter cephalad to the basal turn of the cochlea. Exposure of the labyrinthine segment of cranial nerve VII requires exposure of the internal auditory canal medial and gradual lateral exposure, making sure the anterolateral exposure is cephalad to the labyrinthine segment.

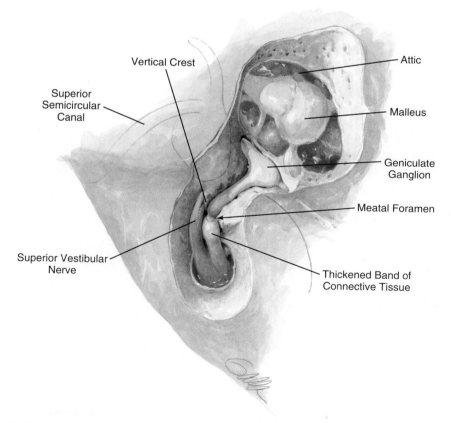

FIG. 37.6 Middle cranial fossa exposure of the facial nerve. The vertical crest separates the superior vestibular nerve and the facial nerve and is the entrance to the meatal foramen. This is the narrowest portion of the fallopian canal (approximately 0.68 mm in diameter). Another important feature of this restricted area is the thickened band of connective tissue that is found at the entrance to the meatal foramen. Removal of the tegmen tympani allows exposure of the head of the malleus and body of incus. The tympanic segment lateral to the geniculate ganglion is exposed.

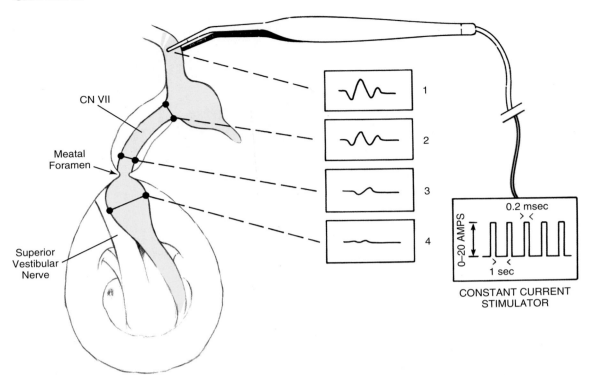

FIG. 37.7 Intraoperative electromyography can be used to identify the site of the nerve conduction block after decompression of the nerve. A bipolar or unipolar nerve stimulator is used to stimulate the nerve first in the tympanic segment. If total neural degeneration has not occurred, a motor unit potential can be recorded (1). In this illustration, stimulation in the internal auditory canal results in failure to record a motor unit potential (4). A conduction block has occurred between these two sites.

ulate ganglion. Bone may now be safely removed from the geniculate ganglion and tegmen tympani (Fig. 37.8).

A 1-mm diamond bur is used to remove the bone over the labyrinthine segment, until a blunt elevator or sharp right-angled hooks can remove the final, eggshell-thin layer of bone. The blue-line of the cochlea should be avoided while performing these maneuvers. A flat 1-mm by 1-mm recording electrode can be placed between the dura of the internal auditory canal and the bone anteriorly for recording near-field auditory whole nerve action potential. The arachnoid band at the entrance to the meatal foramen and periosteum and epineural sheath of the nerve are opened with a disposable microscalpel, from the tympanic segment to the internal auditory canal. After releasing the constraint imposed by these tissue layers, the nerve usually swells to two to three times its normal size.

The site of conduction block along the nerve can be identified using intraoperative electromyography. As long as the nerve has not completely degenerated, stimulation of the nerve lateral to the site of the conduction block will reveal a motor unit potential. Stimulation medial to the block, usually in the internal auditory canal, will fail to evoke a response. The neural activity is demonstrated either by direct observation of the face or a compound muscle action potential on the NIMS device.

Closure is begun by placing a plug of temporalis muscle in the opened internal auditory canal. All opened mastoid air

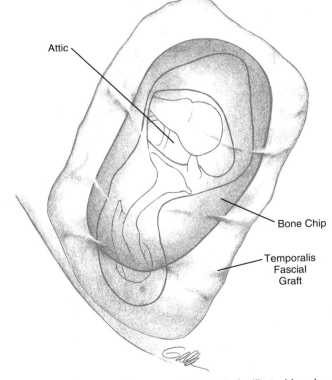

FIG. 37.8 Closure of the operative site is facilitated by placing a large temporalis fascial graft over the temporal bone defect and using a piece of the craniotomy bone flap to prevent herniation of the temporal lobe into the attic.

cells are obliterated with bone wax. The temporalis fascia that was harvested previously is placed over the entire defect, and a corner of the bone flap is used to reinforce the tegmen tympani and internal auditory canal. This ensures that the temporal lobe will not herniate into the internal auditory canal or attic. The retractor is removed, and the temporal lobe is allowed to reexpand. If after several minutes complete reexpansion has not taken place, several 4-0 neuralon sutures are used to tack the dura to the temporalis musculature. The craniotomy flap is replaced, and the temporalis musculature is closed with interrupted 3-0 vicryl sutures. The skin flap is closed with interrupted 4-0 nylon sutures, and a snug mastoid-type dressing is applied.

Postoperatively, the patient is taken to the surgical intensive care unit overnight for neurologic monitoring, and subsequently discharged to the floor the following morning. The patient receives six doses of cefazolin and Decadron, with analgesia limited to codeine. On the third postoperative day, patients are tested for cerebrospinal fluid rhinorrhea by having them place their heads between their knees for 3 minutes. Rarely does a leak occur, but if it does, a lumbar drain should be placed for 5 days. Almost never does one need to revise the surgical defect to stop a leak. Three to 5 days postoperatively, the patient is discharged home.

SUMMARY

The majority of patients who experience Bell's palsy recover either to normal or nearly normal function using medical management alone. Unfortunately, there is a select group of patients who will not recover this level of function and will require further intervention. Electrodiagnostic testing will identify these patients; it must be done in a timely fashion, because decompression does not alter the outcome after 14 days (29). It also must be remembered that nearly every patient will regain some function within 6 months of onset; therefore all patients need to be reevaluated at that time to ensure that a tumor is not present.

Ramsay Hunt syndrome does not have as good a prognosis as Bell's palsy; however, early treatment with steroids and antivirals has dramatically improved the facial nerve outcome in these patients. As previously suggested, the use of antivirals may prolong the dysequilibrium. Decompression does not alter the outcome of this disease and is no longer recommended.

REFERENCES

1. McCormick DP. Herpes-simplex virus as cause of Bell's palsy. *Lancet* 1972;937–939.
2. Burgess RC, Michaels L, Bale JF Jr, et al. Polymerase chain reaction amplification of herpes simplex viral DNA from the geniculate ganglion of a patient with Bell's palsy. *Ann Otol Rhinol Laryngol* 1994; 103:775–779.
3. Furuta Y, Fukuda S, Chida E, et al. Reactivation of herpes simplex virus type 1 in patients with Bell's palsy. *J Med Virol* 1998;54:162–166.
4. Murakami S, Mizobuchi M, Nakashiro Y, et al. Bell palsy and herpes simplex virus: identification of viral DNA in endoneurial fluid and muscle. *Ann Intern Med* 1996;124:27–30.
5. Sugita T, Murakami S, Yanagihara N, et al. Facial nerve paralysis induced by herpes simplex virus in mice: an animal model of acute and transient facial paralysis. *Ann Otol Rhinol Laryngol* 1995;104:574–581.
6. Carreno M, Llorente J, Hidalgo F, et al. Aplicacion de la reaccion en cadena de la polimerase a un modelo experimental de infeccion por el virus del herpes simplex tipo 1. *Acta Otorrinolaryngol Esp* 1998;49:15–18.
7. May M. Facial nerve disorders. Update 1982. *Am J Otol* 1982;4:77–88.
8. Ge XX, Spector GJ. Labyrinthine segment and geniculate ganglion of the facial nerve in fetal and adult human temporal bones. *Ann Otol Rhinol Laryngol* 1981;90:1–12.
9. Fisch U, Felix H. On the pathogenesis of Bell's palsy. *Acta Otolaryngol (Stockh)* 1983;95:532–538.
10. Gantz BJ, Gmur A, Fisch U. Intraoperative evoked electromyography in Bell's palsy. *Am J Otolaryngol* 1982;3:273–278.
11. Fisch U. Prognostic value of electrical tests in acute facial paralysis. *Am J Otol* 1984;5:494–498.
12. Furuta Y, Takasu T, Fukuda S, et al. Detection of varicella-zoster virus DNA in human geniculate ganglia by polymerase chain reaction. *J Infect Dis* 1992;166:1157–1159.
13. Ikeda M, Hiroshige K, Abiko Y, et al. Impaired specific cellular immunity to the varicella-zoster virus in patients with herpes zoster oticus. *J Laryngol Otol* 1996;110:918–921.
14. Wackym PA. Molecular temporal bone pathology: II. Ramsay Hunt syndrome (herpes zoster oticus). *Laryngoscope* 1997;107:1165–1175.
15. Furuta Y, Fukuda S, Suzuki S, et al. Detection of varicella-zoster virus DNA in patients with acute peripheral facial palsy by the polymerase chain reaction, and its use for early diagnosis of zoster sine herpete. *J Med Virol* 1997;52:316–319.
16. Mumenthaler M. Zosterinfektionen des Nervensystems. *Akt Neurol* 1985;12:145–152.
17. Rosler KM, Magistris MR, Glocker FX, et al. Electrophysiological characteristics of lesions in facial palsies of different etiologies. A study using electrical and magnetic stimulation techniques. *Electroencephalogr Clin Neurophysiol* 1995;97:355–368.
18. Adour KK, Byl FM, Hilsinger RL Jr, et al. The true nature of Bell's palsy: analysis of 1,000 consecutive patients. *Laryngoscope* 1978;88:787–801.
19. Peitersen E. Natural history of Bell's palsy. *Acta Otolaryngol Suppl* 1992;492:122–124.
20. Esslen E. Electromyography and electroneurography. In: Fisch U, ed. *Facial nerve surgery.* Birmingham, AL: Aesculapius, 1977:93–100.
21. Fisch U, Esslen E. Total intratemporal exposure of the facial nerve. Pathologic findings in Bell's palsy. *Arch Otolaryngol* 1972;95:335–341.
22. Adour KK, Wingerd J, Bell DN, et al. Prednisone treatment for idiopathic facial paralysis (Bell's palsy). *N Engl J Med* 1972;287:1268–1272.
23. Adour KK, Ruboyianes JM, Von Doersten PG, et al. Bell's palsy treatment with acyclovir and prednisone compared with prednisone alone: a double-blind, randomized, controlled trial. *Ann Otol Rhinol Laryngol* 1996;105:371–378.
24. Katusic SK, Beard CM, Wiederholt WC, et al. Incidence, clinical features, and prognosis in Bell's palsy, Rochester, Minnesota, 1968–1982. *Ann Neurol* 1986;20:622–627.
25. May M, Wette R, Hardin WB Jr, et al. The use of steroids in Bell's palsy: a prospective controlled study. *Laryngoscope* 1976;86:1111–1122.
26. Ramos Macias A, De Miguel Martinez I, Martin Sanchez AM, et al. Incorporacion del aciclovir en el tratamiento de la paralisis periferica. Un estudio en 45 casos. *Acta Otorrinolaringol Esp* 1992;43:117–120.
27. Perry B, Gantz B. Diagnosis and management of acute facial palsies. In: Myers E, Bluestone C, Brackmann D, et al, eds. *Advances in otolaryngology head and neck surgery,* vol 13. St. Louis: Mosby, 1999:127–162.
28. Balance C, Duel AD. The operative treatment of facial palsy by the introduction of nerve grafts into the fallopian canal and by other intratemporal methods. *Arch Otolaryngol* 1932;15:1–70.
29. Gantz BJ, Rubinstein JT, Gidley P, et al. Surgical management of Bell's palsy. *Laryngoscope* 1999;109:1177–1188.
30. Devriese P, Moesker W. The natural history of facial paralysis in herpes zoster. *Clin Otolaryngol* 1988;13:289–298.

31. Dickens JR, Smith JT, Graham SS. Herpes zoster oticus: treatment with intravenous acyclovir. *Laryngoscope* 1988;98:776–779.

32. Murakami S, Hato N, Horiuchi J, et al. Treatment of Ramsay Hunt syndrome with acyclovir-prednisone: significance of early diagnosis and treatment. *Ann Neurol* 1997;41:353–357.

33. Stafford FW, Welch AR. The use of acyclovir in Ramsay Hunt syndrome. *J Laryngol Otol* 1986;100:337–340.

34 Uri N, Greenberg E, Meyer W, et al. Herpes zoster oticus: treatment with acyclovir. *Ann Otol Rhinol Laryngol* 1992;101:161–162.

CHAPTER 38

Facial Reanimation Surgery

Tessa A. Hadlock, Mack L. Cheney, and Michael J. McKenna

Facial nerve disorders encompass a broad spectrum of dysfunction, ranging from subtle dynamic facial asymmetry to complete, dense paralysis. Facial nerve regeneration following injury can vary greatly and may result in hypofunction (persistent weakness or poor excursion of facial muscles), hyperfunction (hypertonicity, spasm), or aberrant regeneration (synkinesis). The impact of a facial nerve disorder can be dramatic. Disabilities encountered include corneal exposure of the affected eye, oral incompetence and articulation difficulties from orbicularis oris weakness, and functional nasal obstruction from dilator nares paralysis. None of these is perhaps as significant as the social isolation these patients often succumb to based on their perceived disfigurement and inability to convey emotion through facial expression. Because of the profound effect of this disorder on patient quality of life, a great deal of effort has been focused toward rehabilitation of the paralyzed face.

When facial nerve discontinuity is encountered, the first approach is to attempt to reestablish direct neural continuity between the facial motor nucleus and the distal facial nerve through either primary repair or autografting techniques. When this is not possible, other methods of reestablishing facial balance and movement may be considered. Facial reanimation procedures refer to interventions that restore facial symmetry, resting tone, voluntary movement, or a combination of these. Several broad categories of facial reanimation techniques exist, each appropriate to a specific set of clinical, anatomic, or outcome-related circumstances. These include reinnervation techniques, muscle transfers, and static procedures. The aim of this chapter is to describe each of these approaches, including appropriate clinical scenarios, technical aspects of the surgery, and adjunctive management strategies to optimize postoperative appearance and function.

REINNERVATION TECHNIQUES

Reinnervation techniques, also termed nerve substitution techniques, are procedures that provide neural input to the distal facial nerve and facial musculature via motor nerves other than the native facial nerve. They are indicated in two situations. The first is when the proximal facial nerve stump is not available but the distal facial nerve and facial musculature are present and functional. This occurs following skull base tumor resections involving sacrifice of the nerve at or very close to the brainstem, where neurorrhaphy is not technically achievable. The second situation occurs following skull base surgery, intracranial injury, or traumatic facial paralysis, when the nerve is thought to be anatomically intact but there is no discernable return of function after a satisfactory waiting period of 12 months. Lack of functional recovery, electrophysiologic demonstration of lack of reinnervation potentials, and the presence of fibrillation potentials at 12 months indicate persistent complete denervation. This suggests insufficient regenerative potential from the proximal facial nerve stump and therefore mandates alternative proximal axonal input to the distal facial nerve and facial musculature.

Hypoglossal–Facial Transfer (XII-VII Crossover)

The nerve most often utilized to reinnervate the distal facial nerve is the hypoglossal nerve. Its proximity to the extratemporal facial nerve, its dense population of myelinated motor axons, the relative acceptability of the resultant hemitongue weakness, and the highly predictable and reliable result make it a logical choice (1–4). In the classic XII-VII transfer, the entire hypoglossal nerve is transected and reflected upward for direct neurorrhaphy to the facial nerve stump (Fig. 38.1A). Several modifications have been described (Fig. 38.1B–D), including the "split" XII-VII transfer (5), in which approximately 30% of the width of the hypoglossal nerve is divided from the main trunk of the nerve for several centimeters and secured to the lower division of the facial nerve (Fig. 38.1B). Another modification, designed to reduce tongue morbidity by avoiding the splicing away of a significant length of the partial hypoglossal trunk, is the XII-VII jump graft. This involves an end-to-side neurorrhaphy between the hypoglossal nerve and a donor cable graft (usually the great auricular nerve), which in turn is sewn to the distal facial trunk (6) (Fig. 38.1C). This modification is based upon improved appreciation of the microanatomy of the hypoglossal nerve, which demonstrates interwoven fascicular architecture; separating a 30% segment away from the main trunk for several centimeters divides a significantly greater number of axons than if the fibers were oriented in parallel (6).

In some circumstances where the facial nerve is able to be mobilized from the second genu within the temporal bone and reflected inferiorly, removal of the mastoid tip allows for direct coaptation of the facial nerve to the hypoglossal without the need for an interposition graft (7) (Fig. 38.1D). Elimination of the cable graft provides a theoretical regenerative advantage by reducing from two neurorrhaphies to one.

Surgical Technique

The classic XII-VII procedure is performed via a modified Blair parotidectomy incision. The main trunk of the facial nerve and the pes anserinus are identified using standard facial nerve landmarks, such as the tragal pointer and the tym-

panomastoid suture line. The hypoglossal nerve is then located in its ascending portion, deep to the posterior belly of the digastric, along the medial surface of the internal jugular vein. The nerve is followed anteriorly and freed of fascial attachments beyond the takeoff of the descendens hypoglossi. The hypoglossal nerve is then sharply transected and reflected superiorly to meet the facial nerve. The facial nerve is transected at the stylomastoid foramen, and the entire distal trunk is reflected inferiorly and secured to the hypoglossal nerve with 5 to 7 10-0 nylon epineurial microsutures.

A modification designed to decrease mass movement of the face involves sectioning the entire facial nerve but performing a neurorrhaphy only to the inferior division of the facial nerve, or ligating the upper division distal to the pes (Fig. 38.1), and employing separate techniques for management of the upper face. The split XII-VII transfer provides many fewer axons and is therefore best utilized only for the lower segment of the face.

In the jump graft or direct XII-VII end-to-side procedure, once the exposure has been obtained the great auricular nerve graft is harvested or the proximal facial nerve is mobilized from the temporal bone, sectioned at the second genu,

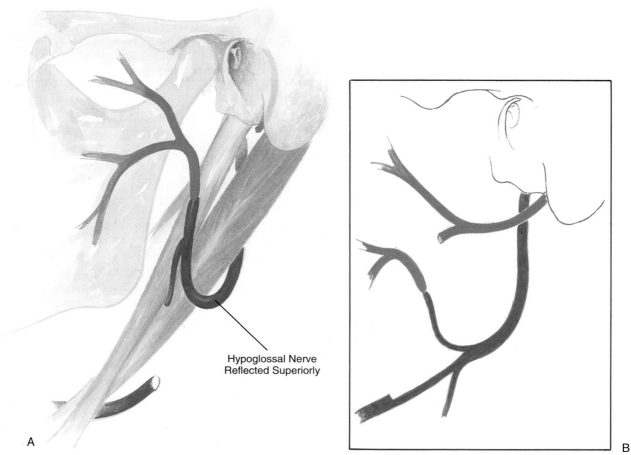

Hypoglossal Nerve
Reflected Superiorly

A

B

FIG. 38.1 Hypoglossal facial nerve transfer. Hypoglossal nerve is shown in *green,* facial nerve in *orange.* **A:** Classic procedure, with entire hypoglossal nerve transected. **B:** Modification with 40% segment of nerve secured to lower division.

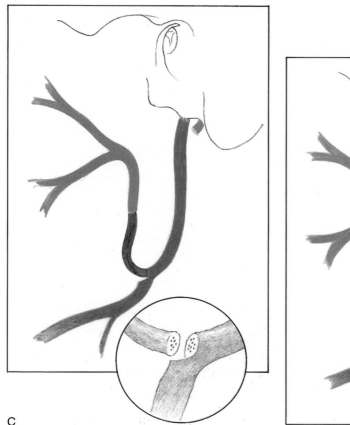

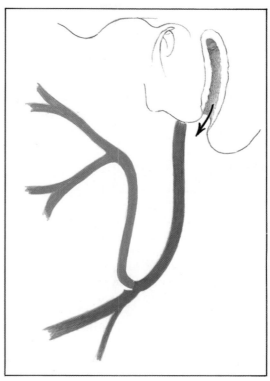

C

D

FIG. 38.1, cont'd. Hypoglossal facial nerve transfer. Hypoglossal nerve is shown in *green*, facial nerve in *orange*. **C:** Jump graft (*purple*) modification. Insert shows how graft is positioned to capture axons extending from the proximal aspect of the opened hypoglossal nerve. **D:** Reflection of the facial nerve out of the mastoid bone to meet the hypoglossal nerve in the neck.

and transposed into the neck by removal of the mastoid tip. The facial nerve can be further mobilized by dissecting it away from the parotid tissue beyond its bifurcation. The end-to-side neurorrhaphy is executed by removing a segment of hypoglossal epineurium, then cutting a 30% opening into the hypoglossal nerve and allowing the defect to open up. The recipient nerve is then laid into the defect, facing the proximal cut surface, and secured with microsutures.

Results, Drawbacks, and Contraindications

With a XII-VII transfer, good resting facial tone is achieved in more than 90% of patients. When successful, the transfer allows deliberate facial movement with intentional manipulation of the tongue. Recovery generally occurs over 6 to 24 months and in some cases has been reported to continue up to 5 years. Results are variable, with time from denervation to transfer playing a key role in outcome. There is general consensus that reinnervation must occur within 2 years following injury, otherwise neuromuscular fibrosis and atrophy progress to a point where meaningful tone and movement are not achievable (6).

The two most significant drawbacks of the procedure are the mass facial movement experienced by many patients and the variable tongue dysfunction, which has been categorized as severe in up to 25% of patients. Articulation and mastication difficulties are commonly cited. The modifications mentioned earlier are aimed at one or the other of these two problems. In addition, botulinum toxin administration in the region of the eye and physical therapy have proven useful adjuncts for patients with clinically significant mass movement.

The procedure is contraindicated in patients who are likely to develop other cranial neuropathies (e.g., neurofibromatosis type II) or who have ipsilateral tenth nerve deficits, as the combined X-XII deficit can lead to profound swallowing dysfunction.

VII-VII CROSS FACIAL GRAFTING

Another potential source of axons for facial reinnervation is the contralateral healthy facial nerve (8). The two distinct advantages of its use are that it is the only donor source with the potential for mimetic function (the involuntary blink and emotive smile) and that it is significantly arborized distally, so several branches may be sacrificed for use in cross facial grafting, usually without adversely affecting the healthy side. The disadvantages include many fewer motor axons than the hypoglossal, with unpredictable results; the need for a lengthy sural nerve jump graft; and the potential for facial weakness on the donor side (9). Most surgeons feel the motor power provided by the hypoglossal nerve is distinctly superior, and the use of the contralateral facial nerve strictly for reinnervation of native facial musculature has largely been replaced by cross face nerve grafting in conjunction with free muscle transfer.

Surgical Technique

The VII-VII cross facial graft technique has a great deal of surgical variability with regard to exposure of the donor and recipient nerves, the length and positioning of jump grafts, and the timing of second stage neurorrhaphy. There are insufficient data to allow specific approaches to emerge as superior to others (10–12). It is ordinarily a staged procedure, where in the first stage a sural nerve graft is harvested from the leg, tunneled subcutaneously from the ipsilateral preauricular region across the face, and sewn to the fresh-cut edges of one or several buccal branches of the functioning facial nerve (Fig. 38.2), via a nasolabial fold or a preauricular incision. The growth of axons into the graft is followed clinically by tapping on the graft (Tinel's sign); tingling indicates the presence of regenerating axons. Once regeneration has occurred across the face, a second stage is performed where the sural nerve graft is sewn to one or several branches of the affected facial nerve. Alternatively, the ipsilateral neurorrhaphy can be performed in the same operative setting.

Results, Drawbacks, and Contraindications

The major disadvantage with cross facial nerve grafting is that results are inconsistent. Some authors report excellent recovery, whereas many others find it entirely unsatisfactory. It appears that it is most useful in association with other reanimation modalities, to address a single territory within the face rather than to reinnervate the entire contralateral facial nerve. Recent studies employing the cross facial graft for isolated marginal mandibular paralysis demonstrate its utility (13).

OTHER REINNERVATION TECHNIQUES

Several other cranial nerves have been employed for reinnervation of the distal facial nerve stump. The spinal accessory nerve (14), glossopharyngeal nerve, and trigeminal nerve have all been described as potential donors, though none has gained great popularity. The donor morbidity and difficulty with surgical exposure far exceed that found with XII-VII and cross facial grafting. Experimentation with uti-

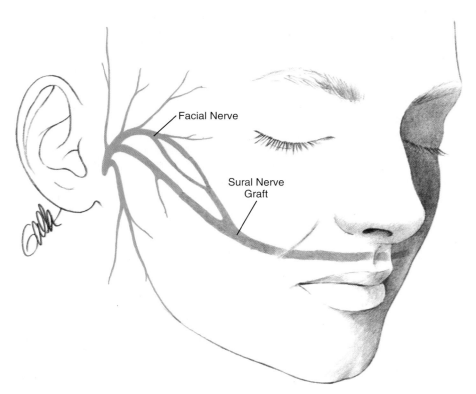

FIG. 38.2 Placement of a cross face nerve graft. Note that several midface branches are sacrificed and routed into the graft.

lizing isolated branches, such as the sternocleidomastoid branch of the spinal accessory nerve (15,16), would decrease donor morbidity, potentially increasing the utility of this technique.

MUSCLE TRANSPOSITION TECHNIQUES

When the distal facial nerve or facial musculature has undergone degeneration to a point of significant atrophy or fibrosis, even the delivery of viable motor axons will not provide adequate excursion to create appreciable facial expression. Occasionally, resection of extensive disease involves removal of facial musculature for adequate tumor extirpation. In these situations, the transfer of functional innervated musculature into the face offers the only possibility of meaningful facial movement. A segment of innervated muscle can be transposed into the appropriate segment of the face from the temporalis, masseter, digastric, or other regional muscles or transferred from a distant site (gracilis, pectoralis minor, serratus anterior, latissimus dorsi) and reinnervated locally.

Effective rehabilitation requires training and physical therapy to achieve optimal function. The literature does support the concept of neural plasticity whereby, after a certain training period, patients with trigeminally driven muscle transfers into the face are able to achieve movement without initiating a clenching of teeth. Whether this is a central nervous system phenomenon or a peripheral phenomenon is not known (17).

Temporalis Muscle Transposition

When intact, the temporalis muscle is the first choice for reanimation of the smile in the chronically paralyzed face. It is also useful as an interim therapy, when the regenerative potential of the facial nerve is in question (e.g., following skull base surgery), during the waiting period for regeneration (18), because it does not interfere with any potential facial nerve regeneration. Further, it may be utilized to manage the upper face in conjunction with a XII-VII transfer to the lower division of the nerve. It serves as a static support to the oral commissure and provides trigeminally controlled dynamic movement.

Before proceeding, it is imperative to establish that the muscle and its nerve and vascular supply are intact, because many neurotologic procedures damage these structures, and several congenital facial palsy syndromes are associated with other cranial nerve abnormalities that may affect temporalis muscle function. Severe atrophy of the musculature, such as in an edentulous patient, would also be a contraindication to this approach.

Surgical Technique (19)

The procedure is performed through an incision from the superior temporal line down to the attachment of the lobule, and sometimes extending postauricularly as with a rhytidectomy. Flaps are then raised both anteriorly and posteriorly in the subdermal plane, just under the hair follicles. Care is taken to preserve the superficial temporal artery and veins, so that the temporoparietal fascial flap can be utilized to obliterate the donor site defect. The temporoparietal fascial flap is then reflected from the true temporalis muscular fascia, working superiorly to inferiorly, leaving the temporoparietal fascial flap pedicled on its vessels. A flap is then raised in the subdermal plane from the zygomatic arch to the oral commissure. The skin flap extends medially all the way to the lateral border of the orbicularis oris muscle to achieve adequate coaptation to the transferred muscle. A 1.5-cm wide strip of temporalis muscle with its underlying pericranium is then elevated from the calvarium. The segment is chosen so that reflection over the zygomatic arch will pull the commissure in a vector appropriate to the patient's smile pattern (20). A double staple line of gastrointestinal anastomosis staples is placed along the superior muscle edge, to provide a firm purchase for the insetting sutures (Fig. 38.3A). Once this is accomplished, the muscle is reflected into the midface and secured with vicryl sutures to the orbicularis oris, with good muscle-to-muscle contact to promote potential neurotization of the orbicularis fibers. The commissure is deliberately overcorrected, so that with relaxation, appropriate position is achieved (Fig. 38.3B). The temporoparietal fascial flap is then placed into the temporalis strip defect (Fig. 38.3C), and the incision is closed over a drain. A mastoid-type dressing is placed for the first postoperative night. The incision is closed with 5-0 nylon interrupted sutures. Physical therapy is vital to achieving satisfactory muscle function and is instituted within weeks after the transfer to develop appropriate control and excursion of the transferred muscle.

Other Regional Muscle Transfers

The masseter muscle transfer, popularized by Rubin (20) and by Baker and Conley (21), can also provide excursion at the oral commissure. The entire muscle is ordinarily freed from its mandibular attachments and secured to the lateral aspect of the orbicularis oris, much the same way as the temporalis muscle. However, given its more lateral vector pull and the contour defect it creates at the commissure, it remains a far second choice to the temporalis muscle transposition. Modifications that address this and simplify the procedure have been reported in a few patients (22), though no substantial improvement has been clearly established.

The digastric muscle transfer is useful in isolated marginal mandibular nerve injuries, but compromises oral competence in the total facial paralysis patient. In the appropriately selected patient with isolated marginal mandibular nerve injury, the procedure can be effective at restoring depressor function to the lower lip. It involves sectioning the digastric muscle at the junction of the posterior belly and its tendon, then freeing the anterior belly and tendon from sur-

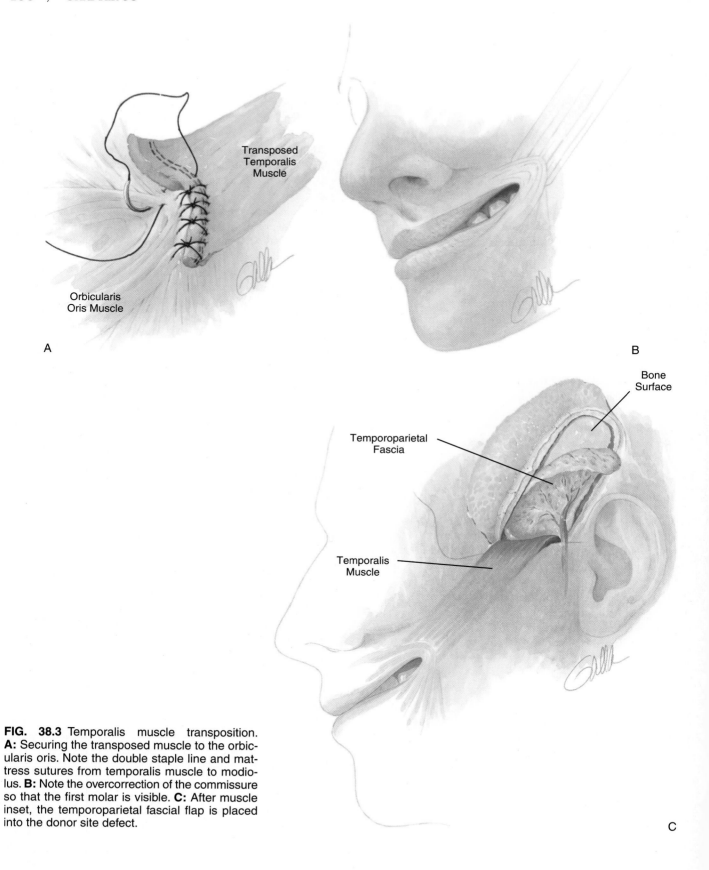

FIG. 38.3 Temporalis muscle transposition. **A:** Securing the transposed muscle to the orbicularis oris. Note the double staple line and mattress sutures from temporalis muscle to modiolus. **B:** Note the overcorrection of the commissure so that the first molar is visible. **C:** After muscle inset, the temporoparietal fascial flap is placed into the donor site defect.

rounding structures and securing it to the orbicularis oris along the ipsilateral inferior border (Fig. 38.4). Mylohyoid nerve innervation to the anterior belly can be maintained (23) or the muscle can be driven by a cross face nerve graft as shown (13).

Other local muscle flaps have been suggested—for example, the innervated platysma musculocutaneous flap (24)—but insufficient numbers of treated patients leave their ultimate utility in question.

Free Muscle Transfer

With the advent of microvascular free tissue transfer, the opportunity to bring functional muscle from a distant site into the face became possible. In a number of clinical scenarios, this approach is preferred. First, if the proximal facial nerve stump is available but the facial musculature has been resected, a free muscle graft can be transferred and driven by the ipsilateral proximal facial nerve. This has the potential of providing involuntary, mimetic movement in the face. Patients with long-standing facial paralysis in whom the temporalis transposition is not an option may achieve superior results from free muscle transfer powered by either the ipsilateral trigeminal nerve or a cross facial nerve graft rather than through an alternative regional muscle transfer.

Congenital facial palsy patients are also good candidates for the procedure because they lack adequate muscles of facial expression or facial nerve trunks for neurorrhaphy and may have other cranial neuropathies (25). The procedure is most commonly performed as a two-stage procedure for

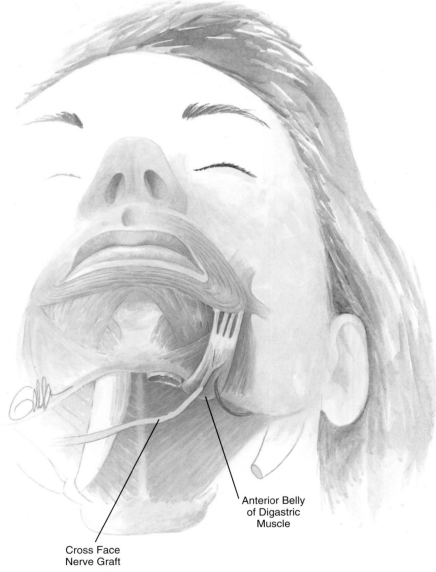

Anterior Belly of Digastric Muscle

Cross Face Nerve Graft

FIG. 38.4 Transfer of the anterior belly of the digastric. The tendon is divided and filleted into separate slips and secured to the orbicularis oris. Note that native innervation can be maintained or replaced by a cross face nerve graft.

unilateral paralysis and a single-stage procedure for bilateral paralysis (i.e., Moebius syndrome). This is because for unilateral paralysis, the muscle is powered by a cross facial graft from a buccal branch of the healthy facial nerve, requiring a 9- to 12-month waiting period for axonal extension through the cable graft before muscle transplantation. For bilateral paralysis, the muscle is driven by the ipsilateral trigeminal or hypoglossal nerve, which eliminates the need for a regeneration phase and second operative procedure.

The gracilis muscle was the first muscle utilized in successful facial reanimation (26), and remains the most popular choice for this purpose. Modifications involving use of subsegments of the muscle and alternative neural sources for the graft have been described (27, 28). The muscle implantation procedure is described next.

Surgical Technique

Preoperatively, the vector of the smile on the healthy side (if present) is noted so that it can be emulated on the affected side. The procedure is begun by harvest of the gracilis muscle from the medial aspect of the thigh. An incision is made 1.5 cm posterior and parallel to a line connecting the pubic tubercle to the medial condyle of the tibia. The soft tissues are divided until the belly of the gracilis muscle is identified. The vascular pedicle is located entering the deep surface of

the muscle, 8 to 10 cm distal to the pubic tubercle, and followed proximally for a length of 6 cm. The obturator nerve is then identified 2 to 3 cm proximal to the vascular pedicle and similarly traced. The muscle is marked at 1-cm increments so that when it is surgically removed and contracted, the resting length can be estimated. The pedicle, nerve, and muscle belly are then divided, using the gastrointestinal anastomosis stapler for the muscle division, and removed from the surgical bed (29).

A preauricular incision is then made and extended to just below the mandible to identify the facial vessels for microvascular anastomosis. An anterior flap is raised, exposing the zygomatic arch and malar eminence, extending medially to expose the orbicularis oris. The stump of the cross face nerve graft is identified for the neurorrhaphy, in the case of a cross face nerve graft, and the masseteric nerve is identified immediately under the zygomatic arch if it is a one-stage procedure. Some surgeons place a temporary static sling from the zygomatic arch to the corner of the mouth so that the newly transferred muscle will not bear the weight of the face for the initial postoperative period (30). The gracilis muscle is then secured to the modiolus, stretched to its resting tension length as determined by the incremental markings, trimmed to the appropriate length, and secured to the zygomatic arch or temporalis fascia to create the appropriate vector pull (Fig. 38.5). The microvascular anastomoses and

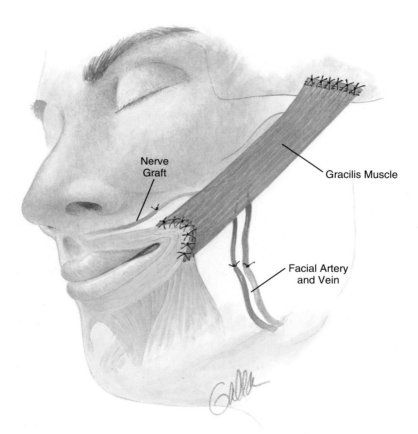

FIG. 38.5 Inset of the gracilis muscle. Note the staple lines at either end of the transferred muscle.

the neurorrhaphy are performed, and the incisions are closed over suction drainage. Chewing is avoided for the first 5 postoperative days.

Alternative free muscle grafts for facial reanimation have been described, including the pectoralis minor, latissimus dorsi, serratus anterior, and abductor hallucis (31–36). The current thrust is to achieve a one-stage reconstruction powered by the contralateral facial nerve (37). This requires a muscle whose nerve supply can be harvested to a length of 15 cm, eliminating the need for a separate cross facial graft. Several pioneers of the initial gracilis transfer now prefer one-stage reconstruction with the latissimus dorsi and its long neural pedicle (30,37). Subjective and objective comparisons of free muscle transfer versus temporalis transfer demonstrate superior excursion in the former but overall poorer aesthetic results based on increased bulk and overlying skin tethering (38). These methods are in a period of rapid evolution, and time will reveal which free muscle transfers yield most optimal long-term facial reanimation results.

STATIC FACIAL REANIMATION PROCEDURES

Some facial paralysis patients are best rehabilitated through static techniques. These include patients who are poor candidates for prolonged general anesthesia for medical reasons, patients with a poor prognosis in whom reanimation over a long time is not appropriate, and dynamic reanimation failures.

Patients with partial recovery following Bell's palsy, Ramsay Hunt syndrome, or other conditions leading to aberrant regeneration are also suitable candidates for static reanimation procedures. Often there is adequate facial movement, and the unsightly facial asymmetry is attributable to hypertonicity, contracture, synkinesis, and subtle cervical and brow positioning abnormalities. These can be addressed via an asymmetric rhytidectomy with unilateral or asymmetric superficial muscular aponeurotic system with possible intraoperative intentional sacrifice of selected branches on the pathologic side to relax an area of hypertonicity. Unilateral brow lift often complements the procedure.

Static procedures can be directed at specific functional and cosmetic issues (19,39) (Figs. 38.6–38.9). For example, nasal obstruction due to nasal valve collapse from dilator nares paralysis can be addressed with standard nasal valve

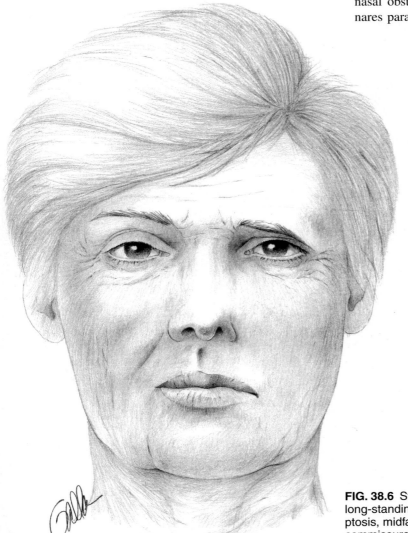

FIG. 38.6 Static technique for facial reanimation. A patient with long-standing left facial paralysis is depicted. Note the brow ptosis, midfacial asymmetry, external nasal valve collapse, and commissure malposition.

repair (Fig. 38.7). If oral incompetence is a significant complaint, lateral lower lip resection (Fig. 38.8) or selective myomectomy may be of benefit; fascia lata slings have been described to improve cosmesis and competence in this area (40). Creation of a nasolabial fold via a two-stitch prolene

suture technique, a modification of the Keller facelift (41), has proven effective as well. Management options for the eye are discussed in detail in a subsequent chapter, though unilateral brow lifting is commonly utilized (Fig. 38.9). Static procedures are also used in conjunction with dynamic re-

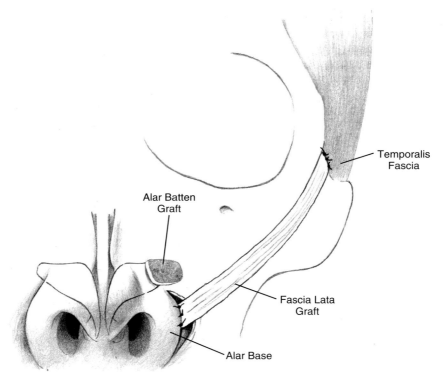

FIG. 38.7 External nasal valve repair via fascia lata sling from alar base to zygoma.

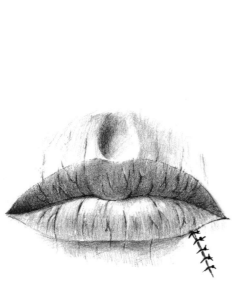

FIG. 38.8 Lower lip wedge resection assists with lower lip competence.

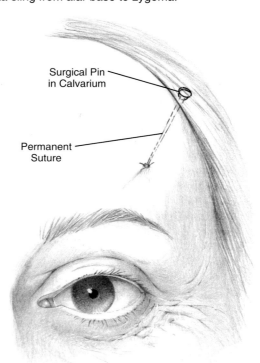

FIG. 38.9 Brow lifting is performed by the placement of a surgical pin in the calvarium and securing of a permanent suture to the pin.

animation techniques as touch-ups or to refine a satisfactory result even further.

SUMMARY

Facial paralysis is a disfiguring and debilitating condition whose management is determined by a large set of clinical variables. A systematic approach to the problem is presented here, employing reinnervation techniques as a first line and muscle transfer for dynamic reanimation as a second line when feasible, reserving static rehabilitation procedures for otherwise poor surgical candidates and those with modest or specific deficits.

Efforts are ongoing to improve or preserve neural function, to evoke better native facial nerve regeneration with nerve grafting techniques, and to optimize static and dynamic transfer for facial expression. The quantification of facial muscle function is another ongoing area of study, so that distinct, measurable changes in function can be recorded following different interventions. Observer-based scales, computer-based image analysis programs, and patient-based outcome surveys will serve as valuable tools in the future to clarify the expected benefit from each of the described interventions.

REFERENCES

1. Gavron JP, Clemis JD. Hypoglossal-facial nerve anastomosis: a review of forty cases caused by facial nerve injuries in the posterior fossa. *Laryngoscope* 1984;94:1447–1450.
2. Conley J. Hypoglossal crossover—122 cases. *Trans Am Acad Ophthalmol Otolaryngol* 1977;84:ORL763–768.
3. Kunihiro T, Kanzaki J, Yoshihara S, et al. Hypoglossal-facial anastomosis after acoustic neuroma resection: influence of the time of anastomosis on recovery of facial movement. *ORL J Otorhinolaryngol Relat Spec* 1996;58:32–35.
4. Stennert E. I. Hypoglossal-facial anastomosis: its significance for modern facial surgery. *Clin Plast Surg* 1979;6:471–486.
5. Conley J, Baker DC. Hypoglossal-facial anastomosis for reinnervation of the paralyzed face. *Plast Reconstr Surg* 1979;63:63–72.
6. May M. Nerve substitution techniques: XII–VII hook-up, XII–VII jump graft, and cross-face graft. In: May M, Schaitkin BM, eds. *The facial nerve, May's second edition.* New York: Thieme, 2000:611–633.
7. Atlas MD, Lowinger DS. A new technique for hypoglossal-facial nerve repair. *Laryngoscope* 1997;107:984–991.
8. Scaramella LF. Cross-face facial nerve anastomosis: historical notes. *Ear Nose Throat J* 1996;75:343–354.
9. Glickman LT, Simpson R. Cross-facial nerve grafting for facial reanimation: effect on normal hemiface movement. *J Reconstr Microsurg* 1996;12:201–202.
10. Fisch U. Facial nerve grafting. *Otolaryngol Clin North Am* 1974;7:517–529.
11. Smith J. A new technique of facial animation. *Transactions of the Fifth International Congress of Plastic Surgery.* Butterworths: Melbourne, Australia, 1971:83.
12. Anderl H. Cross-face nerve grafting—up to 12 months of seventh nerve disruption. In: Rubin LR, ed. *Reanimation of the paralyzed face.* St. Louis: CV Mosby, 1977:241–277.
13. Terzis JK, Kalantarian B. Microsurgical strategies in 74 patients for restoration of dynamic depressor muscle mechanism: a neglected target in facial reanimation. *Plast Reconstr Surg* 2000;105:1917–1934.
14. Ballance C, Duel AD. The operative treatment of facial palsy by the introduction of nerve grafts into the fallopian canal and by other intratemporal methods. *Arch Otolaryngol* 1932;15:1–70.
15. Poe DS, Scher N, Panje WR. Facial reanimation by XI-VII anastomosis without shoulder paralysis. *Laryngoscope* 1989;99:1040–1047.
16. Griebie MS, Huff JS. Selective role of partial XI-VII anastomosis in facial reanimation. *Laryngoscope* 1998;108:1664–1668.
17. Rubin LR, Rubin JP, Simpson RL, et al. Search for the neurocranial pathways to the fifth nerve nucleus in the reanimation of the paralyzed face. *Plast Reconstr Surg* 1999;103:1725–1728.
18. Cheney ML, McKenna MJ, Megerian CA, et al. Early temporalis muscle transposition for the management of facial paralysis. *Laryngoscope* 1995;105:993–1000.
19. Cheney ML, Megerian CA, McKenna MJ. Rehabilitation of the paralyzed face. In: Cheney ML, ed. *Facial surgery: plastic and reconstructive.* Baltimore: Williams & Wilkins, 1997:655–694.
20. Rubin L. *Reanimation of the paralyzed face.* St. Louis: CV Mosby, 1977.
21. Baker DC, Conley J. Regional muscle transposition for rehabilitation of the paralyzed face. *Clin Plast Surg* 1979;6:317–331.
22. Maegawa J, Saijo M, Murasawa S. Muscle bow traction method for dynamic facial reanimation. *Ann Plast Surg* 1999;43:354–358.
23. Aszmann OC, Ebmer JM, Dellon AL. The anatomic basis for the innervated mylohyoid/digastric flap in facial reanimation. *Plast Reconstr Surg* 1998;102:369–372.
24. Fine NA, Pribaz JJ, Orgill DP. Use of the innervated platysma flap in facial reanimation. *Ann Plast Surg* 1995;34:326–330.
25. Carr MM, Ross DD, Zuker RM. Cranial nerve defects in congenital facial palsy. *J Otolaryngol* 1997;26:80–87.
26. Harii K, Ohmori K, Torii S. Free gracilis muscle transplantation, with microneurovascular anastomoses for the treatment of facial paralysis. A preliminary report. *Plast Reconstr Surg* 1976;57:133–143.
27. Manktelow RT, Zuker RM. Muscle transplantation by fascicular territory. *Plast Reconstr Surg* 1984;73:751–757.
28. Zuker RM, Manktelow RT. A smile for the Moebius syndrome patient. *Ann Plast Surg* 1989;22:188–194.
29. Sullivan M, Urken M. Gracilis. In: Urken M, Cheney M, Sullivan M, et al, eds. *Atlas of regional and free flaps for head and neck reconstruction.* New York: Raven Press, 1995:139–148.
30. Swartz WM. Free muscle transfers for facial paralysis. In: May M, Schaitkin BM, eds. *The facial nerve, May's second edition.* New York: Thieme, 2000:667–676.
31. Harrison DH. The pectoralis minor vascularized muscle graft for the treatment of unilateral facial palsy. *Plast Reconstr Surg* 1985;75:206–216.
32. Dellon AL, MacKinnon SE. Segmentally innervated latissimus dorsi muscle. Microsurgical transfer for facial reanimation. *J Reconstr Microsurg* 1985;2:7–12.
33. Terzis JK. Pectoralis minor: a unique muscle for correction of facial paralysis. *Plast Reconstr Surg* 1989;83:767–776.
34. Harrison DH. Current trends in the treatment of established unilateral facial palsy. *Ann R Coll Surg Engl* 1990;72:94–98.
35. Jiang H, Guo ET, Ji ZL, et al. One-stage microvascular free abductor hallucis muscle transplantation for reanimation of facial paralysis. *Plast Reconstr Surg* 1995;96:78–85.
36. Bartlet S. Technical refinements in the use of the serratus anterior for reanimation of the paralyzed face. Presented at the Northeastern Society of Plastic Surgeons, Oct. 12, 1996, Washington D.C.
37. Harii K, Asato H, Yoshimura K, et al. One-stage transfer of the latissimus dorsi muscle for reanimation of a paralyzed face: a new alternative. *Plast Reconstr Surg* 1998;102:941–951.
38. Erni D, Lieger O, Banic A. Comparative objective and subjective analysis of temporalis tendon and microneurovascular transfer for facial reanimation. *Br J Plast Surg* 1999;52:167–172.
39. May M. Regional reanimation: nose and mouth. In: May M, Schaitkin BM, eds. *The facial nerve, May's second edition.* New York: Thieme, 2000:775–795.
40. Spector GJ, Matsuba HM, Killeen TE, et al. Fascial pulley: cross-commissure lip reanimation for inferior division facial nerve paralysis. *Laryngoscope* 1986;96:102–105.
41. Keller GS, Namazie A, Blackwell K, et al. Elevation of the malar fat pad with a percutaneous technique. *Arch Facial Plast Surg* 2002;4:20–25.

CHAPTER 39

Oculoplastic Considerations and Management of Facial Paralysis

Aaron Fay and Peter A.D. Rubin

CAUSES OF FACIAL NERVE DYSFUNCTION

Facial nerve dysfunction may result from infection, inflammation, neoplasm, accidental trauma, or surgery. Each may produce concomitant intraocular disease, which should be excluded in all cases. Ocular surface involvement, however, is closely related to severity and duration of the facial paralysis. Inflammatory conditions, which tend to improve over weeks to months, may be best treated medically and with reversible surgeries. Conversely, permanent facial paralysis resulting from facial nerve transection may require eyelid and lacrimal reconstruction and intensive replacement of aqueous tears. It is therefore imperative to investigate the viability of facial nerve rehabilitation at the time of injury or paralysis. In cases of surgical injury to the facial nerve, it is important to observe intraoperative clues of rehabilitation potential. Intraoperative or postoperative facial nerve stimulation may be of prognostic value in selected cases (Chapters 6, 7, and 35). This chapter will focus primarily on evaluation and treatment alternatives of periocular reconstruction in cases of surgical facial nerve injury.

PERTINENT OPHTHALMIC ANATOMY

Eyelids and Lacrimal Apparatus

An understanding of eyelid and periocular anatomy is essential in evaluating neurologic and myogenic eyelid function and lacrimal secretion (Fig. 39.1). Eyelid anatomy is commonly described in distinct anterior and posterior lamellae. The anterior lamella comprises the skin and pretarsal and preseptal components of the orbicularis oculi; the posterior lamella contains tarsus, the collagenous structural element of the eyelid, and the palpebral conjunctiva. Within the tarsus are meibomian glands, sebaceous glands whose ducts open along the posterior lid margin. Additional sebaceous glands (Zeis) are associated with individual cilia along the anterior lid margin. The anterior and posterior lamellae adjoin along the lid margin to form the visible gray line (Fig. 39.2).

Eyelid elevation and depression are coordinated through a complex neurologic loop that is the critical element in modern surgical approaches to eyelid paralysis (Fig. 39.3). Elevation is produced primarily by stimulation of the levator palpebrae superioris, which is innervated by the superior division of the oculomotor nerve. Eyelid elevation can also be achieved by adjunctive contracture of the ipsilateral frontalis, stimulated by the temporal branch of the facial nerve. Conversely, eyelid closure is produced exclusively by the orbicularis oculi, which is innervated by the temporal and zygomatic branches of the facial nerve. The orbital portion of the orbicularis is under voluntary control and produces forced eyelid closure (wink), whereas the palpebral components (pretarsal and preseptal) produce involuntary reflex closure (blink) (Fig. 39.4). Under physiologic conditions, reflex closure and baseline lacrimation protect the ocular surface from environmental pathogens, debris, and trauma. This spontaneous blinking occurs at a rate of approximately 20 to 30 blinks per minute and increases with age, whereas blink amplitudes range from 25 to 38 degrees and decrease with age. Both are age dependent. Additional reflex closure may be stimulated by bright light (light-blink reflex), exhaustion, photophobia (pain produced by bright light), or the corneal reflex.

Lacrimation is intimately related to eyelid function. The normal tear film comprises three layers: mucinous, aqueous, and lipid. The posterior mucinous layer derives from conjunctival goblet cells, whereas the anterior lipid layer is produced by meibomian glands. Greater than 98% of tear volume, however, is aqueous and derives from both primary and accessory lacrimal glands. Basal secretion is produced by the accessory lacrimal glands of Krause and Wolfring located within the eyelids and conjunctival fornices. The primary lacrimal gland is responsible for reflex tearing and receives autonomic innervation from parasympathetic fibers that travel first with the facial nerve and then with the maxillary division of the trigeminal nerve. Proper lacrimation provides eyelid lubrication and nutrients to the anterior corneal

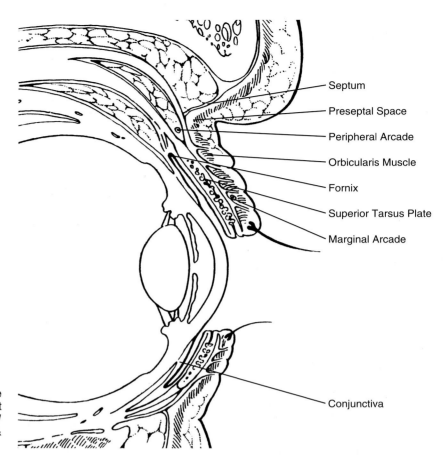

Septum

Preseptal Space

Peripheral Arcade

Orbicularis Muscle

Fornix

Superior Tarsus Plate

Marginal Arcade

Conjunctiva

FIG. 39.1 Cross-sectional anatomy of the eyelids. (From Janfaza P, Nadol JB, Galla R, et al, eds. *Surgical anatomy of the head and neck.* Philadelphia: Lippincott Williams & Wilkins, 2001:169, with permission.)

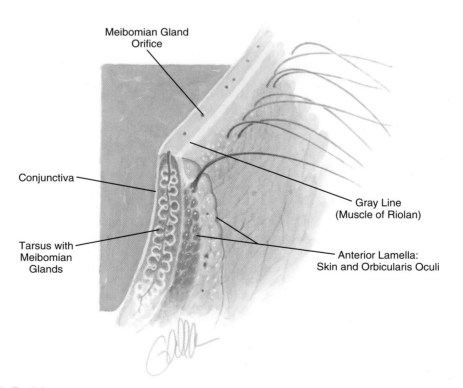

Meibomian Gland Orifice

Conjunctiva

Tarsus with Meibomian Glands

Gray Line (Muscle of Riolan)

Anterior Lamella: Skin and Orbicularis Oculi

FIG. 39.2 Eyelid margin demonstrating distinct posterior and anterior lamellae with intervening gray line (muscle of Riolan).

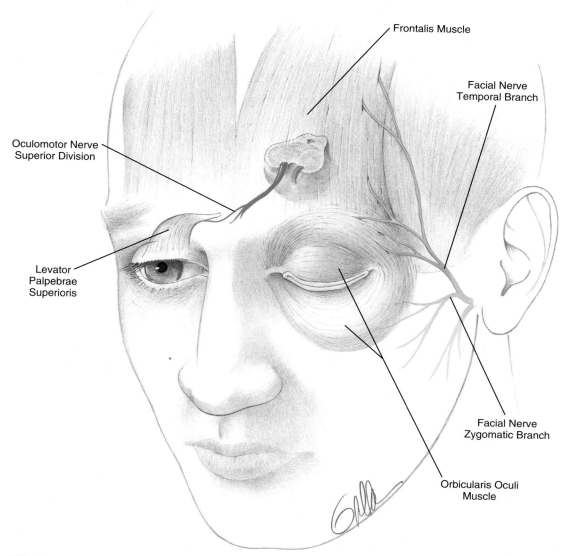

FIG. 39.3 Innervation of the primary eyelid elevators and depressors. The levator palpebrae superioris is innervated by the superior division of the oculomotor nerve, whereas the orbicularis oculi is innervated by the facial nerve.

stroma and epithelium. Tears contain antimicrobial properties (IgA) and serve as the primary refracting surface for the visual system. Once tears are produced, proper eyelid tone and function are required for normal lacrimal drainage.

The tear pump is a physiologic mechanism that sweeps new tears across the ocular surface in a superotemporal to inferonasal direction and assists in drainage through the canaliculi and lacrimal sac. Although the precise mechanism has been debated, the medial heads of the orbicularis oculi (Horner's muscle) encircle the lacrimal sac, producing rhythmic contracture of the sac and a pressure phenomenon that draws the tear lake into the lacrimal puncta while forcing tears into the nasolacrimal duct. Insufficient palpebral tone or function is a common cause of epiphora.

Lower eyelid tone and position rely on facial nerve integrity to mitigate gravitational forces. Orbicularis paresis therefore produces lower lid laxity and frank ectropion, as well as epiphora from lacrimal pump dysfunction. Paradoxically, entropion can also occur as the lax lower eyelid is dislodged from its native apposition to the globe and freely everts or inverts. Entropion produces foreign body sensation, superficial corneal injury, and secondary epiphora.

Cornea

The cornea is approximately 500 microns thick and comprises five distinct layers. The corneal epithelium is a single cell layer that derives its nutrition from the tear film. The ep-

476 / CHAPTER 39

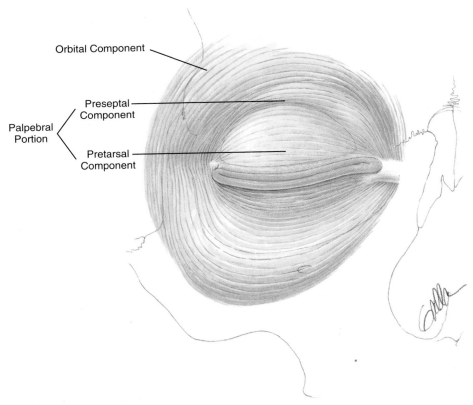

FIG. 39.4 The three segments of the orbicularis oculi. The involuntary blink is produced by the palpebral portions of the muscle, whereas the voluntary wink is produced by the orbital component.

ithelium serves as a primary barrier to microbial infection. Deep to the epithelial basement membrane, Bowman's layer is the anterior condensation of the corneal stroma. Bowman's layer provides a barrier to neoplastic invasion. The corneal stroma consists of highly organized collagen lamellae and keratocytes with intervening terminal trigeminal nerve fibers. Descemet's membrane is the basement membrane of the corneal endothelium, the posterior layer responsible for the continual dehydration that preserves corneal transparency. Corneal perforation produced by severe corneal drying or infection may lead to endophthalmitis and intraocular abscess formation (Fig. 39.5).

Corneal sensation is an important indicator of corneal epithelial vitality and may be critical in maintaining a suitable environment for ocular survival. Corneal sensation is carried by the nasociliary branch of the maxillary division of the trigeminal nerve. In addition to corneal sensation, these trigeminal fibers provide neurotrophic influence to the corneal epithelium. Denervated corneas with epithelial defects heal poorly and may develop neurotrophic ulcers, placing the eye at risk for bacterial infection, perforation, endophthalmitis, and blindness. Furthermore, denervated corneas are at increased risk of trauma due to loss of the corneal blink reflex. When compounded by incomplete eyelid closure, the cornea is extremely vulnerable. In the setting

of corneal denervation, therefore, appropriate eyelid reconstruction is critical, usually requiring tarsorrhaphy.

Corneal exposure may be produced by limited upper eyelid excursion or by lower eyelid retraction. In either situation, pain, foreign body sensation, or tearing may be the initial symptom. Risk of infection is increased by mechanical and chemical deficiencies; perforation, endophthalmitis, and loss of the eye are possible.

OPHTHALMIC EXAMINATION

A full ophthalmic examination is desirable in cases of compromised eyelid or lacrimal function. Many patients, however, may not be ambulatory following head and neck surgery or head trauma. In these cases an abbreviated bedside consultation may suffice as a preliminary screening.

Visual acuity may be recorded as a Snellen equivalent using a near card. It is important to have the patient use his or her reading glasses or to provide an estimated reading spectacle correction in patients nearing presbyopia (+3.00 lenses usually suffice). Visual acuity in the range of 20/40 may be acceptable during bedside examination given the lack of proper lighting, rudimentary testing material, estimated spectacle correction, and likelihood of corneal surface abnormality. Lubricating or antibiotic ointments often

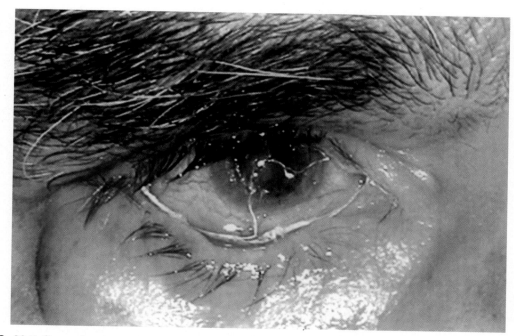

FIG. 39.5 Corneal exposure, drying, and epithelial breakdown place this eye at risk of ulceration and perforation. Note the accompanying paralytic ectropion.

limit visual acuity testing in this setting. The pupils should be examined for relative afferent defects. Extraocular motility should be examined to exclude oculomotor, trochlear, and abducens nerve involvement. A cursory examination of cranial nerves V, VII, and VIII should be performed.

External examination may reveal important indications for particular methods of treatment in cases of facial palsy. Brow position and symmetry, as well as frontalis function, should be noted. Eyelid position should be observed with the patient in both upright and supine positions. Eyelid measurements are typically taken in the upright position. Palpebral fissure height, margin reflex distance, and levator palpebrae superioris function are the cardinal measurements for upper eyelid position and function (Fig. 39.6). Orbicularis tone may be estimated on a scale of one to four. Lower lid ectropion may not be obvious in all cases. Slight punctal ectropion in which the medial lower lid rests away from the globe can produce epiphora and chronic irritation. A prolonged snap-back test may suggest impending ectropion.

When observing eyelid positions, globe protective mechanisms should be evaluated. Lagophthalmos, described in millimeters, measures the height of the palpebral fissure in the closed (resting) position (Fig. 39.7). Bell's phenomenon, or upward deviation of the globe with eyelid closure, should be noted. A fine cotton filament applied to the cornea may be used to test corneal sensation.

Tear production is typically estimated with Schirmer tests. After applying topical anesthetic to the conjunctival cul-de-sac, the tear lake is absorbed and paper test strips are lodged between the lower eyelid and globe (Fig. 39.8). The amount of wetting is measured in millimeters. Schirmer testing measures only the amount of *aqueous* production; mucinous- or lipid-deficient states producing dry eye syndrome may be present despite normal Schirmer tests.

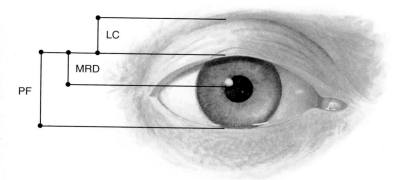

FIG. 39.6 Cardinal measurements of upper eyelid in the resting position. These are taken with the patient seated upright. LC, lid crease height; MRD, margin-reflex distance; PF, palpebral fissure height.

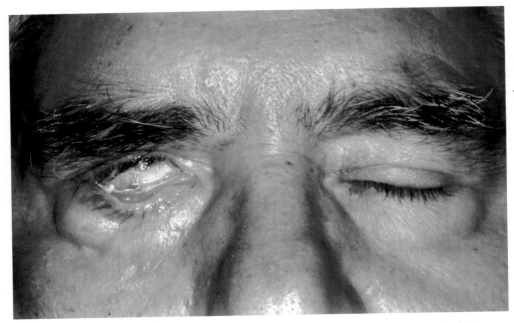

FIG. 39.7 Lagophthalmos. The right upper lid fails to cover the eye during attempted closure.

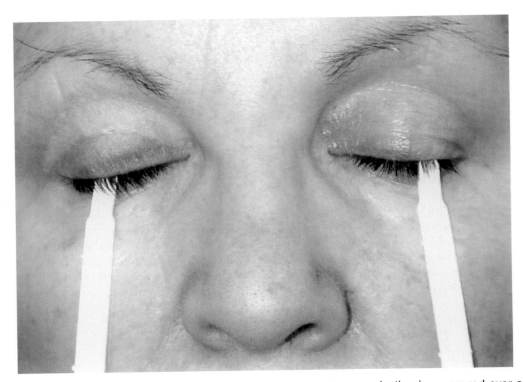

FIG. 39.8 Schirmer testing of the anesthetized eyes. Aqueous tear production is measured over a 5-minute interval.

The anterior segment of the eye may be evaluated with a penlight. The conjunctiva is examined for hyperemia or discharge. The cornea is examined for opacities, neovascularization, focal dry spots with or without thinning (dellen), sensation, and epithelial vitality. After instilling fluorescein solution into the conjunctival fornices, illuminating the cornea with a blue-filtered light may reveal areas of fluorescein staining that correspond to deepithelialized regions. Corneal innervation should be tested before instilling fluorescein solution because the latter may contain anesthetic.

The retinal red reflex can be noted through dilated pupils with a penlight or through undilated pupils with a direct ophthalmoscope held at arm's length from the patient's face. Dilated fundus examination may not be necessary during initial screening.

MANAGEMENT

An array of management alternatives exists for patients with facial paralysis. Management depends primarily on corneal involvement and the likelihood of neuromuscular recovery. Additionally, mental status, overall medical condition, age, and patient motivation must be considered. A comatose or otherwise supine patient will not benefit from gold weight implantation and may indeed experience increased lagoph-

thalmos. These patients are suitable candidates for early tarsorrhaphy (temporary or permanent); it may be reasonable to perform this procedure at the time of initial surgery. Conservative initial management is often more reasonable for alert patients, and an algorithm of interventional possibilities may be useful (Fig. 39.9). More aggressive, albeit reversible intervention, however, may spare the patient discomfort and laborious self-maintenance. In the presence of corneal hypoesthesia, primary surgical intervention is advocated. A more aggressive approach is also advocated in cases of unlikely facial nerve recovery. Although a variety of methods exist to reconstruct periocular anatomy in this setting, only the most common procedures are discussed here in detail. Extensive explanations of other procedures may be found in standard textbooks of oculoplastic surgery.

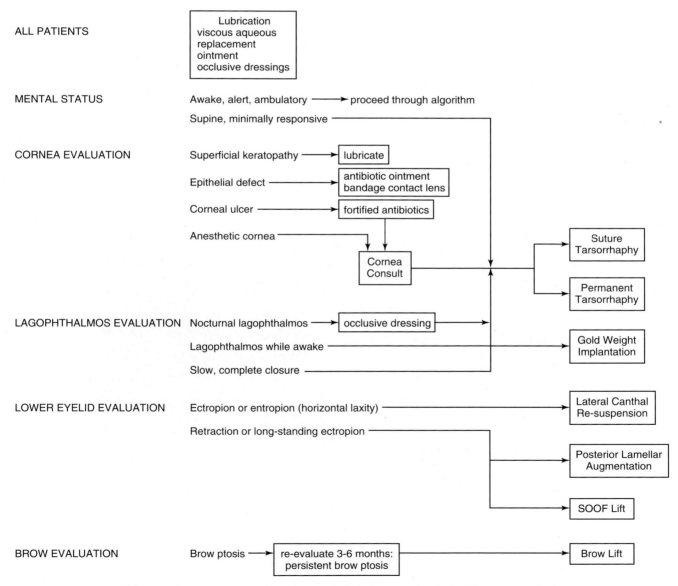

FIG. 39.9 A proposed algorithm for ophthalmic intervention in facial nerve paralysis.

Temporizing Treatments

The goal of temporizing treatments is to ensure corneal hydration until a definitive plan can be implemented. Lacrimal adjuvants are supplied as both drops and ointments. Lubricant drop formulations range from near normal saline to viscous electrolyte solutions. Drops may be applied as frequently as every hour while awake or as infrequently as every 4 hours. Patients with a personal history of chemical sensitivity are advised to use preservative-free artificial tears. These are supplied in single dose vials and must be disposed of after use to avoid bacterial contamination. Patients who develop conjunctivitis after starting artificial tears may benefit from nonpreserved formulations.

Lacrimal ointments provide longer relief from corneal drying but inherently impair vision. They may be somewhat messy, leading to patient noncompliance, and are best used before bedtime. When risk of bacterial infection is increased, such as in inpatient populations, in those with severe blepharitis and poor personal hygiene, or in patients with severe aqueous deficiency, antibiotic ointment such as erythromycin or bacitracin ophthalmic ointments may be substituted.

Other attempts to maintain moisture may be directed toward lacrimal preservation. Punctal occlusion plugs may be placed into the lacrimal puncta at the bedside (Fig. 39.10). These silicone stoppers are inserted into the punctum and are held in place by the punctal sphincter. They may be removed in the event that foreign body sensation develops (rare) or when normal lacrimation is restored. Less common methods of lacrimal preservation include modified specta-

cles (monocular goggle) to prevent ocular cross winds and moisture chambers that can be fitted to the orbital rim with cutaneous adhesive. Patients using the former should be cautioned about the possible loss of peripheral vision. Nonambulatory patients may be best suited for moisture chambers. Ambient humidifiers may be useful in some settings.

Temporary eyelid closure is often required in the acute setting. Closure may be most rapidly achieved by taping the eyelid closed directly. Tegaderm transparent adhesives are often most comfortable. Elderly patients or others with delicate eyelid skin may develop eyelid abrasions or otherwise poorly tolerate tape. In these cases, a pressure bandage may be useful. Two eye pads may be stacked over the closed eyelid while instructing the patient to close the eyelids as forcefully as possible. One-inch-wide tape may then be applied from the central forehead to the zygomatic arch while pulling the buccal fat pad toward the eye. In the relaxed position, pressure is created beneath the bandage. To facilitate frequent examinations, it may be helpful to place a 2-inch segment of tape on the forehead and another along the zygomatic arch that can be left in place for several days to serve as a platform for the bandage.

Medical closure of the eyelids can be achieved using botulinum toxin injections to induce blepharoptosis. Resolution of ptosis can be anticipated in 2 to 4 months. The treatment may be mitigated by further compromise of any residual orbicularis function and is not routinely employed as a treatment for lagophthalmos.

Temporary surgical procedures may often be performed at the bedside. A variety of suture tarsorrhaphy techniques have been described. These temporary sutures are used to

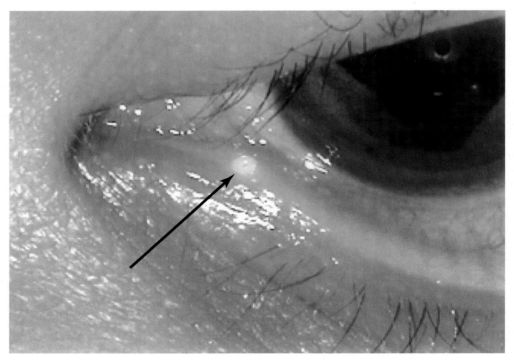

FIG. 39.10 Silicone plug positioned within the lacrimal punctum is used to impede tear outflow.

close the eyelids for a period of days to weeks. The tarsorrhaphy may be placed laterally to permit greater use of the involved eye or centrally to provide greater corneal coverage. In either case, a window is provided for daily corneal examination that may require the patient to gaze in one direction or the other to bring the cornea into view. One method of suture tarsorrhaphy is described next (Fig. 39.11).

Both arms of a double-armed 5-0 nylon suture on a spatulated needle are passed through a previously fashioned sponge or rubber bolster measuring approximately 3 × 5 mm. The first needle enters the skin approximately 4 mm inferior to the lower eyelid margin and exits through the gray line of the lower eyelid. Care must be taken to avoid the posterior lid margin, as any suture approaching this landmark is likely to rub against the cornea while the eye is closed. The needle then enters the gray line of the upper eyelid margin and exits approximately 4 mm superior to the superior lid margin. The second arm is passed in identical fashion parallel to the first. Both arms are passed through a second bolster, the lids are brought into contact, and the suture is knotted. Some authors advocate the use of a 4-0 proline suture passed in serpentine fashion through the eyelid margins. This may produce hematoma formation or cheese-wiring through the lid margin and is generally less reproducible than a bolstered tarsorrhaphy.

Lower lid ectropion may be temporized using ointments, though eyedrops tend not to be effective in these cases. A thin strip of tape can be used to redrape the lower lid in a superotemporal direction. Quarter-inch Steri-Strips are often suitable for this application. Suture tarsorrhaphy may also alleviate lower lid ectropion temporarily.

Permanent Treatments

A permanent tarsorrhaphy is most commonly placed laterally, though medial tarsorrhaphies are created in cases of medial canthal dehiscence and medial exposure. Permanent

tarsorrhaphies are not commonly placed centrally because this essentially negates any potential vision in the involved eye. Surgical tarsorrhaphies are most commonly performed as irreversible procedures utilizing the principle of tarsal transposition. In selected cases, however, the anterior lamella and eyelashes may be spared, creating a "permanent reversible" lateral tarsorrhaphy. In either case, the goal of the surgical tarsorrhaphy is to create a permanent adhesion between the upper and lower eyelid margin, thereby decreasing the horizontal dimension of the palpebral fissure (Fig. 39.12). Surgical tarsorrhaphies have the advantage of requiring no additional personal hygiene, dressing changes, or medications.

The location and length of surgical tarsorrhaphy are determined preoperatively. A surgical marking pen is used to mark the horizontal limits of the intended tarsorrhaphy. Two percent lidocaine with epinephrine 1:100,000 on a 25- to 30-gauge syringe is used to anesthetize the region. The surgical field is sterilized, and a protective corneoscleral shell is used to cover the globe. A no. 15 surgical blade is used to divide the upper and lower eyelids along the respective gray lines, separating the anterior from the posterior lamellae in the region of desired adhesion. Blunt and sharp dissection in the pretarsal plane are carried approximately 3 mm superior and inferior to the lid margins. The dissection should be kept immediately pretarsal to avoid injury to the lash follicles. The superior and inferior tarsal margins are deepithelialized using Westcott scissors. Partial-thickness tarsal sutures are preplaced using 5-0 polyglactin sutures to appose the tarsal margins. Care must be taken to avoid full-thickness passes onto the posterior tarsal surface. (Patients with ongoing cicatricial processes, or others requiring unusually strong tarsal adhesions, may benefit from a tongue-in-groove construction. Relaxing incisions are created in the superior tarsus perpendicular to the lid margin approximately 3 mm in height. The epithelium is removed from the posterior surface

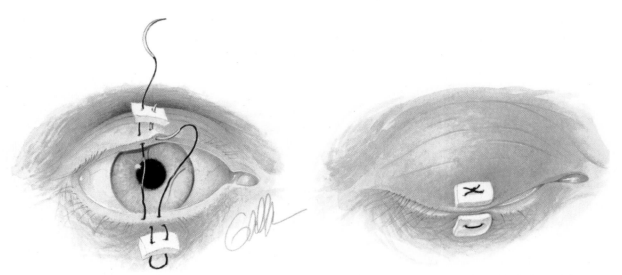

FIG. 39.11 One technique of temporary suture tarsorrhaphy. Care is taken to avoid contact between the sutures and the corneal epithelium.

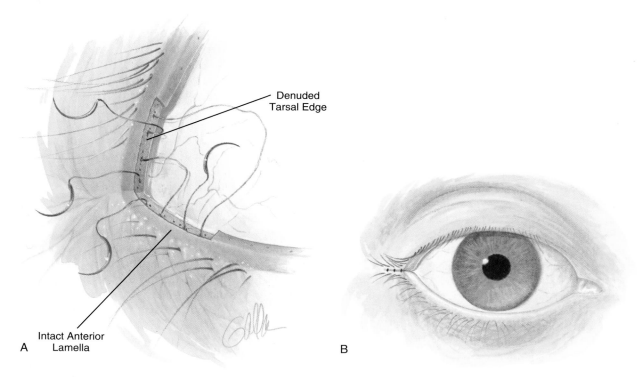

FIG. 39.12 Permanent "reversible" lateral tarsorrhaphy. **A:** Preplaced mattress sutures are placed along exposed tarsal edge. **B:** Anterior lamella, including lashes, remain intact.

in this area using a no. 15 blade. A 5-0 polyglactin mattress suture is passed through the end of this tarsal "tongue." Additional pretarsal dissection is performed inferiorly, creating a "groove" for acceptance of the tarsal advancement. Both arms of the suture are passed into the pretarsal pocket and brought through the skin of the upper lid, where they are tied over a sponge bolster.) Orbicularis may be closed in a separate layer using interrupted 6-0 polyglactin sutures. The skin

is closed with 6-0 fast-absorbing plain gut sutures with sparing of the cilia.

Dynamic methods of surgical eyelid closure may more closely approximate physiologic reconstruction. These procedures may be best suited for ambulatory patients who are capable of maintaining a strict regimen of nightly lubrication. The most common method of orbicularis function augmentation is gold weight insertion (Fig. 39.13). This proce-

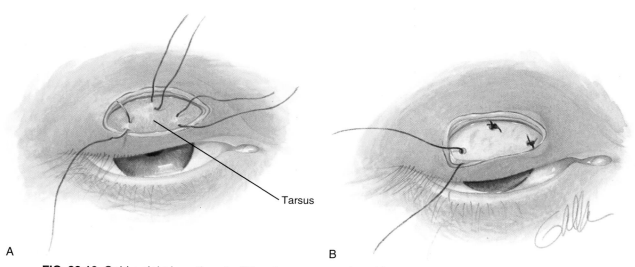

FIG. 39.13 Gold weight insertion. **A:** Silk sutures are preplaced in tarsus. **B:** The weight is immobilized with tarsal fixation, and the orbicularis and skin are meticulously closed in separate layers.

dure is most commonly used to address long-term facial palsy but is easily reversible and is therefore equally suitable for intermediate-term use. A contoured gold implant of between 0.6 and 1.4 g (most commonly 1.2 g) is anchored to the upper eyelid tarsus, producing gravity-dependent eyelid closure. Patients with normal oculomotor function do not experience impaired eyelid elevation with a properly sized gold weight implant.

During preoperative examination, cutaneous adhesive is applied to the upper eyelid skin. Test weights are applied to the external surface. The properly sized weight eliminates lagophthalmos while avoiding mechanical ptosis. After sterile preparation or the eyelid, a protective corneoscleral shell is placed over the globe. A surgical marking pen is used to delineate a 10-mm surgical incision along the primary eyelid crease, or approximately 8 to 10 mm superior to the central eyelid margin. The area is anesthetized with lidocaine 2% with epinephrine 1:100,000. The cutaneous incision is made

with a scalpel, and the anterior tarsal surface is exposed using fine surgical scissors. The implant is laid over the tarsus, and electrical or thermal cautery is used as a marking device to cauterize the tarsus through the eyelets in the implant. The implant is removed, and three 6-0 polyglactin partial thickness interrupted sutures are preplaced into tarsus. The lid is everted to confirm partial thickness placement. The implant is again placed into the host site, and the sutures are knotted. The skin is closed with interrupted 6-0 nylon sutures. The protective corneoscleral shell is removed, and the wound is dressed with ophthalmic antibiotic ointment. Other less commonly performed orbicularis augmentation procedures include Silastic prostheses and an intrapalpebral spring. Both are gravity-independent mechanical methods of facilitating eyelid closure in patients who presumably demonstrate normal levator function.

Definitive correction of paralytic ectropion requires reconstruction of the inferior crus of the lateral canthal tendon. This is best accomplished through the lateral tarsal strip procedure (Fig. 39.14). Long-standing ectropion may be accompanied by lower eyelid retraction, a condition that usually requires an interpositional graft to augment the height of the posterior lamella. Graft materials include autologous

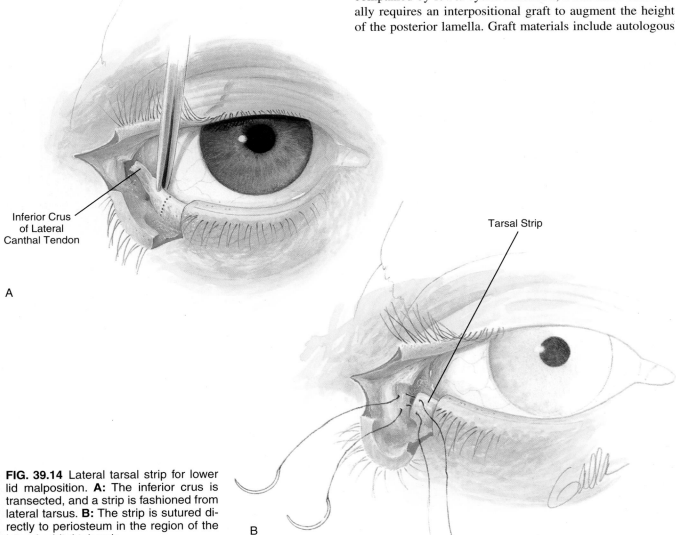

Inferior Crus
of Lateral
Canthal Tendon

A

Tarsal Strip

B

FIG. 39.14 Lateral tarsal strip for lower lid malposition. **A:** The inferior crus is transected, and a strip is fashioned from lateral tarsus. **B:** The strip is sutured directly to periosteum in the region of the lateral orbital tubercle.

cartilage or hard palate mucosa, donor sclera or acellular dermis, or alloplastic compounds. The more common tarsal strip procedure is described here.

The lateral portion of the upper and lower eyelids as well as the lateral orbital rim are anesthetized with 2% lidocaine with epinephrine 1:100,000. The surgical field is sterilized, and a protective corneoscleral shell is placed over the globe. Initially, a lateral canthotomy and cantholysis is performed: a scalpel is used to make a 5 mm skin incision extending laterally from the lateral commissure. Pointed surgical scissors are used to complete the full-thickness canthotomy along the skin incision. Orbicularis is incised to reveal the lateral orbital rim. Anterior traction is placed on the lateral cut edge of the lower lid while pointed surgical scissors are used first to palpate and then to transect the inferior crus of the lateral canthal tendon. This is best accomplished with the scissor tips directed toward the tip of the nose while the handle overlies the lateral orbital rim. The lateral lid should be completely released, and no tethering should remain.

The procedure continues with creation of the tarsal strip: A skin-muscle flap is raised from the anterior tarsal surface over the lateral lower lid. The cut edge of tarsus is pulled laterally to determine the degree of laxity, and a nick is created in the lid margin to delineate the medial limit of the tarsal dissection. A thin strip of epithelium is excised from the lid margin laterally. The posterior lamella is then transected along the inferior tarsal border, thereby creating the tarsal strip. The tarsus is draped over a cotton-tipped applicator, and the posterior surface is denuded using the scalpel.

Suturing of Tarsal Strip and Canthoplasty

Both arms of a 4-0 permanent suture mounted on heavy, tightly curved needles (Polydek, P2 needle) are passed through the base of the newly fashioned tarsal strip in a posterior to anterior orientation, dividing the height of the strip into three equal parts. A Blair retractor (skin rake) is used to retract the skin and orbicularis superotemporally away from the lateral orbital rim. A malleable retractor is used to retract the globe and orbital contents medially, exposing the inner surface of the lateral orbital rim. Both arms of the suture are brought through the periosteum in the region of the lateral orbital tubercle. The sutures should be placed 2 to 3 mm superior to the level of the medial canthus. The ends of the suture are left long. A 2- to 3-mm section is excised from the lateral superior eyelid margin, and a redundant triangle of skin is excised from the lateral lower lid. A 6-0 polyglactin suture is used in buried fashion to recreate the lateral commissure by passing through the cut edge of both lid margins. The protective corneoscleral shell is removed, and the tarsal suture is tied. The orbicularis is closed with two buried, interrupted 6-0 polyglactin sutures, and the skin may be closed with 6-0 nylon interrupted sutures. The wound is dressed with ophthalmic antibiotic ointment.

Brow ptosis correction is best delayed for several months following eyelid reconstruction in paralytic cases. Even minimal elevation of the brow can contribute to recurrent lagophthalmos and may mitigate previous reconstructive and medical interventions. After eyelid and lacrimal normalization have been achieved, brow ptosis may be addressed through direct or endoscopic surgical techniques.

REFERENCES

1. Morel-Fatio D, LaLardrie JP. Palliative surgical treatment of facial paralysis. The palpebral spring. *Plast Reconstr Surg* 1964;33:446–456.
2. Arion HG. Dynamic closure of the lids in paralysis of the orbicularis muscle. *Int Surg* 1972;57:48–50.
3. Beard C. Canthoplasty and brow elevation for facial palsy. *Arch Ophthalmol* 1964;71:386–388.
4. Smellie GD. Restoration of the blinking reflex in facial palsy by a simple lid-load operation. *Br J Plast Surg* 1966;19(3):279–283.
5. Sun WS, Baker RS, Chuke JC, et al. Age-related changes in human blinks. Passive and active changes in eyelid kinematics. *Invest Ophthalmol Vis Sci* 1997;38(1):92–99.

PART IX

Surgery for Tumors
of the Temporal Bone

CHAPTER 40

Management of Malignancies of the Ear

Michael J. McKenna and Hinrich Staecker

Malignant tumors of the temporal bone are among the most challenging and difficult clinical problems encountered by otolaryngologists. Although a variety of malignant tumors may develop within or metastasize to the temporal bone, most tumors in this area are squamous cell carcinomas (1–3). Because these tumors often arise in the setting of chronic infection of the ear canal or tympanomastoid cavity, diagnosis is often delayed until the development of progressive symptoms, which unfortunately correspond with advanced disease and poor prognosis (4–10). The new onset of pain in the face of chronic infection should immediately raise suspicion of an underlying malignancy. Other risk factors for the development of carcinoma of the temporal bone include a history of prior radiation therapy (11,12).

The most common and readily treatable malignancies of the ear are those involving the auricle and include basal cell carcinoma, squamous cell carcinoma, and malignant melanoma. The risks of developing a cutaneous malignancy of the auricle are the same as for other cutaneous sites and are related to ultraviolet radiation and an underlying hereditary predisposition. The principles of management are also the same, requiring local excision with frozen section control of all margins. If managed properly, the cure rate for squamous cell carcinoma and basal cell carcinoma of the auricle exceeds 95%. The cure rate for malignant melanoma is significantly less, because this tumor tends to metastasize at an early stage. One of the greatest challenges in management of these lesions is often related to the auricular repair following excision (5–7,13) (Chapter 46).

Malignant lesions in the pediatric population are usually of mesenchymal origin and include rhabdomyosarcoma, neuroblastoma, and histiocytosis (disorders of Langerhans cells). The treatment varies significantly from the epithelial lesions encountered in adults. The primary treatment modalities usually include chemotherapy and radiation therapy, with surgery reserved for biopsy and occasionally for salvage if chemotherapy and radiation therapy fail to control the disease.

Primary malignant lesions of the middle ear and temporal bone in the adult population are almost always of epithelial origin and most commonly are derived from squamous epithelium. However, other epithelial malignancies do occur and include adenocarcinoma and adenoid cystic carcinoma (14–17). Although the management is fundamentally the same, it is important to keep in mind that lesions of adenoid cystic carcinoma may appear deceptively small based on clinical exam and imaging studies. It is not uncommon for these lesions to extend microscopically far beyond their site of origin and beyond the scope of the planned surgical resection.

EVALUATION AND STAGING OF MALIGNANT LESIONS OF THE EXTERNAL AUDITORY CANAL AND TEMPORAL BONE

Numerous staging systems have been proposed for the staging of malignant tumors of the temporal bone (3,5,7–10, 14,16,18–20). Most of these staging systems are based on the location and the degree of extension, which correlates with long-term survival. As more of the temporal bone is involved, the surgical complexities increase and the chance for cure decreases. Figure 40.1 represents a mid-modiolar view of the temporal bone outlining surgical limits for progressively more extensive lesions. In general, lesions can be divided into four categories: (i) Lesions located solely within the external canal can be successfully managed with surgical resection without postoperative radiation, with cure rates of approximately 90%. (ii) Lesions that involve the middle ear cavity and are found to be confined to the middle ear and external auditory canal at surgery are best managed by surgical resection followed by postoperative radiation therapy. Cure rates for these tumors are approximately 50% to 60%. (iii) Lesions of the external auditory canal and tympanomastoid cavity that demonstrate significant bone erosion are best managed by wide surgical resection with postoperative radiation therapy, with cure rates in the range of 20% to 30%. (iv) Lesions that extend beyond the confines of the external canal and middle ear with involvement of the parotid, temporomandibular joint, jugular vein, carotid artery, facial nerve, and labyrinth have a poor prognosis even with surgi-

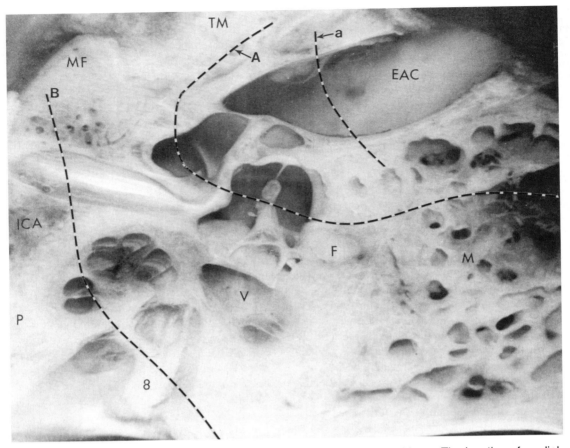

FIG. 40.1 Mid-modiolar horizontal view of a celloidin-embedded temporal bone. The location of medial margins for partial temporal bone resection **(A)**, subtotal temporal bone resection **(B)**, and a subtype of partial temporal bone resection *(a)* for cartilaginous canal lesions are shown by the *broken lines.* MF, middle fossa; TM, temporomandibular joint; EAC, external auditory canal; ICA, internal carotid artery; P, petrous apex; V, vestibule; F, facial nerve; M, mastoid antrum; 8, eighth nerve.

cal resection, radiation therapy, and chemotherapy. Cure rates for these lesions are in the range of approximately 5%. Lesions that extend intracranially to involve the structures of the posterior fossa or middle fossa are essentially incurable, and treatment should be considered palliative. Surgery and radiation are helpful in controlling symptoms of pain and prolonging survival in these cases (4–10,13,14,19–22). Most patients who succumb to malignancies of the temporal bone die from local extension. Regional metastasis is less common than for squamous cell carcinoma in other head and neck locations. Distant metastasis is relatively uncommon.

The initial evaluation of patients with suspected malignancies of the temporal bone should include a complete head and neck exam, a cranial nerve exam, and a high-resolution computed tomographic (CT) scan of the temporal bone, brain, and neck with axial and coronal projections. In cases where there is clinical or radiographic evidence of involvement of the middle fossa plate, posterior fossa plate, or the infratemporal fossa, a magnetic resonance imaging (MRI) scan should be obtained. With MRI it may be possible to demon-

strate involvement of the dura or intracranial extension, which cannot be appreciated on CT alone. Although distant metastases are relatively uncommon, the patient should undergo a metastatic workup with a chest CT and liver function studies. Audiometry is also routinely obtained.

To establish the correct diagnosis, a representative biopsy must be obtained. If malignancy is suspected and a negative biopsy is obtained, a second biopsy should be taken and should include a deep wedge of tissue at the margin of the lesion and normal-appearing tissue. If necessary, this can be done under general anesthesia, but care should be taken that the biopsy does not compromise or interfere with the planned surgical resection.

A confounding problem in the evaluation of lesions of the external auditory canal is the occasional development of pseudoepitheliomatous hyperplasia, which may occur in the setting of both acute chronic inflammation of the external auditory canal (23). The biopsy of the lesions may be indistinguishable from squamous cell carcinoma even when examined by an experienced pathologist. If the clinical presentation and exam are not consistent with malignancy and there is no evidence of bone erosion on CT scan, it is our practice to excise these areas of abnormality with wide local excision and to follow these patients closely. Lesions of pseudoepitheliomatous hyperplasia should heal promptly and completely. Delayed healing or lingering epithelial abnormalities are rebiopsied. If the second biopsy again demonstrates what appears to be squamous cell carcinoma, the lesions are managed accordingly. Even if the canal heals completely without evidence of irregularity, it is imperative that the patients continue to be followed by routine otoscopy and follow-up CT scan for several years.

An unfortunate and not uncommon occurrence is the encountering of a malignant tumor at the time of tympanomastoidectomy that had been planned for the management of chronic otitis media. Usually, neither the surgeon nor the patient is adequately prepared. In many instances, imaging studies have not been obtained preoperatively and the extent of disease is not known. This situation is best managed by obtaining a definitive frozen section diagnosis and a simple one-layer closure of the wound. This patient should then undergo a thorough evaluation to determine the extent of the disease process followed by a definitive surgical procedure as early as possible.

SURGICAL INDICATIONS AND PLANNING

Surgical planning is dependent upon the establishment of a reliable tissue diagnosis, the determination of the extent of the disease process based on clinical exam and radiographic imaging, and the age and general health of the patient.

Adjunctive Therapy

Radiation therapy should be planned as postoperative treatment for all cases of squamous cell carcinoma except those lesions limited to the external canal. Radiation therapy is always given as a planned treatment modality rather than reserved for clinical evidence of recurrence. Primary radiation therapy or combinations of chemotherapy and radiation have not been shown to be as effective as surgery with postoperative radiation (7,21,24).

The role of chemotherapy in the management of temporal bone malignancies has not been clearly established. There does not appear to be a role for primary treatment with chemotherapy or for induction chemotherapy prior to planned surgical resection, because this may delay definitive treatment of a potentially curable lesion. Chemotherapy has been helpful in prolonging survival in patients who have incurable or inoperable tumors and in those patients with positive margins following surgical resection. The role of chemotherapy as an adjunctive treatment modality in patients who undergo resection followed by planned radiation therapy has also not been established. This is in large part related to the fact that these tumors are relatively uncommon, and studies to establish the efficacy of chemotherapy require a relatively large number of patients.

Lesions of the Cartilaginous External Auditory Meatus

Lesions of the external auditory meatus are best managed by en bloc resection of the cartilaginous canal. Specimens should be sent from both the superficial and deep margins to be certain that the tumor has been completely removed. Invasive lesions of the anterior external auditory meatus should also be resected in continuity with the superficial lobe of the parotid gland. The skin of the bony external canal is removed down to the level of the tympanic annulus, and a bony canalplasty is performed. Enlargement of the bony canal facilitates reconstruction, which is accomplished with split-thickness skin grafts that are packed in place. If the pathologic examination of the surgical specimen reveals evidence of involvement of the parotid either by direct extension or lymph node metastasis, full-course radiation therapy should be given in the immediate postoperative period. The cure rates for these tumors is approximately 95% (4–6,20,22).

Lesions of the External Auditory Canal Without Evidence of Bone Erosion on CT

Lesions of the external auditory canal without evidence of bone erosion on CT are highly curable with a partial or lateral temporal bone resection (Fig. 40.2). In this procedure, the cartilaginous and bony ear canal with attached tympanic membrane and malleus is resected en bloc in continuity with the superficial lobe of the parotid (Figs. 40.3 and 40.4). Postoperative radiation therapy is unnecessary unless the final pathology reveals suggestion of positive margins or evidence or parotid invasion or metastasis. The reconstructive technique employed is similar to that for a canal wall–down tympanomastoidectomy with intact stapes. The mastoid is

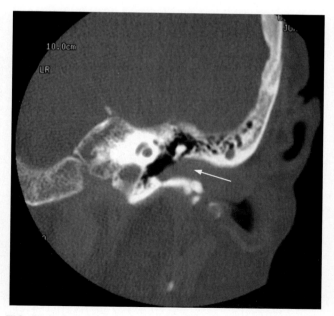

FIG. 40.2 Coronal CT of a 71-year-old female with a T1 adenoid cystic carcinoma *(arrow)* limited to the external auditory canal.

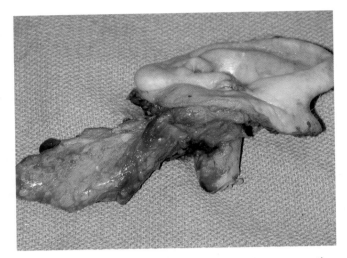

FIG. 40.3 Auriculectomy, lateral temporal bone resection and superficial parotidectomy specimen from a 67-year-old male with squamous cell carcinoma of the auricle and external auditory canal.

obliterated with muscle pedicle flaps. The middle ear is covered with a temporalis fascia graft, which contacts the head of the stapes and placement of split-thickness skin grafts.

Lesions of the External Auditory Canal with Bone Erosion on CT Scanning

These patients are best managed by lateral temporal bone resection with blind sac closure of the external auditory meatus and tympanomastoid obliteration with abdominal fat graft followed by radiation therapy (25). It is generally not worthwhile to attempt to reconstruct the resultant surgical defect because the hearing results following radiation therapy are usually poor, and problems related to mastoid cavity infections and osteoradionecrosis can be avoided by primary obliteration.

Lesions of the External Auditory Canal and Middle Ear Compartment

Although it is technically possible to encompass a small percentage of external auditory canal and middle ear compartment tumors by en bloc resection or subtotal temporal bone resection, it is not clear that the theoretical advantages of such an approach outweigh the morbidity and potential morbidity that results. This includes sacrifice of the facial nerve and labyrinth. These lesions can also be resected through an extended canal wall–down tympanomastoidectomy and resection of the adjacent bone. The reported cure rates of these two techniques are similar (26,27). All these patients are given postoperative full-course radiation therapy. If dural involvement is suspected on CT and MRI, the surgery should include planned neurosurgical collaboration with a subtemporal craniotomy and possible resection of the middle fossa dura. The neurosurgical portion of the procedure should be carried out first. If the tumor is found to involve brain parenchyma, the remainder of the surgical approach should be for palliation without sacrifice of the facial nerve or labyrinthine function (16,28).

Total temporal bone resection, although technically possible, involves planned sacrifice of the internal carotid artery, facial nerve, and inner ear. It is rarely warranted. Lesions with deep skull base involvement are considered incurable, and palliative management should be employed.

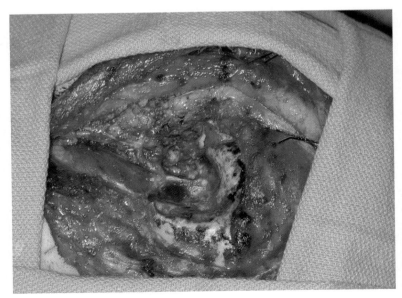

FIG. 40.4 Intraoperative photograph of surgical defect from same patient as in Fig. 40.3.

INFORMED CONSENT

Failure to Cure or Control the Malignancy

Patients should be presented with a treatment plan, including plans for adjunctive therapy with both radiation and chemotherapy. If radiation and chemotherapy are planned, the patient should meet with the radiotherapist and medical oncologist in advance of their procedure so that they have a comprehensive understanding of what their overall treatment involves. They need to be made aware of the need for long-term follow-up and surveillance, including serial MRI and CT scans in the future.

Problems with Hearing, Balance, and Facial Nerve Function

Both conductive and sensorineural hearing loss may result from the proposed procedures. If tympanomastoid obliteration is planned, useful hearing in the affected ear will be lost. Balance problems that result from surgical intervention are usually self-limited. Even if labyrinthine function is lost all together, most patients recover over time.

Most patients with facial nerve involvement of their malignancy have preoperative symptoms of facial nerve dysfunction. However, occasionally the facial nerve may be invaded by tumor without any preoperative deficits. If there are no other signs of unresectability, the involved segment of the facial nerve should be resected and a cable graft placed. All patients undergoing lateral temporal bone resection or more extensive procedures should be informed of the possibility of a complete facial paralysis and the need for possible oculoplastic intervention in the postoperative period. They need to be aware of the possibility for a sural nerve graft and the resultant donor site deficit.

Problems with Speech and Swallowing/Involvement of or Injury of the Lower Cranial Nerves

Preoperative involvement of the jugular foramen carries with it a poor prognosis. If jugular foramen involvement is encountered at surgery, resection of the contents of the jugular foramen may be considered, although the chances for controlling the tumor in this region are very low. The ninth, tenth, and eleventh cranial nerves can be injured as a result of either the resection of the tumor or vigorous packing of the jugular foramen to control venous bleeding once the tumor has been removed. These patients will experience difficulty with aspiration and will have a weak voice and cough. They may require placement of a percutaneous gastrostomy tube to provide the necessary nutritional support, as well as laryngoplasty in the postoperative period to improve their voice and cough and to minimize aspiration.

Intracranial Complications

Patients with advanced malignancy of the temporal bone are at risk for developing problems related to the internal carotid artery, including stroke, as well as problems with venous infarction from occlusion of the venous sinuses. There is also a risk for meningitis in cases where the dura is violated either by tumor invasion or as part of the planned resection.

Cerebrospinal Fluid Leak

Patients with dural involvement who undergo planned resection of the dura universally have problems with spinal fluid leaking into the tympanomastoid space. Usually this can be controlled by obliterating the eustachian tube orifice with bone wax and achieving a watertight closure of the skin and external auditory meatus. However, if evidence of spinal fluid drainage is noted postoperatively, these patients will require placement of a lumbar drain for 3 to 5 days. In a small percentage of cases, this may not prove effective and some patients may require reoperation for control of a spinal fluid leak.

Wound Problems

Wound problems that could possibly result from surgical resection include problems with infection or wound breakdown and liquefaction of the fat graft, which may occur in a delayed manner, especially following radiation therapy.

SURGICAL PROCEDURES

Lateral Temporal Bone Resection (Partial Temporal Bone Resection)

The lateral temporal bone resection is appropriate for lesions confined to the external auditory canal (Figs. 40.5 to 40.12). The surgical limits of a partial temporal bone resection include the stapes medially, the facial nerve posteriorly, the temporomandibular joint anteriorly, and the meatus laterally. These limits are demonstrated in a mid-modiolar temporal bone section (Fig. 40.1). A curved postauricular incision is made approximately 2 cm posterior to the postauricular crease. The anterior extension of the superior rim of the incision extends for approximately 1 cm anterior to the external auditory meatus. The inferior limit of the incision extends approximately 3 cm inferior and anterior to the mastoid tip. This extension will provide the necessary exposure to perform the superficial parotidectomy. A skin flap is developed in the subcutaneous tissue to the level of the external auditory canal, which is transected just inside the meatus. If the lesion involves the concha or the meatus, it is best to make the incisions circumscribing the tumor prior to the postauricular incision such that the lesion is incorporated within the surgical specimen. Once the posterior aspect of the canal has been incised, a direct view of the contents of

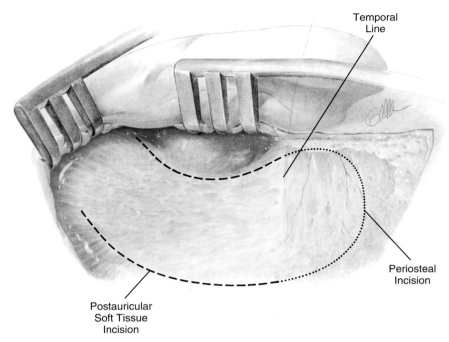

FIG. 40.5 The inferiorly based periosteal flap is developed and preserved for later use in the reconstruction. It can be used to line the surgical defect or to cover a fat graft when tympanomastoid obliteration is required.

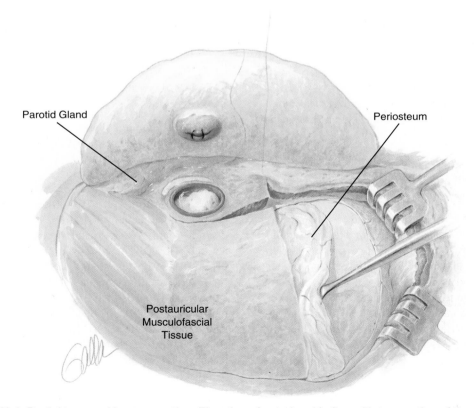

FIG. 40.6 Partial temporal bone resection. Elevation of anterior skin flap with transection of the external auditory canal at the meatus. An inferiorly based periosteal flap with temporal periosteum is elevated from superior to inferior.

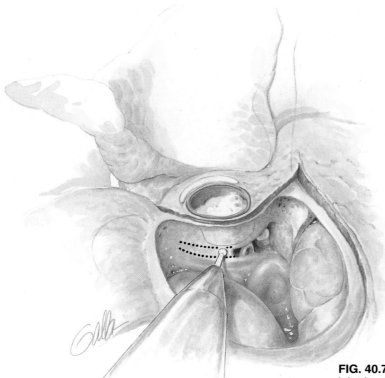

FIG. 40.7 Partial temporal bone resection. The incudostapedial joint has been separated and the incus removed. The facial recess is extended inferiorly with a small diamond bur.

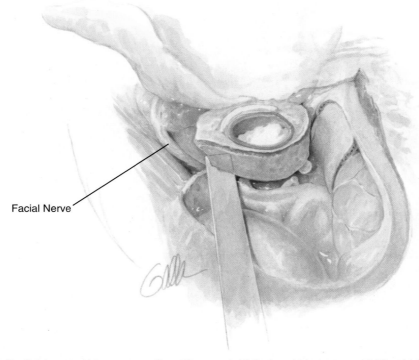

Facial Nerve

FIG. 40.8 Partial temporal bone resection. The mastoid tip has been removed. The facial recess has been opened and extended inferiorly through the limits of the tympanic bone. A medium straight osteotome is used to transect the anterior bony attachment.

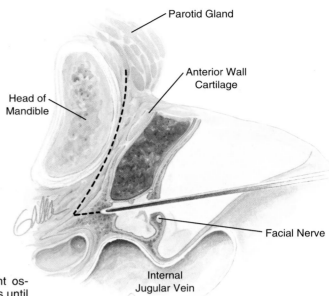

FIG. 40.9 Partial temporal bone resection. A medium straight osteotome is passed anteriorly through the extended facial recess until it abuts the anterior bony attachment.

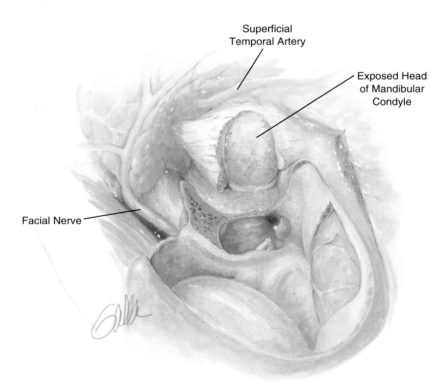

FIG. 40.10 Partial temporal bone resection. The surgical defect created by partial temporal bone resection (Fig. 40.4).

external auditory canal is achieved. The anterior canal incision is then made with direct visualization of the lesion. The tragal cartilage is incised, and the periparotid fascia is identified. The flap is further developed as would be done for a superficial parotidectomy to expose the superficial lobe of the parotid. An inferiorly based muscle-pedicled flap is then developed by sharply incising the postauricular subcuta-neous tissue along the border of the posterior bony canal aperture. The incision is extended superiorly to the level of the temporalis muscle. At the level of the temporal line, the temporalis fascia is incised and the temporalis muscle is elevated, exposing the periosteum of the squamous portion of the temporal bone. Two rake retractors are placed, and the temporalis muscle is elevated from the periosteum using

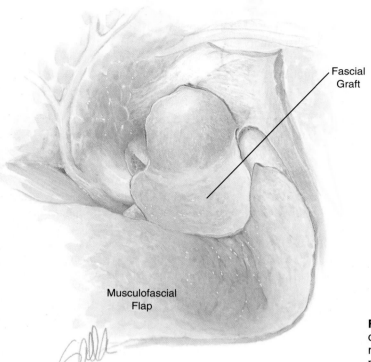

Fascial
Graft

Musculofascial
Flap

FIG. 40.11 Partial temporal bone resection. When postoperative radiation is not planned, the surgical defect is reconstructed similar to a canal wall–down type III tympanomastoidectomy. The inferiorly based periosteal flap is used to line the mastoid cavity.

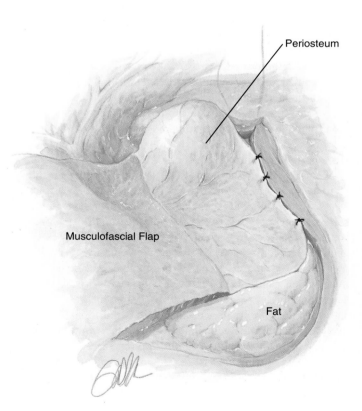

Periosteum

Musculofascial Flap

Fat

FIG. 40.12 Partial temporal bone resection. When postoperative radiation is planned, the surgical defect is obliterated with an abdominal fat graft that is covered by the inferiorly based periosteal flap.

blunt dissection. Bipolar cautery is used to control the bleeding from many small blood vessels, which penetrate from the periosteum into the temporalis muscle. The periosteum is the superior extension of the inferior muscle pedicle flap. A large segment of the periosteum is then incised using the Bovie cautery, leaving the inferior aspect connected to the inferiorly based muscle-pedicled flap. This periosteal extension will ultimately be used to line the mastoid cavity, including, if necessary, the tympanic cavity as would ordinarily be accomplished with the fascia graft. If possible, care should be taken to preserve the superficial temporal artery, which supplies blood to the temporoparietal fascia flap, which may be useful in reconstruction, especially in the future if problems with osteoradionecrosis develop.

The next step in the procedure is to perform a canal wall–up mastoidectomy with an extended facial recess approach. In cases with poorly pneumatized mastoid cavities and low-lying tegmental dura, a small subtemporal craniotomy is performed and the temporal dura is elevated from the floor of the middle cranial fossa so that bone can be removed anterior and superior along the superior aspects of the bony canal to the region of the tympanic bone without injuring the tegmental dura. Once the facial recess has been widely opened, access through the facial recess allows for division of the incudostapedial joint and removal of the incus. The region of the stylomastoid foramen is skeletonized using a diamond bur. The mastoid tip is removed by first removing the bone along the digastric ridge and from the stylomastoid foramen. The remainder of the bone is removed by using sharp dissection with curved iris scissors separating the attachments of the sternocleidomastoid muscle. By keeping the tips of the iris scissors against the bone of the mastoid tip, injury to the facial nerve is prevented. Working through the inferior aspect of the extended facial recess, a cleft is developed between the jugular bulb and the tympanic annulus and extended anteriorly to the region of the glenoid fossa. This dissection is best accomplished using small diamond burs and suction irrigation. Similarly, the bone is removed anteriorly and superiorly along the tegmental plate to the superior attachment of the bony canal in the anterior epitympanum. The facial nerve is then dissected through the stylomastoid foramen into the superficial lobe of the parotid. The superficial lobe is dissected, with its attachment to the surgical specimen preserved. A medium straight osteotome is placed superiorly at the junction of the anterior bony canal and the glenoid fossa. Usually a few gentle taps with a hammer will result in a fracture and disarticulation of the specimen, which can then be removed with curved iris scissors separating the final remaining soft tissue attachments. If the specimen does not fracture easily, additional drilling may be necessary to thin the remaining bony connection between the specimen and the anterior inferior tympanic bone.

Once the specimen has been removed, frozen sections should be taken from the parotid tissue immediately adjacent to the resection margin to be certain that there is no evidence of microscopic invasion. If involvement of the deep lobe of the parotid is encountered, this should be resected as well.

Reconstruction of the surgical defect is determined in part by the requirements for postoperative radiation therapy. If radiation therapy is not required, the mastoid cavity can be obliterated with the inferiorly based periosteal flap and the middle ear reconstructed with either a temporalis fascia graft or a periosteal extension of the inferiorly based pedicle flap, which is then set directly on top of the head of the stapes (type III tympanoplasty). Split-thickness skin grafts are placed circumferentially about the tympanic segment of the cavity, as well as over the medial portions of the inferior muscle pedicle flap. A wide meatoplasty should be performed. Bone paté obliteration of the mastoid cavity should be avoided because bone paté can give the appearance of dystrophic or demineralized bone on CT scan and could possibly be confused for recurrence at a later date.

In cases where radiation therapy is planned in the postoperative period, attempted hearing reconstruction is usually not performed, because the results following radiation therapy are less than gratifying. Problems with the postoperative care of the mastoid cavity, infections of the cavity, and osteoradionecrosis can be avoided by blind sac closure of the external auditory meatus and obliteration of the mastoid cavity with a fat graft, which is then covered by the inferiorly based muscle-pedicled flap and periosteum. The wound is closed in layers with a Penrose drain and covered with a mastoid dressing.

Subtotal Temporal Bone Resection

Subtotal temporal bone resection is indicated for tumors involving the external canal and middle ear with limited mastoid involvement and no evidence of extension to involve the tegmental dura, eustachian tube, parotid gland, or internal carotid artery. The limits of this resection are illustrated in Fig. 40.1. If bone erosion within the middle ear is identified on CT scan and the internal carotid artery is exposed, subtotal temporal bone resection would be a fruitless maneuver with the tumor having escaped resectability through an en bloc approach. Prior to beginning the surgical procedure, patients undergo placement of a lumbar drain to facilitate traction of the temporal dura. A Foley catheter is also placed, and patients are given both mannitol and furosemide (Lasix). An incision is made in the postauricular region that is similar to that for the lateral temporal bone resection. However, the superior limit of the excision is extended to provide the necessary exposure for a subtemporal craniotomy. An anterior skin flap is similarly developed with transection of the ear canal and exposure of the parotid fascia. An inferior pedicled flap with superior periosteal extension is developed. The posterior insertion of the temporalis muscle is incised, and the temporalis muscle is reflected anteriorly with self-retaining retractors to provide exposure for a subtemporal craniotomy. The subtemporal craniotomy is performed with the lower limit of craniotomy at the level of the floor of the middle cranial fossa. The middle fossa dura is then elevated to the petrous ridge, and a House-Urban middle fossa retractor is placed. The canal wall–up mastoidectomy is then performed with skeletization of the sigmoid sinus down to the region of the jugular bulb. Bone is also removed from the sinodural angle with exposure of the superior petrosal sinus. Using a diamond bur and suction irrigation, bone is removed from the floor of the middle cranial fossa to expose the internal carotid artery and the fundus of the internal auditory canal. The labyrinthine segment of the facial nerve is traced up to the region of the geniculate ganglion. The superficial lobe of the parotid gland is dissected free of the facial nerve and left in continuity with the specimen anteriorly. The labyrinth is transected at the distal end of the internal auditory canal using a small diamond bur, and the bone removal is extended posteriorly to the petrous ridge and the dura of the posterior fossa. The lateral wall of the internal carotid artery is then separated from the bony wall of the canal using blunt dissection. Every effort should be made to detach all the attachments between the bony and fibrous wall of the carotid artery so that when the specimen is finally removed, a tear does not result. Similarly, the sigmoid sinus and, if possible, the dome of the jugular bulb should be separated from their overlying bony walls to avoid injury. However, despite the best possible effort, violation of the venous sinuses is common in this procedure. This, however, can be controlled easily with Surgicel packing. Ultimately the specimen must be fractured free using a straight osteotome, which is placed in the bony crevice within the labyrinth that has been created with the diamond drill. The facial nerve is divided at its labyrinthine segment and at the stylomastoid foramen. If possible, a sural cable graft can be placed. If the tegmental dura is involved with tumor, this can be resected and repaired with a fascial graft. A blind sac closure of the external auditory meatus is accomplished, and the cavity is obliterated using a fat graft and the inferiorly based muscle-pedicled flap and superior periosteal extension. The egress cerebrospinal fluid into the wound is common following this procedure, and a watertight closure and obliteration of the eustachian tube without the use of the drain is performed.

Extended Radical Mastoidectomy

At present there are no good data to indicate a significant benefit of subtotal temporal bone resection over extended radical mastoidectomy for the cure and control of squamous cell carcinoma of the middle ear and mastoid. Although some reports suggest that such is the case, the wide diversity in results between reported series regardless of the methodology employed makes comparison between different institutions difficult. At present the morbidity associated with subtotal temporal bone resection, including sacrifice of the facial nerve and labyrinth, and the potential morbidity, which includes injury to the internal carotid artery, is difficult to justify. Ultimately, careful prospective studies will be

necessary to establish the efficacy of each of these treatment modalities and to justify the morbidity of more radical procedures. In reality, only a small percentage of tumors that involve the middle ear and mastoid can be truly removed en bloc by subtotal temporal bone resection without the presence of residual disease in the surgical bed that requires further resection.

With an extended radical mastoidectomy, it is possible to resect the same surgical specimen that can be removed with subtotal temporal bone resection. However, in this approach the specimen is removed piecemeal, with the potential for spreading malignant cells within the operative field. This is more than just a theoretical concern, as anyone who has had significant experience with these tumors has faced problems with multiple satellite recurrences within the skin and presumably within the deep wound as well. Postoperative radiation therapy in the early postoperative period is essential for the management of these tumors and should be employed as early as possible. It has been our recent practice to also employ postoperative chemotherapy with a similar protocol that is used for other head and neck squamous cell carcinomas. However, the utility of chemotherapy in this setting has yet to be established.

Total Temporal Bone Resection

It is technically possible to resect the entire temporal bone, including the petrous apex, internal auditory canal, and internal carotid artery. This procedure has been employed for malignant tumors involving the deep temporal bone and petrous apex. Modifications of this approach, including preservation of the internal carotid artery, have also been described. However, if this approach is considered, patients must be studied preoperatively to determine whether or not they will tolerate sacrifice of their internal carotid artery. This approach carries with it a significantly high morbidity and mortality and, in our view, is rarely ever justified based on the relative incurability of these tumors. Patients with extensive lesions of the temporal bone that extend to involve the petrous apex are best managed with palliative radiation and chemotherapy or surgery for control of pain.

Management of Adenoid Cystic Carcinoma of the Temporal Bone

Adenoid cystic carcinoma of the temporal bone usually occurs within the external auditory canal and presumably arises from the glandular elements of the epithelium. Typically, patients present with pain out of proportion to the relatively small, often indolent-appearing lesion within the canal. A high index of suspicion and early biopsy are essential to establishing the diagnosis. Radiographic imaging is often inadequate in establishing the extent of disease because there is a high propensity for perineural invasion and microscopic local infiltration that cannot be appreciated either on exam or with imaging studies. These lesions are best managed by lateral temporal bone resection with tympanomastoid obliteration followed by postoperative radiation therapy. Although the efficacy of radiation therapy has not been well established for adenoid cystic carcinoma, the degree of local infiltration and the near certainty of positive margins makes this a prudent undertaking. Local control can be achieved in approximately 50% of cases. However, most of these patients ultimately succumb to distant metastases, often many years following the primary resection.

Management of Low-Grade Malignancies of the Temporal Bone

Adenocarcinoma and carcinoid tumors of the middle ear space may arise de novo within the middle ear and present as a middle ear mass. Imaging studies usually fail to demonstrate evidence of bone erosion. Often the diagnosis is established at surgery with frozen-section analysis of the specimen. These lesions are best managed by canal wall–down tympanomastoidectomy with obliteration of the cavity and reconstruction of the middle ear space with a fascial graft and split-thickness skin grafting. With carcinoid tumors of the middle ear, recurrence may develop many years following resection of the primary and can be appreciated on otoscopic exam of the cavity. Local and regional metastases may also occur many years following resection of the primary. The role for radiation therapy in the treatment of these lesions has not been established for temporal bone primaries. Similar lesions that occur elsewhere have not been cured with radiation therapy; however, radiation as a palliative modality has been employed.

POSTOPERATIVE MANAGEMENT

Critical to the management of patients with malignancies of the temporal bone is planned postoperative adjunctive therapy in the early postoperative period, including most commonly radiation therapy and in some cases chemotherapy. Optimally, radiation should be begun within 1 month of the surgical procedure. Patients generally receive the maximum amount of tolerated radiation, which is in the range of 65 gray. Fractionated protocols are most commonly employed. The efficacy of b.i.d. radiation and stereotactic radiation for these lesions has not been established.

There is no evidence at present to support the efficacy of adjunctive chemotherapy in patients with malignancies of the temporal bone. However, as evidence arises to support the use of this modality for other squamous cell carcinomas of the head and neck, it is reasonable to employ similar methods for management of temporal bone lesions. As is the case with radiation therapy, the use of chemotherapy once a clinical recurrence has occurred is only of palliative value.

Patients who undergo resection of temporal bone malignancies should undergo early radiographic imaging to establish baseline studies with which future comparisons can be made. It has been our practice to use both CT and MRI for this purpose. If a patient develops a suspected local recurrence within the tympanomastoid cavity, reoperation, exploration, and resection should be done. Although recurrence is an ominous sign under any circumstances, it is still possible to achieve a cure if the recurrence is confined to the tympanomastoid cavity. The role for salvage surgery in patients who develop local recurrence outside the tympanomastoid cavity, including the parotid gland, temporomandibular joint, jugular foramen, or middle fossa, is of questionable utility. A recent report would suggest that even some of these patients may be ultimately curable with radical surgery (27,28).

Patients with recurrent carcinoma of the temporal bone or incurable primary malignancies often suffer from intractable pain, which increases over time. The satisfactory management of pain in this setting has proven to be a difficult problem. Early tachyphylaxis to narcotic medications may make them ineffective over time. Radiation therapy, chemotherapy, and palliative surgery have all proved to be of some effectiveness in this regard. It is prudent to enlist the expertise of a pain specialist early in the management of these patients to help achieve the best possible long-term palliation.

Surgical Complications

Complications following lateral temporal bone resection are similar to those that result from tympanomastoidectomy for chronic otitis media. Wound infections are relatively uncommon. However, it is important to identify signs of infection early in the postoperative course so that intravenous antibiotics can be employed to eradicate the infection and prevent unnecessary delays before instituting radiation therapy when necessary. Liquefaction of fat grafts, which are used for obliteration of the mastoid cavity, occurs in approximately 10% of cases in the early postoperative period or following delivery of radiation therapy. This often results in a draining postauricular sinus and may require 2 to 3 weeks before it completely resolves and the wound heals. In some cases, a residual sinus tract remains following complete evacuation of the fat graft. It is better to institute radiation therapy prior to a planned repair of the wound. These wounds have been successfully repaired following radiation therapy by rotating a temporoparietal fascial flap with its abundant blood supply into the wound, which facilitates closure of the wound. If necessary, the margins of the wound can be sutured directly to the temporoparietal fascial flap and the split-thickness skin graft applied.

Major complications following more radical procedures, including subtotal temporal bone resection, are managed with the help of neurosurgical consultation. Of these complications, injury to the internal carotid artery is often the most significant and most difficult complication to manage intraoperatively. Patients who can tolerate occlusion of the internal carotid artery are best managed by tight extraluminal packing of the carotid canal. In some cases, the carotid can be repaired primarily or with a vein or synthetic graft.

These patients are at increased risk for delayed complications following radiation therapy, including carotid artery rupture and intraluminal thrombus formation with embolic infarction.

CONCLUSIONS

In summary, management of malignancies of the temporal bone is challenging. Prognosis is predicated most of all on the basis of the extent of the disease process. Because pain is the cardinal feature of these lesions, a high index of suspicion will facilitate early diagnosis and ultimately improve outcome. Patients who have potentially curable lesions should be carefully studied preoperatively with CT scanning and in some cases MRI to determine the extent of their disease. The surgical planning should include a procedure that can encompass the lesion and, if at all possible, an en bloc procedure. When en bloc resection is not feasible or possible, a wide-field radical mastoidectomy approach should be employed. Patients with more extensive lesions should always receive planned postoperative radiation therapy early in the postoperative period. If in the future it is established that more radical procedures with their associated morbidity and increased mortality offer a true advantage for survival, their role in the management of more advanced lesions may become warranted.

REFERENCES

1. Clairmont AA, Conley JJ. Primary carcinoma of the mastoid bone. *Ann Otol Rhinol Laryngol* 1977;86:306–309.
2. Conley J, Schuller DE. Malignancies of the ear. *Laryngoscope* 1976;86:1147–1163.
3. Gacek RR, Goodman M. Management of malignancy of the temporal bone. *Laryngoscope* 1977;87:1622–1634.
4. Goodman ML. Middle ear and mastoid neoplasms. *Ann Otol Rhinol Laryngol* 1971;80:419–424.
5. Goodwin WJ, Jesse RH. Malignant neoplasms of the external auditory canal and temporal bone. *Arch Otolaryngol* 1980;106:675–679.
6. Greer JA, Cody TR, Weiland LH. Neoplasms of the temporal bone. *J Otolaryngol* 1976;5:391–398.
7. Kenyon GS, Marks PV, Scholtz CL, et al. Squamous cell carcinoma of the middle ear. A 25-year retrospective study. *Ann Otol Rhinol Laryngol* 1985;94:273–277.
8. Kinney SE, Wood BG. Malignancies of the external ear canal and temporal bone: surgical techniques and results. *Laryngoscope* 1987;97:158–164.
9. Kinney SE. Squamous cell carcinoma of the external auditory canal. *Am J Otol* 1989;10:111–116.
10. Kuhel WI, Hume CR, Selesnick SH. Cancer of the external auditory canal and temporal bone. *Otolaryngol Clin North Am* 1996;29:827–852.
11. Applebaum EL. Radiation-induced carcinoma of the temporal bone. *Otolaryngol Head Neck Surg* 1979;87:604–609.
12. Lustig LR, Jackler RK, Lanser MJ. Radiation-induced tumors of the temporal bone. *Am J Otol* 1997;18:230–235.
13. Austin, JR, Stewart KL, Fawzi N. Squamous cell carcinoma of the external auditory canal. Therapeutic prognosis based on a proposed staging system. *Arch Otolaryngol Head Neck Surg* 1994;120:1228–1232.
14. Lewis JS. Temporal bone resection. Review of 100 cases. *Arch Otolaryngol* 1975;101:23–25.
15. Liu FF, Keane TJ, Davidson J. Primary carcinoma involving the petrous temporal bone. *Head Neck* 1993;15:39–43.
16. Manolidis S, Pappas D Jr, Von Doersten P, et al. Temporal bone and lateral skull base malignancy: experience and results with 81 patients. *Am J Otol* 1998;19:S1–15.
17. Michaels L, Wells M. Squamous cell carcinoma of the middle ear. *Clin Otolaryngol* 1980;5:235–248.
18. Arriaga M, Curtin H, Takahashi H, et al. Staging proposal for external auditory meatus carcinoma based on preoperative clinical examination and computed tomography findings. *Ann Otol Rhinol Laryngol* 1990;99:714–721.
19. Arriaga M, Curtin HD, Takahashi H, et al. The role of preoperative CT scans in staging external auditory meatus carcinoma: radiologic-pathologic correlation study. *Otolaryngol Head Neck Surg* 1991;105:6–11.
20. Leonetti JP, Smith PG, Kletzker GR, et al. Invasion patterns of advanced temporal bone malignancies. *Am J Otol* 1996;17:438–442.
21. Birzgalis AR, Keith AO, Farrington WT. Radiotherapy in the treatment of middle ear and mastoid carcinoma. *Clin Otolaryngol* 1992;17:113–116.
22. Lesser RW, Spector GJ, Devineni VR. Malignant tumors of the middle ear and external auditory canal: a 20-year review. *Otolaryngol Head Neck Surg* 1987;96:43–47.
23. Sauerwein W, Feldmann HJ. [Radiotherapy of carcinoma of the auditory canal]. *Strahlenther Onkol* 1988;164:567–573.
24. Nadol JB Jr, Schuknecht HF. Obliteration of the mastoid in the treatment of tumors of the temporal bone. *Ann Otol Rhinol Laryngol* 1984;93:6–12.
25. Pensak ML, Gleich LL, Gluckman JL, et al. Temporal bone carcinoma: contemporary perspectives in the skull base surgical era. *Laryngoscope* 1996;106:1234–1237.
26. Prasad S, Janecka IP. Efficacy of surgical treatments for squamous cell carcinoma of the temporal bone: a literature review. *Otolaryngol Head Neck Surg* 1994;110:270–280.
27. Moffat DA, Grey P, Ballagh RH, et al. Extended temporal bone resection for squamous cell carcinoma. *Otolaryngol Head Neck Surg* 1997;116:617–623.
28. Somekawa Y, Asano K, Hata M. [En bloc resection of the temporal bone for middle ear carcinoma extending to the cranial base]. *Nippon Jibiinkoka Gakkai Kaiho* 1997;100:782–789.

CHAPTER 41

Paragangliomas of the Temporal Bone

Robert W. Jyung

Paragangliomas are highly vascular, slow-growing neoplasms that can occur within the temporal bone, as well as other sites in the head and neck. They develop from paraganglia, which are neurosecretory structures derived from the neural crest. Paraganglia are distributed in the middle ear and jugular bulb but are also found in the carotid and aortic bodies, where they have an established chemosensory function. Paragangliomas are distinguished by their extreme vascularity, which facilitates their diagnosis yet complicates their management. Although typically benign, these tumors can cause significant morbidity by bone erosion, cranial nerve paralysis, and intracranial invasion.

Paraganglia were first described as glomus body–like structures in the carotid body by Von Haller (1) in 1762, but it was not until 1840 that Valentin (2) identified these structures in the temporal bone, using the term *ganglionum tympanicum*. In 1878 Krause (3) described a carotid body–like structure in the tympanic canaliculus. Similar structures were also identified in the nodose ganglion and subsequently in a number of sites in the head and neck, including the nasal cavity, the orbit, and the larynx. In 1941 Guild (4) provided the first modern description of temporal bone paraganglia, and in 1945 Rosenwasser (5) reported a vascular tumor of the hypotympanum that he concluded must have originated from the *glomus jugularis* described by Guild.

Glenner and Grimley (6) classified paraganglia into four categories: (i) branchiomeric, (ii) juxtavagal, (iii) aorticosympathetic, and (iv) visceral autonomic. Within the branchiomeric category they included jugulotympanic, intercarotid, subclavian, laryngeal, coronary, aorticopulmonary, and pulmonary subtypes. From a clinical standpoint, however, the primary distinction needs to be made among paragangliomas arising from the middle ear (glomus tympan-icum), the jugular bulb (glomus jugulare), the vagus nerve (glomus vagale), and the carotid body (carotid body tumor or glomus caroticum). Although in strict terms the designation *glomus tumor* should be reserved for neoplasms of glomus bodies contained in skin, the term *glomus* in conjunction with an identifying site is well understood in the literature to indicate a paraganglioma.

Several schemes for surgical classification of paragangliomas have been devised. Although one scheme has not been universally applied, the Fisch system is widely accepted, logical, and easily remembered (Table 41.1) (7).

TABLE 41.1 *Fisch classification of temporal paragangliomas*

Class A	Tumors arising from the promontory and confined to the middle ear
Class B	Tumors arising from the hypotympanum, with or without mastoid involvement, with intact cortical bone over the jugular bulb
Class C	Tumors eroding bone of the infralabyrinthine, retrolabyrinthine, or apical compartments, with erosion of cortical bone over the jugular bulb
C1	Tumors with no carotid canal involvement or only involving the carotid foramen
C2	Tumors involving the vertical carotid canal
C3	Tumors involving the vertical and horizontal carotid canal
C4	Tumors with extension to the foramen lacerum and cavernous sinus
Class D	Tumors with intracranial extension
De1	Tumors with intracranial, extradural extension up to 2 cm in diameter
De2	Tumors with intracranial, extradural extension greater than 2 cm in diameter
Di1	Tumors with intracranial, intradural extension up to 2 cm in diameter
Di2	Tumors with intracranial, intradural extension greater than 2 cm in diameter
D3	Tumors with inoperable intracranial extension

(Adapted from Hawthorne MR, Makek MS, Harris JP, et al. The histopathological and clinical features of irradiated and nonirradiated temporal paragangliomas. *Laryngoscope* 1988; 98:325–331.)

The author acknowledges J. Gershon Spector, M.D., Professor, Department of Otolaryngology—Head and Neck Surgery, Washington University School of Medicine, as a mentor and authority on paragangliomas of the head and neck. His advice and generous contribution of photomicrographs, illustrations, and clinical photographs to this chapter are sincerely appreciated.

EPIDEMIOLOGY

Paragangliomas of the head and neck occur with an approximate incidence of 1 in 30,000. Overall, carotid body tumors are the most common, comprising 60% of all head and neck paragangliomas. However, in the temporal bone the glomus jugulare tumor is the most common, followed by the glomus tympanicum tumor. The relative frequency of tumor sites within the temporal bone reflects the distribution of normal paraganglia as quantified by Guild. In his study of 88 temporal bones, about 50% were found in the adventitia of the jugular bulb, 20% in the inferior tympanic canaliculus, and 10% on the cochlear promontory (4).

Approximately 10% of all head and neck paragangliomas are familial, but in some populations this proportion has been estimated as high as 50% (8). Multicentricity occurs in about 10% of all sporadic paragangliomas cases. However, in familial cases, the rate of multicentricity ranges from 25% to 55% (9).

Paragangliomas are more commonly found in Caucasians and in populations living at high altitude. In addition, there is a striking threefold to sixfold (or greater, depending on the series) predominance of female patients with paragangliomas, despite an equal complement of temporal bone paraganglia between women and men in Guild's study. Tumors are rarely detected before age 18 years, and most patients are diagnosed in the fifth to sixth decade. Typically, there is a delay in diagnosis of several years from the onset of symptoms. Patients with familial paragangliomas can often be diagnosed in the second or third decade due to heightened awareness and proactive screening.

PATHOGENESIS

Important clues to the pathogenesis of paragangliomas include (i) familial occurrence, (ii) extreme vascularity, (iii) association with hypoxic states, and (iv) an increased incidence in women. Therefore any mechanism postulated for their pathogenesis should account for these clinical features. An important impediment to progress in understanding the pathogenesis of paragangliomas has been the lack of a reliable animal model, despite efforts such as tumor implantation into the subrenal capsule of nude mice (10).

Familial cases account for at least 10% and possibly a much larger percentage of patients with head and neck paragangliomas (11). The genes for familial paragangliomas, termed PGL1 and PGL2, are transmitted in an autosomal dominant manner; therefore each child of an affected individual will have a 50% chance of inheriting the gene. However, only individuals who have inherited the gene from their father will eventually develop tumors, demonstrating greater expression with increasing age (8). This occurs through the process of genomic imprinting, where an allele is altered (possibly by DNA methylation) based on the sex of the transmitting parent (12). It has been postulated that PGL is inactivated during oogenesis and reactivated in spermatogenesis. Therefore "skipped" generations can occur, because transmitting fathers who have inherited the gene from their mothers will not develop tumors.

Through linkage studies using large Dutch kindreds, PGL1 was originally mapped to two regions of the long arm of chromosome 11, one between loci 22.3 and 23.2 (PGL1) (13) and another at locus 13.1 (PGL2) (14). In screening North American kindreds, PGL1 appeared to be the more common (15,16). Using these and Dutch kindreds, Baysal and coworkers (17) made a breakthrough discovery by demonstrating point mutations in SDHD, a gene that encodes the small subunit protein (cybS) of cytochrome B in mitochondrial complex II. These mutations were shown to result in either premature stop codons that could block synthesis of cybS protein or amino acid substitutions that could alter cybS conformation and function (17). Interestingly, no evidence for imprinting of SDHD was found, and the reasons for the discrepancy remain unclear. Because electron transport by mitochondrial complex II has been proposed as a mechanism for oxygen sensing in chemoreceptor organs such as the carotid body, mutations in SDHD may explain paraganglioma development as a consequence of inappropriate signaling of hypoxia (17).

Hypoxia has been implicated in the development of these tumors both in animals and humans. For example, bovines experiencing chronic hypoxia due to altitude are predisposed to hyperplasia and subsequently neoplasia of the carotid bodies (18). Brachycephalic breeds of dogs, including the boxer and the Boston terrier, are predisposed to obstructed airways and also have an increased incidence of paragangliomas of the aortic body (19).

In humans exposed to chronic hypoxia due to high altitude, the incidence of carotid body tumors increases progressively with higher altitude; ultimately the incidence is about 10 times greater than populations at sea level (20). There may be differences between paragangliomas that develop at high altitude versus sea level in terms of a greater female predominance and a lower rate of multicentricity and familial tumors (21). Hyperplasia of the carotid body occurs as a result of chronic hypoxia due to conditions such as emphysema, cyanotic congenital heart disease, and cystic fibrosis (22,23). Some investigators have argued that carotid body tumors generated at high altitude are in fact examples of extreme hyperplasia, not neoplasia. However, because hyperplasia can be the precursor of actual neoplasia, these hypoxic states may provide a permissive environment for the development of paragangliomas. Interestingly, patients with hypoxia secondary to chronic obstructive pulmonary disease may be at increased risk for paragangliomas (24).

Not surprisingly, comparisons have been drawn between PGL and the causative gene for Von Hippel–Lindau disease (VHL), in which a negative regulator of hypoxia-inducible genes is disrupted (25). In VHL, a number of highly vascular tumors develop, including renal cell carcinomas, central nervous system hemangioblastomas, retinal angiomas, endolymphatic sac tumors, and sometimes paragangliomas

(26,27). However, VHL mutations have been examined in a large pedigree of familial paragangliomas, with no mutations found (28).

The influence of hormones such as estrogens has also been implicated in the development of paragangliomas. Many clinical series show a clear preponderance of female patients by a ratio of 3:1, and the highest disparity reported is 19:1. The disparity is best documented in carotid body tumors: At sea level there is a 2:1 female-to-male ratio, but in high-altitude populations, this ratio increases to 12:1 (20,29). In a large clinical series of paragangliomas from multiple sites in the head and neck, the female-to-male ratio was 6:1 (30). Interestingly, many of the patients in this series may have lived at high altitude. The magnified female-to-male ratio in populations at high altitude suggests an interaction between hypoxia and estrogens in the genesis of these lesions.

Expression of angiogenic peptide growth factors might represent a common mechanism triggered by these external influences. It is established that angiogenesis is a critical step in the progression of solid tumors (31). Cell-to-cell signaling by angiogenic growth factors, including vascular endothelial growth factor (VEGF), platelet-derived endothelial cell growth factor (PD-ECGF), and basic fibroblast growth factor (bFGF), is essential to the angiogenic process. In a rat model of chronic hypoxia induced by hypobaric conditions, exuberant angiogenesis and hyperplasia of the carotid body was accompanied by a dramatic upregulation of messenger RNA for VEGF and one of its receptors, flk-1 (32). Furthermore,

there is evidence that paragangliomas of the temporal bone and other sites in the head and neck express both VEGF and PD-ECGF protein (33). Because the expression of VEGF and PD-ECGF are both upregulated by hypoxia and estrogens, synthesis of these growth factors by paragangliomas can contribute to the increased incidence and progression of these tumors in hypoxic states and in women. Expression of these angiogenic growth factors by paragangliomas again draws comparison to Von Hippel–Lindau disease, because many of the hypervascular tumors associated with VHL express hypoxia-inducible factors such as VEGF (27). Finally, the recently identified mutations in *SDHD* may cause inappropriate signaling of hypoxia, which culminates in overexpression of proteins such as VEGF. In addition to driving angiogenesis, which would indirectly support tumor growth, VEGF might interact with its receptors on tumor cells as part of an autocrine (self-sustaining) mechanism (33).

HISTOLOGY

As seen in light microscopy, paragangliomas recapitulate the endocrinologic organization of normal paraganglia. These tumors consist of organoid clusters of type I ("chief") and type II ("sustentacular") cells, which have been described as "Zellballen." These clusters are surrounded by a highly vascular stroma containing numerous capillary-sized vessels (Fig. 41.1). Chief cells are polygonal, epithelioid cells that comprise the bulk of the Zellballen and are considered to be modified neurons. Their cy-

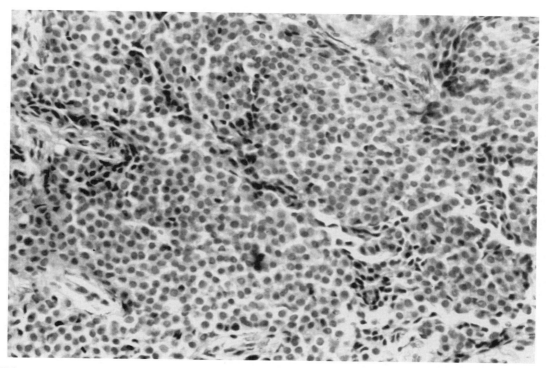

FIG. 41.1 Paraganglioma with predominance of chief cells. Note there are no mitoses. H&E, 127X. (Courtesy of Dr. J. Gershon Spector, Department of Otorhinolaryngology—Head and Neck Surgery, Washington University, St. Louis.)

toplasm has a granular quality due to the presence of numerous vacuoles and catecholamine-containing granules, which are best demonstrated with electron microscopy (Fig. 41.2). Elongated sustentacular cells envelop the chief cells but are difficult to observe on standard light microscopy. Their function may be analogous to Schwann cells or pericytes, and a decrease in their number relative to normal paraganglia is a feature of paragangliomas (34). Identification of sustentacular cells is important, because their presence allows differentiation of paragangliomas from other neuroendocrine lesions such as carcinoid tumors (35). Most jugulotympanic paragangliomas have a highly cellular pattern; in contrast, hyalinized collagenous septae separating clusters of tumor cells are associated with glomus vagale lesions (6).

Immunohistochemically, chief cells can be identified by chromogranin staining, whereas sustentacular cells are highlighted by neural markers such as S-100 or neuron-specific enolase. A host of substances, including substance P, vasoactive intestinal peptide, and somatostatin, have also been identified in paragangliomas with immunohistochemistry (36).

The overall rate of malignancy in paragangliomas is about 5%, considering all sites in the head and neck, and the incidence of malignancy in temporal bone lesions is slightly less (37). The highest rate of malignancy has been associated with glomus vagale lesions, up to 19% (38). The exact criteria for "malignancy" have been debated. For example, extensive local invasion and bone destruction have been considered indicators of malignancy. There is also immunohistochemical evidence that malignant paragangliomas express fewer neuropeptides than benign tumors (36). However, it is now accepted that histologic features such as mitotic figures and nuclear pleomorphism do not reliably distinguish malignant from benign paragangliomas. Even frank DNA aneuploidy is not correlated with either aggressive local extension or metastatic disease (39). Ultimately, the only clear indicator of malignancy in these lesions is metastatic spread to lymph nodes or distant sites that do not contain paraganglia, such as lung, bone, and liver. Using this criterion, metastases can be easily distinguished from multicentric lesions, which should be presumed if the coexisting lesions are found in sites known to contain paraganglia. It should be noted that evidence of malignancy in the form of bone metastases has been reported up to 6 years after surgical removal of the primary tumor (40).

Cranial nerve involvement by paragangliomas occurs through infiltration along neural microvasculature, not simple compression. A grading system has been proposed based on involvement of epineurium, perineurium, and endoneurium (41). Unfortunately, clinical assessment of cranial nerve palsies underestimates the rate of neural invasion observed intraoperatively and confirmed with histopathology; clinically, the facial nerve is most often impaired, whereas intraoperatively the vagus nerve is most often invaded (41).

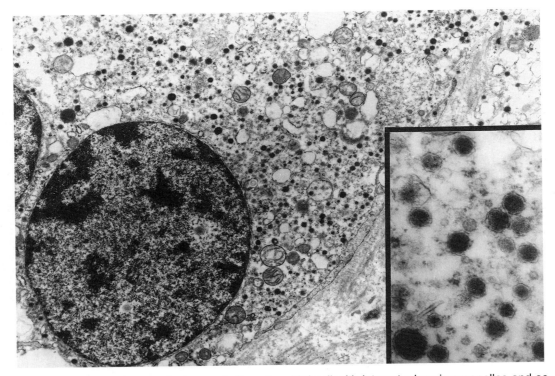

FIG. 41.2 Electron microscopic demonstration of a chief cell with intracytoplasmic organelles and secretory granules. 12,000X. *Insert:* higher magnification of secretory granules. 44,000X. (Courtesy of Dr. Paul E. Swanson, Department of Pathology, Washington University School of Medicine, St. Louis.)

CLINICAL PRESENTATION

Glomus tympanicum tumors typically present with pulsatile tinnitus and unilateral hearing loss, which is usually conductive in nature. However, sensorineural hearing loss accompanying these lesions has been observed, which occasionally improves after surgical removal. Otoscopic examination reveals a reddish mass, often in the anteroinferior quadrant of an otherwise normal middle ear, forming a meniscus where the mass contacts the tympanic membrane. However, because the tumors are roughly spherical, the meniscus underestimates the size of the tumor. Occasionally, extension of a glomus tympanicum into the eustachian tube orifice results in secondary serous otitis media. When the entire circumference or at least maximum diameter of the mass is visible above the tympanic annulus, the diagnosis of a glomus tympanicum can be made (Fig. 41.3). With positive pressure pneumatoscopy, Brown's sign can be elicited, consisting of an initial phase of blanching (by displacement of venous congestion), followed by arterial pulsations (43).

Glomus jugulare tumors are more varied in presentation due to their capacity to involve lower cranial nerves and to extend intracranially. Nonetheless, otologic symptoms predominate early, with lower cranial nerve deficits occurring later. Pulsatile tinnitus is the most common presenting symptom, followed by conductive hearing loss (44). Symptoms of lower cranial nerve dysfunction, including hoarseness, dysphagia, aspiration, or dysarthria, are the next most common form of presentation, followed by otalgia and either bloody or purulent otorrhea. Bleeding from the ear can be provoked by coughing, sneezing, or straining. Vertigo can be a presenting symptom in about 20% of cases of glomus jugulare. Presentation with a neck mass is uncommon.

On otoscopy, the appearance of a glomus jugulare tumor can range from the barely visible dome of a vascular mass to complete tumor obliteration of the middle ear space with erosion through the tympanic membrane and formation of a polyp. With any glomus jugulare tumor, the maximum diameter of the mass is hidden below the fibrous annulus. Neovascularization in the form of dilated arterial vessels can be seen along the external auditory canal and tympanic membrane, demonstrating the angiogenic nature of these lesions (Fig. 41.4).

A thorough cranial nerve exam may demonstrate additional palsies that have not troubled the patient, but in most cases the exam will merely confirm symptomatic deficits. On exam, the most common cranial nerve involved by glomus jugulare tumors is the facial nerve (Fig. 41.5), with the most common site of involvement being the vertical segment (41). Deficits of cranial nerves IX, X, XI, and XII can occur in isolation or various combinations, and classic jugular foramen syndromes can occur, which are easily recognized. Unfortunately, tumors can also invade these nerves without clinical signs, creating a dilemma when discovered intraoperatively. Deficits of cranial nerves V and VI are unusual, due to the infrequency of middle fossa extension (45). Involvement of the adventitia of the carotid artery can present as Horner's syndrome.

By themselves, symptoms and signs cannot reliably predict the extent of glomus jugulare tumors, and it is well known that very extensive tumors can occur with minimal symptoms and sometimes no demonstrable cranial nerve deficits. However, Spector and colleagues (45) have identified findings that are associated with intracranial extension. In their series, 50% of patients with Horner's syndrome had evidence of middle fossa invasion, 50% of patients with

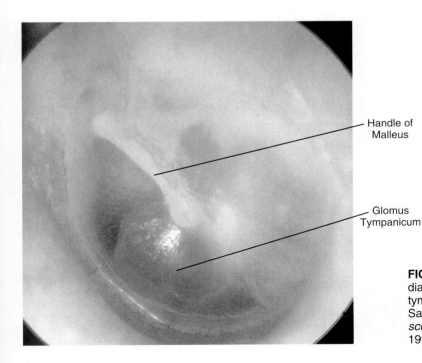

Handle of Malleus

Glomus Tympanicum

FIG. 41.3 Glomus tympanicum. Note that the greatest diameter of the lesion is superior to the level of the tympanic annulus. (Reprinted with permission from Sanna M, Russo A, De Donato G. *Color atlas of otoscopy: from diagnosis to surgery.* New York: Thieme, 1999:85, 91.)

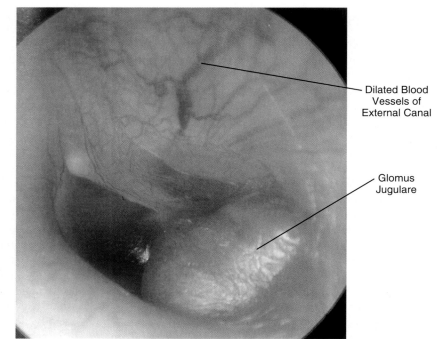

Dilated Blood
Vessels of
External Canal

Glomus
Jugulare

FIG. 41.4 Glomus jugulare. Note that the greatest diameter of the lesion cannot be visualized superior to the tympanic annulus. Dilated blood vessels extend toward the tumor along the posterosuperior canal wall. (Reprinted with permission from Sanna M, Russo A, De Donato G. *Color atlas of otoscopy: from diagnosis to surgery.* New York: Thieme, 1999:85, 91.)

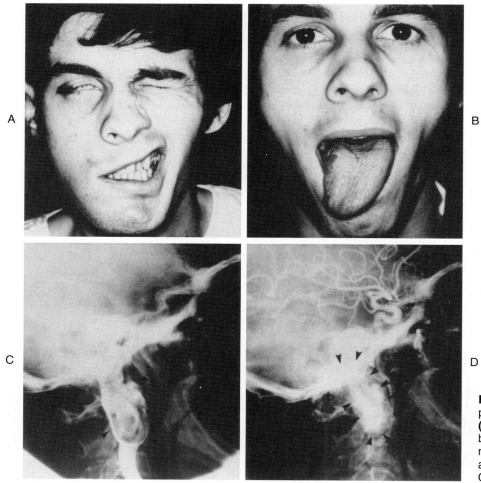

FIG. 41.5 A 23-year-old man with facial paralysis **(A)** and hypoglossal paralysis **(B).** The internal jugular vein is occluded by tumor **(C),** and the arteriogram denotes tumor boundaries *(arrowheads)* and vascularity **(D).** (Courtesy of Dr. J. Gershon Spector.)

jugular foramen symptoms had posterior fossa invasion, and 75% of patients with hypoglossal nerve paralysis had posterior fossa extension (44). Patterns of temporal bone invasion have been described by Spector and colleagues (45) and are illustrated in Fig. 41.6.

Facial nerve paralysis can be a presenting symptom of a paraganglioma, most commonly due to involvement of the mastoid segment by direct extension of a glomus jugulare tumor (41). Rarely, a primary paraganglioma of the fallopian canal, which produces smooth expansion of the canal similar to a schwannoma, can present with a facial palsy or pulsatile tinnitus without facial paralysis (46). As with most neoplastic involvement of the facial nerve, the paralysis is usually progressive in onset, but it can occur suddenly or even be heralded by twitching or hemifacial spasm.

DIFFERENTIAL DIAGNOSIS

The differential diagnosis of a vascular mass in the middle ear includes paragangliomas and other neoplasms, vascular anomalies, and inflammatory lesions. Other tumors of the temporal bone, including meningioma, facial nerve schwannoma, and adenomatous tumors with or without neuroendocrine differentiation (carcinoid tumor), should be considered. Rare lesions such as hemangiopericytoma, extramedullary plasmacytoma, and giant cell tumor can be in-

distinguishable from glomus jugulare tumors, clinically and radiographically (47,48). Metastatic tumors have also been confused with glomus tympanicum and glomus jugulare tumors (49). However, with the exception of endolymphatic sac tumors, few other neoplasms of the temporal bone display the same degree of vascularity as paragangliomas. On otoscopy, a vascular anomaly, especially an aberrant or aneurysmal carotid artery or a persistent stapedial artery, can be easily confused with a paraganglioma by its arterial coloration and pulsatile nature (50). A high-riding jugular bulb may be easier to distinguish from a paraganglioma by its more posterior location in the middle ear, lack of pulsations, and bluish hue. An inflammatory polyp due to chronic otitis media can mimic a paraganglioma that has eroded through the tympanic membrane and become secondarily infected.

Of all the lesions that could be potentially misconstrued as a glomus tumor, the aberrant internal carotid artery carries the greatest potential for a catastrophic error. The failure to preoperatively distinguish an aberrant internal carotid artery from other vascular lessons of the middle ear can result in grave consequences, including stroke and death. For this reason, it is essential that all patients, including those with suspected glomus tympanicum, be evaluated with a high-resolution computed tomographic (CT) scan to ensure that the carotid artery resides in its normal location and is not in continuity with the middle ear mass.

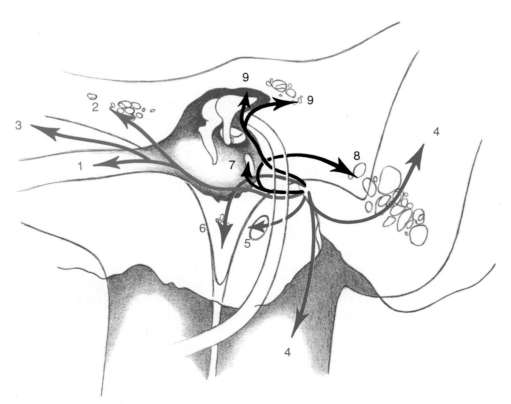

FIG. 41.6 Schema of tumor spread from the protympanum to eustachian tube *(1),* peritubal cells *(2),* and internal carotid artery *(3);* from the hypotympanum and jugular bulb into the internal jugular vein and sigmoid sinus *(4),* inferior petrosal sinus *(5),* carotid sheath in the parapharyngeal space *(6),* and direct invasion of the jugular and hypoglossal canal; and from the mesotympanum to invade the round window *(7),* under the facial nerve *(8),* tegmen tympani, and aditus ad antrum *(9).*

Paraneoplastic Syndromes and Associated Lesions

The most commonly recognized paraneoplastic syndrome of paragangliomas is excess catecholamine production (1% to 4% of all paragangliomas). Based on their neuroendocrine derivation, paragangliomas possess the necessary enzymes to synthesize norepinephrine, but in most cases they lack phenylethanolamine N-methyl transferase (PNMT) and therefore cannot synthesize epinephrine. However, one case report indicated that a glomus jugulare tumor can contain PNMT and secrete epinephrine (51). Although all paragangliomas are capable of catecholamine synthesis, only tumors that elevate serum levels at least fourfold to fivefold above normal will produce symptoms (52). Rarely, tumors secreting catecholamines above this threshold will remain asymptomatic. Symptoms of excess catecholamine production include headaches, nausea, palpitations, perspiration, and pallor, as well as angina, anxiety, and episodic flushing; these symptoms may be evoked with tumor manipulation during physical examination. Although hypertension is the most common physical sign, it can be episodic, leaving only signs of chronic hypertension, such as cardiac hypertrophy (52). It is important to search for these symptoms and signs in the preoperative evaluation of any patient, because surgery on a secreting tumor can induce a hypertensive crisis, with intraoperative risks of myocardial infarction or stroke. Vasomotor crisis usually does not occur after routine embolization, but it has been reported after embolization of a secreting tumor (53).

Diagnosis of a secreting tumor depends on serum catecholamine levels and a 24-hour urine collection for norepinephrine breakdown products, normetanephrine and vanillylmandelic acid. Certain medications, such as monoamine oxidase inhibitors and dopamine derivatives, can produce false-positive results and therefore must be discontinued prior to testing. If serum and urine testing are negative but a history consistent with catecholamine excess has been obtained, direct sampling of the venous return from the tumor site should be performed by an interventional radiologist. If specific elevation of epinephrine is documented, the presence of a synchronous adrenal pheochromocytoma must be considered and ruled out. Once a secreting tumor has been diagnosed, pharmacologic blockade of alpha- and beta-adrenergic receptors must be established for 2 weeks prior to surgery. Postoperative intensive care monitoring is mandatory, because hypotension can follow the removal of a catecholamine-secreting paraganglioma.

Excess secretion of other hormones, including serotonin, cholecystokinin, somatostatin, vasoactive intestinal peptide, and dopamine, have been reported (52). Other syndromes, such as unexplained anemia, have been associated with metastatic paragangliomas (54). Most recently, the association of sensorineural hearing loss with carotid body tumors has been reported; however, this association was ascribed to co-inheritance of sensorineural hearing loss with familial paragangliomas, not a paraneoplastic syndrome (55).

A number of other neoplasms are associated with paragangliomas of the head and neck. These tumors have been associated with the multiple endocrine neoplasia-1 (MEN-1) syndrome, but they are not by themselves a cardinal feature of any of the MEN syndromes. A significant association between paragangliomas and thyroid carcinomas has also been identified. The rare combination of a pulmonary chondroma, gastric leiomyosarcoma, and catecholamine-secreting paraganglioma is known as Carney's triad (56).

Radiology

CT and magnetic resonance imaging (MRI) with gadolinium enhancement are complementary techniques in the diagnosis and evaluation of temporal bone paragangliomas. Because the hypotympanum and jugular foramen are inaccessible to physical examination, both modalities are invaluable for defining the extent of a suspected paraganglioma. However, as an initial modality, a high-resolution CT scan of the temporal bones (with fine cuts in the axial and coronal planes) provides excellent anatomic information, demonstrating proximity of the tumor to the cochlea, the facial nerve, and the carotid artery. By itself, CT is adequate for assessment of local extension of small lesions involving only the middle ear or confined to the hypotympanum and mastoid (Fisch type A and B). However, even for small tumors, an MR scan is useful to confirm tumor vascularity and to screen for multicentric lesions.

On CT, a glomus tympanicum lesion is often seen as a rounded soft-tissue density on the promontory of the middle ear, limited laterally by the tympanic membrane, and often not associated with any ossicular erosion (Fig. 41.7). A CT also allows clear differentiation of a glomus tympanicum from a vascular anomaly such as an aberrant carotid artery, preventing a potential catastrophe on middle ear exploration. The classic CT finding for a glomus jugulare is loss of the sharp cortical margin at the lateral aspect of the jugular foramen, creating a "moth-eaten" appearance (Fig. 41.8).

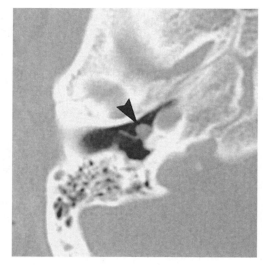

FIG. 41.7 Axial CT of right glomus tympanicum demonstrating rounded soft-tissue density on the promontory of the middle ear.

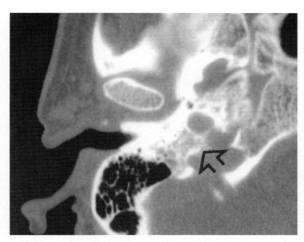

FIG. 41.8 Axial CT of right glomus jugulare demonstrating loss of the sharp cortical bony margin at the lateral aspect of the jugular foramen.

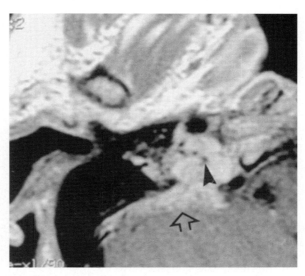

FIG. 41.9 Axial MRI of right glomus jugulare (same case as in Fig. 41.4), demonstrating "salt-and-pepper" consistency with flow voids in the center of the tumor *(arrowhead)*. Also note that the tumor extends retrograde into the sigmoid sinus *(open arrow).*

This contrasts with the smooth bony expansion of the jugular foramen seen with schwannomas. On MRI a glomus jugulare typically has a "salt-and-pepper" pattern, along with serpiginous flow voids (57). Because of its superior soft tissue resolution, MRI better demonstrates the overall size of the tumor, degree of intracranial extension, and relationship to structures of the central nervous system and the carotid artery (Fig. 41.9). Even with these characteristic findings on CT and MRI, the diagnosis of a paraganglioma is not always assured, and, rarely, other neoplasms requiring different management considerations can masquerade as glomus jugulare tumors (47,48).

Angiography

A preoperative angiogram serves several purposes: (i) to confirm the vascular nature of the lesion to support the diagnosis of a paraganglioma (Fig. 41.10); (ii) to define the feeding vessels and to provide an opportunity for embolization (Fig. 41.11); (iii) to display collateral vessels with the internal carotid and vertebral arteries, which must be avoided during embolization (Fig. 41.12); (iv) to help define the size of the lesion; (v) to establish whether the contralateral venous system is patent, informing the surgeon if sacrifice of the ipsilateral sigmoid sinus and jugular vein will compromise cerebral venous outflow (Fig. 41.13); (vi) to demonstrate tumor extension into the sigmoid sinus or jugular vein; and (vii) to identify multicentric tumors, where it remains the gold standard (Fig. 41.14). Definition of feeding vessels can be helpful in determining the site of origin, and the presence of feeding vessels from intracranial circulation can alert the surgeon to the likelihood of intracranial extension. Magnetic resonance angiography (MRA) and MR venography (MRV) can provide some of the same information noninvasively but cannot yet match the resolution of conventional angiography.

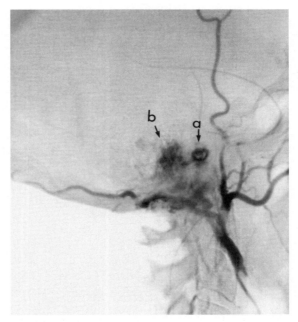

FIG. 41.10 Glomus tympanicum in the middle ear *(a)* invading the mastoid via the antrum *(b)*. Arterial phase of subtraction angiogram of the external carotid artery. (Courtesy of Dr. J. Gershon Spector.)

Moret and colleagues (58) have divided the vascular supply of temporal bone paragangliomas into four "compartments," based on (i) the inferior tympanic branch of the ascending pharyngeal artery, (ii) the stylomastoid artery (arising from either the occipital or the posterior auricular artery), (iii) the anterior tympanic branch of the internal maxillary artery (or a direct caroticotympanic branch of the inter-

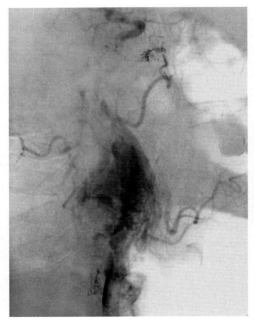

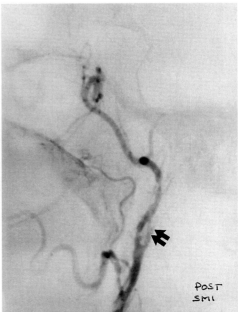

FIG. 41.11 The use of subtraction angiography in tumor embolization. **A:** Capillary phase determines tumor size and feeding vessels. **B:** Tumor completely embolized and vessel occluded *(arrows).* (Courtesy of Dr. J. Gershon Spector.)

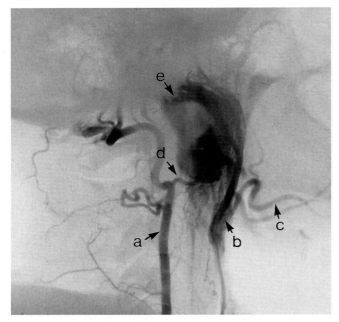

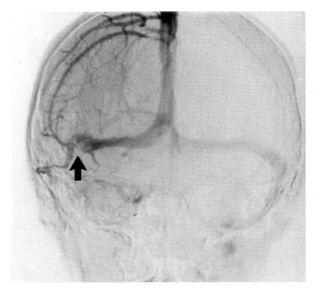

FIG. 41.12 Lateral view of a glomus jugulare tumor by a four-vessel subtraction angiogram. Extension to the carotid sheath between the vertebral artery *(a)* and the carotid artery *(b).* The blood supply is also derived from the internal maxillary artery *(c)* and aberrant vessels from the vertebral artery *(d).* The cephalic border is clearly delineated *(e).* (Courtesy of Dr. J. Gershon Spector.)

FIG. 41.13 Venogram demonstrates growth within the vein lumen to the level of the lateral sinus *(arrow).* The outflow is via the larger dural veins. (Courtesy of Dr. J. Gershon Spector.)

nal carotid artery), and (iv) the superior tympanic branch of the middle meningeal artery. As tumors enlarge, they encompass more compartments; because the compartments are hemodynamically independent, the vessels must be individually embolized to effectively devascularize the tumor.

Although paragangliomas are characteristically hypervascular, two cases of "avascular" tumors have been reported (59,60). These lesions did not display the expected tumor "blush" seen on angiography, but Zellballen and hypervascularity were observed histologically. Therefore the absence

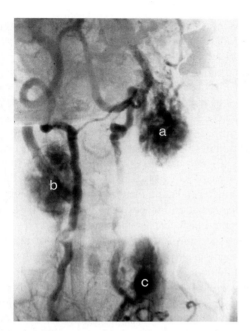

FIG. 41.14 Multiple paragangliomas in a 65-year-old woman. Her two brothers and a sister had carotid body tumors. A four-vessel subtraction carotid arteriogram demonstrates one glomus jugulare (*a*) and two carotid body tumors (*b* and *c*). (Courtesy of Dr. J. Gershon Spector.)

of classic angiographic findings does not always exclude consideration of a paraganglioma in anatomic regions associated with these tumors.

Embolization is a valuable aid in minimizing blood loss during resection of these highly vascular tumors, although it may not be necessary in most glomus tympanicum tumors. Using polyvinyl alcohol or Gelfoam material, the major arterial supply to the tumor can be temporarily interrupted, and the abolition of tumor blush can be confirmed at the completion of the procedure. Reduction of blood loss to less than one-half of nonembolized cases has been documented (61). Depending on the embolization material used, surgery must be performed within 2 or 3 days due to eventual recanalization of embolized vessels. Otalgia and fever are commonly reported after successful devascularization of the tumor and typically resolve spontaneously (62). However, significant complications, including stroke and cranial nerve paralysis, can occur; these can potentially be avoided by testing candidate vessels with lidocaine infusion prior to embolization.

When the carotid artery is involved, angiography and balloon occlusion studies are utilized to confirm adequate collateral flow across the circle of Willis should carotid sacrifice be necessary. At the same time that adequate cross-flow is confirmed angiographically, serial neurologic examination and xenon blood flow measurements are necessary to confirm the safety of carotid occlusion. These additional measures are important, because in the past approximately 14% of patients cleared by angiographic

means alone ultimately did not tolerate carotid occlusion (63). A more recent review documented permanent strokes in 9 of 192 (4.7%) patients undergoing sacrifice of the internal carotid artery after passing a balloon occlusion test (64).

Evaluation of Multicentricity

Which radiologic technique is best to screen for multicentricity in the head and neck remains controvsersial. Currently, an angiogram is the gold standard that other techniques must be measured by. However, from a practical standpoint the angiogram is usually deferred until the time of admission so that embolization can be performed 1 or 2 days prior to surgery. In a minority of cases, this can lead to alteration of treatment plans if one or more unsuspected temporal bone or neck paragangliomas are identified. A sensitive, noninvasive technique for screening multicentric lesions would ideally detect all paragangliomas of the temporal bone and neck in the early phases of treatment planning. An MRI is currently recommended as the most sensitive screening modality, detecting tumors as small as 5 mm in diameter, and it is especially useful for screening patients at risk for familial paragangliomas (65).

Radionuclide scanning with octreotides such as ^{123}iodine-labeled Tyr^3-octreotide is less sensitive, demonstrating lesions 1 cm in diameter or larger (66). However, asymptomatic glomus tympanicum lesions have been identified with this technique, and one study indicated that tumors 5 mm in diameter could be detected (67). One advantage with this technique is that the entire body, with attention to the mediastinum and abdomen, can be screened. In addition, because octreotide imaging takes advantage of somatostatin receptor expression by paragangliomas, this modality may be more specific and therefore potentially useful in distinguishing tumor recurrence from scar formation in previous treatment sites (68). Finally, octreotide imaging is reported to have no side effects. In a series of 21 suspected head and neck paragangliomas, octreotide scanning demonstrated a sensitivity of 94% and a specificity of 75% (69). Some authors recommend initial screening of high-risk individuals with this technique, followed by MRI dedicated to areas of abnormal uptake and a follow-up octreotide scan in 5 years if the initial image is negative (70).

Treatment

As with other lesions of the skull base, for glomus jugulare tumors a biopsy may not be readily available prior to starting treatment. When there is an easily accessed component of the tumor, such as polypoid extension into the middle ear or external auditory canal, a biopsy should be performed in the operating room. Similarly, if there is an accessible component in the mastoid, a cortical mastoidectomy with biopsy can prevent misdiagnosis of other lesions mimicking a glomus jugulare tumor.

Radiation Therapy for Paragangliomas

Radiation therapy can be used as a single treatment modality, as adjunctive treatment following surgery, or as salvage after surgical failure. The decision to select radiation therapy as the primary treatment modality must be made by the surgeon and the patient after considering several factors, including (i) the necessity for treatment after serial imaging, (ii) the patient's age and general medical health, (iii) the size and location of the tumor, and (iv) the number of existing cranial nerve deficits. It must be kept in mind that most paragangliomas are benign; therefore when nonsurgical treatment has been chosen, initial observation with serial MRI scans may be a reasonable option in selected cases (9). If observation has been chosen, the decision to treat can be prompted later by (i) observed growth or (ii) onset of new cranial nerve deficits. In considering age, a patient's physiologic state should be weighed more heavily than simple chronologic age.

Radiation therapy is not recommended for glomus tympanicum lesions, because these can be resected with minimal risks to hearing and facial nerve function. As a sole modality, radiation therapy is also inadvisable for young patients with glomus jugulare lesions, given their long-term potential for regrowth and the subsequent risks of surgery in an irradiated field. Radiotherapy can be useful for large glomus jugulare lesions without any cranial nerve findings, because surgery for these cases might result in multiple, acute cranial nerve deficits. Radiation therapy is also indicated for elderly or medically unstable patients, provided the necessity for treatment has been established. Specific situations in which radiotherapy is warranted include (i) progressive disease in patients refusing surgery, (ii) extensive central nervous system (CNS) involvement, (iii) preexisting contralateral vagal or hypoglossal deficits where surgery might incur bilateral lower cranial nerve palsies, (iv) residual disease after attempted resection, such as tumor investing the internal carotid artery, and (v) salvage treatment following incomplete surgical resection.

The total dose of radiotherapy usually is 40 to 50 Gy, given over a 4- to 5-week schedule. In the past, cobalt-60 gamma radiation was typically delivered using a pair of ipsilateral, oblique fields through wedge filters. More recently, techniques using photons (megavoltage radiographs) and electrons (linear accelerator), as well as the gamma "knife," have been utilized (71,72). Treatment guidelines have evolved after protocols using higher doses were associated with higher complication rates but not greater control rates. After review of more than 200 radiated glomus tympanicum and jugulare tumors reported in the literature, Kim et al. concluded that the optimum dosage was between 40 and 50 Gy, because below 40 Gy, the recurrence rate increased significantly, and above 50 Gy, the incidence of complications increased (73). Complications of doses greater than 50 Gy included facial nerve paralysis, osteoradionecrosis of the temporal bone, stenosis of the external auditory canal, and chronic otitis media. Late local recurrence with distant metastases after radiotherapy has also been reported (74). Of concern, radiation-induced malignancies can occur years after doses of 50 Gy or less (75,76).

Whether radiation causes direct damage to paraganglioma tumor cells has been questioned. In a study of five radiated, then resected, paragangliomas, Spector and coworkers (77) demonstrated a decrease in the number of small vessels (less than 100 μm) and persistence of viable type I tumor cells that were encased in reactive fibrosis (Fig. 41.15). Hawthorne and coworkers (7) also described intact tumor cells without evidence of necrosis in eight cases requiring surgery for tumor progression after radiation therapy. Based on this evidence, it appears that radiation induces vasculitis and fibrosis without much specific injury to the type I cells themselves. Interestingly, after short-term follow-up, the degree of tumor blush seen angiographically can vary considerably after gamma "knife" radiotherapy with or without a corresponding change in tumor volume (78). The mechanism for radiation control of paraganglioma growth, then, may depend more on an antiangiogenic effect rather than any direct effect on type I cells.

Success rates for radiotherapy ranging from 80% to 100% have been reported (79,80). However, the criteria that are used to define "success" or "local control" need to be clearly stated, such as arrest of tumor growth or actual reduction in size or improvement of cranial nerve symptoms. After radiation, most patients have reported significant improvement in symptoms such as pulsatile tinnitus and otalgia but little change in pretreatment cranial nerve deficits. In one series of 38 patients treated with primary radiotherapy (n = 14), combined therapy (n = 13), or salvage radiotherapy (n = 11), 38% had symptomatic improvement and 10% demonstrated partial or complete reversal of cranial nerve deficits; however, local control rates for the three groups were 79%, 100%, and 91%, respectively (71). A recent report on gamma knife treatment indicated reduction of tumor size in 40% of 47 patients, within a median follow-up of 2 years with the remaining cases showing no growth (78). Another report of eight patients with glomus jugulare tumors indicated that improvement of cranial nerve symptoms such as pulsatile tinnitus occurred within 6 months after stereotactic radiotherapy (81).

If arrest of tumor growth is used as a criterion for success, then ideally, tumor progression should have been documented by serial MRI prior to radiotherapy. Ultimately, control of tumor progression over 10 to 20 years needs to be assessed, given the indolent growth of paragangliomas. Indeed, postradiation tumor progression requiring surgical salvage can occur at any time, with a reported range of 4 months to 22 years (7).

Medical Treatment

It has been suggested that long-term administration of octreotides may cause reduction of paragangliomas of the head and neck, but very limited MRI volumetry data have been provided (67). Using subcutaneous injections of octreotides,

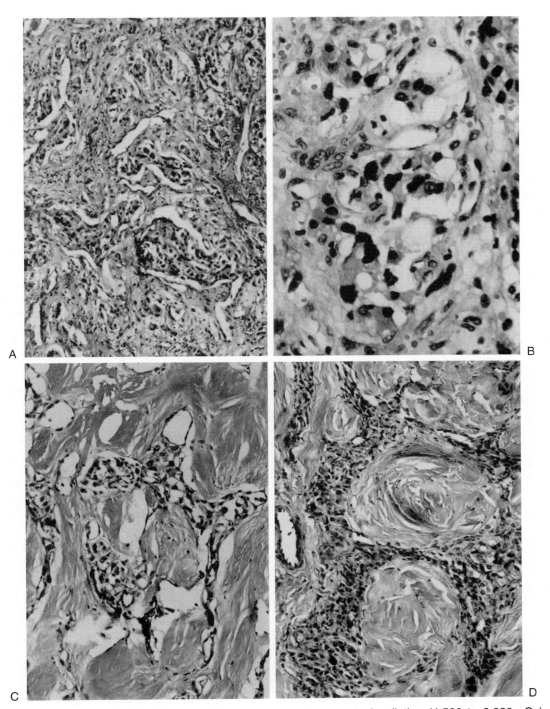

FIG. 41.15 Four histologic patterns of glomus tumor responses to irradiation (4,500 to 6,020 cGy). **A:** Fibrosis with persistent vasculature and tumor cells. H&E, 81X. **B:** Higher magnification demonstrating variable response by the chief cells to irradiation. H&E, 180X. **C:** Fibrosis of the perineoplastic stroma with persistent chief cells. H&E, 135X. **D:** Endarteritis obliterans in some vessels with fibrosis and persistent tumor cells and vessels. H&E, 135X. (Courtesy of Dr. J. Gershon Spector.)

short-term palliation of a patient with a metastatic adrenal paraganglioma has also been reported (82). Chemotherapy for paragangliomas using cyclophosphamide, doxorubicin, and dacarbazine has been described, but it has been reserved for patients with metastatic disease or an unresectable primary (83). As more is learned about the angiogenic biology of these tumors, pharmacologic inhibition of angiogenesis may provide an alternate form of treatment.

Observation

The natural history of paragangliomas has been examined by following untreated patients over an average of 13.5 years (9). In that series of 17 untreated patients with hereditary tumors and 9 patients with sporadic lesions, there was no worsening of the mortality rate due to local or metastatic disease compared with patient groups undergoing surgery, radiation therapy, or combined treatment (9). Keeping in mind the typically benign histopathology of these tumors, observation with serial MRI scans must be discussed as an initial option, especially if the patient has few symptoms or no cranial nerve deficits. Although guidelines for timing of repeat imaging are not well established, it is reasonable to reimage at 6 months from initial diagnosis with subsequent images every 6 to 12 months given the slow growth of most lesions. Ultimately, the option of observation or "watchful waiting" must be weighed against treatment with radiation therapy, which has very low morbidity, does not preclude future surgery, and may prevent further progression.

Surgical Treatment

Surgical removal of glomus tympanicum and jugulare tumors has been significantly improved with descriptions of the anterior hypotympanic and infratemporal fossa approaches by Farrior and Fisch, respectively (84,85). In addition, better delineation of tumor boundaries with CT and MRI and improved tumor devascularization with angiographic techniques have contributed to higher success rates. The establishment of skull base teams, including neurosurgeons and head and neck surgeons experienced in neurotologic procedures, has also been invaluable.

Glomus Tympanicum Tumors

Small type A tumors can be removed through a transcanal tympanotomy approach, provided the external canal is sufficiently wide. Canal incisions must be adjusted to allow more anterior and inferior middle ear exposure relative to a standard stapedectomy flap, because the tumors are often based anteriorly, along the course of Jacobson's nerve. An argon laser delivered through a fiber-optic handpiece can be helpful to coagulate feeding vessels and to ablate any residual tumor on the underlying bone. This can be accomplished simultaneously, lasing at the junction of the tumor and the promontory as the mass is elevated anteriorly.

Larger type A tumors with hypotympanic extension should be removed using the anterior hypotympanic approach of Farrior with facial nerve monitoring. Through a postauricular incision, bony canal exposure is established, with the inferior cut for the Korner's canal flap biased more anteriorly to allow full exposure of the floor of the canal. From approximately 2 o'clock to 10 o'clock, the tympanic membrane, the annulus, and a short segment of canal skin are elevated and folded onto the manubrium of the malleus. Using diamond burs, the anterior, posterior, and inferior bony annulus and canal floor are drilled to expose the hypotympanum, taking care to avoid the mastoid segment of the facial nerve posteriorly. Once the inferior border of the tumor is visualized, feeding vessels from the inferior tympanic artery are controlled either with bipolar cautery or a slightly defocused laser. Tumor removal can proceed as described for smaller type A tumors, again using bipolar cautery or a laser as an adjunct. The middle ear is packed with Gelfoam, and the gap between the fibrous annulus and the lowered canal floor is bridged by a temporalis fascia graft. Any exposed areas of the bony canal can be covered with split-thickness skin grafts. The tympanic membrane and graft are held in place with a rosebud pack of nylon mesh strips around cotton packing, and the remainder of the external canal is packed with an outer layer of antibiotic ointment–filled gauze. The postauricular wound is closed with subcutaneous absorbable sutures and Steri-strips.

For tumors extending into the mastoid but *not* infiltrating bone around the jugular bulb or carotid artery (type B), a canal wall–up mastoidectomy with an extended facial recess approach is optimal. Postauricular exposure is established as described earlier. The same maneuvers in the anterior hypotympanic approach can be utilized to maximize exposure of the middle ear component of the tumor prior to performing a canal wall–up mastoidectomy. The facial nerve is skeletonized down to the stylomastoid foramen, and an extended facial recess is developed, sacrificing the chorda tympani and following the contour of the bony annulus inferiorly and anteriorly. Care should be taken to avoid overly thinning any part of the bony canal wall. Retrofacial air cells are removed, demonstrating the limits of the mastoid component of the tumor and its proximity to the jugular bulb. The tumor can be mobilized from multiple angles with laser assistance if needed. Early control of feeding vessels from the anterior and inferior tympanic arteries during tumor dissection may reduce bleeding, facilitating removal.

Type B tumors with erosion of the posterior canal wall, extensive middle ear involvement, or facial nerve invasion may require a canal wall–down approach with removal of the tympanic membrane, malleus, and incus, and decompression or cable grafting of the facial nerve. Hearing reconstruction can be performed as for chronic ear surgery. An adequate meatoplasty will allow surveillance for tumor recurrence postoperatively. However, if the resulting cavity is too large or if postoperative radiation is planned, tympanomastoid obliteration with abdominal fat and blind sac closure of the external auditory canal is preferable to avoid epithelial breakdown and chronic drainage from a radiated mastoid cavity (86).

Glomus Jugulare Tumors

The classic method for removal of glomus jugulare lesions is the infratemporal fossa approach of Fisch (87). To maximize hearing and facial nerve function postoperatively, new approaches have been developed, including the hearing preservation approach described by Glasscock and Jackson

(88) and the fallopian bridge technique of Pensak and Jackler (89). The primary determinants of whether these other approaches can be used are tumor size and level of carotid artery involvement.

In the classic infratemporal fossa approach, facial nerve and lower cranial nerve monitoring are utilized. A wide C-shaped incision is created, with its midpoint about 8 cm posterior to the postauricular sulcus and its inferior limb extending into a cervical skin crease two fingerbreadths inferior to the angle of the mandible (Fig. 41.16). This delineates a broad anteriorly based flap incorporating the pinna; the flap is elevated in a plane just superficial to the temporalis fascia and mastoid periosteum and in a subplatysmal plane inferiorly. Alternatively, the superior plane of dissection can be developed just deep to the hair follicle roots if a temporoparietal fascial flap is required. The temporalis muscle and its vascular pedicle should be preserved for potential use in reconstruction or facial reanimation. The external auditory canal is transected at the bony cartilaginous junction and the skin of the cartilaginous canal is dissected circumferentially, everted as a sleeve through the meatus, and closed as a blind sac. A square flap of soft tissue can be harvested from the undersurface of the pinna and rotated forward to reinforce the canal closure (Fig. 41.17). Retractors

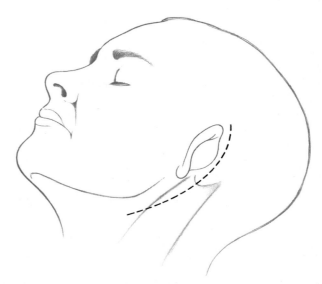

FIG. 41.16 Infratemporal fossa approach for removal of glomus tumor of the jugular foramen. A postauricular incision is carried into the neck for exposure of the great vessels and cranial nerves.

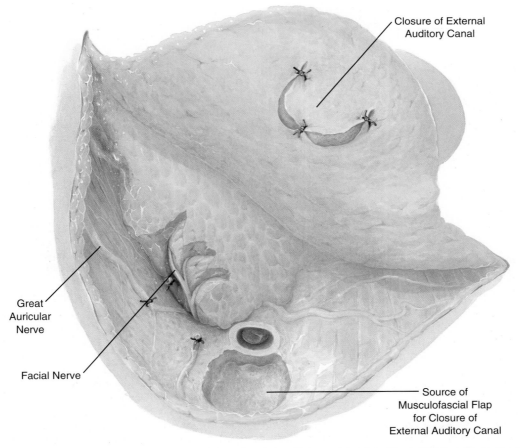

Closure of External Auditory Canal

Great Auricular Nerve

Facial Nerve

Source of Musculofascial Flap for Closure of External Auditory Canal

FIG. 41.17 A postauricular incision has been elevated and the external auditory canal closed primarily employing a musculofascial flap from the lateral mastoid cortex. The greater auricular nerve is identified and preserved for later grafting if necessary. The facial nerve has been exposed.

are positioned with the parotid fascia forming the anterior limit of exposure.

A canal wall–down mastoidectomy is performed, defining the tegmen mastoideum, sigmoid sinus, posterior fossa plate, and digastric ridge. All squamous epithelium is meticulously removed from the bony canal along with the tympanic membrane, malleus, and incus. The superior margin of the tumor is assessed. The posterior bony canal wall is lowered to the level of the mastoid segment of the facial nerve, which is skeletonized from the geniculate ganglion down to the stylomastoid foramen (Fig. 41.18). The tympanic bone is drilled away, proceeding anteriorly until the capsule of the temporomandibular joint and parotid fascia are encountered. The anterosuperior limit of the tumor is now visualized. Bone over the carotid genu is thinned, following the carotid into the medial wall of the eustachian tube orifice. The orifice is widened to allow thorough obliteration at completion of the operation. At this point, after thinning the digastric ridge to an "eggshell" and disattaching the sternocleidomastoid muscle, the mastoid tip is removed, taking care to preserve the periosteal sheath around the facial nerve at the sty-

lomastoid foramen. All bone is removed from the sigmoid sinus and the posterior fossa plate, and the sinus is followed inferiorly to the level of the jugular bulb. The sinus is doubly ligated, preferably below the level of the mastoid emissary vein, by making dural incisions anterior and posterior to the sinus and passing 2-0 silk sutures.

A carotid sheath dissection is performed, identifying cranial nerves X, XI, and XII. The internal jugular vein is ligated and divided inferior to any intraluminal tumor extension. With the stump of the jugular vein reflected superiorly, the internal carotid artery is followed to the skull base and vessel loops are loosely placed around the internal, external, and common carotid arteries (Fig. 41.19).

Facial nerve mobilization can proceed after meticulously removing eggshell-thin bone over the mastoid and tympanic segments of the nerve, including the geniculate ganglion. A groove can be drilled into the remaining bone at the root of the zygoma to accept the transposed facial nerve. The posterior belly of the digastric muscle is elevated in continuity with the periosteum investing the stylomastoid foramen. The entire complex is rotated anteriorly, with the facial nerve re-

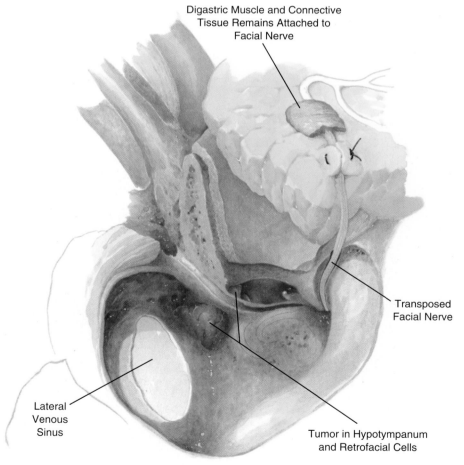

Digastric Muscle and Connective
Tissue Remains Attached to
Facial Nerve

Transposed
Facial Nerve

Lateral
Venous
Sinus

Tumor in Hypotympanum
and Retrofacial Cells

FIG. 41.18 An extended canal wall–down mastoidectomy has been performed. The lateral venous sinus has been exposed by removal of a portion of the posterior fossa plate. The facial nerve has been mobilized in its descending segment and transposed anteriorly. At the stylomastoid foramen, a small piece of digastric muscle and surrounding fascia is left attached to the facial nerve to avoid trauma at this location.

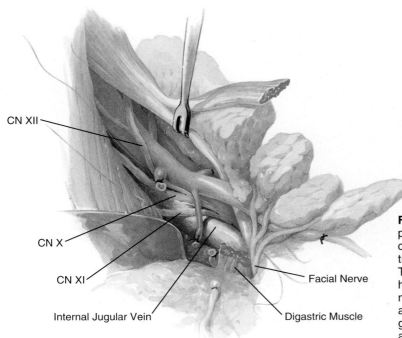

CN XII

CN X

CN XI

Internal Jugular Vein

Facial Nerve

Digastric Muscle

FIG. 41.19 Exposure of the upper neck for infratemporal fossa procedure. The sternocleidomastoid muscle has been separated from the mastoid tip and retracted posteriorly and the digastric muscle divided. The internal jugular vein, common carotid artery, and hypoglossal (XII), vagus (X), and accessory (XI) cranial nerves are identified. The external carotid artery and its branches (facial, occipital, ascending pharyngeal, and postauricular) are ligated above the lingual artery. Sutures are passed, but not tied, around the internal jugular vein and internal carotid artery.

flected at the level of the geniculate ganglion; the digastric muscle is sutured anteriorly to maintain the nerve in a tension-free, transposed position. With this technique, extrinsic vascular supply to the distal facial nerve may be better preserved with improved functional results. Moist Gelfoam is placed over the transposed facial nerve to prevent desiccation. In addition, the substance of the parotid gland can be incised and closed over the facial nerve trunk to protect it.

With the jugular foramen now maximally exposed, all remaining bone and fibrous bands are removed from the jugular bulb (Fig. 41.20). The lower cranial nerves are followed as far superiorly as allowed by the exposure and protected during the final extirpation. The tumor is mobilized from the promontory, hypotympanum, and retrofacial air cells, and attention is then directed to separating the tumor from the carotid, if necessary. Careful subadventitial dissection can often be successful if the tumor does not directly invade the vessel wall (Fig. 41.21). Final tumor excision requires a series of incisions around the base of the tumor on the dome of the jugular bulb, rapidly packing the lumen with Surgicel as the incisions are extended (Fig. 41.22). Incisions may have to be extended along the lateral aspect of the sigmoid sinus and jugular vein to retrieve intraluminal extensions of the tumor. Because the bulb has been isolated proximally and distally, the remaining venous inflow from the inferior petrosal sinus must be controlled with direct packing of its lumen on the medial wall of the bulb. Overly aggressive packing can lead to postoperative cranial nerve palsies. The stump of the jugular vein and the remaining lateral wall of the jugular bulb are removed with the tumor.

Wound closure commences by harvesting an abdominal fat graft with a new set of instruments. To avoid necrosis, liquefaction, and volume loss, the fat graft should be harvested en bloc with minimal fragmentation or use of electrocautery; the donor site is closed in layers over a suction drain. The surgical field is irrigated and meticulous hemostasis is achieved. The eustachian tube is thoroughly obliterated with bone wax after inverting the mucosa deep within the expanded lumen. Any microneural repair that is required is performed at this time. The fat graft is modified to conform to the surgical defect, and the incisional wound is closed in layers. A small suction drain can be placed in the cervical portion of the wound away from the carotid artery and the cranial nerves.

Intracranial Extension

When intracranial extension occurs, the posterior fossa is most commonly involved. Whether to resect in two stages or a single stage is debated, but given the broad exposure available at the completion of the infratemporal fossa approach, it is logical to proceed with removing limited intracranial tumor at one stage. When massive intracranial extension exists, a two-stage approach allows a rested neurosurgical team to proceed on the second day.

Complete bone removal from the posterior fossa dura anterior and posterior to the sigmoid sinus is performed, and the dural incisions cross the sigmoid sinus at or below the ligation site. Using bipolar cautery, the neurosurgeon can microdissect the tumor from the adjacent cerebellum, and a

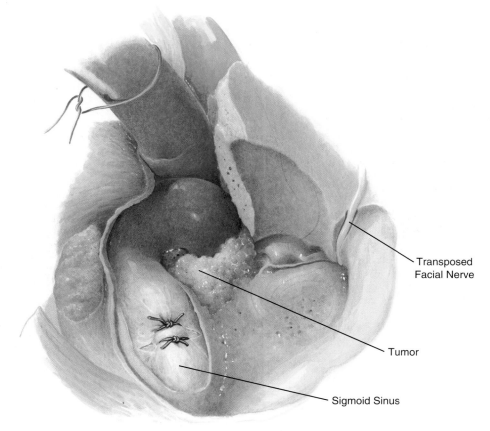

Transposed
Facial Nerve

Tumor

Sigmoid Sinus

FIG. 41.20 The jugular foramen has been exposed by removal of the mastoid tip bone overlying the sigmoid sinus. Additional bone anterior to the jugular vein may also be removed to expose the internal carotid artery. The sigmoid sinus may be occluded by extraluminal or intraluminal packing or by suture ligature after incising the posterior fossa dura as indicated.

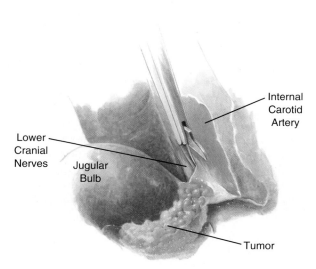

Internal
Carotid
Artery

Lower
Cranial
Nerves

Jugular
Bulb

Tumor

FIG. 41.21 Final en block removal of the dome of the jugular bulb by sharp dissection along lower cranial nerves and internal carotid artery to prevent avulsion injuries to these nerves.

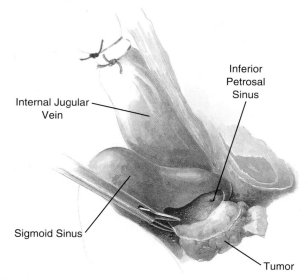

Inferior
Petrosal
Sinus

Internal Jugular
Vein

Sigmoid Sinus

Tumor

FIG. 41.22 After ligation of the internal jugular vein in the neck and occlusion of the sigmoid sinus, dissection is carried intraluminally to preserve the anterior wall of the jugular bulb to protect lower cranial nerves. The ostium of the inferior petrosal sinus is occluded with Surgicel.

plane of separation is often readily established. The tumor is resected with a cuff of dura, and the resultant defect is repaired in a watertight fashion with temporalis fascia. The cerebrospinal fluid pressure is lowered using a lumbar drain for 5 to 7 days.

Surgical Results

Results of surgery, as with radiotherapy, must be assessed over the long term. In general, the surgical results for glomus tympanicum tumors are very favorable, with a low rate of complications and a cure rate approximating 90% (90). The exact results of surgical treatment for glomus jugulare tumors have been obscured by reporting primary surgical cases and surgical salvage after radiation in combination. However, in a series of 52 previously untreated glomus jugulare tumors resected at the House Ear Clinic, 85% were completely excised and 85% of the patients returned to their preoperative level of activity; 29% reported persistent hoarseness or dysphagia, and 95% demonstrated normal or nearly normal facial nerve function on median follow-up of 3 to 4 years (91). In the experience of the University of Zurich in 136 advanced glomus jugulare tumors (Fisch class C or D), total excision with the infratemporal fossa approach was possible in 109 (80%) cases; intradural extension was the primary reason for subtotal resection (92). When total removal was possible, follow-up ranging from 2 to 11 years demonstrated 98% disease-specific survival (92). Using a questionnaire, 36 patients from the same series were surveyed 10 to 15 years postoperatively: 97% felt that their cranial nerve deficits were acceptable, 75% stated they had regained their preoperative quality of life, and 97% had returned to their prior occupation (93).

Complications

Complications of surgery can be divided into intraoperative, immediate postoperative, and delayed postoperative categories. Intraoperative complications include excessive bleeding, cranial nerve injury, and injury to the carotid artery, as well as hypertensive crisis from manipulation of a secreting tumor. Immediate postoperative complications include hematoma formation, infection, spinal fluid leak, and problems related to anesthesia. Delayed postoperative complications include excessive scar formation; complications directly related to cranial nerve deficits, such as corneal exposure after facial nerve paralysis or aspiration pneumonia following vagal nerve injury; or recurrence due to incomplete resection.

Postoperative Care

After resection of a glomus jugulare tumor, the patient is extubated in the operating room or in the intensive care unit the following morning, depending on the duration of the procedure. The patient should be observed in the unit for 24 hours with continuous monitoring using pulse oximetry, electrocardiogram, and an arterial line. Complete blood counts are assessed as the hematocrit equilibrates, and transfusions are selectively given to maintain adequate oxygenation, blood pressure, and heart rate. Decompression of spinal fluid through a lumbar drain at 10 ml per hour may be needed if the procedure required dural repair. A thorough cranial nerve exam is performed, including fiber-optic laryngoscopy to assess vocal cord mobility. If facial paralysis has occurred, early corneal protection with taping of the eyelid, ointment, and artificial tears is mandatory. A nasogastric tube is maintained if there are existing or anticipated swallowing difficulties, which are assessed with a modified barium swallow study when the patient is stable. A Foley catheter and compression stockings are maintained until the patient can ambulate. The number and severity of cranial nerve deficits will dictate much of the postoperative course. Consultation with ophthalmology, speech pathology, and physical therapy services is important for optimal care.

If complete facial paralysis exists, a gold weight implant of the upper eyelid can be performed prior to discharge, with ophthalmologic follow-up as an outpatient. Severe swallowing difficulties and aspiration usually require placement of a percutaneous gastrostomy. Vocal cord medialization with or without cricopharyngeal myotomy can be performed either in the same hospitalization or as a second stage.

CONCLUSION

Paragangliomas are relatively uncommon, highly vascular tumors of the temporal bone with distinct clinical and histopathologic features, as well as an underlying genetic mutation that should soon be identified. Because of their vascularity, propensity to involve cranial nerves, and late potential for CNS invasion, these tumors can pose significant risks to the patient and challenges to the otologic surgeon. Quality of life should be considered when weighing treatment options, because a patient's life expectancy can be relatively unaltered even with persistent disease. Innovative techniques for surgical removal and more precise control of radiation delivery have significantly improved success rates of treatment, but complications are still associated with both methods. Ultimately, new pharmacologic strategies that take advantage of the angiogenic and endocrine nature of paragangliomas may augment the time-honored approaches.

REFERENCES

1. Von Haller A. *Elementa physiologiae corporis humani Lausannae: Fr. Grasset.* Tom IV, Lib X/6-Nervi. Section 41. Nervus sympathicus maximus, vel intercostalis nervus. Ganglion cevicale superius. 1762: 254–257.
2. Valentin G. Über eine gangliöse Anschwellung in der Jacobsonchen Anastomose des Menschen. *Arch Pathol Physiol Lpz* 1840;2:287–290.
3. Krause W. Die Glandula tympanica des Menschen. *Zbl Med Wiss* 1878; 16:737.
4. Guild SR. A hitherto unrecognized structure, the glomus jugularis in man. *Anat Rec* 1941;[Suppl 79]:28.

5. Rosenwasser H. Carotid body tumor of the middl ear and mastoid. *Arch Otolaryngol* 1945;41:64–67.

6. Glenner GG, Grimley PM. Tumors of the extra-adrenal paraganglion system (including chemoreceptors). *Atlas of tumor pathology,* second series, fascicle 9. Armed Forces Institute of Pathology, Washington, DC, 1974.

7. Hawthorne MR, Makek MS, Harris JP, et al. The histopathological and clinical features of irradiated and nonirradiated temporal paragangliomas. *Laryngoscope* 1988;98:325–331.

8. Van der Mey AG, Maaswinkel-Mooy PD, Cornelisse CJ, et al. Genomic imprinting in hereditary glomus tumors: evidence for new genetic theory. *Lancet* 1989;2:1291–1294.

9. Van der Mey AG, Frijns JH, Cornelisse CJ, et al. Does intervention improve the natural course of glomus tumors? A series of 108 patients seen in a 32-year period. *Ann Otol Rhinol Laryngol* 1992;101: 635–642.

10. Gulya AJ. Growth of human paragangliomas in the subrenal capsule of the nude mouse. *Otolaryngol Head Neck Surg* 1998;118:309–311.

11. McCaffrey TV, Meyer FB, Michels VV, et al. Familial paragangliomas of the head and neck. *Arch Otolaryngol Head Neck Surg* 1994;120: 1211–1216.

12. Rainier S, Feinberg AP. Genomic imprinting, DNA methylation, and cancer. *J Natl Cancer Inst* 1994;86:753–759.

13. Heutink P, Van der Mey AG, Sandkuijl LA, et al. A gene subject to genomic imprinting and responsible for hereditary paragangliomas maps to chromosome 11q23-qter. *Hum Mol Genet* 1992;1:7–10.

14. Mariman EC, Van Beersum SE, Cremers CW, et al. Analysis of a second family with hereditary non-chromaffin paragangliomas locates the underlying gene at the proximal region of chromosome 11q. *Hum Genet* 1993;91:357–361.

15. Baysal BE, Farr JE, Rubinstein WS, et al. Fine mapping of an imprinted gene for familial nonchromaffin paragangliomas, on chromosome 11q23. *Am J Hum Genet* 1997;60:121–132.

16. Milunsky J, DeStefano AL, Huang XL, et al. Familial paragangliomas: linkage to chromosome 11q23 and clinical implications. *Am J Med Genet* 1997;72:66–70.

17. Baysal BE, Ferrell RE, Willett-Brozick JE, et al. Mutations in SDHD, a mitochondrial complex II gene, in hereditary paraganglioma. *Science* 2000;287:848–851.

18. Arias-Stella J, Bustos F. Chronic hypoxia and chemodectomas in bovines at high altitudes. *Arch Pathol Lab Med* 1976;100:636–639.

19. Hayes HM Jr, Fraumeni JF Jr. Chemodectomas in dogs: epidemiologic comparisons with man. *J Natl Cancer Inst* 1974;52:1455–1458.

20. Saldana MJ, Salem LE, Travezan R. High altitude hypoxia and chemodectomas. *Hum Pathol* 1973;4:251–263.

21. Rodriguez-Cuevas S, Lopez-Garza J, Labastida-Almendaro S. Carotid body tumors in inhabitants of altitudes higher than 2000 meters above sea level. *Head Neck* 1998;20:374–378.

22. Edwards C, Heath D, Harris P. The carotid body in emphysema and left ventricular hypertrophy. *J Pathol* 1971;104:1–13.

23. Lack EE. Carotid body hypertrophy in patients with cystic fibrosis and cyanotic congenital heart disease. *Hum Pathol* 1976;8: 39–51.

24. Chedid A, Jao W. Hereditary tumors of the carotid bodies and chronic obstructive pulmonary disease. *Cancer* 1974;33:1635–1641.

25. Iliopoulos O, Levy AP, Jiang C, et al. Negative regulation of hypoxia-inducible genes by the von Hippel-Lindau protein. *Proc Natl Acad Sci U S A* 1996;93:10595–10599.

26. Manski TJ, Heffner DK, Glenn GM, et al. Endolymphatic sac tumors. A source of morbid hearing loss in von Hippel-Lindau disease. *JAMA* 1997;277:1461–1466.

27. Zanelli M, Van der Walt JD. Carotid body paraganglioma in von Hippel-Lindau disease: a rare association. *Histopathology* 1996;29: 178–181.

28. Skoldberg F, Grimelius L, Woodward ER, et al. A family with hereditary extra-adrenal paragangliomas without evidence for mutations in the von Hippel-Lindau disease or ret genes. *Clin Endocrinol* 1998;48:11–16.

29. Parry DM, Li FP, Strong LC, et al. Carotid body tumors in humans: genetics and epidemiology. *J Natl Cancer Inst* 1982;68:573–578.

30. Brown JS. Glomus jugulare tumors revisited: a ten-year statistical follow-up of 231 cases. *Laryngoscope* 1985;95:284–288.

31. Folkman J. Tumor angiogenesis: therapeutic implications. *N Engl J Med* 1971;285:1182–1186.

32. Chen J, Dinger B, Jyung RW, et al. Altered expression of vascular endothelial growth factor and flk-1 receptor in chronically hypoxic rat carotid bodies. *Adv Exp Med Biol* 2003;536:583–391.

33. Jyung RW, LeClair EE, Bernat RA, et al. Expression of angiogenic growth factors in paragangliomas. *Laryngoscope* 2000;110:164–167.

34. Kliewer KE, Cochran AJ. A review of the histology, ultrastructure, immunohistology, and molecular biology of extra-adrenal paragangliomas. *Arch Pathol Lab Med* 1989;113:1209–1218.

35. Min KW. Diagnostic usefulness of sustentacular cells in paragangliomas: immunocytochemical and ultrastructural investigation. *Ultrastruct Pathol* 1998;22:369–376.

36. Linnoila RI, Lack EE, Steinberg SM, et al. Decreased expression of neuropeptides in malignant paragangliomas: an immunohistochemical study. *Hum Pathol* 1988;19:41–50.

37. Manolidis S, Shohet JA, Jackson CG, et al. Malignant glomus tumors. *Laryngoscope* 1999;109:30–34.

38. Druck NS, Spector GJ, Ciralsky RH, et al. Malignant glomus vagale: report of a case and review of the literature. *Arch Otolaryngol* 1976; 102:534–536.

39. Van der Mey AG, Cornelisse CJ, Hermans J, et al. DNA flow cytometry of hereditary and sporadic paragangliomas (glomus tumors). *Br J Cancer* 1991;63:298–302.

40. Kawai A, Healey JH, Wilson SC, et al. Carotid body paraganglioma metastatic to bone: report of two cases. *Skeletal Radiol* 1998;27: 103–107.

41. Makek M, Franklin DJ, Zhao JC, et al. Neural infiltration of glomus temporale tumors. *Am J Otol* 1990;11:1–5.

42. Sanna M, Russo A, De Donato G. *Color atlas of otoscopy: from diagnosis to surgery.* New York: Thieme, 1999;85, 91.

43. Brown LA. Glomus jugulare tumor of the middle ear; clinical aspects. *Laryngoscope* 1953;63:281–292.

44. Ogura JH, Spector GJ, Gado M. Glomus jugulare and vagale. *Ann Otol Rhinol Laryngol* 1978;87:622–629.

45. Spector GJ, Druck NS, Gado M. Neurologic manifestations of glomus tumors in the head and neck. *Arch Neurol* 1976;33:270–274.

46. Petrus LV, Lo WM. Primary paraganglioma of the facial nerve canal. *Am J Neuroradiol* 1996;17:171–174.

47. Megerian CA, McKenna MJ, Nadol JB Jr. Non-paraganglioma jugular foramen lesions masquerading as glomus jugulare tumors. *Am J Otol* 1995;16:94–98.

48. Rosenbloom JS, Storper IS, Aviv JE, et al. Giant cell tumors of the jugular foramen. *Am J Otol* 1999;20:176–179.

49. Hellier WP, Crockard HA, Cheesman AD. Metastatic carcinoma of the temporal bone presenting as glomus jugulare and glomus tympanicum tumours: a description of two cases. *J Laryngol Otol* 1997;111: 963–966.

50. Morantz RA, Kirchner FR, Kishore P. Aneurysms of the petrous portion of the internal carotid artery. *Surg Neurol* 1976;6:313–318.

51. Blumenfeld J, Cohen N, Anwar M, et al. Hypertension and a tumor of the glomus jugulare region. Evidence for epinephrine biosynthesis. *Am J Hypertens* 1993;6:382–387.

52. Schwaber MK, Glasscock ME, Nissen AJ, et al. Diagnosis and management of catecholamine secreting glomus tumors. *Laryngoscope* 1984;94:1008–1015.

53. Kremer R, Michel RP, Posner B, et al. Catecholamine-secreting paraganglioma of glomus jugulare region. *Am J Med Sci* 1989;297:46–48.

54. Schwartz ML, Israel HL. Severe anemia as a manifestation of metastatic jugular paraganglioma. *Arch Otolaryngol* 1983;109:269–272.

55. Lord RS, Chambers AJ. Familial carotid body paragangliomas and sensorineural hearing loss: a new syndrome. *Cardiovasc Surg* 1999;7: 134–138.

56. Carney JA. The triad of gastric epithelioid leiomyosarcoma, functioning extra-adrenal paraganglioma, and pulmonary chondroma. *Cancer* 1979;43:374–382.

57. Olsen WL, Dillon WP, Kelly WM, et al. MR imaging of paragangliomas. *Am J Roentgenol* 1987;148:201–204.

58. Moret J, Lasjaunias P, Theron J. Vascular compartments and territories of tympano-jugular glomic tumors. *J Belge Radiol* 1980;63:321–337.

59. Balli R, Dallari S, Bergamini G, et al. Avascular tympanojugular paraganglioma. *Laryngoscope* 1996;106:721–723.

60. Trimas SJ, Mancuso A, De Vries EJ, Cassisi NJ. Avascular carotid body tumor. *Otolaryngol Head Neck Surg* 1994;110:131–135.

61. Murphy TP, Brackmann DE. Effects of preoperative embolization on glomus jugulare tumors. *Laryngoscope* 1989;99:1244–1247.

62. Lasjaunias P, Menu Y, Bonnel D, et al. Non chromaffin paragangliomas of the head and neck. Diagnostic and therapeutic angiography in 19 cases explored from 1977 to 1980. *J Neuroradiol* 1981;8:281–299.

63. Beatty RA, Richardson AE. Predicting intolerance to common artery ligation by carotid angiography. *J Neurosurg* 1968;28:9–13.
64. Mathis JM, Barr JD, Jungreis CA, et al. Temporary balloon test occlusion of the internal carotid artery: experience in 500 cases. *Am J Neuroradiol* 1995;16:749–754.
65. Van Gils AP, Van der Mey AG, Hoogma RP, et al. MRI screening of kindred at risk of developing paragangliomas: support for genomic imprinting in hereditary glomus tumors. *Br J Cancer* 1992;65:903–907.
66. Lamberts SW, Bakker WH, Reubi JC, et al. Somatostatin-receptor imaging in the localization of endocrine tumors. *N Engl J Med* 1990;323:1246–1249.
67. Kau R, Arnold W. Somatostatin receptor scintigraphy and therapy of neuroendocrine (APUD) tumors of the head and neck. *Acta Otolaryngol* 1996;116:345–349.
68. Whiteman ML, Serafini AN, Telischi FF, et al. 111In octreotide scintigraphy in the evaluation of head and neck lesions. *Am J Neuroradiol* 1997;18:1073–1080.
69. Telischi FF, Bustillo A, Whiteman ML, et al. Octreotide scintigraphy for the detection of paragangliomas. *Otolaryngol Head Neck Surg* 2000;122:358–362.
70. Myssiorek D, Palestro CJ. 111 Indium pentetreotide scan detection of familial paragangliomas. *Laryngoscope* 1998;108:228–231.
71. De Jong AL, Coker NJ, Jenkins HA, et al. Radiation therapy in the management of paragangliomas of the temporal bone. *Am J Otol* 1995;16:283–289.
72. Liscak R, Vladyka V, Simonova G, et al. Leksell gamma knife radiosurgery of the tumor glomus jugulare and tympanicum. *Stereotact Funct Neurosurg* 1998;70:152–160.
73. Kim JA, Elkon D, Lim ML, et al. Optimum dose of radiotherapy for chemodectomas of the middle ear. *Int J Radiat Oncol Biol Phys* 1980;6:815–819.
74. Gabriel EM, Sampson JH, Dodd LG, et al. Glomus jugulare tumor metastatic to the sacrum after high-dose radiation therapy: case report. *Neurosurgery* 1995;37:1001–1005.
75. Preissig SH, Bohmfalk GL, Reichel GW, et al. Anaplastic astrocytoma following radiation for glomus jugular tumor. *Cancer* 1979;43:2243–2247.
76. Lalwani AK, Jackler RK, Gutin PH. Lethal fibrosarcoma complicating radiation therapy for a benign glomus jugular tumor. *Am J Otol* 1993;14:398–402.
77. Spector GJ, Compagno J, Perez CA, et al. Glomus jugulare tumors: effects of radiotherapy. *Cancer* 1975;35:1316–1321.
78. Liscak R, Vladyka V, Wowra B, et al. Gamma knife radiosurgery of the glomus jugulare tumour: early multicentre experience. *Acta Neurochir* 1999;141:1141–1146.
79. Verniers DA, Keus RB, Schouwenburg PF, et al. Radiation therapy, an important mode of treatment for head and neck chemodectomas. *Eur J Cancer* 1992;28A:1028–1033.
80. Cole JM, Beiler D. Long-term results of treatment for glomus jugulare and glomus vagale tumors with radiotherapy. *Laryngoscope* 1994;104:1461–1465.
81. Jordan JA, Roland PS, McManus C, et al. Stereotatic radiosurgery for glomus jugulare tumors. *Laryngoscope* 2000;110:35–38.
82. Tenenbaum F, Schlumberger M, Lumbroso J, et al. Beneficial effects of octreotide in a patient with a metastatic paraganglioma. *Eur J Cancer* 1996;32A:737.
83. Patel SR, Winchester DJ, Benjamin RS. A 15-year experience with chemotherapy of patents with paraganglioma. *Cancer* 1995;76:1476–1480.
84. Farrior JB. Anterior hypotympanic approach for glomus tumor of the infratemporal fossa. *Laryngoscope* 1984;94:1016–1021.
85. Fisch U. Infratemporal fossa approach for glomus tumors of the temporal bone. *Ann Otol Rhinol Laryngol* 1982;91:474–479.
86. Nadol JB Jr, Schuknecht HF. Obliteration of the mastoid in the treatment of tumors of the temporal bone. *Ann Otol Rhinol Laryngol* 1984;93:6–12.
87. Jenkins HA, Fisch U. Glomus tumors of the temporal region. Technique of surgical resection. *Arch Otolaryngol* 1981;107:209–214.
88. Glasscock ME III, Jackson CG. Section V. Basic surgical principles of neurotologic skull base surgery. *Laryngoscope* 1993;103[Suppl 60]:29–44.
89. Pensak ML, Jackler RK. Removal of jugular foramen tumors: the fallopian bridge technique. *Otolaryngol Head Neck Surg* 1997;117:586–591.
90. Spector GJ, Fierstein J, Ogura JH. A comparison of therapeutic modalities of glomus tumors in the temporal bone. *Laryngoscope* 1976;86:690–696.
91. Green JD Jr, Brackmann DE, Nguyen CD, et al. Surgical management of previously untreated glomus jugulare tumors. *Laryngoscope* 1994;104:917–921.
92. Moe KS, Li DQ, Linder TE, et al. An update on the surgical treatment of temporal bone paraganglioma. *Skull Base Surgery* 1999;9:185–194.
93. Briner HR, Linder TE, Pauw B, et al. Long-term results of surgery for temporal bone paragangliomas. *Laryngoscope* 1999;109:577–583.

CHAPTER 42

Cerebellopontine Angle Tumors

Joseph B. Nadol, Jr. and Robert L. Martuza

Because lesions of the cerebellopontine angle most commonly cause hearing loss and vestibular disturbance as their earliest symptoms, the otologist is often consulted for diagnosis and treatment. Although an acoustic neurinoma (vestibular schwannoma, acoustic neuroma, acoustic neurilemoma) is the most common lesion found in the cerebellopontine angle, the otologist should be aware that a variety of primary benign and metastatic malignant lesions may present in the cerebellopontine angle. Management of these lesions has undergone revolutionary change in the last decade. The introduction of diagnostic modalities, such as auditory evoked response audiometry and magnetic resonance imaging, allows demonstration of lesions at much earlier stages. Also, improvements in surgical technique have markedly reduced morbidity and mortality and have made preservation of hearing possible in resection of some of these lesions.

INCIDENCE OF SPECIFIC LESIONS OF THE CEREBELLOPONTINE ANGLE

Although acoustic neurinomas comprise between 75% and 90% of all tumors of the cerebellopontine angle, a variety of other primary and other metastatic lesions may mimic acoustic neurinomas clinically and radiographically. The most common lesions of the cerebellopontine angle and their approximate incidence are shown in Table 42.1. Approximately 98% of all lesions of the cerebellopontine angle are benign and 2% are malignant, either primary or metastatic. The clinical and diagnostic findings that will help differentiate these lesions preoperatively are discussed later (see Differential Diagnosis of Lesions of the Cerebellopontine Angle).

PRESENTING SIGNS AND SYMPTOMS OF CEREBELLOPONTINE ANGLE TUMORS

Unilateral progressive sensorineural loss with retrocochlear signs is the most common first symptom in tumors of the cerebellopontine angle. However, tumors may reach diameters of several centimeters without any substantial hearing loss. Although a down-sloping sensorineural pattern with poor discrimination is the most common audiometric pattern, low-frequency, midfrequency, fluctuating, and sudden sensorineural losses have also been described. Although the presenting symptoms may vary depending upon the origin and type of tumor, the most common presenting symptoms at initial diagnosis of cerebellopontine angle lesions are shown in Table 42.2. Given the fact that between 75% and 90% of all cerebellopontine angle lesions are acoustic neurinomas, the statistics in Table 42.2 are most descriptive of this lesion. More unusual lesions of the cerebellopontine angle may have a higher incidence of nonauditory and vestibular disturbances. For example, facial nerve schwannomas (Chapter 43) may present with slowly progressive facial nerve paresis as the initial neurologic deficit.

DIAGNOSTIC STRATEGY IN THE EVALUATION OF CEREBELLOPONTINE ANGLE LESIONS

The diagnosis of lesions of the cerebellopontine angle is based on neurotologic evaluation; audiometry, including auditory evoked response testing; vestibular testing; and radiographic imaging.

Neurotologic Evaluation

A complete neurotologic evaluation should include a history, particularly seeking the common symptoms presented in Table 42.2, such as auditory, vestibular dysfunction; headache; twitching or weakness of the facial muscles; and numbness of the face. A complete examination should include testing for facial hypesthesia to pin and light touch, evaluation of the corneal reflex using a wisp of cotton on the cornea, clinical evaluation of the facial nerve, cerebellar testing including rapid alternating movements, evaluation of gait disturbances, and testing of the function of the other cranial nerves (14,15).

Audiometry and Auditory Evoked Response Testing

Behavioral audiometry should include bilateral testing of pure-tone thresholds and evaluation of speech discrimina-

TABLE 42.1 *Lesions of the cerebellopontine angle*

Lesions	Approximate incidence	References
Primary	98%	
Benign	75%–90%	1,2
Acoustic neurinoma	5%–13%	1–5
Meningioma	3%–6%	1–3
Primary cholesteatoma	1%–2%	2,6
Schwannoma of cranial nerve VII or other cranial nerves	2%	—
Other	1%	3
Arachnoid cyst	—	—
Hemangioma	—	—
Aneurysm, glomus tumor	—	—
Lipoma	—	—
Abscess, fungal lesion	—	—
Tuberculoma	1%	—
Malignant	—	—
Malignant schwannomas	—	—
Sarcoma	—	—
Glioma	1%	—
Metastatic	—	—
From breast, kidney, lung, stomach, larynx, prostate, and thyroid		

TABLE 42.2 *Presenting symptoms in cerebellopontine angle lesions*

Symptom	Approximate prevalence at diagnosis
Hearing loss	95% (2,7–10)[a]
Tinnitus	80% (6)
Vestibular disturbance	50%–75% (2,11,12)
Head pain (occipitofrontal or suboccipital)	25% (6)
Facial hypesthesia	35%–50% (1,6)
Facial nerve dysfunction	20% (13), 50% (11)
Cerebellar or brainstem dysfunction	—
Lower cranial nerve dysfunction	—
Diplopia	—
Hydrocephalus	10%

[a]Numbers in parentheses refer to references.

tion. The most common audiometric pattern is a high-tone sensorineural loss, although flat loss, midfrequency loss, and low-frequency loss have been described (7). Although in most cases the hearing loss is slowly progressive, sudden or even fluctuant sensorineural loss may be seen. Decrement in speech discrimination tests is common, although there is little relationship between the size of the tumor and either pure-tone or discrimination results. Thus patients with intracanalicular lesions may present with profound sensorineural loss, whereas patients with lesions several centimeters in diameter in the cerebellopontine angle may have nearly normal hearing (Fig. 42.1).

The classical tests of retrocochlear involvement, such as tone decay, have been largely replaced by auditory evoked response testing. Brainstem evoked response audiometry is the single most reliable audiometric diagnostic procedure in the diagnosis of cerebellopontine angle lesions. Depending on the parameters used to analyze the evoked response test-

ing, the false-positive and false-negative rates are consistently less than 10% (16).

Vestibular Testing

Approximately 50% of the patients complain of vestibular symptomatology, most commonly mild unsteadiness. However, vestibular hypofunction, as demonstrated by electronystagmography, is seen in most patients with cerebellopontine angle lesions. In a review of 500 patients for unilateral acoustic neurinomas, Brackmann (6) reported that vestibular hypofunction was found in 82%. Similarly, Ojemann et al. (8) reported that 96% of their patients demonstrated vestibular hypofunction by caloric testing. Positional nystagmus was present in approximately 80% of cases, and in more than half of these the positional nystagmus was of the persistent variety (types 1 and 2).

Radiographic Imaging

In no area of diagnostic evaluation has there been more dramatic change in the last decade than in radiographic imaging of the cerebellopontine angle. Laminograms of the internal auditory canal and Pantopaque cisternograms, common 10 years ago, have now been replaced with modern computed tomography (CT) and magnetic resonance imaging (MRI). CT scans with contrast enhancement can reliably image lesions in excess of 1 cm in diameter. MRI, particularly with the introduction of gadolinium contrast enhancement, has provided a reliable method for diagnosing acoustic neurinomas that are purely intracanalicular and provides a technique of low morbidity to evaluate tumor growth or monitor for postoperative recurrence (Fig. 42.2). Gadolinium-enhanced MRI is currently the most sensitive test to evaluate for a suspected cerebellopontine angle tumor and should be

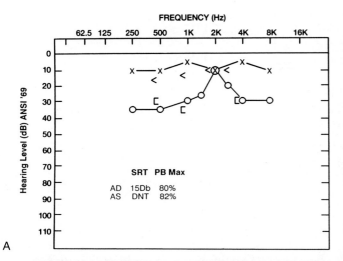

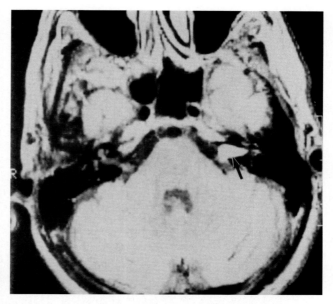

FIG. 42.2 MRI with gadolinium enhancement demonstrating an intracanalicular acoustic neurinoma on the left *(arrow).* This lesion was not visualized by CT or MRI without contrast enhancement.

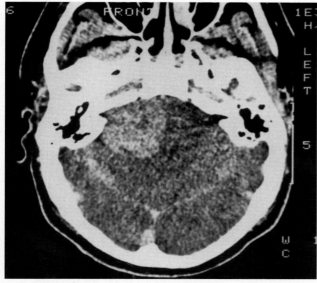

FIG. 42.1 A: Audiogram of a 26-year-old man whose only symptoms were slight hearing loss and tinnitus in the right ear. **B:** Computed tomographic (CT) scan of the patient demonstrating a 5-cm tumor of the right cerebellopontine angle, histologically demonstrated to be an acoustic neurinoma.

performed in cases of unilateral hearing loss in which the etiology is unclear.

DIFFERENTIAL DIAGNOSIS OF LESIONS OF THE CEREBELLOPONTINE ANGLE

Although between 75% and 90% of all lesions of the cerebellopontine angle are benign acoustic neurinomas, a variety of other lesions may be found in this location (Table 42.1). The results of the neurotologic and diagnostic evaluations may provide hints as to the presence of a lesion other than an acoustic neurinoma. Differential features of the most common lesions other than acoustic neurinomas are therefore presented.

Meningiomas

The presenting symptoms of meningioma differ only slightly from those of acoustic neurinoma. Hearing loss seems to be less common and trigeminal symptomatology more common in meningiomas (17). In addition, dysfunction of the ninth and lower cranial nerves is more common in meningioma than in acoustic neurinoma. Radiologic evaluation with MRI or CT often aids in the differential diagnosis (Fig. 42.3). Meningiomas are less likely to show enlargement of the internal auditory canal. Features on the noncontrast CT scan that suggest meningioma include a lesion that is hyperdense relative to the cerebellum or the presence of calcifications within or at the edge of the tumor. Enhanced MRI or CT may show the presence of a broad attachment to the petrous ridge and may also show involvement of the tentorium or enhancement of the adjacent dura ("dural tail") (Fig. 42.3C).

Epidermoid Lesions

These lesions, although uncommon and slow growing, tend to envelop rather than displace vascular and neural structures of the cerebellopontine angle. Thus abnormalities of multiple cranial nerves and cerebellar dysfunction are more common in these lesions. The CT scan will show a lesion of lower density than the surrounding brain and with irregular borders. The lesion generally will not enhance with contrast. A combination of CT and MRI greatly facilitates the differential diagnosis (Chapters 4 and 44).

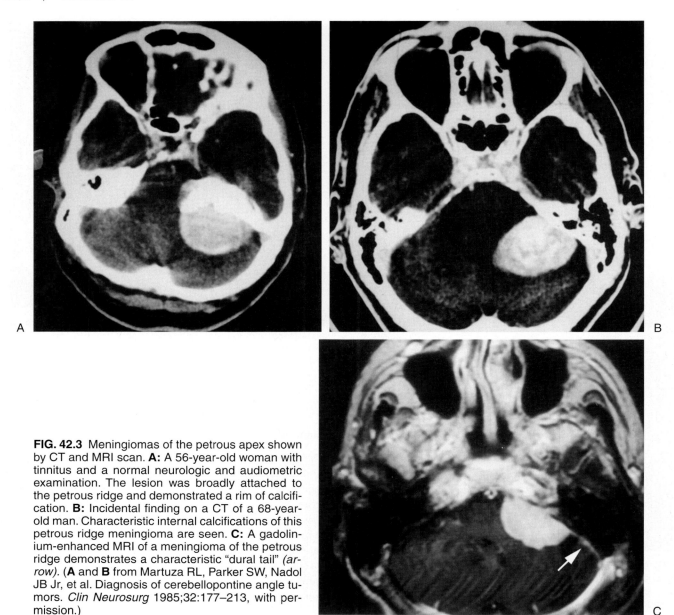

FIG. 42.3 Meningiomas of the petrous apex shown by CT and MRI scan. **A:** A 56-year-old woman with tinnitus and a normal neurologic and audiometric examination. The lesion was broadly attached to the petrous ridge and demonstrated a rim of calcification. **B:** Incidental finding on a CT of a 68-year-old man. Characteristic internal calcifications of this petrous ridge meningioma are seen. **C:** A gadolinium-enhanced MRI of a meningioma of the petrous ridge demonstrates a characteristic "dural tail" *(arrow)*. (**A** and **B** from Martuza RL, Parker SW, Nadol JB Jr, et al. Diagnosis of cerebellopontine angle tumors. *Clin Neurosurg* 1985;32:177–213, with permission.)

Arachnoid Cyst

The CT scan generally demonstrates a low-density lesion with smooth edges within the internal auditory canal or in the cerebellopontine angle (Figs. 42.4 and 42.5). The density of the lesion is dependent upon the protein content, and enhancement on CT scanning does not occur.

Other Lesions

The differential diagnosis of more unusual lesions of the cerebellopontine angle are well described by Martuza et al. (17). Schwannomas arising from the seventh cranial nerve may present with facial nerve symptoms earlier than in acoustic neurinomas. However, up to 20% of patients with acoustic neurinomas will have facial nerve symptoms and the differential diagnosis may not be made without surgical

confirmation of the origin of the lesion. Malignant lesions of the cerebellopontine angle, either primary or metastatic, generally demonstrate rapid progressive symptoms with early cranial nerve involvement and destructive rather than expansile lesions on CT scanning.

BIOLOGY AND NATURAL HISTORY OF ACOUSTIC NEURINOMAS

Pathogenesis

Acoustic neurinomas arise in two clinical settings: the genetic syndrome of neurofibromatosis type 2 and sporadic unilateral acoustic neurinoma. Neurofibromatosis type 2 has now been clearly differentiated from neurofibromatosis type 1 (Von Recklinghausen's disease) (18).

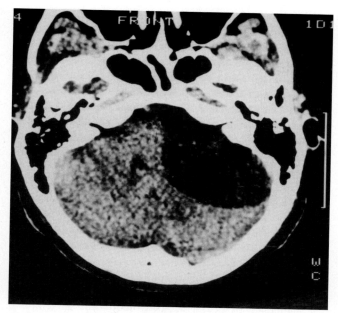

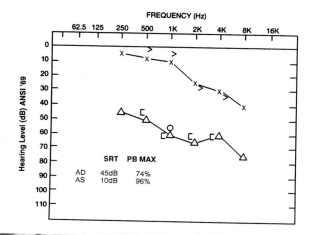

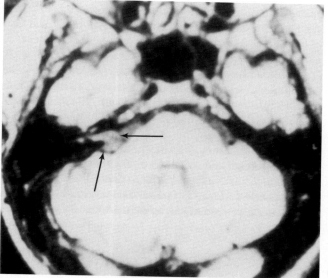

FIG. 42.4 Large arachnoid cyst of the posterior fossa demonstrated by contrast-enhanced CT scan in this 49-year-old woman whose only symptom was tinnitus in the left ear. An audiogram showed slight, low-frequency, conductive loss in the left ear. Auditory evoked response testing was diagnostic of a retrocochlear lesion on the left. (Reprinted with permission from Martuza RL, Parker SW, Nadol JB Jr, et al. Diagnosis of cerebellopontine angle tumors. *Clin Neurosurg* 1985;32:177–213.)

Role of the Neurofibromatosis Type 2 Gene in Vestibular Schwannoma Formation

Vestibular schwannomas (acoustic neuromas) occur from mutations in the neurofibromatosis type 2 (NF2) gene (19). The formation of a tumor requires the inactivation of both copies of this gene, either through a chromosomal deletion or through an inactivating mutation. At the molecular level, the genetic abnormalities are at the same locus whether they occur in the unilateral nonhereditary vestibular schwannoma or in the bilateral vestibular schwannoma of the patient with NF2 (20). The difference is at the level of the patient. The patient with NF2 is born with one of the NF2 genes already inactive or missing in every cell of the body. The chance is high—in fact, it is virtually certain—that at some point in his or her lifetime a second inactivating mutation will occur at the same genetic locus; thus bilateral vestibular schwannomas (as well as other tumors, such as meningiomas, schwannomas, and ependymomas) are common and multifocal in NF2 patients (21). Moreover, because one copy of the NF2 gene is abnormal in each germ cell and thus in 50% of each sperm or egg cell, there is a 50% chance of transmitting this disorder to any offspring. In contrast, the patient with a unilateral acoustic neuroma is born with both NF2 genes intact. The odds that both NF2 genes would mutate in the same Schwann cell are so low that the incidence of unilateral acoustic neuroma is low in the general population, and within any individual, he or she is only likely to develop

FIG. 42.5 **A:** Audiogram showing sensorineural loss on the right with reduced speech discrimination. **B:** MRI scan demonstrating a lesion in the right cerebellopontine angle centered at the internal auditory canal *(arrows)*. This was interpreted radiographically as consistent with acoustic neuroma but on surgical exploration proved to be an arachnoid cyst.

one vestibular schwannoma. Moreover, because the NF2 gene copies are normal in the sperm and egg cells of a patient with a nonhereditary unilateral acoustic neuroma, there is no transmission to offspring.

Located on the long arm of chromosome 22, the NF2 gene contains 17 exons and produces the protein merlin, a 60- to 70-kDa protein related to the ERM family of proteins, which includes ezrin, radixin, and moesin (22,23). In vitro, the expression of merlin has been shown to be able to inhibit the growth of human meningioma cells (24), to inhibit the growth of NIH-3T3 fibroblasts, (25) and, with overexpression, even to be able to reverse the effects of ras-mediated cell transformation (26). Therefore, functionally, merlin acts like other tumor suppressor genes and its loss would be expected to lead to increased cell growth.

Merlin, like other members of the ERM family, may interact with the cell membrane and thus may relay information from the external surface of the cell to the interior (27). Within merlin, the so-called FERM domain has a membrane-localizing function and is involved with attachment of protein 4.1 to the plasma membrane by binding to cytoplasmic domains of several transmembrane molecules (28). Alternate splicing of exon 16 of merlin can produce two different isoforms of merlin. The exact mechanism of the tumor suppressor properties of Isoform 1 is not understood but likely is involved with the interactions of the cell membrane with the cytoskeleton and mediating cellular responses to the environment at the outer surface of the cell membrane. Isoform 2 can interact with ßII spectrin (29), but its full function within the cell is not yet understood. However, changes in the amounts of these two isoforms may offer insight into normal Schwann cell growth regulation and also into potential therapeutic approaches for the treatment of schwannomas.

At present there is no medical therapy known to slow the growth of either unilateral nonhereditary vestibular schwannomas or of the tumors of the patient with NF2. The mechanisms of growth control by the category of tumor suppressors that include merlin are poorly understood. The interactions of merlin with other cellular proteins have only recently been studied (30). More research is needed to define the molecular pathways of Schwann cell growth regulation by merlin isoforms before rational targeted therapies of vestibular schwannomas can be envisioned.

The term *acoustic neuroma* is a misnomer in that the cell of origin of this lesion appears to be the Schwann cell of the vestibular nerve. It arises most commonly from the inferior division of the vestibular nerve (Fig. 42.6) and next most commonly from the superior division (Fig. 42.7) (31,32). In rare cases it may arise from the cochlear nerve (33). It may arise along the vestibular nerve between the Schwann-glial junction and the cribrose area. Intralabyrinthine origin has been reported in neurofibromatosis type 2 (Fig. 42.8), and it also may occur in the isolated sporadic form (34–36). To date there is no explanation for the site of predilection of the superior branch of the vestibular nerve, although Skinner (37) suggests that it may be a consequence of embryogenesis. The histopathology of acoustic neurinoma is consistent with the Antoni type A and type B patterns (38), although there is no clear correlation between biologic behavior and the histologic subtypes.

Incidence and Prevalence of Acoustic Neurinoma

The incidence of occult acoustic neurinoma in temporal bone studies is approximately 0.85% (39,40). In each of these series, an acoustic neurinoma was found that had not caused clinical symptoms during life. Thus the prevalence of acoustic neurinoma is at least 850 individuals per 100,000 population. From clinical series (41,42), the frequency of intracranial tumors in the general population has been estimated as 0.15 per 1,000 population, and of these, vestibular schwannomas represent approximately 10%. Thus it is reasonable to deduce that clinically symptomatic acoustic

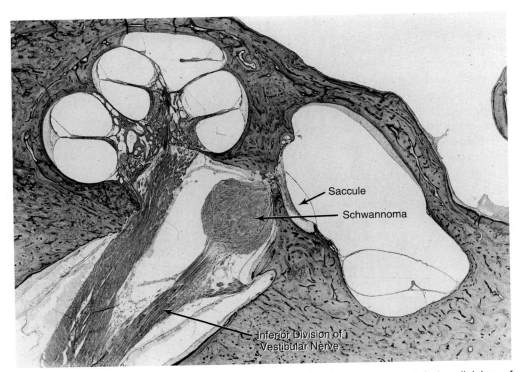

Saccule
Schwannoma
Inferior Division of Vestibular Nerve

FIG. 42.6 A vestibular schwannoma (acoustic neurinoma) arising from the inferior division of the vestibular nerve in a 49-year-old man with no known symptoms referable to the lesion.

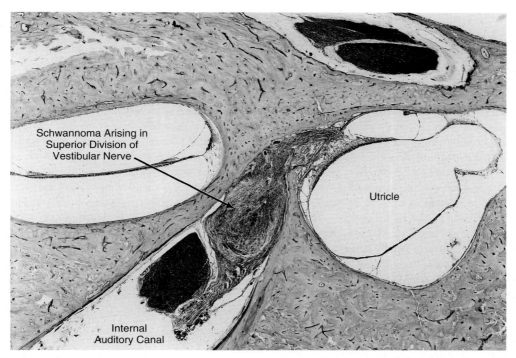

FIG. 42.7 A vestibular schwannoma (acoustic neurinoma) arising in the superior division of the vestibular nerve. This was an incidental finding in an 84-year-old man with no known symptoms referable to the tumor.

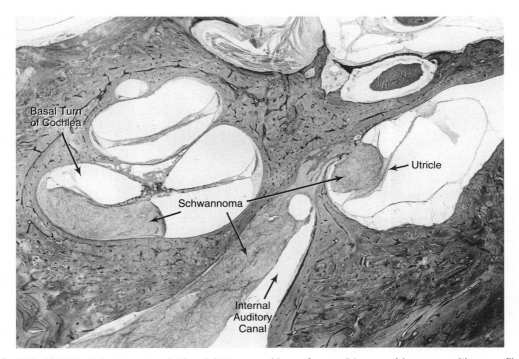

FIG. 42.8 Multiple schwannomas in the right temporal bone from a 31-year-old woman with neurofibromatosis type 2. Schwannomas are seen in the basal turn of the cochlea, within the utricle, and in the internal auditory canal.

neurinomas are seen at an incidence of 1.5 per 100,000 population. From these calculations it is apparent that most of the 850 schwannomas per 100,000 population remain clinically asymptomatic during life and approximately 0.2%

demonstrate biologic or growth behavior resulting in clinical symptomatology and detection. The recent dramatic improvement in radiographic imaging of acoustic neurinomas has allowed a clinical assessment of the growth rate of these lesions (43–45) and has similarly shown either a very slow growth rate or no detectable growth in most tumors.

Pathophysiology of Symptoms

Although there is poor correlation of the auditory and vestibular symptoms with the size of the tumor (46,47), it is proposed by Schuknecht (48) that there may be at least three mechanisms of compromise of auditory and vestibular function: (i) compressive degeneration of auditory and vestibular nerve trunks in the internal auditory canal, (ii) vascular compromise and subsequent degeneration of end organs of the inner ear, and (iii) a toxic metabolic effect of "choking" of the internal auditory canal by the neurinoma. Tumor invasion and compression of the auditory and vestibular nerves have been shown in large (49) and small (50) acoustic neurinomas. A cochlear nerve conduction block induced by compression has also been hypothesized by Kveton et al. (51). In contrast, a highly significant linear relationship between tumor size and vestibular hypofunction as measured by the caloric response has been demonstrated (52). This contrasts with the lack of correlation with auditory symptoms. In addition, because various audiometric patterns of hearing loss have been described in cases of acoustic neurinoma, including down-sloping, flat, and even fluctuant sensorineural loss, there may be different mechanisms of interference of cochlear and vestibular function. Johnsson et al. (53) demonstrated severe degeneration of the vestibular nerve but insufficient degeneration of the auditory end organ and nerve to explain the degree of sensorineural hearing loss. In a microdissected specimen of a human temporal bone with an acoustic neurinoma, these authors also suggest other mechanisms such as conduction block (54) within the inner ear as a consequence of abnormal cochlear capillary permeability. It is possible that the protein products of upregulated genes may play a role in auditory dysfunction (47).

Treatment Strategies and Patient Selection

Because the growth rate of acoustic neurinomas is generally slow and fewer than 1% of acoustic neurinomas may come to surgery (55), the otologic surgeon must have a strategy for selection of patients for surgical excision. Stratification of patients by using the indicators of bilateral versus unilateral, age of patient, size of tumor, and status of hearing in both ears provides a useful basis for this purpose.

Unilateral Tumors

For small tumors (less than 2.0 cm diameter) with good hearing, two options may be offered: (i) surgical removal in an attempt to save hearing or (ii) radiographic follow-up, reserving surgery for tumors that demonstrate enlargement. The age, medical status, wishes, and temperament of the patient and the status of the nonaffected ear are determinants that must be considered.

For small tumors with poor or no hearing, either surgical removal or radiographic follow-up, reserving surgery or radiotherapy for enlarging tumors, may be offered. Again, the age, medical status, wishes, and temperament of the patient should be considered.

For large tumors (greater than 2.0 cm) in healthy young and middle-aged patients (less than 65 years), surgical removal is generally recommended, given the fact that the morbidity of surgical removal is directly correlated with the size of the tumor and that enlargement in healthy patients younger than 65 years is more likely.

For tumors in older patients (65 years and older) with auditory and vestibular symptoms only and no evidence of brainstem compression, radiographic follow-up is recommended, reserving surgery or radiotherapy for enlarging tumors and progressive symptoms. However, in patients with evidence of brainstem compression or hydrocephalus, total removal or subtotal decompression are recommended despite advanced age.

Bilateral Tumors

In patients with neurofibromatosis type 2, given the high incidence of other lesions of the central nervous system, the major treatment objective is to avoid bilateral deafness and nonauditory or vestibular symptomatology due to the acoustic neurinoma. Thus if a patient has bilateral tumors, both with good hearing, it is reasonable to proceed immediately to surgical removal of one tumor in an attempt to preserve hearing. If hearing is preserved on the first side, the second lesion may be followed, reserving surgery for radiographic evidence of enlargement. If surgery on the first side results in loss of hearing, surgery on the second side is done only with evidence of an enlarging tumor or evidence of decreased hearing, and an intracapsular decompression is performed to minimize the chance of creating bilateral deafness. Fractionated stereotaxic radiosurgery is also being explored as a method to stop growth of the tumor and also preserve hearing.

In patients with bilateral tumors who have become deaf, treatment strategy is similar to that described for large tumors in the unilateral cases.

Nonsurgical Options in the Treatment of Acoustic Neurinoma

Stereotaxic radiosurgery has been used since 1969 for acoustic neurinomas in Sweden (56–58). Success, as measured by failure of tumor enlargement, has been reported in up to 86% (59). It is important to recognize that contemporary radiation doses are lower than those reported in earlier reports and hence no more than 10-year follow-up is available to determine recurrence rates for these lower radiation dosages. However, 14% of tumors subsequently increased in size and required surgical removal. Although failure of radiation therapy to prevent further growth does not preclude subsequent surgical salvage, surgical morbidity following radiotherapy may be increased (60). Paresis of the facial nerve was described in 15% but may be transitory. Although hearing may be initially preserved by such treatment, progressive sensorineural loss was commonly observed (61). In addition, approximately 5% of patients developed "peritumoral swelling" and evidence of ischemia in the distribution of the anterior inferior cerebellar artery. At present, surgical removal or radiographic follow-up with surgical removal reserved for evidence of enlargement are the treatments of choice for most patients younger than age 65 years and in good health.

SURGICAL APPROACHES AND TECHNIQUES

Modern surgical options for removal of acoustic neurinomas include the translabyrinthine (62), middle fossa (1,9), and retrosigmoid or suboccipital approaches (63–65) and variations on them. A combination of the suboccipital and translabyrinthine procedures, either staged (66) or as a one-stage procedure (1), is a useful approach for large tumors with anterior extension in the cerebellopontine angle. Each of the three major approaches (translabyrinthine, middle cranial fossa, suboccipital) have several advantages and disadvantages as outlined in Table 42.3; hence, each surgeon must develop a strategy for selection of an appropriate approach given the objectives of surgery and size of tumor. Thus if an attempt is to be made to preserve hearing, only the middle cranial fossa and suboccipital approaches are appropriate. The middle cranial fossa approach should be reserved for intracanalicular tumors, given the relatively poor exposure of the posterior fossa.

If no attempt will be made to preserve hearing, the translabyrinthine or suboccipital approaches are most appropriate. Although advocates of the translabyrinthine approach claim that acoustic neurinomas of any size may be removed by this approach, there is little question that the suboccipital approach provides a wider exposure of the posterior fossa and, hence, easier dissection of the tumor from its attachments to the cerebellum and brainstem. Thus for small tumors (less than 2 cm) with cerebrospinal fluid (CSF) demonstrated between the tumor and the brainstem on CT scanning or MRI and in the presence of good pneumatization of the mastoid, the translabyrinthine approach is preferred. However, with larger tumors, particularly with radiographic evidence of distortion of the brainstem, absence of CSF space between the brainstem or cerebellum and the tumor, or in cases of poor pneumatization of the mastoid, the suboccipital approach is preferred.

The transsigmoid approach, which combines the translabyrinthine and suboccipital techniques, provides excellent exposure for very large tumors (greater than 4.0 cm), particularly with extension anterior to the brainstem or with large tumors with extensive erosion of the internal auditory canal. The suboccipital approach is presented here, and the details of surgical approaches and techniques are presented in Chapter 12.

Suboccipital Approach

Positioning and Soft Tissue Incision

The suboccipital craniotomy may be performed with the patient in the sitting or recumbent position. The latter is preferred because of the risk of air embolism in the sitting position. The Mayfield-Kees three-point head holder is useful in

TABLE 42.3 *Selection of surgical approach for acoustic neurinoma*

Surgical approach	Advantages	Disadvantages
Translabyrinthine	Excellent exposure of fundus of internal auditory canal, labyrinthine segment of facial nerve	Relatively limited exposure of posterior fossa
	Most direct, shortest working distance to cerebellopontine angle	Requires sacrifice of auditory and vestibular function
	Little or no cerebellar retraction for small tumors	Exposure of internal auditory canal may be compromised by high jugular bulb
	Low incidence of postoperative CSF leak	Relatively complex and time-consuming approach
		Variable exposure dependent on pneumatization of mastoid
Middle cranial fossa	Excellent exposure of fundus of internal auditory canal and labyrinthine segment of facial nerve	Requires significant retraction of temporal lobe
	Auditory function may be preserved	Incidence of facial nerve paresis
		Poor exposure of posterior fossa
		Acoustic neurinoma deep to facial nerve
Suboccipital	Auditory function may be preserved	Relatively difficult exposure of fundus of internal auditory canal, especially when hearing to be preserved
		Oblique angle (longer working distance)
	Excellent exposure of posterior fossa, cerebellum, and brainstem	Higher incidence of CSF leak
	Relatively rapid approach	Requires retraction of cerebellum

stabilizing the head during this approach. The soft tissue incision is made just posterior to the occipitomastoid suture line (Fig. 42.9A). The galea and periosteum of the mastoid and occipital bones and the insertions of the trapezius and splenius capitis are elevated.

An occipital craniotomy is performed using the transverse and lateral venous sinuses as the superior and anterior margins (Fig. 42.9B). The dura is opened to form flaps that are sutured to the elevated and retracted subcutaneous tissue (Fig. 42.9C) to protect the venous sinuses. A self-retaining retractor using extracranial fixation is placed to retract the cerebellum and expose the cerebellopontine angle and posterior fossa surface of the temporal bone and lateral aspect of the brainstem. Opening of the lateral cerebellomedullary cistern will release spinal fluid to facilitate and minimize retraction of the cerebellum. An internal decompression of the tumor is performed for biopsy and to enhance exposure. The tumor is mobilized from the cerebellum and brainstem and the facial and eighth nerve complex identified if possible.

Exposure of the Internal Auditory Canal (Fig. 42.9D)

A medially based dural flap is outlined with a no. 11 blade centered at the internal auditory meatus. This is elevated with a Rhoton canal knife and the dural flap reflected over the tumor to protect the contents of the internal auditory canal from

subsequent drilling. The lateral extent of the bony aperture is difficult to judge preoperatively. Normative data on the distance between the bony meatus and the crus commune are impractical to use, particularly in cases in which significant erosion and distortion of the internal auditory canal have occurred. The endolymphatic sac and duct, which can be identified on the posterior fossa surface, provide a more reliable landmark to the underlying membranous labyrinth (67,68) (Fig. 42.9D). Bony removal lateral to the endolymphatic duct will result in entrance into the posterior semicircular canal or the crus commune and sensorineural hearing loss.

When hearing preservation is not to be attempted, the distal end of the internal auditory canal can be easily visualized. However, if hearing preservation is attempted, dissection lateral to the endolymphatic duct cannot be accomplished and the distal 1 to 3 mm of the internal auditory canal may not be directly visualized.

The facial nerve is generally found in the superior aspect of the internal auditory canal as it enters its labyrinthine segment. For smaller tumors, the seventh and eighth cranial nerves are also identified medial to the tumor at the brainstem. For larger tumors, internal decompression within the tumor capsule will facilitate mobilization of the tumor and identification of the facial and auditory nerves. After identification of the facial nerve has been ascertained, internal decompression of the meatal portion of the

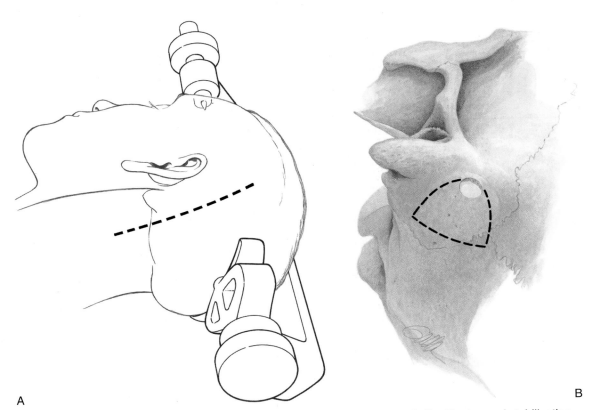

A   B

FIG. 42.9 Suboccipital approach to the resection of acoustic neurinoma. **A:** Positioning and stabilization of the head is accomplished using the Mayfield-Kees three-point head holder. The incision for suboccipital craniotomy is indicated by the *dashed line.* **B:** Location of the osteotomy and bur hole for suboccipital craniotomy.

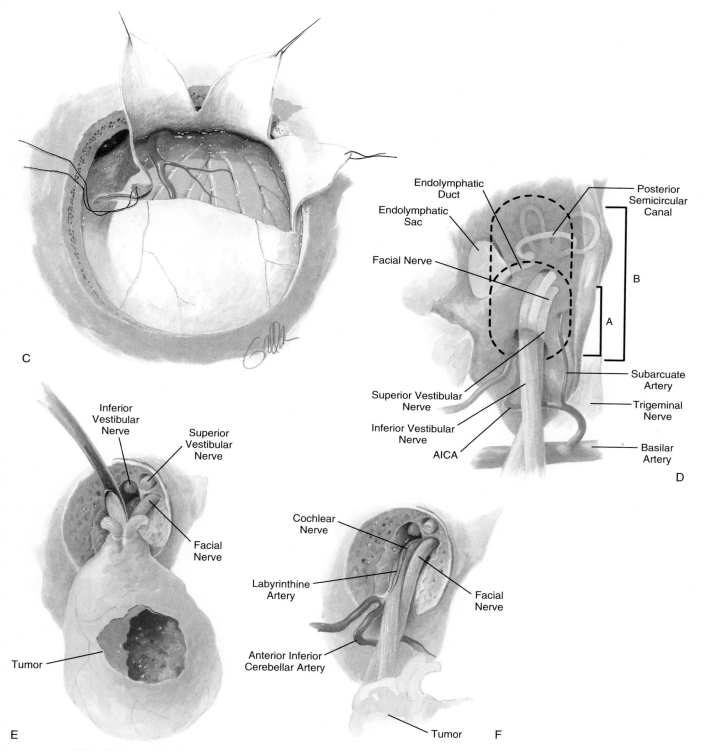

FIG. 42.9, cont'd. Suboccipital approach to the resection of acoustic neurinoma. **C:** The dura is reflected and held in place with silk sutures to protect the venous sinus. **D:** Anatomy of the posterior fossa surface of the internal auditory canal. The tumor has been eliminated for the purposes of anatomic clarity. The *dashed lines* indicate the area of bone removal if an attempt to save hearing is made *(A)* and if hearing preservation is not attempted *(B)*. AICA, anterior inferior cerebellar artery. **E:** After internal intracapsular decompression of the tumor and opening of the posterior aspect of the internal auditory canal and its covering dura, the facial nerve is identified as it passes through the superior aspect of the internal auditory canal to enter the labyrinthine segment. For small- to medium-sized tumors, the seventh and eighth cranial nerves are identified medially near the brainstem prior to tumor dissection. The superior and inferior vestibular nerve trunks are severed, and the tumor is reflected medially to expose the cochlear nerve and more proximal portion of the meatal segment of the facial nerve. **F:** The tumor has been elevated from the cochlear and facial nerves, revealing the labyrinthine artery.

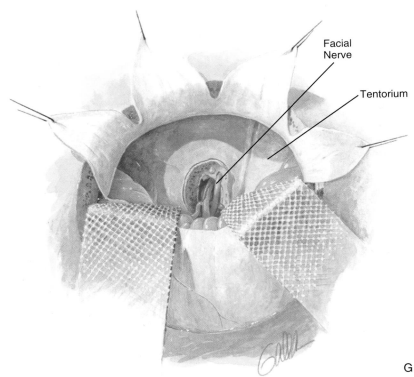

Facial
Nerve

Tentorium

G

FIG. 42.9, cont'd. Suboccipital approach to the resection of acoustic neurinoma. **G:** Anatomy of the cerebellopontine angle after removal of acoustic neurinoma.

tumor is helpful in identifying the course of the facial and cochlear nerves. Dissection of the tumor in the internal auditory canal begins distally by sharply dividing remnants of the vestibular nerve and allowing the tumor to "roll off" in a medial direction from the facial and underlying cochlear nerves (Fig. 42.9E–G). Preservation of an arachnoid layer between the tumor and auditory nerve will help to protect the vasculature of the cochlea. This dissection is extended to the meatus, and the attachments at the bony meatus are separated. Tumor removal proceeds anterograde from the brainstem and retrograde from the fundus of the canal to maximize the opportunity for preservation of cochlea and facial function.

Closure

Openings into the mastoid air cells are sealed with bone wax, and a free graft of abdominal fat is placed in the bony aperture to reduce the incidence of postoperative CSF leakage. After dural closure, the craniotomy is closed by replacing the previously removed calvarial segment and by the use of miniplates, methyl methacrylate, or bone chips.

Intraoperative Complications

Facial Nerve Injury

Preservation of the facial nerve is greatly facilitated by intraoperative electromyographic monitoring. Video monitoring and the placement of a motion detector over the central

aspect of the face supplements electromyographic monitoring, which is suspended during electrocautery. Identification of the facial nerve at the brainstem and at the most distal portion of the internal auditory canal facilitates a combination of anterograde and retrograde dissection. Although the facial nerve is usually anterior to the tumor and lies in the superior and anterior aspects of the internal auditory canal, this relationship is not constant. In fact, in unusual cases the facial nerve may be located posterior to the tumor mass.

Cardiac Slowing

Excessive retraction of the cerebellum or the brainstem or cool irrigating solutions may result in cardiac slowing or standstill.

Injury to Anterior Inferior Cerebellar Artery

The location of the anterior inferior cerebellar artery is variable in the cerebellopontine angle. Occasionally a loop of the anterior inferior cerebellar artery will extend into the internal auditory canal. In unilateral sporadic acoustic neurinoma, this vessel will not be encompassed within the tumor mass, and intracapsular removal of tumor with preservation of arachnoid layers will help to prevent injury to this vessel. However, in neurofibromatosis type 2 in which the schwannoma may be multicentric and in cases of meningioma, the anterior inferior cerebellar artery or one of its branches may be incorporated within the tumor mass.

Laceration of Lateral Venous Sinus

Preoperative assessment of the temporal bone with CT scan is useful to identify the proximity of the jugular bulb and lateral venous sinus to the posterior aspect of the internal auditory canal. Magnetic resonance imaging is not useful in providing the necessary bony landmarks. The jugular bulb may abut or actually overlap the posterior aspect of the internal canal (Figs. 42.10 and 42.11). Careful bone removal with suction irrigation and a watchful eye to the blue appearance of a jugular bulb within the posteroinferior wall of the internal auditory canal is essential. Laceration of the jugular bulb is controlled with Surgicel and Gelfoam and cottonoid tampon.

Laceration of the Facial Nerve

Despite careful dissection and electrophysiologic monitoring, attachment to or invasion of the facial nerve by tumor may result in loss of neural integrity. End-to-end anastomosis or cable grafting may be accomplished if the proximal stump can be clearly identified.

Postoperative Complications

Hematoma

Careful monitoring in an intensive care nursing unit is essential, particularly in the first 24 hours. Failure to awaken from anesthesia in a timely fashion, fluctuating levels of awareness, contralateral hemiparesis or posturing, and ele-vated blood pressure should all raise the suspicion of developing hematoma and demand emergency imaging. A rapidly deteriorating neurologic course may require opening the wound to relieve the pressure of the hematoma before imaging can be performed.

Cerebrospinal Fluid Otorhinorrhea

Careful sealing of open air cells, either in the area of the mastoid or internal auditory canal, with bone wax and free fat grafts is helpful in reducing the incidence of postoperative CSF otorhinorrhea.

If CSF leak is noted postoperatively, elevation of the head and repeated lumbar punctures or placement of lumbar CSF drain for 3 days to reduce spinal fluid pressure may allow healing to occur. A noncontrast CT of the head should be performed prior to lumbar puncture to rule out intracranial hemorrhage and hydrocephalus. Vigorous leakage despite or after these measures requires a transmastoid approach to identify the site of leakage and obliteration of the mastoid with free fat grafts. Leakage usually occurs through the perisinal cells near the lateral venous sinus or in the posterosuperior or posteromedial cell tracts near the internal auditory canal.

Subgaleal Effusion

Collection of spinal fluid in the subgaleal space is common postoperatively and will resolve spontaneously over several weeks postoperatively. No drainage is necessary unless in-

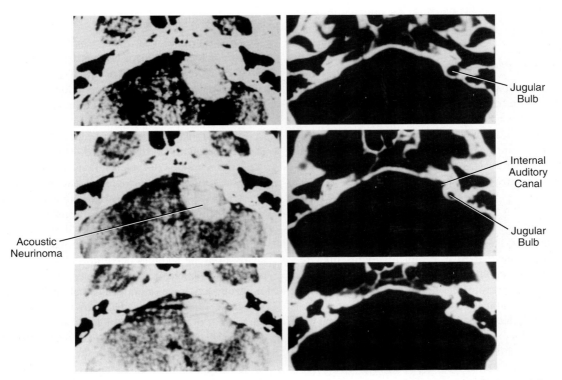

FIG. 42.10 Soft tissue and bone windows on serial CT scans demonstrate the proximity of the jugular bulb to the internal auditory canal and acoustic neurinoma of the cerebellopontine angle.

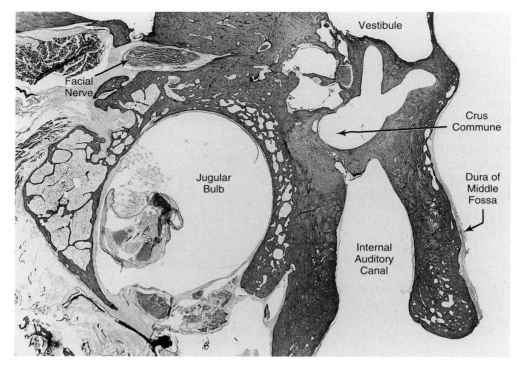

FIG. 42.11 Histologic section of a human temporal bone in a plane parallel to that of the posterior fossa. The proximity of the jugular bulb to the internal auditory canal is seen.

creased pressure of this effusion threatens the wound. In such cases, lumbar puncture or lumbar drain is useful. Development of hydrocephalus perpetuating effusion requires a ventricular shunt.

Exposure Keratitis and Corneal Ulcer

Patients with facial paresis or paralysis postoperatively, particularly those with trigeminal hypesthesia, are at high risk for keratitis and corneal ulceration. The frequent use of artificial tears while awake and an eye patch with lubricating ointment at night are useful preventative measures. If extended paresis or paralysis is expected, a lateral tarsorrhaphy will protect the cornea from injury.

Recurrent Tumor

Despite the fact that an acoustic neurinoma is removed by a "shell-out" technique, when a complete microscopic removal has been accomplished, recurrence is extremely rare. Occasionally, small portions of the tumor may be left deliberately because of attachment to the brainstem or facial nerve and result in recurrence. A postoperative baseline MR scan is usually done 4 to 6 months postoperatively. If no residual or recurrent tumor is identified, follow-up MRI is done 2, 4, 8, and 16 years thereafter. If residual or recurrent tumor is identified, MRI is done yearly unless subsequent intervention is performed.

HEARING PRESERVATION IN ACOUSTIC NEURINOMA

Surgical Technique

When useful hearing is present preoperatively, an attempt may be made to preserve hearing by the use of the middle fossa (subtemporal) or suboccipital approaches. There is a statistically significant correlation between the ability to save hearing and the size of the tumor (69), and salvage of hearing in patients with tumors larger than 2.5 cm is rare.

Intraoperative monitoring of auditory evoked potentials (69,70) is helpful in this surgical effort. Three mechanisms have been offered for the etiology of hearing loss during acoustic neurinoma removal. First, entrance into the labyrinth during the creation of a bony aperture in the posterior aspect of the internal auditory canal will result in sensorineural loss prior to manipulation of the tumor. Second, dissection of the tumor in the internal auditory canal may result in traction or avulsion of the auditory nerve fibers (69,71,72). Careful dissection with intraoperative monitoring and care to prevent significant traction are essential. Dissection in a medial to lateral direction, insofar as possible, will help to prevent avulsion injury. Third, interruption of the blood supply to the cochlea by vasospasm or avulsion may occur (69,71–73). The labyrinthine artery is variable in origin and in number (74), which creates significant variations in the expected anatomy. The local application of papaverine may help restore auditory responses when lost due to vasospasm.

SPECIAL CONSIDERATIONS FOR BILATERAL TUMORS

The presence of bilateral acoustic neurinomas caused by neurofibromatosis type 2 may require alteration of the usual therapeutic protocol (75). Clinical experience would suggest that preservation of hearing and total removal of the tumor are much more difficult in neurofibromatosis type 2 than in a sporadic unilateral tumor. This may be due to the multicentric origin in neurofibromatosis type 2, resulting in encompassment of nerve roots within the tumor mass. In addition, the common occurrence of schwannomas elsewhere in the

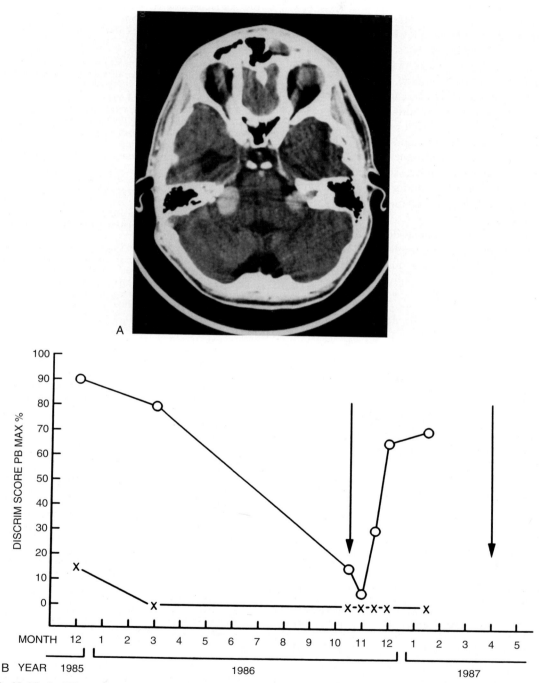

FIG. 42.12 A: CT scan of a 19-year-old man with neurofibromatosis type 2. **B:** Graphic representation of hearing before and after a suboccipital internal decompression of acoustic neurinoma of the right internal auditory. There was a progressive loss of speech discrimination in both ears (right = O; left = X). A suboccipital decompression was done, with significant improvement and preservation of hearing until death from unrelated causes 5 months later.

neuraxis in neurofibromatosis type 2 dictates a more reactive than proactive therapeutic response to the presence of such tumors. If removal of an acoustic neuroma is planned, preoperative MRI of the cervical spine should be done to rule out a neuroma at that site, which could cause compression of the spinal cord during rotation of the neck required for posterior fossa surgery. In general, if bilateral tumors are identified prior to loss of useful hearing, an attempt should be made to remove the tumor on one side with preservation of hearing. The opposite side is followed until such time as growth or decreased hearing dictates contralateral surgery. Total removal on the second side is attempted only if hearing has been preserved on the first side. In cases of acoustic neurinoma of the only hearing ear, careful monitoring with MRI scans and audiometry is essential. Surgery is reserved for evidence of decrease in hearing or sufficient growth to compromise or threaten other neural function. In cases where the tumor involves the only hearing ear, subtotal internal decompression and decompression of the internal auditory canal by removing the posterior aspect of the bone of the internal auditory canal may prolong or actually improve useful hearing (Fig. 42.12).

In some cases in which bilateral deafness has occurred, the use of an auditory brainstem implant (ABI) may restore some auditory function (76). If the auditory nerve has been preserved, conventional cochlear implants may be used (2,10).

REFERENCES

1. House WF, ed. Monograph II. Acoustic neuroma. *Arch Otolaryngol* 1968;88:576–715.
2. Graham J, Lynch C, Weber B, Stollwerck L, et al. The magnetless Clarion cochlear implant in a patient with neurofibromatosis 2. *J Laryngol Otol* 1999;113:458–463.
3. Pool JL, Pava AA. *The early diagnosis and treatment of acoustic nerve tumors.* Springfield, IL: Charles C. Thomas, 1957.
4. Dandy WE. The brain. In: Lewis DD, Walters W, eds. *Practice of surgery,* vol 12. Hagerstown, Maryland: WF Prior, 1955.
5. Brackmann DE, Bartels LJ. Rare tumors of the cerebellopontine angle. *Otolaryngol Head Neck Surg* 1980;88:555–559.
6. Brackmann DE. Acoustic neuroma surgery: Otologic Medical Group results. In: Silverstein H, Norrell H, eds. *Neurological surgery of the ear,* vol 2. Birmingham, AL: Aesculapius, 1979:248–259.
7. Johnson EW. Auditory test results in 500 cases of acoustic neuroma. *Arch Otolaryngol* 1977;103:152–158.
8. Ojemann RG, Montgomery WW, Weiss AD. Evaluation and surgical treatment of acoustic neuroma. *N Engl J Med* 1972;287:895–899.
9. House WF. Middle cranial fossa approach to the petrous pyramid. Report of 50 cases. *Arch Otolaryngol* 1963;78:460–469.
10. Hoffman RA, Kohan D, Cohen NL. Cochlear implants in the management of bilateral acoustic neuromas. *Am J Otol* 1992;13:525–528.
11. Basauri L, Riesco MacClure JS. Cerebellopontine angle syndrome: diagnostic problems and surgical indication. *Acta Neurol Latinoamer* 1959;5:220–232.
12. Gonzalez Revilla A. Differential diagnosis of tumors of the cerebellopontine recess. *Bull Johns Hopkins Hosp* 1948;83:187–212.
13. Moller AR, Hatam A, Olivecrona H. The differential diagnosis of pontine angle meningioma of acoustic neuroma with computed tomography. *Neuroradiol* 1978;17:21–23.
14. Norrell H. Neurologic examination in patients with suspected cerebellopontine angle tumors. In: Silverstein H, Norrell H, eds. *Neurological surgery of the ear,* vol 2. Birmingham, AL: Aesculapius, 1979:237–240.
15. Sheehy JL. Acoustic neuroma. The neuro-otologic evaluation. *Arch Otolaryngol* 1968;88:592–597.
16. Joseph J, West CA, Thornton AR, et al. Improved decision criteria for evaluation of clinical ABRs. *Proc Int Electric Response Audiometry Study Group,* Abstract 73, 1987.
17. Martuza RL, Parker SW, Nadol JB Jr, et al. Diagnosis of cerebellopontine angle tumors. *Clin Neurosurg* 1985;32:177–213.
18. Martuza RL, Eldridge R. Neurofibromatosis 2 (bilateral acoustic neurofibromatosis). *N Engl J Med* 1988;318:684–688.
19. Seizinger BR, Martuza RL, Gusella JF. Loss of genes on chromosome 22 in tumorigenesis of human acoustic neuroma. *Nature* 1986;322:644–647.
20. Wu CL, Thakker N, Neary W, et al. Differential diagnosis of type 2 neurofibromatosis: molecular discrimination of NF2 and sporadic vestibular schwannomas. *J Med Genet* 1998;35:973–977.
21. Seizinger BR, Rouleau G, Ozelius LJ, et al. Common pathogenetic mechanism for three tumor types in bilateral acoustic neurofibromatosis. *Science* 1987;236:317–319.
22. Trofatter JA, MacCollin MM, Rutter JL, et al. A novel moesin-, ezrin-, radixin-like gene is a candidate for the neurofibromatosis 2 tumor suppressor. *Cell* 1993;72:791–800.
23. Rouleau GA, Merel P, Lutchman M, et al. Alteration in a new gene encoding a putative membrane-organizing protein causes neuro-fibromatosis type 2. *Nature* 1993;363:515–521.
24. Ikeda K, Saeki Y, Gonzalez-Agosti C, et al. Inhibition of NF2-negative and NF2-positive primary human meningioma cell proliferation by overexpression of merlin due to vector-mediated gene transfer. *J Neurosurg* 1999;91:85–92.
25. Lutchman M, Rouleau GA. The neurofibromatosis type 2 gene product, schwannomin, suppresses growth of NIH 3T3 cells. *Cancer Res* 1995;55:2270–2274.
26. Tikoo A, Varga M, Ramesh V, et al. An anti-Ras function of neurofibromatosis type 2 gene product (NF2/Merlin). *J Biol Chem* 1994;269:23387–23390.
27. Algrain M, Turunen O, Vaheri A, et al. Ezrin contains cytoskeleton and membrane binding domains accounting for its proposed role as a membrane-cytoskeleton linker. *J Cell Biol* 1993;120:129–139.
28. Chishti AH, Kim AC, Marfatia SM. The FERM domain: a unique module involved in the linkage of cytoplasmic proteins to the membrane. *Trends Biochem Sci* 1998;23:281–282.
29. Scoles DR, Huynh DP, Morcos PA, et al. Neurofibromatosis 2 tumour suppressor schwannomin interacts with βII-spectrin. *Nat Genet* 1998;18:354–359.
30. Kimura Y, Koga H, Araki N, et al. The involvement of calpain-dependent proteolysis of the tumor suppressor NF2 (merlin) in schwannomas and meningiomas. *Nat Med* 1998;4:915–922.
31. Ylikoski J, Palva T, Collan Y. Eighth nerve in acoustic neuromas. Special reference to superior vestibular nerve function and histopathology. *Arch Otolaryngol* 1978;104:532–537.
32. Komatsuzaki A, Tsunoda A. Nerve origin of the acoustic neuroma. *J Laryngol Otol* 2001;115:376–379.
33. Nager G. Association of bilateral VIIIth nerve tumors with meningiomas in von Recklinghausen's disease. *Laryngoscope* 1964;74:1220–1261.
34. Perez De Moura LF, Hayden RC Jr, Connor GH. Further observations on acoustic neurinoma. *Trans Am Acad Ophthalmol Otolaryngol* 1969;73:60–70.
35. Karlan MS, Basek M, Potter GB. Intracochlear neurilemoma. *Arch Otolaryngol* 1972;96:573–575.
36. Wanamaker HH. Acoustic neuroma: primary arising in the vestibule. *Laryngoscope* 1972;82:1040–1044.
37. Skinner H. Origin of acoustic nerve tumors. *Br J Surg* 1929;16:440.
38. Nager GT. Acoustic neurinomas. *Acta Otolaryngol (Stockh)* 1985;99:245–261.
39. Stewart TJ, Liland J, Schuknecht HF. Occult schwannomas of the vestibular nerve. *Arch Otolaryngol* 1975;101:91–95.
40. Leonard JR, Talbot ML. Asymptomatic acoustic neurilemoma. *Arch Otolaryngol* 1970;91:117–124.
41. Brooks WH. Geographic clustering of brain tumors in Kentucky. *Cancer* 1972;30:923–926.
42. Olivecrona H. Acoustic tumours. *J Neurol Psychiatr* 1940;3:141–146.
43. Valvassori GE, Guzman M. Growth rate of acoustic neuromas. *Am J Otol* 1989;10:174–176.
44. Laasonen EM, Troupp H. Volume growth rate of acoustic neurinomas. *Neuroradiology* 1986;28:203–207.
45. Gardner G, Moretz WH Jr, Robertson JH, et al. Nonsurgical management of small and intracanalicular acoustic tumors. *Otolaryngol Head Neck Surg* 1986;94:328–333.

46. Nadol JB Jr, Diamond PF, Thornton AR. Correlation of hearing loss and radiologic dimensions of vestibular schwannomas (acoustic neuromas). *Am J Otol* 1996;17:312–316.

47. Mahmud MR, Khan AM, Nadol JB Jr. Histopathology of the inner ear in unoperated acoustic neuroma. *Ann Otol Rhinol Laryngol* 2003;112: 979–986.

48. Schuknecht HF. Pathology of vestibular schwannoma (acoustic neurinoma). In: Silverstein H, Norrell H, eds. *Neurological surgery of the ear.* Birmingham, AL: Aesculapius, 1977:193–197.

49. Eckermeier L, Pirsig W, Mueller D. Histopathology of 30 non-operated acoustic schwannomas. *Arch Otorhinolaryngol* 1979;222:1–9.

50. Neely JG, Hough J. Histologic findings in two very small intracanalicular solitary schwannomas of the eighth nerve. *Ann Otol Rhinol Laryngol* 1986;95:460–465.

51. Kveton JF, Tarlov EC, Drumheller G, et al. Cochlear nerve conduction block: an explanation for spontaneous hearing return after acoustic tumor surgery. *Otolaryngol Head Neck Surg* 1989;100:594–601.

52. Bergenius J, Magnusson M. The relationship between caloric response, oculomotor dysfunction and size of cerebello-pontine angle tumours. *Acta Otolaryngol (Stockh)* 1988;106:361–367.

53. Johnsson L-G, Hawkins JE Jr, Rouse RC. Sensorineural and vascular changes in an ear with acoustic neurinoma. *Am J Otolaryngol* 1984;5: 49–59.

54. Ylikoski J, Collan Y, Palva T, et al. Cochlear nerve in neurilemomas. Audiology and histopathology. *Arch Otolaryngol* 1978;104:679–684.

55. Thomsen J, Tos M. Acoustic neuroma: clinical aspects, audiovestibular assessment, diagnostic delay, and growth rate. *Am J Otol* 1990;11: 12–19.

56. Newman H, Sheline GE, Boldrey EB. Radiation therapy of tumors of the eighth nerve sheath. *Am J Roentgenol Radium Ther Nucl Med*1974;120:562–567.

57. Hirsch A, Norén G, Anderson H. Audiologic findings after stereotactic radiosurgery in nine cases of acoustic neurinomas. *Acta Otolaryngol (Stockh)* 1979;88:155–160.

58. Hirsch A, Norén G. Audiological findings after stereotactic radiosurgery in acoustic neurinomas. *Acta Otolaryngol (Stockh)* 1988;106: 244–251.

59. Kamerer DB, Lunsford LD, Moller M. Gamma knife: an alternative treatment for acoustic neurinomas. *Ann Otol Rhinol Laryngol* 1988;97: 631–635.

60. Slattery WH III, Brackmann DE. Results of surgery following stereotactic irradiation for acoustic neuromas. *Am J Otol* 1995;16:315–319.

61. Brackmann D, Kwartler JA. Treatment of acoustic tumors with radiotherapy. *Arch Otolaryngol Head Neck Surg* 1990;116:161–162.

62. House WF. Monograph. Transtemporal bone microsurgical removal of acoustic neuromas. *Arch Otolaryngol* 1964;80:599–756.

63. Gushing H. *Tumors of the nervus acousticus and the syndrome of the cerebellopontine angle.* Philadelphia: WB Saunders, 1917.

64. Krause F. Zur Feilegung der lirnteren Felsenbeinflache and des-Kleinhims. *Beitr Klin Clur* 1903-37:728–764.

65. Dandy WE. An operation for the total removal of cerebellopontine (acoustic) tumors. *Surg Gynecol Obstet* 1925;41:129–148.

66. Montgomery WW, Ojemann RG, Weiss AD. Suboccipital-translabyrinthine approach for acoustic neuroma. *Arch Otolaryngol* 1966;83:566–569.

67. Parisier SC. The middle cranial fossa approach to the internal auditory canal—an anatomical study stressing critical distances between surgical landmarks. *Laryngoscope* 1977;87[Suppl 4]:1–20.

68. Domb GH, Chole RA. Anatomical studies of the posterior petrous apex with regard to hearing preservation in acoustic neuroma removal. *Laryngoscope* 1980;90:1769–1776.

69. Nadol JB Jr, Levine R, Ojemann RG, et al. Preservation of hearing in surgical removal of acoustic neuromas of the internal auditory canal and cerebellar pontine angle. *Laryngoscope* 1987;97:1287–1294.

70. Levine RA, Ojemann RG, Montgomery WW, et al. Monitoring auditory evoked potentials during acoustic neuroma surgery. Insights into the mechanism of the hearing loss. *Ann Otol Rhinol Laryngol* 1984;93: 116–123.

71. Sekiya T, Moller AR. Effects of cerebellar retractions on the cochlear nerve: an experimental study on rhesus monkeys. *Acta Neurochir (Wien)* 1988;90:45–52.

72. Sekiya T, Moller AR, Jannetta PJ. Pathophysiological mechanisms of intraoperative and postoperative hearing deficits in cerebellopontine angle surgery: an experimental study. *Acta Neurochir (Wien)* 1986;81: 142–151.

73. Sekiya T, Iwabuchi T, Kamata S, et al. Deterioration of auditory evoked potentials during cerebellopontine angle manipulations. An interpretation based on an experimental model in dogs. *J Neurosurg* 1985;63: 598–607.

74. Fisch U. The surgical anatomy of the so-called internal auditory artery. In: Hamberger CA, Wersall J, eds. *Proceedings of the tenth Nobel symposium.* Stockholm, Sweden: Almquist & Wiksell, 1968;121–130.

75. Martuza RL, Ojemann RG. Bilateral acoustic neuromas: clinical aspects, pathogenesis, and treatment. *Neurosurgery* 1982;10:1–12.

76. Otto SR, Brackmann DE, Hitselberger WE, et al. Brainstem electronic implants for bilateral anacusis following surgical removal of cerebello pontine angle lesions. *Otolaryngol Clin North Am* 2001;34:485–499.

CHAPTER 43

Tumors of the Facial Nerve

Michael J. McKenna and K. Paul Boyev

The facial nerve may be involved by both benign and malignant neoplasms. Although the resulting symptoms maybe similar, the management and prognosis are different. The successful management is dependent upon an accurate and early diagnosis.

The most common benign neoplasms that arise from the facial nerve are schwannoma, neurofibroma, and hemangioma. Other benign neoplasms that may affect the facial nerve include paraganglioma, meningioma, endolymphatic sac tumor, epidermoid tumor, and vestibular schwannoma. The facial nerve may also be involved by a variety of malignant processes, including squamous cell carcinoma, adenocarcinoma, sarcomas, adenoid cystic carcinoma, mucoepidermoid carcinoma, and hemangiopericytoma. The successful treatment is dependent upon establishing an accurate diagnosis, acquiring a knowledge of the natural history of the disease process, determining the extent of involvement, and determining the age and general health of the affected individual. In general, the management of malignant tumors involving the facial nerve is based upon oncologic principles of control or cure of the underlying malignancy. Early surgical intervention with sacrifice of the facial nerve is indicated when a possible cure can be accomplished. The management of benign neoplasm involving the facial nerve requires a more thoughtful consideration. Ultimately the best approach depends upon the natural history of neoplasm, the degree of symptomatology, and the patient's own desire following a discussion of realistic expectations for recovery of function with intervention, both immediate and delayed.

DIAGNOSIS

The most common presenting symptom of both benign and malignant tumors involving the facial nerve is a gradual progressive paresis and paralysis occurring over a period of weeks to months. Approximately 5% of all lower motor neuron facial palsies are secondary to facial nerve tumors (1). The time course over which the paresis or paralysis occurs is often the most important clinical feature in differentiating a neoplastic process from the more sudden paresis characteristic of Bell's palsy. The gradual onset of paresis is the presenting symptom in approximately 60% of patients. However, a sudden paralysis similar to Bell's palsy may also occur in 10% to 20% of cases (2,3). In addition, some benign neoplasms may present with transient paresis. Approximately 30% of patients with facial nerve schwannomas have normal facial function at the time of diagnosis (3). An accurate and timely diagnosis is dependent upon an index of suspicion and a careful and complete clinical evaluation.

The presence of auditory or vestibular symptoms should raise the index of suspicion. A history of malignant disease, either local or distant, could indicate possible metastatic involvement of the facial nerve. This is especially true for cutaneous malignancies involving the face, head, and neck, which may readily metastasize or spread to involve the facial nerve by perineural extension.

A complete head and neck, otologic, and neurotologic evaluation is paramount in the evaluation of patients with facial paralysis. Involvement of a single branch of the facial nerve, with sparing of others, should also raise concern of an underlying neoplasm.

Audiometry may be useful in establishing the presence of an ipsilateral conductive or sensorineural hearing loss. Hearing loss of either type is present in 28.5% (4) to 49% (3) of patients with schwannomas of the facial nerve. Electroneuronography is also useful both from a diagnostic and prognostic standpoint once a diagnosis is established and surgery is being considered.

RADIOGRAPHIC EVALUATION (FIG. 43.1)

Any patient who is suspected of having a neoplasm of the facial nerve should undergo radiographic evaluation with both high-resolution temporal bone computed tomographic (CT) scan and gadolinium-contrast magnetic resonance imaging (MRI) (5). The MRI scan with gadolinium can demonstrate abnormal enhancement of the facial nerve from the brainstem to the periphery. Because patients with idiopathic facial paralysis often have abnormal enhancement of the facial nerve

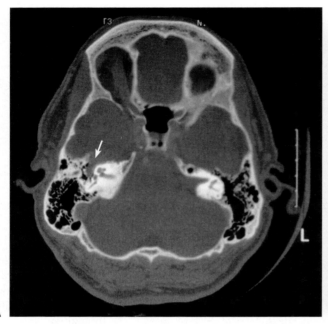
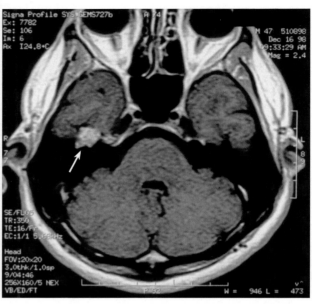

FIG. 43.1 A: Axial CT scan with bone window technique demonstrating an expansile lesion in the area of the geniculate ganglion on the left *(arrow)*. Patient had a history of progressive facial paresis. The cause was hemangioma. **B:** Axial T1 gadolinium-enhanced image of the same patient shows enhancement of the lesion *(arrow)*.

centered in the geniculate area and extending both antero-grade and retrograde into the tympanic cavity and internal auditory canal, it may be difficult on the MRI scan alone to differentiate this enhancement from that which is seen in cases of facial nerve schwannomas. The CT scan is often useful in evaluating for the presence of bone erosion in the region of geniculate fossa and labyrinthine segment, which may occur with a facial nerve schwannoma or geniculate hemangioma.

Ultimately the diagnosis of a primary facial nerve tumor is made on the basis of clinical evaluation and radiographic studies. Although it might be tempting to biopsy a primary facial nerve tumor to establish the histologic diagnosis, this will often result in immediate facial paralysis and should be avoided if possible (6). Facial nerve tumors involving the tympanic segment of the facial nerve may present initially as a mass within the middle ear, with conductive hearing loss. Although not a common postmortem finding, Zhang et al. (7) found 12 asymptomatic tympanic segment schwannomas in a collection of 1,526 temporal bones. Often the diagnosis is difficult to establish solely on the basis of exam and radiographic studies, especially when there is no evidence of preoperative facial nerve dysfunction. An accurate diagnosis may be further clouded by a concurrent problem with chronic otitis media secondary to eustachian tube dysfunction.

DIFFERENTIAL DIAGNOSIS

The most common tumors of the facial nerve are schwannoma, followed by hemangioma. These benign lesions must be differentiated from other benign and malignant lesions of

the temporal bone, such as meningioma, vestibular schwannoma, primary epidermoid tumor, paraganglioma, and metastatic lesions. To some extent, schwannomas and hemangiomas exhibit distinct proclivities for certain anatomic sites along the facial nerve (3,4,8–10) (Fig. 43.2). Characteristic radiographic features of each are often helpful in establishing a differential diagnosis (11). However, definitive diagnosis can only be established at surgical exploration.

MANAGEMENT

At present there is no role for medical management of benign neoplasms of the facial nerve. However, in the future, the use of antiangiogenetic factors may possibly play a role for vascular neoplasms affecting the facial nerve, such as paragangliomas and hemangiomas. There is no evidence at present to support the use of radiation therapy as a primary treatment modality for benign facial nerve tumors (12).

The surgical management of malignant lesions can be divided into palliative and curative procedures. The preservation of facial nerve integrity and function may be a primary goal of palliative procedures. Curative procedures for malignant lesions involving the facial nerve may require sacrifice of the facial nerve. Because many malignant lesions have a tendency for perineural invasion and spread, reconstructive efforts with cable grafting should make use of intraoperative frozen sections to be certain that both the proximal and distal segments of the nerve are free of disease. Often, extensive malignant disease precludes the use of cable grafting, and other alternative forms of facial reanimation may be

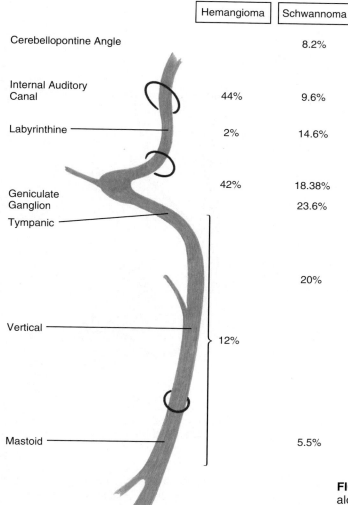

	Hemangioma	Schwannoma
Cerebellopontine Angle		8.2%
Internal Auditory Canal	44%	9.6%
Labyrinthine	2%	14.6%
Geniculate Ganglion	42%	18.38%
Tympanic		23.6%
		20%
Vertical	12%	
Mastoid		5.5%

FIG. 43.2 Distribution of hemangiomas and schwannomas along the facial nerve. Approximately 90% of hemangiomas occur between the internal auditory canal and tympanic segment, whereas schwannomas tend to be more evenly distributed.

necessary. Adjunctive therapy with either chemotherapy or radiation should not be delayed even if a cable graft is used. These patients should undergo a baseline imaging study with CT, MRI, or both in the early postoperative course, which will serve as a baseline for surveillance for possible recurrence.

The most critical aspect of preoperative planning for surgical management of benign facial nerve tumors surrounds the timing for intervention and should be individualized based on the degree of preoperative impairment, amount of neuronal degeneration as determined by electroneuronography, progression of auditory and vestibular dysfunction, and the patient's own desires. Although some facial nerve hemangiomas can be resected in a manner that maintains facial nerve integrity and continuity, it is more common that a portion of the facial nerve must be resected, which necessitates a cable graft (8). The central dilemma of planning surgical intervention is timing: The operation needs to take place while conditions for maximizing postoperative cable graft function are optimal; however, during this window, the patient's level of function is usually better than the best expected cable graft outcome. It has been our philosophy to wait until there is evidence of noticeable progression of symptoms but to recommend surgical intervention before residual facial neuronal function drops below 40% on electroneuronography. Our results and the results reported by others indicate that the best possible recovery is a House-Brackmann grade III, with most patients ending up with House-Brackmann grade IV (13). Because the final recovery is often poorer than the preoperative facial function, the patients need to have a clear understanding of the goals of the proposed surgical procedure and realistic expectations prior to surgery. Patients should undergo both still and video photography prior to surgery. We have also found it helpful for patients to view photographs and videos of other patients who have undergone similar procedures so that they can gain a realistic expectation of the degree of recovery that might be expected in their case.

SURGICAL PLANNING

Planning the appropriate surgical approach is dependent upon an accurate preoperative diagnosis, especially with regard to the exact location and extent of involvement of the facial nerve. The surgical approach selected should provide the surgeon with the greatest technical ease of placing and securing the cable graft. Primary anastomosis of nerves is the more desirable method of repairing facial nerve defects, but this is often not possible (14). Although in some cases of small schwannomas and hemangiomas, it is technically possible to strip the tumor away without resecting the nerve, the planned procedure should provide exposure necessary for placement of the cable graft, which is more often required.

Choice of Cable Graft

In choosing a cable graft, the two important features are the length of graft required and the branching pattern necessary to accommodate the number of distal anastomoses. With the great auricular nerve, it is possible to bridge gaps up to 5 cm (Fig. 43.3). The great auricular nerve offers the distinct advantage that it can be harvested from within the same operative field. The sural nerve offers the advantage of greater length. It also has a branching pattern in its distal segment, which can accommodate up to three distal anastomoses (Fig. 43.4). We have utilized the medial antebrachial cutaneous

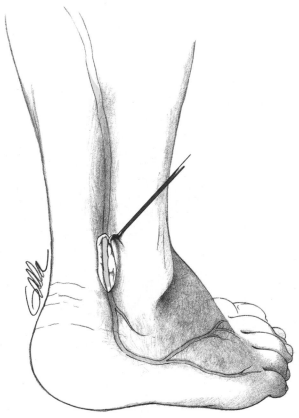

FIG. 43.4 The sural nerve can be located superficially in the subcutaneous plane posterior to the lateral malleolus.

nerve graft for tumors that involve the facial nerve beyond the pes anserinus, where multiple distant anastomoses are required. With the medial antebrachial cutaneous nerve, it is possible to obtain a nerve graft up to 24 cm in length with up to five distal branches (Fig. 43.5).

Harvesting of Cable Graft

The great auricular nerve can be found overlying the sternocleidomastoid muscle at a point midway between the mastoid tip and the angle of the mandible and lying just posterior to the external jugular vein. This nerve may be harvested through an extension of a postauricular incision or a small separate incision in the neck.

The sural nerve is found on the lateral aspect of the foot approximately 2 cm posterior to the lateral (fibular) malleolus just deep to branches of the saphenous vein. Often, two operative fields can be set up such that harvest of the nerve can be performed by one surgeon while the other surgeon is working in the temporal bone.

The medial antebrachial cutaneous nerve, another sensory nerve, passes through the brachial fascia near the basilic vein to become superficial on the medial aspect of the arm. It then divides into posterior and anterior branches, which further ramify (15).

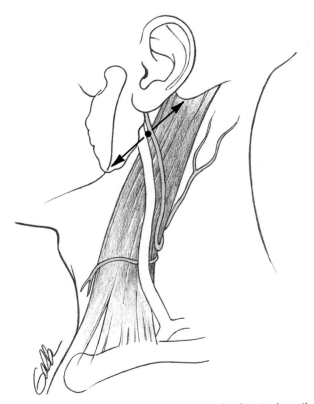

FIG. 43.3 The great auricular nerve can be located on the lateral surface of the sternocleidomastoid muscle at the midpoint of a line drawn between the mastoid tip and the angle of the mandible.

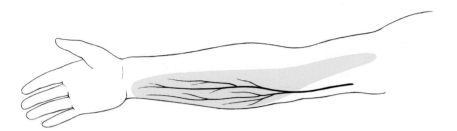

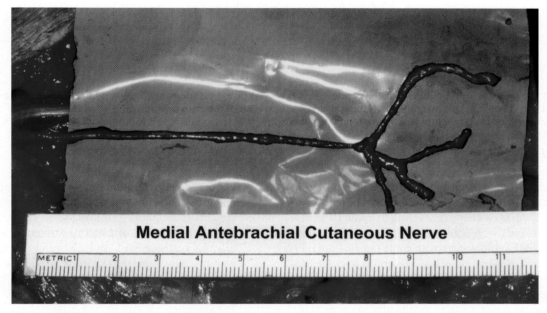

Medial Antebrachial Cutaneous Nerve

FIG. 43.5 A: The medial antebrachial cutaneous nerve, a sensory nerve located on the medial surface of the arm (sensory distribution in *yellow*), is useful for repairing large facial nerve defects. **B:** The length and branching pattern of the medial antebrachial cutaneous nerve make possible a repair with multiple anastomoses to remaining distal segments of the facial nerve.

Selection of a Surgical Approach to the Tumor

Translabyrinthine Approach

The translabyrinthine approach is utilized for tumors involving the facial nerve in the posterior fossa; internal auditory canal; labyrinthine segment; geniculate area, with or without involvement of the middle ear; and mastoid segments of the facial nerve when hearing is poor and hearing preservation is not a goal of the procedure.

Middle Fossa Approach

The middle fossa approach is selected for tumors involving the internal auditory canal with minimal extension into the posterior fossa, labyrinthine segment, and geniculate when the hearing is good and hearing preservation is a goal of the procedure.

Transmastoid Approach

The transmastoid approach is used for tumors that involve the middle ear and mastoid segment of the facial nerve without extension to the geniculate ganglion.

Combined Middle Fossa/Transmastoid

The combined middle fossa/transmastoid approach is utilized for tumors that involve the facial nerve within the internal auditory canal, labyrinthine segment, geniculate, middle ear, and mastoid when hearing preservation is a goal of the procedure (Fig. 43.6).

INFORMED CONSENT

Patients who undergo surgery for both benign and malignant facial nerve tumors should be presented with realistic expectations for recovery, as well as a detailed discussion of the possible risks and complications specific for the proposed surgical approach.

1. *Failure of cable graft.* The best results with cable grafting are achieved for grafts confined to the tympanomastoid cavity, with greater than 95% of patients recovering some movement when some facial function is present preoperatively. Approximately 70% recover to grade IV, 20% to grade III. For patients who have preoperative facial paralysis, the results are less predictable. Generally,

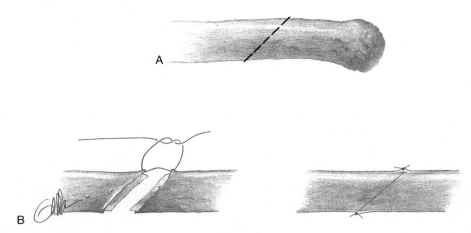

FIG. 43.6 A: The facial nerve stump and cable graft are prepared for anastomosis by sectioning with a sharp blade at approximately 45 degrees to the long axis of the nerve trunk. **B:** The epineurium is removed for a distance of approximately 1 mm from the anastomotic site to promote apposition of nerve fibers.

if the paralysis has been present for less than 1 year, 70% recover some function, most of whom recover to grade IV, with no patients recovering to grade III or better. For patients with paralysis of greater than 2 years' duration, the overall results with cable grafting are poor and better results can be achieved with hypoglossal facial anastomosis combined with temporalis transposition. Securing a cable graft with a proximal anastomosis within the posterior fossa is technically more difficult, and the percentage of patients who achieve a grade III result is significantly less, with most patients recovering to grade IV. In our experience, approximately 15% to 20% do not recover to grade IV and eventually require ancillary facial reanimation procedures.

Patients who require sacrifice of their facial nerve, with or without cable grafting, will require oculoplastic intervention to protect the affected eye. These patients are at risk for exposure keratitis from inadequate corneal coverage resulting from weakness of the orbicularis oculi.

Postoperative aberrant regeneration with synkinesis and hypertonicity at rest is a common feature of even successful cable grafts. Most patients have not experienced this aspect of facial dysfunction preoperatively and should be educated regarding this expected result. Synkinesis affecting the eye may be relieved using botulinum (Oculinum) injections, which necessitate reinjection every 3 to 6 months. Other ancillary procedures for improving facial symmetry after the final recovery should also be discussed, including endoscopic brow lift and unilateral or asymmetric rhytidectomy.

2. *The loss of some or all hearing in the operated ear and problems with tinnitus.* Both conductive and sensorineural hearing loss can result from resection of facial nerve tumors. The presence of preoperative sensorineural hearing loss is a poor prognostic factor. Patients with facial nerve tumors involving the middle

ear may require a future procedure to correct a residual conductive hearing loss when it persists postoperatively.

3. *Deficits in balance.* In most cases, vestibular problems related to resection of facial nerve tumors improve significantly or resolve with time. A small percentage of patients may require additional procedures, including labyrinthectomy or vestibular neurectomy if vestibular compensation does not occur.

4. *Postoperative spinal fluid leakage and meningitis.* In cases that require craniotomy, such as resection of facial nerve tumors proximal to the labyrinthine segment, spinal fluid leakage may occur. Most of these cases resolve with postoperative lumbar drainage for 3 to 5 days. If the spinal fluid leak persists following removal of the lumbar drain, an additional procedure for repair of the leak will be required. This could conceivably result in hearing loss even if the hearing was preserved following the initial procedure.

5. *Injury to other cranial nerves and possible stroke.* Patients who undergo surgical resection of tumors within the posterior fossa are subject to the same risks as patients who undergo resection of acoustic neuromas and should be counseled accordingly. In addition to the aforementioned risk of cerebrospinal fluid (CSF) fistula, lower cranial nerves such as IX and X are within the surgical field and may be affected.

6. *Donor site deficits.* Patients who undergo cable grafting will incur a sensory deficit from resection of the donor graft. For the great auricular nerve graft, the sensory deficit will include the ipsilateral auricle. Patients who undergo harvesting of sural nerve graft will have numbness of the top of the foot. Patients who have a medial antebrachial cutaneous nerve graft will experience numbness of the forearm. Nearly all patients will experience some degree of recovery of sensation in theses areas in subsequent years.

7. *Tumor recurrence.* Patients should be counseled as to the risk of tumor recurrence, which is based primarily on the histology of the primary neoplasm and the ability to achieve a complete resection. Subtotal resection, to which surgeons may resort if total resection would result in unacceptable morbidity, would obviously raise the possibility of recurrence. This issue should be addressed based on the surgeon's judgment of the likelihood of subtotal resection.

SURGICAL TECHNIQUE

Transmastoid Approach

The transmastoid approach is selected for tumors that involve the tympanic segment of the facial nerve, the mastoid segment, or both. It should not be utilized for tumors that involve the geniculate ganglion. Although the geniculate ganglion can be dissected through a transmastoid approach, this approach does not afford the exposure necessary for securing the proximal anastomosis of the cable graft if one is necessary.

The transmastoid approach is accomplished through a postauricular incision, which is 1 to 2 cm posterior to the postauricular crease. The soft tissues over the mastoid cortex are elevated using a periosteal elevator to the level of the external auditory canal. Following placement of self-retaining retractors, a canal wall–up mastoidectomy is performed with an extended posterior tympanotomy. Both the lateral semicircular canal and mastoid segment of the facial nerve are skeletonized. For tumors involving the tympanic segment, the incudostapedial joint is separated through the posterior tympanotomy and the incus is removed. Exposure of the tumor within the epitympanum can also be improved by removal of the head of the malleus using a malleus nipper and cutting the malleus at its neck. Ultimately, at the conclusion of procedure, the incus may be refashioned into a minor columellar strut and a type III tympanoplasty performed. Care should be taken to preserve the fallopian canal, within which will ultimately lie the interposed cable graft. For tumors that extend through the stylomastoid foramen, the mastoid tip is removed, allowing dissection of the tumor into the proximal portion of the parotid gland. The proximal and distal segments of facial nerve are sharply resected using a Wheeler ophthalmic blade. A portion of the proximal and distal segment of the specimen is sent for frozen section to be certain that the tumor has been completely excised. An adequate cable graft can almost always be fashioned using the great auricular nerve, harvested either by extending the incision inferiorly and anteriorly over the sternocleidomastoid muscle or through a separate incision. A measurement of length necessary for the cable graft is made using either umbilical tape or a 2-0 silk suture placed at the proximal and distal anastomosis sites and within the hemicanal of the facial nerve. This then serves as a template for establishing the length of the cable graft, the ends of which are cut at 45-degree angle using the Wheeler blade. Both the umbilical

tape template and the cable graft are placed side by side on a sterile wooden tongue blade moistened with saline. The graft is cut at both ends at a 45% obliquity to increase the surface area of contact with the similarly prepared nerve stumps (Fig. 43.6). The graft can then be positioned in the hemicanal. Because there will be no motion to disturb either the proximal or distal anastomosis, no suture is necessary to secure the anastomosis. Instead, a small piece of Surgicel is placed over the anastomosis. The type III tympanoplasty with the incus minor columella strut should be completed prior to placement of the graft so that the anastomoses are not disturbed during this portion of the procedure. The wound is closed in layers with a Penrose drain, which is brought out through the inferior aspect of the incision.

Translabyrinthine Approach

The translabyrinthine approach is selected for cases where hearing preservation is not a goal (Fig. 43.7). Tumors involving the posterior fossa, internal auditory canal, labyrinthine segment, geniculate, middle ear, and mastoid can all be resected and grafted through this approach. A postauricular incision is made approximately 3 cm posterior to the postauricular crease. Because hearing preservation is not a goal, the external canal is transected, the canal skin undermined, and a blind sac closure accomplished. The residual squamous epithelium of the distal canal and drum are removed. A canal wall–down tympanomastoidectomy is then performed. The eustachian tube orifice is widened with a diamond drill, and the eustachian tube is obliterated with fascia and bone wax impacted using the tip of a cotton-tipped applicator. A labyrinthectomy is then performed, and the internal auditory canal and posterior fossa dura are skeletonized. The overlying eggshell of bone is removed. The dura is then opened, and the tumor is resected. The proximal segment of the facial nerve should be divided using neurectomy scissors. Complete surgical resection is confirmed using frozen sections. If possible, the eighth nerve complex should be preserved to provide structural support for the facial nerve cable graft. The length of graft is measured using umbilical tape or a 2-0 silk suture. If greater than 4.0 cm of nerve graft is required, often the sural nerve will provide a better match in both length and diameter. The proximal anastomosis should be accomplished using 9-0 proline suture with at least two well-placed sutures. The distal anastomosis should also be secured using a suture anastomosis. This will prevent distraction of the anastomosis when abdominal fat is packed in to seal the durotomy and to obliterate the cavity. The wound is closed in layers with a watertight closure of the skin.

Middle Fossa and Combined Transmastoid/Middle Fossa Approaches (Fig. 43.8)

This approach is used for tumors involving the facial at the geniculate, proximal to the geniculate, and with or without distal extension into the middle ear and mastoid. It has been

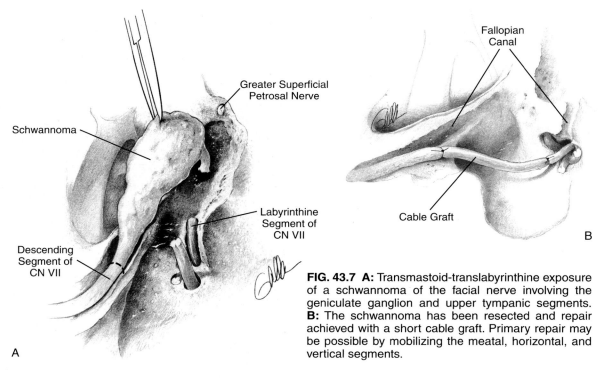

FIG. 43.7 A: Transmastoid-translabyrinthine exposure of a schwannoma of the facial nerve involving the geniculate ganglion and upper tympanic segments. **B:** The schwannoma has been resected and repair achieved with a short cable graft. Primary repair may be possible by mobilizing the meatal, horizontal, and vertical segments.

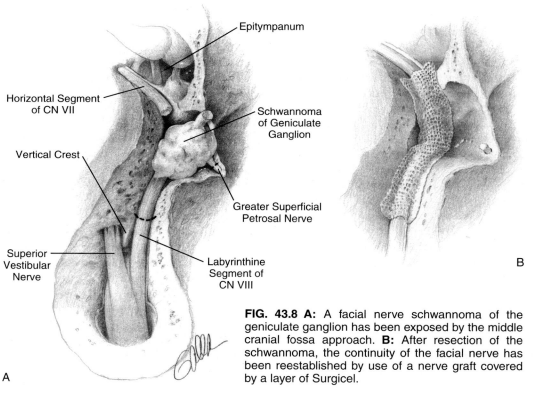

FIG. 43.8 A: A facial nerve schwannoma of the geniculate ganglion has been exposed by the middle cranial fossa approach. **B:** After resection of the schwannoma, the continuity of the facial nerve has been reestablished by use of a nerve graft covered by a layer of Surgicel.

our practice to place a preoperative lumbar drain at the time of surgery once the patient has been anesthetized. This is helpful during the procedure in lowering the spinal fluid pressure and facilitating placement of the middle fossa retractor, as well as in the prevention of CSF fistula in the postoperative period. The superior limb of the mastoid inci-

sion is extended anteriorly and superiorly to provide exposure of the temporal fossa. Care must be taken not to interrupt the temporalis muscle because this might possibly be required for future facial reanimation. The temporalis muscle is incised near its insertion and reflected inferiorly. A 5-by 6-cm rectangular craniotomy is created, centered two-thirds anterior and one-third posterior to the external auditory canal. Additional bone is then removed inferiorly using a diamond bur so that the inferior limb of the craniotomy is flush with the floor of middle cranial fossa. The middle fossa dura is then elevated medially to the level of the petrous ridge. A House-Urban middle fossa retractor is then placed with the retractor blade perched at the petrous ridge. Using diamond burs and suction irrigation, the internal auditory canal is first exposed medially in the region of the porus acousticus. The roof of the internal auditory canal is then followed laterally to the level of the labyrinthine segment and geniculate ganglion in a manner similar to that used for resection of acoustic neuromas through the middle fossa approach. Bone of the tegmen tympani is removed, exposing the upper tympanic segment of the facial nerve. The dura of the internal auditory canal and posterior fossa are then opened, and the proximal segment of the facial nerve is divided using neurectomy scissors. It is not uncommon for tumors involving the geniculate area to have eroded into the cochlea or to have resulted in exposure of the cochlear endosteum. Therefore care should be taken not to disturb or penetrate the cochlea when the geniculate segment of the tumor is resected. Once the distal segment of the facial nerve has been resected sharply, frozen sections should be sent from both the proximal and distal segments of the specimen to be certain that they are free of tumor. Prior to placement of a cable graft, the air cells within the petrous apex are obliterated with bone wax. The length of graft necessary is measured using either umbilical tape or a 2-0 silk suture. The graft is secured at both its proximal and distal anastomoses with 9-0 prolene suture. Once secured, small pieces of abdominal fat are then placed within the bony defect in the petrous apex and over the internal auditory canal. The wound is closed in layers with a watertight closure of the skin. Postoperatively, the lumbar drain is left in place draining for up to 5 days to prevent a CSF fistula.

POSTOPERATIVE CARE

Management of the Paralyzed Eye

Patients who undergo resection of facial nerve tumors, with or without cable grafting, will require ongoing oculoplastic management of the paralyzed eyelid. Initially, ocular lubricants in the form of artificial tears and Lacrilube are prescribed. The eyelid is taped closed during periods of sleep. An oculoplastic consult is obtained in all cases. Under most circumstances, these patients can be managed with combination of a gold weight implant in the upper lid and a minimal lateral canthoplasty. Both these procedures are reversible if adequate recovery of facial function in the region of the eye ensues. These patients require continuous monitoring and oculoplastic follow-up over time.

At the onset of recovery of facial function, patients may benefit from intensive facial nerve physical therapy. This usually consists of a series of exercises that are structured to both maximize recovery of the paralyzed side of the face and to achieve improved symmetry by modifying the movement of the contralateral normal face. To date, there has been no good evidence to support the role for electrical stimulation in facilitating recovery of the paralyzed face.

Patients who undergo resection of facial nerve tumors with cable grafting may require ancillary procedures even when the outcome from the cable nerve graft is considered excellent. One such procedure, which has proven helpful in many of our patients, has been the endoscopic brow lift. Because most patients fail to recover function of the brow, symmetry in this region can be improved. It may also provide some benefit for patients in whom a ptotic brow obstructs their superior visual field. The use of botulinum type A toxin (Oculinum) has proven extremely helpful in the management of patients who develop synkinesis in the region of the eye when facial nerve function is restored (16). It is also helpful in patients with hypertonicity and dimpling in the region of the chin and platysma. The disadvantage of Oculinum therapy is that it requires ongoing treatment with injections given as often as three to four times yearly.

If no recovery of function is noted at 1 year following placement of the cable graft, some consideration should be given to other reanimation procedures. For cable grafts with the proximal segment within the posterior fossa, recovery may require up to 18 months. However, delays beyond 18 months may adversely impact the outcome of other nerve transfer procedures, such as a hypoglossal facial anastomosis, because of muscular atrophy. The use of electromyography may be sometimes helpful in determining the presence of reinnervation before clinical evidence of return is apparent. However, presence of reinnervation potentials can also be misleading because they are sometimes detected in cases where no significant clinical return of function occurs.

SURGICAL COMPLICATIONS

Infectious complications following resection of facial nerve tumors and cable grafting are rare but can have deleterious effects on the eventual function of cable grafts. For this reason, it has been our practice to place patients on perioperative antibiotics for 5 to 7 days following surgery. Patients who have CSF leakage following surgery are at risk for developing meningitis. Prior to the patient's discharge, provocative testing to exclude the possibility of CSF fistula should be performed. The patient is seated upright and asked to lean forward with hands on knees. This posture is maintained for 3 minutes while the surgeon watches for CSF rhinorrhea. Because the incidence of CSF leakage following middle fossa surgery for resection of facial nerve tumors is relatively high, it has been our practice to maintain prophylactic lumbar drainage in these patients for 5 days following surgery. It is also our practice to maintain antibiotic coverage for patients who have CSF fistula, because a recent meta-analysis suggests that the incidence of meningitis can be decreased (17).

Many serious and often overlooked potential complications following management of patients with facial nerve tumors are related to corneal exposure from inadequate closure of the lid. Patients who develop problems with corneal irritation may progress to exposure keratitis and, in some cases, to corneal ulceration. They may suffer permanent pain and visual loss despite eventual recovery of facial function. A sequela of corneal inflammation is corneal opacification, treatable only by corneal transplantation. Therefore these patients require careful and planned systematic follow-up by an oculoplastic specialist who can offer the patient a range of options from ocular lubrication to eyelid surgery or botulinum injections. Patients need to be educated regarding the significance of increased pain and redness of the eye upon discharge and should seek help immediately if such symptoms develop. We have found that the use of protective, clear shield humidification chambers in the immediate perioperative period has been helpful in reducing such symptoms.

REFERENCES

1. Shambaugh G, Alford BR, Devriese PP, et al. Panel discussion No. 12. Treatment of facial palsy of infectious origin. In: Fisch U, ed. *Facial nerve surgery.* Birmingham, AL: Aesculapius, 1977:419–424.
2. Fisch U, Rüttner J. Pathology of intratemporal tumors involving the facial nerve. In: Fisch U, ed. *Facial nerve surgery.* Birmingham, AL: Aesculapius, 1977:448–456.
3. Lipkin AF, Coker NJ, Jenkins HA, et al. Intracranial and intratemporal facial neuroma. *Otolaryngol Head Neck Surg* 1987;96:71–79.
4. Saleh EM, Achilli V, Naguib M, et al. Facial nerve neuromas: diagnosis and management. *Am J Otol* 1995;16:521–526.
5. Lo WW, Shelton C, Waluch V, et al. Intratemporal vascular tumors: detection with CT and MR imaging. *Radiology* 1989;171:445–448.
6. Pillsbury HC, Price HC, Gardiner LJ. Primary tumors of the facial nerve: diagnosis and management. *Laryngoscope* 1983;93:1045–1048.
7. Zhang Q, Jessurun J, Schachern PA, et al. Outgrowing schwannomas arising from tympanic segments of the facial nerve. *Am J Otolaryngol* 1996;17:311–315.
8. Eby TL, Fisch U, Makek MS. Facial nerve management in temporal bone hemangiomas. *Am J Otol* 1992;13:223–232.
9. O'Donoghue GM, Brackmann DE, House JW, et al. Neuromas of the facial nerve. *Am J Otol* 1989;10:49–54.
10. Shelton C, Brackmann DE, Lo WW, et al. Intratemporal facial nerve hemangiomas. *Otolaryngol Head Neck Surg* 1991;104:116–121.
11. Curtin HD, Jensen JE, Barnes L Jr, et al. Ossifying hemangiomas of the temporal bone: evaluation with CT. *Radiology* 1987;164:831–835.
12. Mabanta SR, Buatti JM, Friedman WA, et al. Linear accelerator radiosurgery for nonacoustic schwannomas. *Int J Radiat Oncol Biol Phys* 1999;43:545–548.
13. Arriaga MA, Brackmann DE. Facial nerve repair techniques in cerebellopontine angle tumor surgery. *Am J Otol* 1992;13:356–359.
14. Coker NJ. Management of traumatic injury to the facial nerve. *Otolaryngol Clin North Am* 1991;24:215–227.
15. Cheney ML, Megerian CA, McKenna MJ. Rehabilitation of the paralyzed face. In: Cheney ML, ed. *Facial surgery: plastic and reconstructive.* Baltimore: Williams & Wilkins, 1997:655–684.
16. Sadiq SA, Downes RN. A clinical algorithm for the management of facial nerve palsy from an oculoplastic perspective. *Eye* 1998;12:219–223.
17. Brodie HA. Prophylactic antibiotics for posttraumatic cerebrospinal fluid fistulae. A meta-analysis. *Arch Otolaryngol Head Neck Surg* 1997;123:749–752.

CHAPTER 44

Cystic Lesions of the Petrous Apex

Richard R. Gacek and Mark R. Gacek

The subtle clinical presentations of petrous apex lesions are related to the regional anatomy of the apical segment of the temporal bone (Fig. 44.1). The usual presenting symptoms of an expanding lesion in the petrous apex are a conductive hearing loss from the serous effusion caused by eustachian tube obstruction, headache from pressure on the dural covering, diplopia related to involvement of the third and sixth cranial nerves, facial hypesthesia caused by compression of the fifth cranial nerve, and varying degrees of faintness or vertigo probably caused by changes in vascular flow (1). Various pathologies may arise within this small region of the temporal bone because of the complex anatomic composition of the petrous apex, consisting of air cells, bone marrow, cartilage, nerve bundles, and vascular structures (internal carotid artery, jugular bulb) (2). Sophisticated imaging techniques (e.g., computed tomography [CT], magnetic resonance imaging [MRI]) now permit early recognition of a petrous apex lesion. The pathologies involving the petrous apex may be divided into solid and cystic lesions (Table 44.1).

DIAGNOSIS

The clinical suspicion of a progressive lesion in the petrous apex is based on recognition of one or more of the signs and symptoms related to adjacent anatomic structures (eustachian tube, cranial nerves III through VIII, dura, and internal carotid artery). In the premodern imaging era (before CT and MRI), lesions in this area were probably underrecognized because of the difficulty in clearly demonstrating bone erosion with the conventional base of skull radiographs or polytomography. Extensive bone erosion could be detected with such studies, followed by confirmation of an extradural mass by supplementary studies such as arteriography and pneumoencephalography. Presently, thin-section (1 to 1.5 mm) CT scanning and MRI are capable of identifying such lesions in the petrous apex much earlier in their development with minimal risk (Fig. 44.2). The evaluation of a suspected lesion in the petrous apex should require CT scanning and MRI (3,4). The nature of a lesion as solid or cystic

is usually revealed by the enhancement on CT and signal picture on T1 and T2 images with MRI. Arteriography may be added to define a vascular lesion or to locate displacement of the internal carotid artery.

MANAGEMENT

Solid Tumors

The management of solid tumors requires identification of the histopathology prior to definitive treatment (1). Several factors determine the approach to biopsy of solid petrous apex lesions. If the tumor has extended into an area that is easily accessible without risk to labyrinthine function, such as the infralabyrinthine and hypotympanic cell tracts, or into the sphenoid sinus, these compartments should be accessed for sampling the tumor. However, if the tumor is contained

---

TABLE 44.1 *Petrous apex pathologies categorized by lesion type*

Solid Lesions
Benign
  Neurofibroma or schwannoma
  Chondroma
  Meningioma
  Paraganglioma
  Dermoid
Malignant
  Chondrosarcoma
  Eosinophilic granuloma
  Lymphoma
  Metastatic malignancies (breast, lung, kidney, prostate)

Cystic Lesions
Vascular
  Internal carotid aneurysm
  Venous lake
Nonvascular
  Apicitis (abscess)
  Congenital epidermoid cyst
  Cholesterol granuloma (mucocele)
  Arachnoid cyst

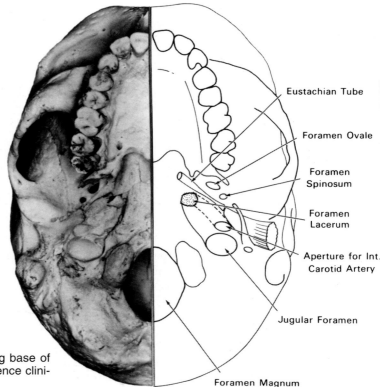

FIG. 44.1 Composite drawing and photograph showing base of skull structures adjacent to the petrous apex that influence clinical presentation.

Eustachian Tube

Foramen Ovale

Foramen Spinosum

Foramen Lacerum

Aperture for Int. Carotid Artery

Jugular Foramen

Foramen Magnum

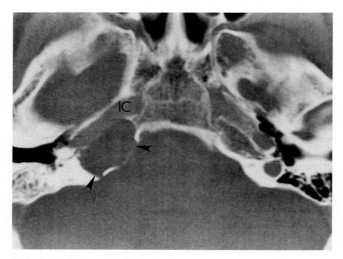

FIG. 44.2 Bone erosion from a petrous apex epidermoid *(arrowheads)* as seen in a CT scan. IC, internal carotid artery.

within the petrous apex and labyrinth function is normal, a middle cranial fossa extradural approach skirting the temporal bone is the most direct approach to the tumor while preserving seventh and eighth cranial nerve function.

Definitive management is guided by the histologic nature of the lesion. A benign lesion may be excised totally or subtotally depending on the progressive nature of the clinical symptoms and the patient's age and medical status. Postoperative surveillance of the petrous apex tumor may be car-

ried out with imaging studies to determine possible recurrence and progression. A malignant tumor will require nonsurgical management (radiation therapy, chemotherapy) because en bloc resection of this portion of the temporal bone is not feasible for cure, particularly if one considers the morbidity associated with the surgery. However, low-grade malignancy such as eosinophilic granuloma may be treated more effectively by extensive subtotal removal using curettage followed by radiation therapy.

Cystic Lesions

Cystic lesions may be vascular or nonvascular, and their management will vary from case to case. If imaging studies are not able to demonstrate the vascular nature of a lesion with certainty, then arteriography is required. The major vascular lesion of the petrous apex is an internal carotid aneurysm (Fig. 44.3). If the lesion is causing minimal nonprogressive clinical symptoms, then the aneurysm should be conservatively followed clinically and neuroradiologically. If the aneurysm becomes progressive and is responsible for significant neurologic symptoms, a team approach (neurosurgery and otolaryngology) to management of the aneurysm is necessary. Progressive preoperative occlusion followed by resection is one method of management if the patient tolerates the occlusive maneuver.

Occasionally, imaging studies are misleading. We have seen two patients presenting with episodic vertigo that revealed on T2 MRI a high-signal-intensity mass resembling a

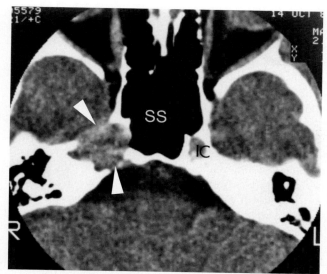

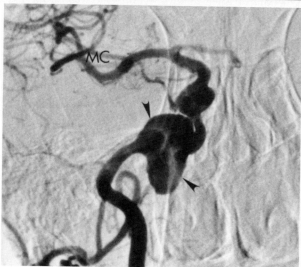

FIG. 44.3 A: CT scan of a 60-year-old woman with occasional episodes of vertigo (several hours' duration) over a 10-year period demonstrates an erosive lesion *(arrowheads)* in the petrous apex. There was a normal auditory, vestibular, and neurologic examination. The bony ridge on the posterior wall of sphenoid sinus serves as a landmark for internal carotid artery *(IC)*. SS, sphenoid sinus. **B:** Arteriogram in the same patient shows the internal carotid artery aneurysm *(arrowheads)*. Neurosurgical consultation advised observation because of the lack of neurological deficits. MC, middle cerebral artery.

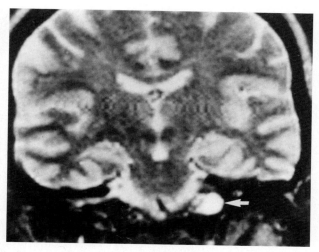

FIG. 44.4 MRI scan of a 56-year-old woman with episodic vertigo and dysequilibrium but without headache or other neurologic symptoms for 6 months. Her neurologic examination and auditory-vestibular assessment was normal. *Arrow* points to a high-signal collection in the petrous apex.

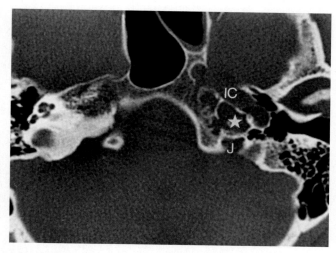

FIG. 44.5 CT scan on same patient in Fig. 44.6 shows a thin-walled compartment *(star)* medial to the internal carotid artery *(IC)* in the petrous apex but separate from the jugular bulb *(J)*.

cholesterol cyst in the petrous apex (Fig. 44.4). CT scan did not reveal bone erosion, but a compartment in the petrous apex was present (Fig. 44.5). It has been suggested that this may represent bone marrow. However, exploration of the petrous apex in these cases with severe sensorineural hearing loss in the involved ear revealed a thin-walled space with brisk venous bleeding requiring firm packing to control (Fig. 44.6). It is possible that these lesions represent venous anomalies (venous lakes). The sigmoid sinus and the jugular bulb were anatomically separated from this vascular compartment.

The importance of this entity is that if it is properly recognized with the positive MRI but with no evidence of bone erosion on CT scanning, surgical exploration should be withheld and the patients only followed with clinical and radiologic methods to detect the possibility of a progressive lesion. Documentation of progression justifies surgical exploration.

Nonvascular Cystic Lesions

Petrositis

In the preantibiotic era, the most common cystic lesion of the petrous apex was infection, either chronic or acute, as a result of extension of the inflammatory process from the

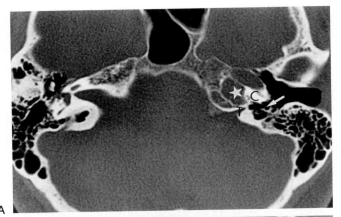

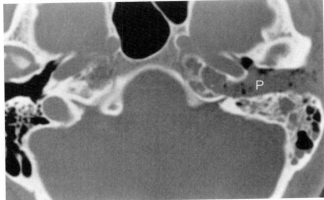

middle ear and mastoid compartments. Progression of an epidural abscess in the air cell system of the petrous apex resulting in bone destruction with dural irritation and involvement of the cranial nerves adjacent to the petrous apex represents Gradenigo's syndrome (Fig. 44.7). The advent of antibiotics and thorough mastoid surgery have virtually eliminated this complication of suppurative otitis media. Nevertheless, this complication does occasionally occur and presents a similar constellation of cranial nerve deficits and symptoms (pain) associated with signs of infection. Surgical exenteration and drainage of the epidural petrous apex abscess cavity is urgently indicated (5,6). Wide-field mastoid and middle ear exploration with identification of the cell tract leading to the apex is necessary to correctly locate and manage the abscess cavity (Fig. 44.8). Most commonly this tract will be located in the infralabyrinthine or perilabyrinthine cell groups (posteromedial, posterosuperior). The extent of bone removal required to expose the cavity

FIG. 44.6 Same patient as Fig. 44.5. **A:** The petrous apex compartment *(star)* was adjacent to the tympanomeningeal fissure *(T)* and the otic capsule *(C)*. The *arrow* shows the infralabyrinthine cell tract. **B:** The compartment was exposed by a transcochlear approach and required firm packing *(P)* to control brisk venous hemorrhage.

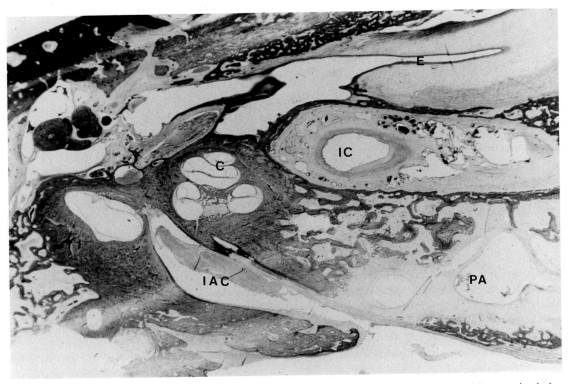

FIG. 44.7 Photomicrograph of a petrous apex abscess cavity *(PA)*. If the cavity cannot be reached via an existing air cell tract, the transcochlear approach is direct and offers adequate fistulization of the abscess. E, eustachian tube; C, cochlea; IC, internal carotid artery; IAC, internal auditory canal.

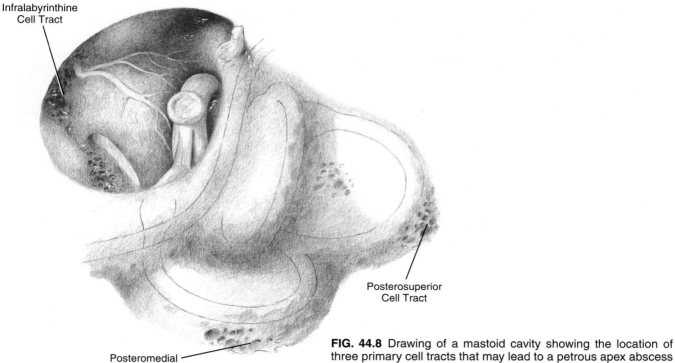

Infralabyrinthine Cell Tract

Posterosuperior Cell Tract

Posteromedial Cell Tract

FIG. 44.8 Drawing of a mastoid cavity showing the location of three primary cell tracts that may lead to a petrous apex abscess cavity.

will depend on the presence or absence of function in the involved ear. If labyrinthine function is normal, exenteration of the diseased air cells should be performed with preservation of the otic capsule. Insertion of a drainage tube for the instillation of antibiotics into the abscess cavity is recommended for complete treatment of the infected cavity. Resolution of the inflammatory process results in obliteration of the defect with fibrous and osseous tissue. If labyrinthine function is significantly depressed, a transcochlear translabyrinthine approach to the petrous apex abscess is chosen (1,7).

Congenital Epidermoid Cyst

Although involvement of the petrous apex may occur as an extension of congenital epidermoid or acquired cholesteatoma arising in the middle ear, a congenital epidermoid cyst limited to the petrous apex is a cystic lesion caused by retention of epithelial remnants embryonically in the region of the foramen lacerum. The cartilage in this space is a remnant of the embryonic mesenchyme in the cephalic flexure, which may entrap epithelial remnants from the foregut as they recede before the shrinking cephalic flexure during development. The pattern of growth and clinical symptoms are similar to other progressive petrous apex lesions. Congenital epidermoid cysts of the petrous apex usually become manifest in young adulthood or early middle age (7,8). At this point the epidermoid has reached a size where surrounding structures are affected and significant bone loss permits

identification with modern CT and MRI techniques. The expanding pattern of bone erosion typical of a congenital cystic lesion is demonstrated best with CT scanning (Fig. 44.9A). An MRI study (Fig. 44.9B) showing a low to medium signal intensity on T1 image and a high signal intensity on the T2 image is characteristic of an epidermoid cyst (3) (Fig. 44.10). Because of the progressive pressure exerted by retained keratin within a stratified squamous epithelial cyst wall, compression of the cranial nerves and vascular and ventilatory structures of the temporal bone eventually requires surgical treatment of this epidural tumor. Because removal of the stratified squamous epithelial lining from surrounding structures (internal carotid artery, dura, jugular bulb, cranial nerves) is not possible without significant morbidity, the principle of management recommended is decompression and exteriorization of the epidermoid cyst (1,7,9,10). The surgical considerations of this maneuver are essentially the same as with other nonvascular cystic lesions of the petrous apex such as cholesterol cyst (granuloma). Therefore the technical considerations will be discussed together with management of cholesterol cysts or granuloma of the petrous apex.

Extension of cholesteatoma toward the petrous apex through perilabyrinthine cell tracts or through the labyrinth is managed by surgical removal of the cholesteatoma membrane after wide exposure of the extension through an open mastoidectomy approach. The epithelial membrane responsible for congenital cholesteatoma (epidermoid) cysts of the petrous apex, however, is firmly adherent to the dura, inter-

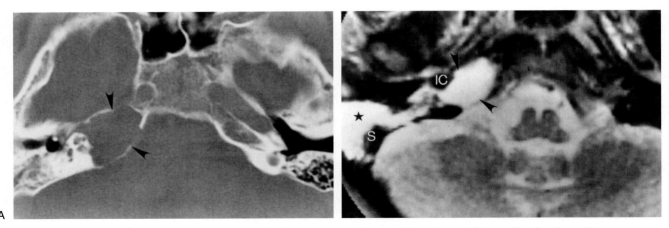

A   B

FIG. 44.9 A CT scan **(A)** and MRI **(B)** of a 37-year-old man with a 1-year history of episodic vertigo, headaches, and blurred vision. He had undergone two unsuccessful ear procedures for conductive hearing loss with an atelectatic middle ear. Note opacification of middle ear and mastoid air cell system *(star)* secondary to eustachian tube compression by the epidermoid cyst *(arrowheads)*. IC, internal carotid artery; S, sigmoid sinus.

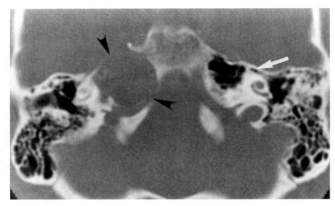

FIG. 44.10 A CT scan of a 42-year-old man with a 5-month history of episodic vertigo, deep-seated headaches, and right dental pain. A transcochlear exposure was necessary to successfully fistulize this cholesterol cyst *(black arrowheads)* after two attempts to fistulize through the infralabyrinthine cell tract failed. *White arrow* points to a narrow cell tract that pneumatizes the contralateral petrous apex.

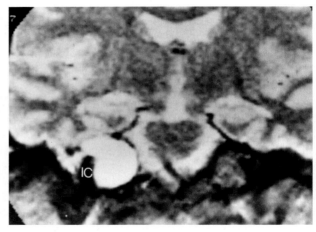

FIG. 44.11 This coronal view of MRI demonstrates how the epidermoid cyst almost surrounds the internal carotid artery *(IC)* and covers the dural surface of the petrous apex, rendering removal of the epithelial matrix virtually impossible.

nal carotid artery, and nerve bundles, requiring an extraordinary surgical exposure associated with significant morbidity (Fig. 44.11). It is questionable whether this membrane can be completely excised to safely permit a closed technique for repair (obliteration) (11). However, it has been suggested that once a congenital epidermoid cyst has been evacuated, it may require 10 to 20 years for sufficient reaccumulation to produce clinical symptoms (12). Nevertheless, the technique of decompression and exteriorization is favored because it has proven to carry low morbidity and mortality while restricting enlargement of the cyst (1,7,10). There is evidence that such decompression leads to decrease in cyst size (1) (Fig. 44.12).

Cholesterol Granuloma (Mucocele, Cholesterol Cyst)

Cholesterol granuloma is the most common cystic lesion of the petrous apex and represents the end result of complete obstruction of an air cell tract to the petrous apex early in life (2). The contralateral petrous apex in patients with cholesterol cysts of the petrous apex is usually well pneumatized, suggesting that the involved petrous apex was similarly pneumatized early in development. MRI characteristically demonstrates a high-signal lesion on both T1 and T2 images (Fig. 44.13). A fibrous and bony obliteration occurs in a narrow cell tract that provides the pneumatization to the apex (2). Complete obstruction leads to the sequence of events that is responsible for mucocele formation in aer-

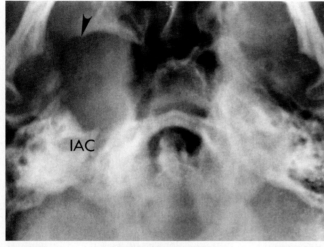

A

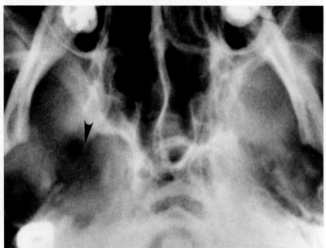

B

FIG. 44.12 A: A petrous apex cholesterol cyst demonstrated by bone erosion abutting the foramen ovale *(arrowhead)* in a 32-year-old woman. IAC, internal auditory canal. **B:** One year after decompression the medial margin of the foramen ovale has remineralized *(arrowhead)*.

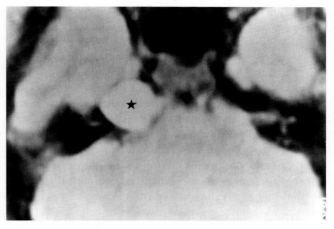

FIG. 44.13 An MRI on the same patient as in Fig. 44.12 demonstrates high signal intensity on a T2-weighted image consistent with a cholesterol cyst *(star)*.

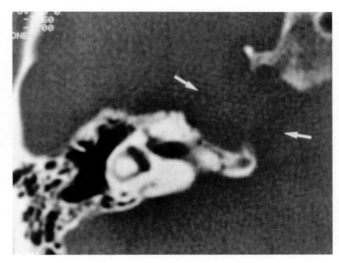

FIG. 44.14 This CT scan demonstrates the extensive bone erosion and exposed dura produced by a large cholesterol cyst *(arrows)*.

ated compartments of the paranasal sinuses, as well as in the temporal bone (13–15). Resorption of the normal gas component leads to obliteration of the space with mucoid fluid and breakdown products of blood from the capillary network of mucoperiosteal lining. The breakdown products of hemoglobin (hemosiderin) eventually produce a foreign body reaction with macrophage accumulation, giant cells, and the distribution of cholesterol crystals within the soft tissue lining of the cyst. The continued accumulation of fluid is responsible for progressively increased pressure on the bony walls of the space, resulting in breakdown of bone composition and compression of the adjacent soft tissue structures (Fig. 44.14). This lesion has been referred to in various terms that reflect either the mechanisms of the lesion or the various stages of reaction to the obstruction. *Mucocele, cholesterol granuloma,* and *cholesterol cyst* have been used syn-

onymously for this lesion. Because this lesion has been documented with increased frequency by the new imaging techniques, it is surprising that it was not described in early literature. Petrous apex cystic lesions fitting this description were reported in 1975 (1) and 1979 (2), although the true nature of pathogenesis was not appreciated. The 1979 report described in a young man a cystic petrous apex lesion demonstrated by polytomography that was shown at surgery to be a mucocele. It was suggested that this lesion resulted from an obstructed air cell tract in the petrous apex because the contralateral petrous apex was well pneumatized.

Because it is unlikely that this is a new form of pathology in the petrous apex, it is reasonable to assume that it has been overlooked in the past, eluding diagnosis and treatment. Radiologic techniques prior to the modern era of temporal bone imaging failed to detect bone erosion in the petrous apex unless it reached extensive proportions. The fate of patients with undiagnosed congenital epidermoids or cholesterol cysts of the petrous apex can only be guessed. It is possible that untreated progressive enlargement of these lesions resulted in a defect of thinned dura with communication into the adjoining intracranial space at the base of the skull. Leakage of the cyst's contents could produce a chemical or bacterial meningitis and unexplained death. The temporal bone and the paranasal sinuses are often overlooked in routine postmortem examination of such cases unless that portion of the skull is examined carefully after brain removal. This scenario is suggested in the report of Canfield (16) describing a young man with a chronically retracted tympanic membrane, several episodes of unexplained coma, somnolence, and fatal meningitis. Despite drainage and treatment of the meningitis, the patient died and postmortem examination revealed a large cystic space in the petrous apex with a dural defect near the middle fossa.

Therefore decompression and permanent exteriorization is recommended for cystic lesions in the petrous apex region that manifest progression by (i) bone erosion and exposed dura, (ii) unresolved or recurrent cranial nerve deficits, and (iii) persistent or recurrent headache. The justification for surgical decompression is the prevention of a lethal complication into the subarachnoid space. If the cystic lesion demonstrates bone erosion short of dural exposure, observation with monitoring by CT scan periodically (every 6 months to 1 year) is permissible.

SURGICAL TECHNIQUE

The technique of fistulization of the cystic lesion in the petrous apex depends on (i) pneumatization of the temporal bone and surrounding pneumatized structures such as the sphenoid sinus, (ii) the function of the labyrinth in the involved and uninvolved ears, and (iii) the presence of infection in spaces that may be used to approach the lesion, such as in the paranasal sinuses and the location of the cyst within the petrous apex (17).

If the involved ear has severely depressed auditory function, the transcochlear approach with or without mastoidectomy, depending on the presence of mastoid disease, is recommended (Figs. 44.15 to 44.18). Removal of bone between the internal carotid artery, jugular bulb, and middle fossa will permit the largest exposure of the petrous apex cyst. Bone should be removed anteriorly as far as the internal carotid artery, superiorly to the dura of the floor of the middle cranial fossa and/or fallopian canal, inferiorly to the dome of the jugular bulb, and posteriorly to the level of the vertical portion of the facial canal and cribrose portion of the cochlea. Excision of all vestibular sense organs should be completed so that optimal recovery from the labyrinthectomy is permitted.

Wide fistulization of the petrous apex may require skin grafts or stents to ensure patency. Split-thickness skin grafts should be applied to the surfaces of the bony tract leading from the cystic space to the skin of the external auditory

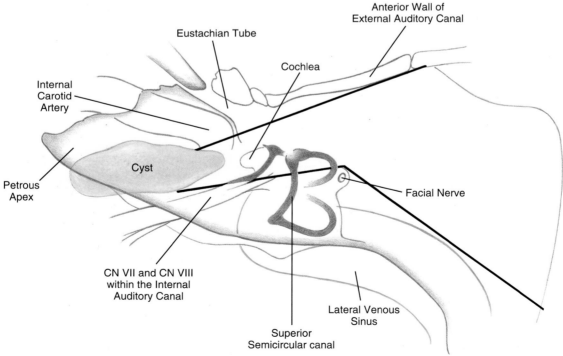

FIG. 44.15 Drawing of the pertinent anatomic landmarks that allow transcochlear fistulization of the petrous apex for decompression of a cystic lesion.

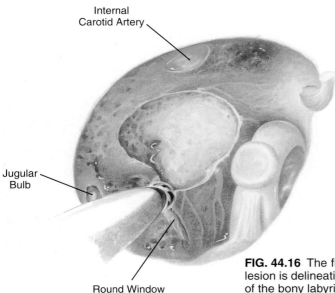

Internal
Carotid Artery

Jugular
Bulb

Round Window

FIG. 44.16 The first step in transcochlear fistulization on the petrous apex cystic lesion is delineation of internal carotid artery and jugular bulb followed by removal of the bony labyrinth.

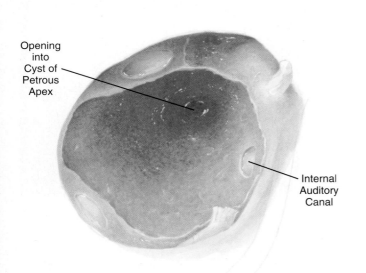

Opening
into
Cyst of
Petrous
Apex

Internal
Auditory
Canal

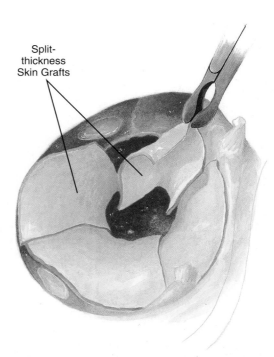

Split-
thickness
Skin Grafts

FIG. 44.17 The second step in transcochlear fistulization consists of extending the cavity medial to the internal carotid artery into the petrous apex.

FIG. 44.18 The third step in transcochlear fistulization is lining the bony fistula wall with split-thickness skin grafts.

canal. Such skin grafts should be maintained in place for at least 10 days with packing until a proper vascular bed has provided viability for the grafts. After removal of packing, close follow-up is necessary to prevent fibrous stenosis of the fistulous tract. Granulation tissue must be controlled with chemical cautery and the insertion of an expandable wick saturated with a steroidal antibiotic solution. The wick should be replaced with a fresh wick on a weekly basis until the tract has been epithelialized. The transcochlear approach for fistulization of the petrous apex has the advantage of low risk from a

potentially contaminated area such as the paranasal sinuses and a short working distance for periodic aspiration and debridement of the cystic space (Figs. 44.19 to 44.22).

If labyrinthine function is normal in both ears, consideration should be given to other anatomic routes for establishing a fistulous tract into the petrous apex cyst. If the sphenoid sinus is extensively pneumatized and the cystic lesion encroaches upon the posterior wall of the sphenoid sinus, transethmoid transsphenoid decompression of the cyst through the posterior wall of the sphenoid is favored (Fig. 44.23) (9).

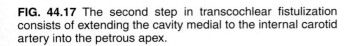

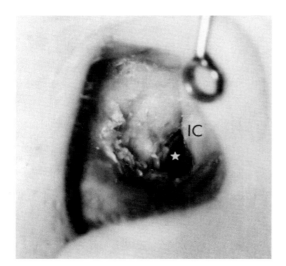

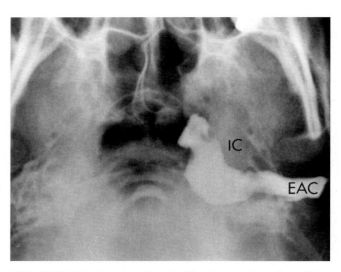

FIG. 44.19 Appearance of the middle ear orifice *(star)* of the fistulous tract into a petrous apex cyst (right ear). IC, internal carotid artery.

FIG. 44.20 Radiopaque dye instilled into external auditory canal *(EAC)* outlines the fistulous tract into a petrous apex epidermoid cyst. IC, internal carotid artery.

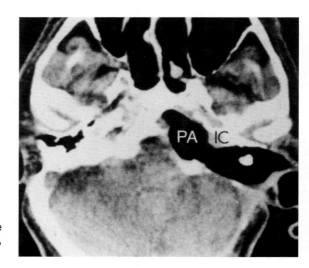

FIG. 44.21 A CT scan demonstrating a fistulized epidermoid cyst of the petrous apex *(PA)*. IC, internal carotid artery. (Courtesy of S. Parisier, M.D.)

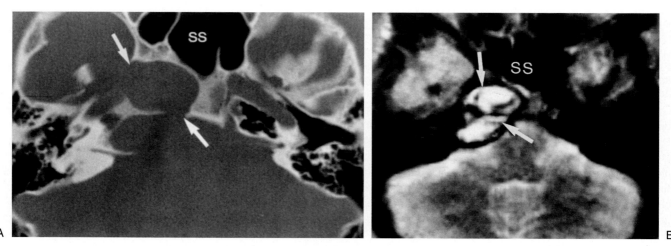

FIG. 44.22 A CT scan **(A)** and MRI **(B)** demonstrate a cholesterol cyst *(arrows)* in a 19-year-old woman with a 3-month history of headache and diplopia. Notice pneumatized contralateral petrous apex. SS, sphenoid sinus.

Insertion of a Silastic stent in the form of a collar button may be used to maintain patency of this method of fistulization (9). A second route for perilabyrinthine fistulization of the petrous apex may utilize a well-developed infralabyrinthine cell tract (18) posterior to the internal carotid artery canal, inferior to the basal turn of the cochlea, and superior to the jugular bulb communicating with the mastoid (18) or directly to the middle ear (Fig. 44.24). However, the size of the infralabyrinthine tract depends on the location of the jugular bulb. Often the diameter that is permitted by this cell tract is limited and requires long-term or permanent stenting to achieve successful fistulization. The tract may be exteriorized (Fig. 44.25) or fistulization via the infralabyrinthine cell tract may be created between the petrous apex and the middle ear and with preservation of the tympanic membrane, ossicular chain, and cochlear function. This may be done employing a Farrior hypotympanotomy approach without mastoidectomy (19). Stenting of the tract with Silastic tubing may be necessary, and periodic MRI is used to rule out reaccumulation of the cyst. If neither of these two routes is an available option in a patient with bilateral normal labyrinth function, it is justified to destroy labyrinthine function in one ear by a transcochlear approach to limit progressive enlargement of cystic lesions, which is responsible for clinical deficits.

In the rare instance where there is no function in the contralateral ear and the involved ear is an only hearing ear, an

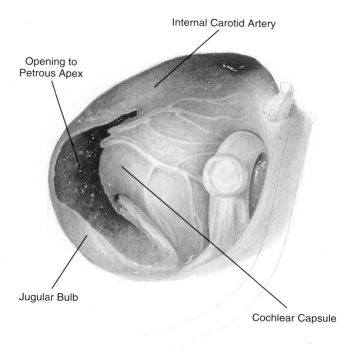

FIG. 44.24 If a generous infralabyrinthine tract is present, it may be enlarged between the internal carotid artery, jugular bulb, and cochlear capsule to expose and fistulize a petrous apex cyst. Split-thickness skin grafts are used to line the bony surfaces of the tract.

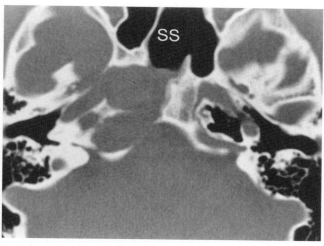

FIG. 44.23 Because hearing was normal in the patient shown in Fig. 44.22, a transsphenoid approach was used to fistulize the cyst. Although the fistula closed, the cyst has been decompressed and the patient is free of symptoms 1 year after surgery. SS, sphenoid sinus.

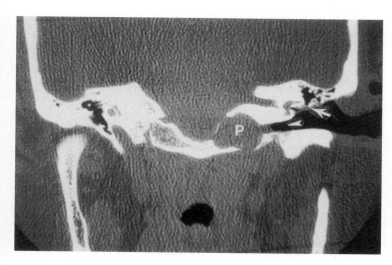

FIG. 44.25 CT scan of a 36-year-old woman with a petrous apex cholesterol cyst (P) that was fistulized (arrowhead) through an infralabyrinthine cell tract with preservation of labyrinth function. A temporalis muscle fascial graft (arrow) was placed on the promontory to reconstruct sound transmission. Granulation tissue occludes the deep end of the fistula.

approach should be selected that allows preservation of that function. Fistulization through an infralabyrinthine cell tract or sphenoid sinus carried out with permanent stenting should be used to maintain decompression of the cyst.

REFERENCES

1. Gacek RR. Diagnosis and management of primary tumors of the petrous apex. *Ann Otol Rhinol Laryngol* 1975;84[Suppl 18]:1–20.
2. DeLozier HL, Parkins CW, Gacek RR. Mucocele of the petrous apex. *J Laryngol Otol* 1979;93:177–180.
3. Valvassori GE, Guzman M. Magnetic resonance imaging of the posterior cranial fossa. *Ann Otol Rhinol Laryngol* 1988;97:594–598.
4. Valvassori GE. Diagnosis of retrocochlear and central vestibular disease by magnetic resonance imaging. *Ann Otol Rhinol Laryngol* 1988;97:19–22.
5. Dearmin RM. A logical surgical approach to the tip cells of the petrous pyramid. *Arch Otolaryngol* 1937;26:314–320.
6. Kopetzky SJ, Almour R. The suppuration of the petrous pyramid: Pathology, symptomatology and surgical treatment. Part III. Surgical therapy. *Ann Otol Rhinol Laryngol* 1931;40:396–414.
7. Gacek RR. Evaluation and management of primary petrous apex cholesteatoma. *Otolaryngol Head Neck Surg* 1980;88:519–523.
8. Cole TB, McCoy G. Congenial cholesteatoma of temporal bone and sphenoid sinus. Report of a case. *Arch Otolaryngol* 1968;87:576–579.
9. Montgomery WW. Cystic lesions of the petrous apex: transsphenoid approach. *Ann Otol Rhinol Laryngol* 1977;86:429–435.
10. Sataloff RT, Myers DL, Roberts B-R, et al. Giant cholesterol cysts of the petrous apex. *Arch Otolaryngol Head Neck Surg* 1988;114:451–453.
11. Franklin DJ, Jenkins HA, Horowitz, BL, et al. Management of petrous apex lesions. *Arch Otolaryngol Head Neck Surg* 1989;115:1121–1125.
12. House WF, Doyle JB Jr. Early diagnosis and removal of primary cholesteatoma causing pressure to the VIIIth nerve. *Laryngoscope* 1962;72:1053–1063.
13. Friedmann I. Epidermoid cholesteatoma and cholesterol granuloma. Experimental and human. *Ann Otol Rhino Laryngol* 1959;68:57–79.
14. Dota T, Nakamura K, Shaheki M, et al. Cholesterol granuloma. Experimental observations. *Ann Otol Rhinol Laryngol* 1963;72:346–356.
15. Main TS, Shimada T, Lim DJ. Experimental cholesterol granuloma. *Arch Otolaryngol* 1970;91:356–359.
16. Canfield RB. Some conditions associated with the loss of cerebrospinal fluid. *Ann Otol Rhinol Laryngol* 1913;22:604–622.
17. Chole RA. Petrous apicitis: surgical anatomy. *Ann Otol Rhino Laryngol* 1985;94:251–257.
18. Gherini SG, Brackmann DE, Lo WWM, et al. Cholesterol granuloma of the petrous apex. *Laryngoscope* 1985;95:659–664.
19. Farrior JB. Anterior hypotympanic approach for glomus tumor of the infratemporal fossa. *Laryngoscope* 1984;94:1016–1021.

Plastic and Reconstructive Surgery of the Auricle

CHAPTER 45

Reconstruction of Congenital Auricular Malformations

Roland D. Eavey

GENERAL CONSIDERATIONS

The form of the external ear is so closely associated with otorhinolaryngology that a simple line drawing of the auricle serves as a symbol of the specialty. Paradoxically, however, effective correction of malformations of the auricle has not been possible until recently. The otolaryngologist who trains to correct this malformation is in a fine position to serve the patient, because both hearing and aesthetic issues, as well as associated conditions such as facial paralysis, can be addressed. The counseling and treatment that must be provided are long term, starting shortly after birth.

Embryologic development of the ear is extremely complex (1–5), involving multiple types of tissue such as skin, fat, cartilage, bone, blood vessels, nerve, and mucous membrane. Ectoderm and mesoderm are involved in the development of the auricle. In addition to these basic tissue elements, the temporal bone also contains endodermal primordia. The auricle is the product of the maturation of six hillocks originating from the mandibular and hyoid arches. These hillocks coalesce by the third fetal month. The first branchial (mandibular) arch is the origin of the tragus. The second (hyoid) arch produces the other five hillocks that then generate the remainder of the auricle. The branchial groove between the two arches invaginates to produce the external auditory canal.

The range of auricular malformations is extensive. For example, the ears merely can be malpositioned or low set. Other minor malformations can occur as noted in Fig. 45.1 (6). More severe malformations of the auricle may be present that exhibit extensive cartilage deformity but preserve a meatus and canal (Fig. 45.2). In the typical microtia malformation, the external ear is severely deformed, with no canal, meatus, or tragus. The auricle is most commonly reduced in size and vertically oriented in an abnormal position. In the typical case, there is an amorphous rudimentary cartilaginous mass superiorly and a lobule-like tissue mass inferiorly (Fig. 45.3). Anotia can also occur and is generally associated with a low-lying hairline. Although unusual, stenosis or

atresia of the external auditory canal may be found in the presence of a well-developed auricle (7).

Microtia occurs commonly as an isolated condition. However, specific syndromes have been associated with microtia and atresia. Treacher Collins syndrome, a result of a mutation in the gene TCOF1 (8), is associated with bilateral microtia, whereas unilateral microtia is more common in Goldenhar's syndrome. Other syndromes less commonly associated with auricular dysmorphic features have been detailed by Konigsmark and Gorlin (9) and include the following: microtia, hypertelorism, cervical fistula and nodules, and mixed hearing loss; thickened earlobes and incudostapedial abnormalities; lacrimoauriculodentodigital syndrome; malformed low-set ears and conductive hearing loss; and lop ears, micrognathia, and deafness. An excellent monograph by Melnick and Myrianthopoulos (10) provides other listings of congenital conditions associated with malformations of the auricle. Trisomy 13–15, 18, and 22 have been reported with microtia as one of multiple anomalies (11–13). Antenatal detection of microtia by ultrasonography could alert physicians to other anomalies (14).

The incidence of microtia has been estimated to be 1 in 10,000 births according to the Center for Disease Control and Prevention data for metropolitan Atlanta (J. Cordero, personal communication). This rate includes syndromic forms of microtia. A higher incidence has been noted in other geographic populations (15–20), as well as in infants born of diabetic mothers (21,22) and infants exposed to intrauterine varicella (23). The inheritance pattern theoretically can be calculated if microtia is part of a dominant or recessive pattern; however, even if familial, the inheritance pattern can vary (22,24–28). Twins do not necessarily both develop microtia, suggesting that the intrauterine environment is not solely responsible (29). Genetic animal models are being developed or exist in nature (30–33). In isolated microtia, the genetic probability is not easily computed; however, there is quite possibly an increased incidence for subsequent siblings (24–28). I have seen microtia occur in four individuals of the same family.

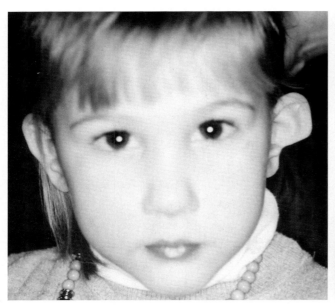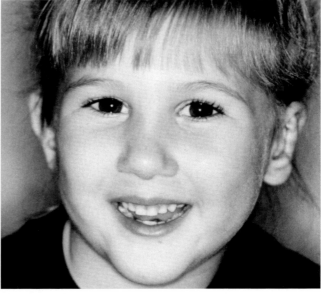

A

B

FIG. 45.1 Minor auricular malformation; the auricle is prominent with partial congenital absence of the lower helix, scapha, anthelix, conchal bowl, and lobule. **A:** Preoperative. **B:** Postoperative appearance.

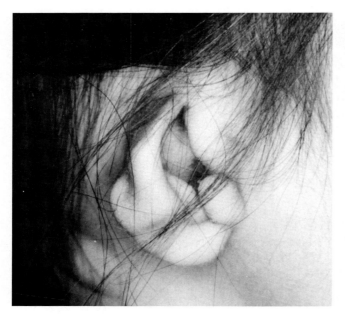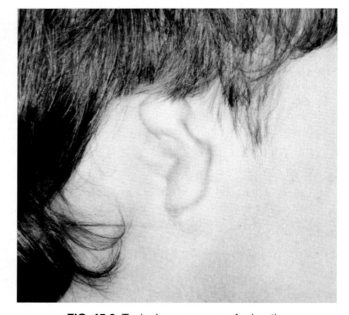

FIG. 45.2 Despite severity of malformation, a meatus, canal, and tympanic membrane are present.

FIG. 45.3 Typical appearance of microtia.

Animal models suggest possible embryologic mechanisms for microtia and atresia. Poswillo (34) has provided a mouse model to demonstrate a similar malformation caused by rupture of the stapedial artery during development. Unfortunately, no mechanism to confirm this hypothesis yet exists (34,35). As an alternative mechanism of abnormal development, the failure of neural crest migration has been implicated in the pathogenesis. This hypothesis has been circumstantially strengthened by the known teratogenic effect of maternal ingestion of vitamin A (36). The selectivity of vitamin A toxicity on the

second branchial arch is hypothesized to be the reason that microtia due to vitamin A teratogenicity is characterized by a preserved tragus (Fig. 45.4). Animal models have shown that the second branchial arch in mice does not develop when migration of the neural crest is retarded by vitamin A (4). However, because in most cases of microtia the tragus is not preserved, this theory has not been widely applicable.

Intrauterine deformation (37) may also cause auricular malformation. As an example, from personal experience, in one patient the ipsilateral hand was deformed presumably

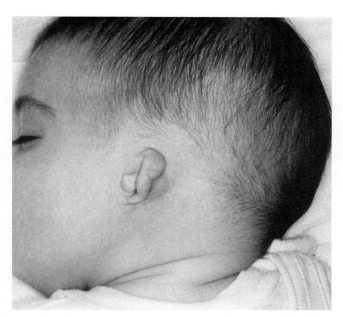

FIG. 45.4 Vitamin A teratogenicity. Note the presence of a tragus, which usually is absent in microtia.

due to an abnormal intrauterine position in which the hand rested against the ear. Of clinical interest is the fact that this infant selected a peculiar posture for several weeks postpartum, holding the deformed hand against the deformed ear.

Classification systems have been devised to grade the degree of severity of auricular malformation; however, these subjective grading schemata of types I, II, and III or of mild, moderate, and severe malformation are of little practical use. Instead, individual analysis of the specific anatomic features is more important for decisions concerning reconstruction. Specific considerations from the physical examination follow.

The Presence of a Meatus and Canal

In cases of severe malformation, the meatus and canal are usually absent. However, their presence raises several issues. First, if the auricle is not severely malformed and if a canal exists, the potential for hearing preservation or reconstruction is enhanced (38). Second, the presence of a canal, especially if narrow, makes the patient susceptible to secondary cholesteatoma. Third, auricular reconstruction will need to accommodate to this fixed canal position yet be symmetrically located in relation to the contralateral ear. Fourth, for hearing habilitation in bilateral microtia, an air- rather than bone-conduction hearing aid may be preferred. Fifth, the otologic surgeon must not be tempted to reconstruct a canal stenosis until after the external ear has been repaired.

The Presence of a Tympanic Membrane

The presence of a tympanic membrane raises the possibility that hearing levels may be acceptable or a conductive loss more easily corrected. Additionally, the tympanic membrane

allows otoscopic monitoring because the microtic ear is at risk for otitis media and extended complications (39).

The Hairless Zone Around the Auricle

Even with severe microtia, a hairless cutaneous rim persists in most cases. With anotia, on the other hand, the hairline can be extremely low. The significance of a hairless zone is apparent during the first stage of rib reconstruction because the superior portion of the cartilaginous framework of necessity will reside under hair-bearing skin. In the patient who has an adequate zone of hairless skin, fewer hair removal techniques, such as skin grafting or hair lasering, will be needed later.

The Cartilaginous Appendage

The cartilaginous appendage varies in appearance and orientation. Importantly, in less severe malformations, the superior cartilaginous portion of the auricle may have only a moderate deformity and may be reconstructed using less morbid techniques adapted from otoplasty (40). In severe microtia, the volume of cartilaginous remnant determines the degree of overlying soft tissue cover. If rib reconstruction is elected, skin coverage is critical. The greater the size of the cartilaginous remnant, the greater will be the amount of pliable soft tissue cover with which the surgeon can work. Another important point is whether the auricle remnant has a smooth covering or whether the skin convolutes to fit the contours of the auricular remnant. Should the convolutions be very deep and pitted, preservation of intact skin will be more difficult. Also, at times a rudimentary conchal bowl and tragus will exist. Auricular features that are well formed can be incorporated into the reconstruction. Conversely, an abnormally located conchal bowl and tragus may add to the challenge of removing the cartilaginous remnants during the reconstruction phase, because the location of the cartilaginous framework as it relates to the contralateral auricle is a priority in the repair of microtia.

Lobular Remnant

A lobular remnant is present in the typical case, even with severe malformation. During reconstruction, this tissue is rotated posteriorly and inferiorly to abut the costal framework at its inferior margin. The presence of lobular tissue provides for some flexibility in establishing the overall vertical height of the new auricle as it is normally transferred at a secondary stage and allows for accurate design at this point. Additionally, this lobule-like tissue hopefully will be adequate to place an earring, which some patients desire and which assists with eventual aesthetic appeal.

The Position of the Auricle

On lateral view, the microtic ear is smaller in vertical height than the contralateral, normal ear. The most cephalad portion of the normal ear lies approximately at the level of the lateral brow, whereas the microtic ear is caudad to this level. Microtic ears also exhibit a more vertical axis of orientation than a normal auricle. In the normally oriented auricle, an imaginary line drawn from the most superior portion of the helix through the lobule is roughly parallel with the dorsum of nose. This relationship is very helpful in properly placing the cartilage framework during surgery. Another common finding is that in the frontal view, the lobule tends to be 3 to 5 mm higher on the microtic side than on the contralateral normal side and is coupled with a lack of tragal prominence.

Skin Tags

Skin tags are often present. Their removal should be delayed until after placement of the reconstructed cartilaginous framework to avoid vascular compromise of the overlying skin. Occasionally, a skin tag can be used in the reconstructive effort.

The Mandible

Especially in Goldenhar's syndrome (oculoauriculovertebral syndrome or hemifacial microsomia), the mandible may be smaller on the microtic side. This finding carries implications for the aesthetics of ear reconstruction because the mandible may be reconstructed at another time. Depending on the reconstruction technique, rib grafting may be used for mandibular augmentation, as well as for auricular repair. Should distraction osteogenesis be planned, the mandible will expand quickly and the position of the ear will appear to change rapidly. If mandibular reconstruction is not planned, the presence of an asymmetric mandible makes it necessary for the surgeon to rely upon aesthetic judgment rather than strict measurement in determining the proper location of the newly created auricle. I see patients in conjunction with an oral surgeon so that simultaneous ear and jaw reconstruction can be planned.

The Contralateral Ear

It is very important to evaluate the contralateral ear prior to the reconstruction. Good hearing is more likely in a normal-appearing ear; however, the hearing of both ears must be tested. Further, minor otologic anomalies are often present in the contralateral ear. In addition to these concerns, the normal contralateral ear serves as the model for reconstruction and associated otoplasty techniques are often necessary to enhance the overall symmetry of the repair.

EVALUATION AND CARE OF THE PATIENT PRIOR TO SURGERY

Infancy

Because auricular malformation is less common and less familiar than other congenital malformations such as cleft lip or club foot, the parents will require extensive counseling.

Compounding the situation, the malformed auricle is a visible condition during the first several months or even years of life because of the lack of hair to camouflage the condition. After the initial concern about the auricular appearance, parental attention then focuses on hearing. A thorough brainstem evoked response audiometric test, not merely an auditory brainstem response (ABR) screening, should be performed as soon after birth as possible. During the first few weeks of life, brainstem evoked response audiometry can be performed under natural sleep conditions rather than under sedation. Even in cases with unilateral microtia, the hearing must be evaluated. Although the contralateral normal-appearing ear has normal hearing in most cases, this must be proven. The abnormal ear usually has a maximum conductive hearing loss of about 60 dB. However, a lesser conductive loss or associated sensorineural loss may be present (41).

In bilateral microtia with conductive hearing loss, the use of a bone-conduction aid allows normal speech and language development (41). The parents should also be aware that a bone-conduction aid need not be fixed solely by a headband. In fact, the use of double-sided sticky tape can be effective in fixing the oscillator to the mastoid region in the zone of hairless skin (Fig. 45.5). Another form of bone-conduction device contains all components in the headband so that no body pack is required. Where an ear canal is present, a standard air-conduction hearing aid can be utilized.

The patient can be evaluated for other associated congenital malformations while in infancy. Commonly associated abnormalities would include epibulbar dermoids on the side of the microtia, facial nerve malfunction, mandibular hypoplasia, vertebral body abnormality, and cardiac anomalies (41).

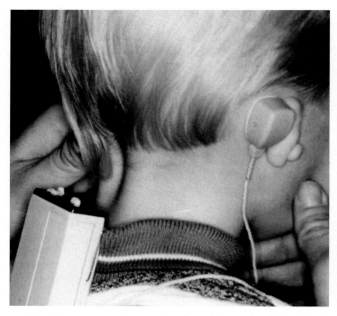

FIG. 45.5 Bone-conduction hearing aid attached in this patient by double-sided tape.

Genetic counseling is helpful. Even the parents of patients with isolated microtia should be aware that their subsequent children and grandchildren may be at slightly greater risk than average for similar anomalies.

Early Childhood

The child with microtia is at no less risk for otitis media than the child in whom the tympanic membrane can be visualized, because the mucosal continuity from the nasopharynx along the eustachian tube to the middle ear and mastoid region is intact. In fact, complications such as mastoiditis have been reported in children with microtia and atresia (39). Therefore antibiotics can be prescribed in cases of suspected acute otitis media, despite the lack of otoscopic confirmation.

Another reason for diligence regarding acute otitis media or serous otitis media with effusion is that the patient might accumulate an effusion in the normal ear. With the contralateral reduction of hearing, the patient is at risk of bilateral loss. Persistent effusion with substantial conductive loss on the normal side may require tube placement or a hearing aid (6,41).

During early childhood, the microtic auricle grows and the stiffness of the cartilage remnant increases. The overall proportions and appearance of the auricle will not change in the typical case. Hair growth allows the microtic vestige to be concealed and is the only cosmetic change that the patient will experience.

The child who also has a diminutive canal should be monitored for the development of an acquired cholesteatoma. Although visualization can be difficult, otorrhea, a tiny polyp in the small canal, or even mastoiditis may be the first signs of cholesteatoma.

An important consideration in the management of these patients is the timing of surgical reconstruction. The mildly to moderately malformed ear may be corrected at an earlier age using procedures to remove extraneous tags or otoplasty type techniques. However, a major deformity that requires costal cartilage harvest should be delayed until age 6 years.

RECONSTRUCTIVE OPTIONS

The potential nonoperative correction of a slightly malformed auricle in newborns by application of tape has been reported (42). It is free of risks and may be applicable in selected cases.

Several anatomic options exist for surgical reconstruction in childhood. A major consideration is whether to attempt surgical reconstruction of hearing or to concentrate solely on auricular reconstruction. There are two major reasons why auricular reconstruction should precede aural atresia reconstruction. First, any hearing reconstruction effort will cause substantial scarring. This will severely limit the ability to utilize the skin in the region, necessitate more extensive auricular surgery, and perhaps condemn the patient to a compromised cosmetic result. Second, in unilateral cases,

the external appendage is perceived as a severe congenital malformation, whereas the hearing tends to be somewhat less pressing because the patient will usually have normal speech and language development due to the normal-hearing contralateral ear. It is important that no major surgical decision be considered until the surgeon (if capable of both components of the operation) or surgeons responsible for reconstruction of both the auricle and middle ear have coordinated plans. Should the patient also have a malformed mandible, coordination of surgical reconstruction with an oral surgeon should be orchestrated.

The simplest reconstructive decision is to elect no reconstruction. In this situation, the parents would choose merely to allow hair growth to conceal the appendage. Because surgical correction of the severely microtic ear (43–47) requires several stages, the parents should be appraised of the potential risks, as well as benefits.

A technique popularized in Europe utilizes a prosthetic auricle anchored by osseointegrated titanium implants (48). The technique is applied at a somewhat older age to allow the skull cortex to become sufficiently thick to anchor the implants. Advantages include fewer surgeries with less morbidity, a fine "arm's-length" result if the prosthesis is well made, and no donor site scars. Disadvantages include a prosthesis that requires daily hygiene, an unsightly appearance when the prosthesis is not in place, an abnormal feel when the prosthesis is touched by another, the need for a lifetime of summer and winter prosthetic replacements, and the permanent loss by amputation of the original microtic ear. Various centers have evolved different philosophies about the use of autogenous or prosthetic reconstruction. We currently favor autogenous reconstruction for a child who has not undergone a previous reconstructive effort. A prosthetic ear provides fine backup technique if the auricular area has, for example, been irretrievably altered by trauma, previous unsuccessful surgery, or, possibly, regional burns.

Another reconstruction technique quite satisfactorily applied (RDE) for an ear with a moderate degree of deformity is a modification of techniques demonstrated by Davis (40). Although each such ear is unique, typically the condition is unilateral, which allows for the reconstruction materials to be contralateral ear conchal cartilage and postauricular skin. These ears usually are about 50% of the appropriate width and 75% of the vertical height of the normal contralateral ear. Such an auricle typically has a missing or diminutive tragus, no conchal bowl, a reasonable but shortened helix, a minimal to nonexistent anthelix, a near normal lobule, and a small postauricular sulcus. Each ear must be custom crafted. The final enhanced result is accomplished in one or two stages with minimal morbidity and no visible donor scars. The touch of the ear is obviously normal because the donor materials are autogenous auricular elastic cartilage and skin (Fig. 45.6). Such soft tissue reconstructive surgery is much more demanding than classical rib reconstruction and should not be undertaken by an inexperienced microtia surgeon.

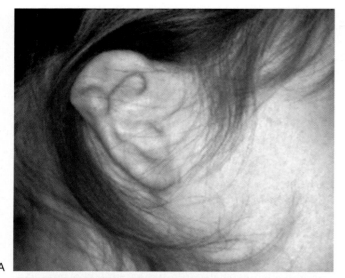

A

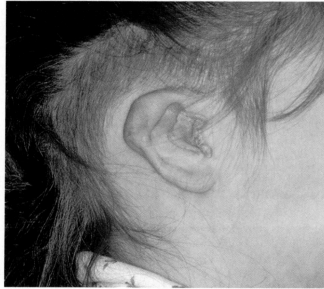

B

FIG. 45.6 A moderate ear deformity has been improved in a single stage from contralateral ear postauricular skin and cartilage with no visible scars elsewhere on the body. **A:** Preoperative. **B:** Postoperative. Note enhanced size and contours.

TECHNIQUE OF SURGICAL CORRECTION USING RIB

Patient Selection

Patients are surgical candidates if they are of adequate body size so that rib length likely will be sufficiently generous to sculpt into an auricular framework of adult size. As a general rule, this occurs at age 6 years. On occasion, in a thin child the surgeon can palpate the costochondral junctions and the synchondrosis and estimate the available cartilage in advance of surgery. However, the cartilage rib determination usually is not possible by either physical or X-ray examination, so that waiting for a child to grow is the safest option.

Lack of available rib due to congenital rib malformation or previous bilateral rib harvest may preclude successful reconstruction. It should be noted that the rib from either side can be used for creation of the auricle, but it is preferable to use the contralateral rib due to more favorable curvature.

Severe local trauma or an extensive burn in the temporal area may preclude surgical candidacy because of extensive scarring and absence of hair. Chronic infection of a malformed canal or in the site of a previous canalplasty should delay surgery until this can be controlled. If unrealistic expectations persist by the patient or parent after careful counseling, surgery should not be performed.

Preoperative Evaluation

The preoperative evaluation consists of measurements of both the malformed and the normal auricle; a step-by-step illustrated guide is provided elsewhere for the motivated reader (47). Lateral measurements include vertical height of the auricle, distance between the outer canthus of the eye to the anterior root of the helix, and distance from the outer canthus of the eye to the anterior insertion of the lobule. The axis of the normal ear in relation to the long axis of the nose should be noted. In the anterior view, the superior portion of the auricles are compared at the level of the eyebrows and the lobules inferiorly.

A piece of unexposed X-ray film is placed over the normal auricle. An outline of the ear is drawn (Fig. 45.7). This template should include the helix, anthelix, scapha and fossa triangularis, lobule, tragus, and posterior margin of the conchal bowl. This template is then reversed and used to create a block template that is used during harvest of rib cartilage. In bilateral microtia, a template is created using a family member's ear as a model.

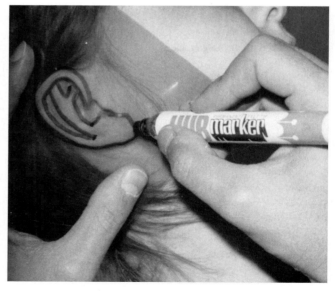

FIG. 45.7 The template that will serve as the auricular model is designed from the patient's own contralateral normal ear.

Operative Procedure

The patient is placed in a supine position on the operating table. Prophylactic intravenous antibiotics are administered. Contralateral ribs are preferred for reconstruction due to their more favorable convex curvature. A linear incision is drawn above the inferior costal margin and extended through the skin and subcutaneous tissues. The rectus muscle is retracted (49). The cartilaginous ribs must be preserved without damage to either the cartilage or perichondrium. It is necessary to harvest segments of two ribs with a synchondrosis for the auricular framework, as well as a third segment for reconstruction of the helix. In younger patients, about 6 years, it can be necessary to obtain a fourth piece of rib in case the floating rib is insufficiently long to create the helix (Fig. 45.8). The block X-ray template is placed over the synchondrosis to determine if there is sufficient cartilage. In younger patients, this requires removal of the entire cartilaginous rib from the sternum medially to the costochondral junction laterally. Care should also be taken not to thermally injure the rib with a cautery device because this may jeopardize the long-term reconstruction. The ribs can be resected either en bloc with the intercostal musculature still attached or a cautery device can be used to divide the intercostal muscles. Care should be taken to avoid damage to the underlying pleura. Should the pleura be entered, the puncture site is oversewn with a purse-string suture and a red Robinson catheter is used to evacuate air as the purse string is tightened and the catheter is removed. Once the three ribs are harvested, it is sometimes possible to harvest the tip of a fourth rib inferiorly to augment the helix if necessary. Prior to closure of the incision, a Marcaine intercostal nerve block will reduce postoperative pain. A chest X-ray examination should be obtained while the patient is still in the operating room to check for the development of a pneumothorax.

A side table is used to prepare the cartilage. The cartilage is placed in saline with added antibiotic prior to use. The instruments for carving are quite simple (Fig. 45.9). Adherent muscle is removed from the rib segment with a sharp scissors. The long rib for the helix is cleaned of musculofascial tissue (Fig. 45.10). Perichondrium should be preserved on the concave surface of the rib. Cartilage will naturally curve with perichondrium on the concave side; the curve should be smooth and demonstrate a natural, bowlike tension.

The ribs with the synchondrosis are then cleaned of attached muscle. The X-ray template is used to determine the most useful segment of the graft. The X-ray template is fixed firmly either by finger pressure or by needles impaling the X-ray film to the rib. A no. 11 or no. 15 blade is used to carve the periphery of the X-ray template to produce the curved shape of the base of the auricular framework (Fig. 45.11). The helix can now be sutured to the base. Care should be taken to preserve sufficient length of the long rib to allow the helix to project into the conchal bowl while allowing a natural descending extension of the helix as well. A second stitch, which attaches the inferior aspect of the helix to the framework, is important because the position of this stitch will determine the size and shape of the helix. Clear nylon (4.0) suture is used in a horizontal mattress fashion starting first from the undersurface of the base and then through the helix. Wire suture can also be used but is less easily manipulated. The framework is inspected to ensure that the anteriormost aspect of the helix has a satisfactory curve toward the conchal bowl. A suture can be used to create a more natural curvature at the root of the helix.

It is necessary to sculpture the base cartilage to simulate the anthelix as a peak and the fossa triangularis and scapha

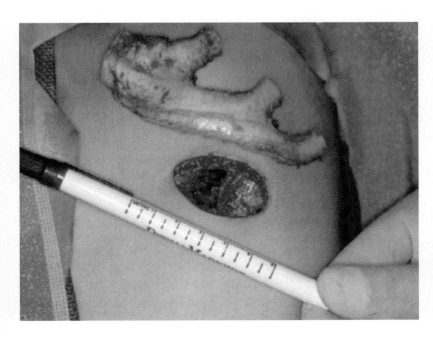

FIG. 45.8 Removal of four cartilaginous ribs. Using retraction, a relatively small incision is adequate. (From Eavey RD. Microtia repair: creation of a functional postauricular sulcus. *Otolaryngol Head Neck Surg* 1999;120:789–793, reprinted with permission.)

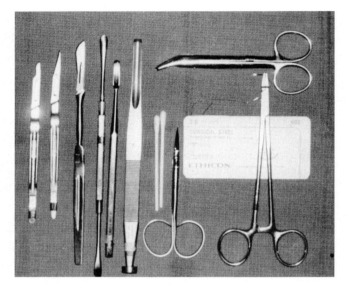

FIG. 45.9 Instruments utilized for rib carving and auricular framework design.

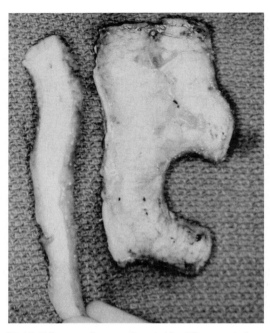

FIG. 45.10 Ribs on the carving table. The partially carved long rib *(left)* will become the helix. The synchondrosis of two ribs will serve as the underlying framework.

as valleys. The area is outlined with marking ink, and a no. 15 blade is used to outline the region. A dissection gouge is used to develop the details of the cartilage framework (Fig. 45.12). It is not necessary to produce a through-and-through defect; in fact, the framework has more stability when a thin layer of base cartilage remains. Should more projection of the anthelix be necessary, in an unusual situation, extra rib can be sutured into position as a superior and inferior crus.

Care should also be taken inferiorly to develop a robust antitragal prominence. In patients with excess rib cartilage, a tragus can be constructed at this stage by fixing a cartilage bridge between the helical root and caudad aspect of the framework (Fig. 45.13).

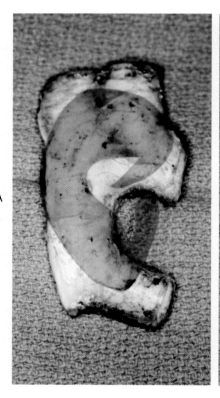

A

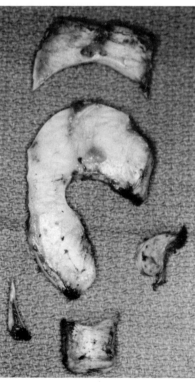

B

FIG. 45.11 The shape of the auricle is carved from the synchondrosis. **A:** Template placed over ribs. **B:** Excess rib cartilage carved away.

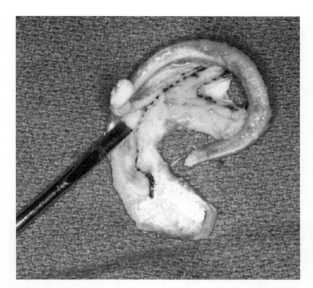

FIG. 45.12 A dissection gouge carves three-dimensional detail.

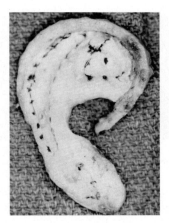

FIG. 45.13 Example of a completed framework. The helix has been attached and the fossa triangularis and scapha deepened by a gouge. Note the curl of the anterior helix.

Additional augmentation can provide further projection from the side of the head if necessary to achieve symmetry. This additional relief can be produced with an extra cartilage block placed under the mid-framework. Care should be taken that such a block does not project beyond the perimeter of the helix because it will increase the width of the new auricle and disturb the smooth curve.

Creation of the skin pocket is at least as critical as the framework construction. Preoperatively, the hair should be shaved by an electrical haircutting clippers. After adequate preparation and draping, the preoperative measurements of the distance from the outer canthus of the eye to the anterior helix and to the lobule should be marked. The template should be positioned in the proper position and a marker used to outline the region where the auricle will be placed. As checks, the axis of the ear should be compared with the dorsum of the nose and the cephalad extent of the framework compared with the lateral aspect of the eyebrow.

The surgeon should avoid locating the skin incision over the area where the framework is to be placed because the three-dimensional demands exerted upon the soft tissue pocket can cause wound breakdown (Fig. 45.14). A 2- to 3-cm vertical incision anterior to the framework position is sufficient. An alternative incision can be placed in the scalp. The skin thickness at the level of the cartilage remnant in the microtic vestige serves as a guide to the appropriate plane of subcutaneous dissection. A good rule of thumb is that the skin should be sufficiently thin to allow visualization of the scissor points tenting under the skin during the development of the soft tissue pocket. Hemostasis can be obtained surprisingly easily by pressure and occasionally by bipolar cautery. To test the adequacy of the pocket, the framework can be installed. The framework is introduced into the pocket after hemostasis is obtained and the two suction drains (butterfly) evacuate additional blood and coapts the soft tissue pocket to the sculptured details of the costal cartilage (Fig. 45.14B). Should the surgeon desire a final check for symmetry, the patient's head can be rotated. The incision is closed with a running suture. Any excess cartilage can be banked under the scalp using a separate incision depending on potential future need. The framework is packed with moistened conforming gauze or lubricated cotton, and a sterile mastoid dressing is placed.

The patient is hospitalized for approximately 2 to 3 days. During this time, drainage from the soft tissue pocket is continued via the suction drains by vacuum tubes, which are saved to quantify the drainage. Patients experience pain at the site of rib harvest; however, patient-assisted intravenous analgesia has been used quite successfully even in children as young as 6 years.

It is personal practice to change the mastoid dressing daily until discharge. Dressing change is facilitated by use of a neoprene and Velcro external wrap instead of the standard gauze mastoid dressing. The suction drain is removed usually on the second postoperative day based on the diminishing volume of drainage. When the patient returns to the office in 7 to 10 days, the dressing and sutures are removed. As the edema of the overlying skin subsides in subsequent months, the underlying cartilaginous contours will become more apparent. The second stage of reconstruction can be scheduled at approximately 3 months, but the actual date of surgery depends often on family scheduling convenience.

At the second surgical stage, the lobular remnant is rotated posteriorly and inferiorly (47). The new internal surface of the lobule must be deepithelialized, defatted, and placed over a matching deepithelialized area at the inferior aspect of the cartilaginous framework (Fig.45.14C). The donor site is closed primarily. A careful check for symmetry is important at this point because the newly positioned lobule tends to project laterally unless the lobule or the underlying cartilaginous framework is thinned appropriately. The new lobule should be able to hold an earring if desired later. A hoop design is preferable.

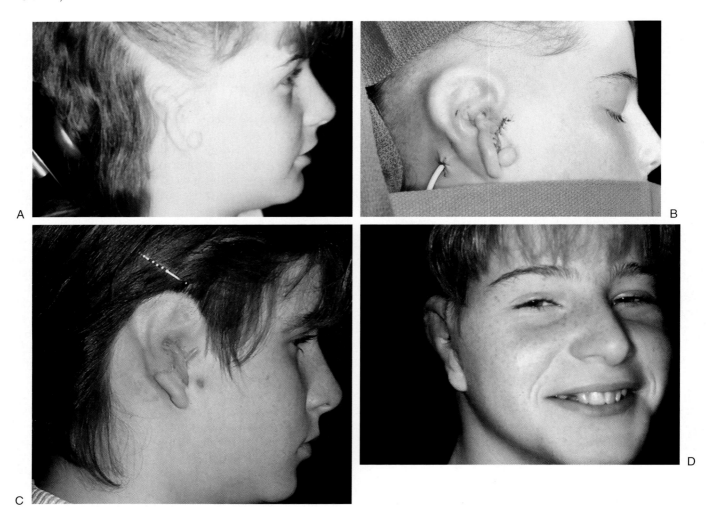

FIG. 45.14 A: Preoperative appearance. **B:** Postoperative view. The framework has been placed under the skin and a suction drain placed. Note the small incision. **C:** Later stage after lobular transposition and skin graft to donor site. **D:** Last stage of skin graft to upper auricle to provide hairless skin and curve to superior auricle.

A postauricular skin graft at the next stage will be placed to give a rounded contour to the peripheral helical rim, to provide coverage with hairless skin, and, importantly, to provide a functional postauricular space for eyeglasses or a hearing aid (Fig. 45.14D). A split-thickness skin graft can be taken from the buttock, but personal preference is a full-thickness graft from the lower midline back; the donor site is closed in a linear fashion (50). The recipient site is prepared by making an incision along the inferior aspect of the hair-bearing skin. If this is near the superior margin of the auricle, the skin grafting will be done in one stage. If the lateral aspect of the auricle has a particularly shaggy appearance, it is preferable to have the lateral auricular hair lasered postoperatively. The incision extends through the skin; however, the thin, fibrous connective tissue covering over the cartilage is preserved as the skin is removed. The split-thickness skin graft is then sutured into position and reinforced with a bol-

ster dressing. The sulcus should be deep enough to permit eyeglasses to fit (Figs. 45.15 and 45.16).

If a patient desires a tragus, an additional procedure can be performed if the tragus could not be incorporated into the first-stage framework. This is also an opportunity to modify the contralateral ear so that the projections can be approximated. To construct the tragus, contralateral conchal bowl cartilage and postauricular skin is removed and the donor site is closed primarily. The graft is then placed into and under a wide peninsula-shaped incision at the location of the new tragus; a small skin graft is attached to surface the equivalent of a meatal and conchal bowl lining. The reconstructed tragus adds a more realistic appearance to the ear, as well as acting to shadow the indentation of the neoconchal bowl, thus giving the illusion of a meatus and external auditory canal. An alternative tragal reconstruction technique is to utilize rib cartilage at either the first or a subsequent stage (Fig. 45.15B,C)

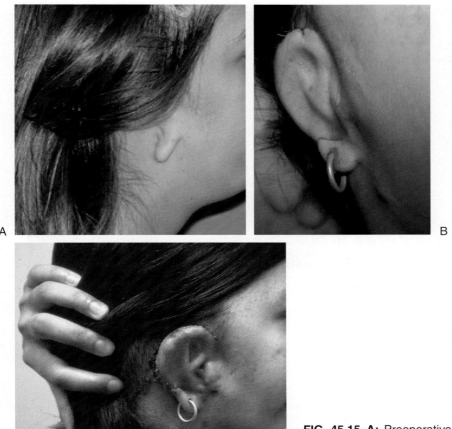

FIG. 45.15 A: Preoperative appearance. **B:** Oblique view on operating table after three stages, including mandibular distraction performed by the Otorhinolaryngology and Maxillofacial Service. **C:** Lateral view 1 week after third stage.

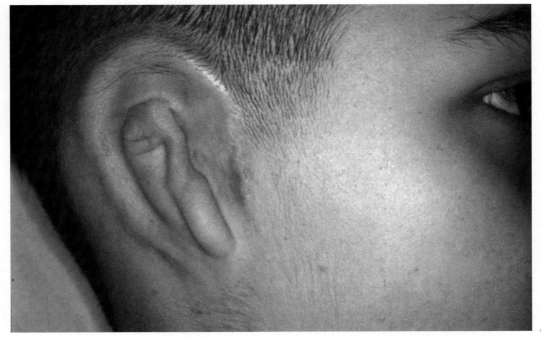

FIG. 45.16 Creation of a postauricular sulcus. **A:** Microtic ear after first-stage rib implant.

Continued

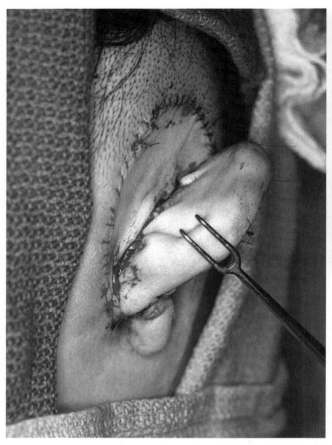

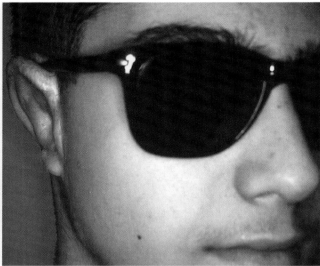

B

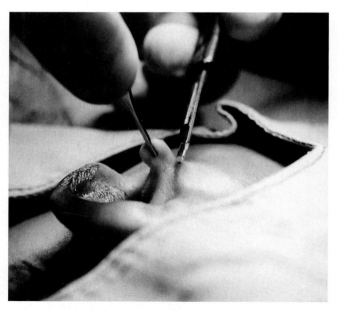

FIG. 45.16, cont'd. Creation of a postauricular sulcus. **B:** Elevation and grafting of sulcus. **C:** Final result with the patient wearing sunglasses.

ASSOCIATED SURGICAL CONSIDERATIONS

Removal of Tags

Preauricular tags are not difficult to remove. However, it should be remembered that such tags are three-dimensional anatomic entities that occasionally can be used by the reconstructive surgeon and should not be excised automatically. A time-honored method of treating a preauricular tag is to tie a loop around it at birth and allow necrosis over the next few days. This technique, however, leaves a residual, palpable cartilaginous remnant. To eliminate this persistent remnant, it is necessary to perform an elliptically shaped incision around the base. This maneuver can be facilitated by retraction of the tag itself to expose the subcutaneous remnant. The subcutaneous cartilage is removed by beveling the blade. The skin is closed primarily (Fig. 45.17). Such a tag can be removed during infancy if it will not jeopardize later reconstruction. Otherwise the tag can be removed or used at the time of definitive repair.

FIG. 45.17 Tag removal. Note that the blade must bevel down below the skin surface.

Ear Surgery for Cholesteatoma

The child who has a malformed canal is at increased risk for acquired canal cholesteatoma. Although in general it is preferable to do auricular reconstruction prior to any canal or middle ear surgery, the presence of a cholesteatoma may require modification of the surgical plan. It may be possible to treat a patient with an intermittently draining ear, without cholesteatoma, with topical eardrops until a stable, uninfected ear canal is achieved, allowing auricular reconstruction before canal or middle ear surgery. However, obvious cholesteatoma could be managed prior to auricular reconstruction, although subsequent auricular reconstruction in such a case may require the use of a temporoparietal fascial flap (51–53). More detail on the temporoparietal fascial flap is available in Chapter 46.

Reconstructive Middle Ear Surgery

Aural atresia repair is discussed in Chapter 24 (54). Once the auricle is recreated, there is no contraindication to a postauricular incision and creation of a canal as long as the middle ear and mastoid anatomy seems suitable by CT imaging. Atresia repair can be done between phases of auricular reconstruction or after auricular reconstruction is completed (41,55). Another potential method of hearing rehabilitation is the implantable bone-conducting hearing aid in bilateral microtia cases (56).

UNPREDICTABLE OUTCOMES OF AURICULAR RECONSTRUCTION

Early

Prophylactic antibiotics, irrigation, and drainage of the wound may help to prevent infection. However, should infection occur, drainage of an abscess may not require sacrifice of the cartilaginous graft.

A small area of skin necrosis may spontaneously reepithelialize. However, should soft tissue coverage be required, the compromised area can be covered early or be allowed to demarcate and stabilize. A rotation flap from the scalp can be used because the usual location of exposure is the anterior helical rim. At this time, any dried, exposed cartilage can be shaved to underlying healthy cartilage. It is possible to delay flap coverage until the time of a planned later stage. A split-thickness skin graft, rotation flap, or a temporoparietal fascial flap can be used to close such defects.

Late

Hypertrophic scars can occur near the ear or even at sites distant from the auricular reconstruction such as the skin graft site or rib donor incision. Steroid injection can be used. If periauricular scars are particularly unsightly, they can be excised during subsequent stages of the auricular reconstruction. For example, a hypertrophic scar from the first stage can be excised at the time of transposition of the lobule. Additionally, rather than performing a primary closure for the lobular transposition, a split-thickness skin graft can

be placed in this site. With less tension on the closure, there is less likelihood of the creation of an unsightly scar.

TISSUE ENGINEERING

Although not yet possible in humans, creation of an ear from the patient's own tissue is a plausible goal. This model has moved from the xenograft model of "the mouse with the ear on its back" to the robust production of healthy autogenous auricular cartilage in an immunocompetent animal model. Should this technique become reality, fewer procedures will be necessary, patients will experience less morbidity, and the finished ear will have a more natural feel (57–61).

REFERENCES

1. Wolff D, Bellucci RJ, Eggston A. *Surgical and microscopic anatomy of the temporal bone.* New York: Hafner, 1971:1–26.
2. Schuknecht H. *Pathology of the ear.* Cambridge, MA: Harvard University Press, 1974:184–186.
3. Pearson A. *The development of the ear: a manual prepared for the use of graduates in medicine.* Rochester, MN: American Academy of Ophthalmology and Otolaryngology, 1967.
4. Jarvis BL, Johnston MC, Sulik KK. Congenital malformations of the external, middle, and inner ear produced by isotretinoin exposure in mouse embryos. *Otolaryngol Head Neck Surg* 1990;102:391–401.
5. Anson BJ, Donaldson JA. *Surgical anatomy of the temporal bone.* Philadelphia: WB Saunders, 1981:23–31.
6. Eavey RD. Management strategies for congenital ear malformations. *Pediatr Clin North Am* 1989;36:1521–1534.
7. Grundfast KM, Camilan F. External auditory canal stenosis and partial atresia with associated anomalies. *Ann Otol Rhinol Laryngol* 1986;95:505–509.
8. Isaac C, Marsh KL, Paznekas WA, et al. Characterization of the nucleolar gene product, treacle, in Treacher Collins syndrome. *Mol Biol Cell* 2000;11:3061–3071.
9. Konigsmark BW, Gorlin RJ. *Genetic and metabolic deafness.* Philadelphia: WB Saunders, 1976:49–73.
10. Melnick M, Myrianthopoulos NC. *External ear malformations: epidemiology, genetics, and natural history,* vol 15. The National Foundation-March of Dimes Birth Defects. Original article series. New York: Alan R Liss, 1979:122–123.
11. Saito R, Fujimoto A, Fujita A, et al. Temporal bone histopathology of atresia auris congenita with chromosome aberration. *Acta Otolaryngol (Stockh) Suppl* 1983;393:96–104.
12. Verloes A, Seret N, Bernier V, et al. Branchial arch anomalies in Trisomy 18. *Ann Genet* 1991;34:22–24.
13. Bacino CA, Schreck R, Fischel-Ghodsian N, et al. Clinical and molecular studies in full Trisomy 22: Further delineation of the phenotype and review of the literature. *Am J Med Gen* 1995;56:359–365.
14. Shih JC, Shyu MK, Lee CN, et al. Antenatal depiction of the fetal ear with three-dimensional ultrasonography. *Obstet Gynecol* 1998;91:500–505.
15. Castilla EE, Lopez-Camelo JS, Campana H. Altitude as a risk factor for congenital anomalies. *Am J Med Genet* 1999;86:9–14.
16. Harris J, Kallen B, Robert E. The epidemiology of anotia and microtia. *J Med Genet* 1996;33:809–813.
17. Lopez-Camelo JS, Oriolio IM. Heterogeneous rates for birth defects in Latin America: hints on causality. *Genet Epidemiol* 1996;13:469–481.
18. Nelson SM, Berry RI. Ear disease and hearing loss among Navajo children—a mass survey. *Laryngoscope* 1984;94:316–323.
19. Castilla EE, Orioli IM. Prevalence rates of microtia in South America. *Int J Epidemiol* 1986;15:364–368.
20. Aase JM. Microtia: clinical observations. *Birth Defects* 1980;16:289–297.
21. Ewart-Toland A, Yankowitz J, Winder A, et al. Oculoauriculovertebral abnormalities in children of diabetic mothers. *Am J Med Genet* 2000;90:303–309.
22. Mastroiacovo P, Corchia C, Botto LD, et al. Epidemiology of genetics and microtia-anotia: A registry based study on over one million births. *J Med Genetics* 1995;32:453–457.

23. Jones KL, Johnson KA, Chambers CD. Offspring of women infected with varicella during pregnancy: a prospective study. *Teratology* 1994;49:29–32.

24. Cremers C. Meatal atresia and hearing loss. Autosomal dominant and autosomal recessive inheritance. *Int J Pediatr Otorhinolaryngol* 1985;8:211–213.

25. Kessler L. Observation of an over 6 generations simple dominant inheritance of microtia of the first degree. *HNO* 1967;15:113–116.

26. Orstavik KH, Medbo S, Mair IW. Right-sided microtia and conductive hearing loss with variable expressivity in three generations. *Clin Genet* 1990;38:117–120.

27. Gupta A, Patton MA. Familial microtia with meatal atresia and conductive deafness in five generations. *Am J Med Genetics* 1995;59:238–241.

28. Llano-Rivas I, Gonzalez-del Angel A, del Castillo V, et al. Microtia: a clinical and genetic study at the National Institute of Pediatrics in Mexico City. *Arch Med Res* 1999;30:120–124.

29. Neal GS, Hankins GD. Left microtia in one monozygotic twin. A case report. *J Reprod Med* 1992;37:375–377.

30. Naora H, Kimura M, Otani H, et al. Transgenic mouse model of hemifacial microsomia: cloning and characterization of insertional mutation region on chromosome 10. *Genomics* 1994;3:515–519.

31. Kaur S, Singh G, Stock JL, et al. Dominant mutation of the murine Hox-2.2 gene results in developmental abnormalities. *J Exp Zool* 1992;264:323–336.

32. Bleyl DW. Microtia in a Wistar rat. *Z Versuchstier kd* 1983;25:285–286.

33. Basrur PK, Vadau BR. Genetic disorders of sheep and goats. *Vet Clin North Am Food Anim Pract* 1990;6:779–802.

34. Poswillo D. The pathogenesis of the first and second branchial arch syndrome. *Oral Surg* 1973;35:302–328.

35. Phelps PD, Poswillo D, Lloyd GA. The ear deformities in mandibulofacial dysostosis (Treacher Collins syndrome). *Clin Otolaryngol* 1981;6:15–28.

36. Lammer EJ, Chen DJ, Hoar RM, et al. Retinoic acid embryopathy. *N Engl J Med* 1985;313:837–841.

37. Jones KL, ed. *Smith's recognizable patterns of malformation*, 4th ed. Philadelphia: WB Saunders, 1988:634.

38. Kountakis SE, Helidonis E, Jahrsdoerfer RA. Microtia grade as an indicator of middle ear development in aural atresia. *Arch Otolaryngol Head Neck Surg* 1995;121:885–886.

39. Zalzal GH. Acute mastoiditis complicated by sigmoid sinus thrombosis in congenital aural atresia. *Int J Pediatr Otorhinolaryngol* 1987;14:31–39.

40. Davis J, ed. *Otoplasty: aesthetic and reconstruction techniques.* New York: Thieme-Verlag, 1997.

41. Eavey RD. Microtia and significant auricular malformation: ninety-two pediatric patients. *Arch Otolaryngol Head Neck Surg* 1995;121:57–62.

42. Muraoka M, Nakai Y, Ohashi Y, et al. Tape attachment therapy for correction of congenital malformations of the auricle: clinical and experimental studies. *Laryngoscope* 1985;95:167–176.

43. Tanzer RC. Total reconstruction of the external ear. *Plast Reconstr Surg* 1959;23:1–15.

44. Brent B. The correction of microtia with autogenous cartilage grafts. I. The classic deformity. *Plast Reconstr Surg* 1980;66:1–12.

45. Brent B. Total auricular reconstruction with sculpted costal cartilage. In: *The artistry of reconstructive surgery.* St. Louis: Mosby, 1987:113–127.

46. Nagata S. New method of total reconstruction of the auricle for microtia. *Plast Reconstr Surg* 1993;92:187–201.

47. Eavey RD. Surgical repair of the auricle for microtia. In: Bluestone CD, Stool SE, eds. *Atlas of pediatric otolaryngology.* Philadelphia: WB Saunders, 1994.

48. Tjellstrom A. Osseointegrated implants for replacement of absent or defective ears. *Clin Plast Surg* 1990;17:355–366.

49. Eavey RD, Ryan DP. Refinements in microtia surgery. *Arch Otolaryngol Head Neck Surg* 1996;122:617–620.

50. Eavey RD. Microtia repair: creation of a functional postauricular sulcus. *Otolaryngol Head Neck Surg* 1999;120:789–793.

51. Brent B, Byrd HS. Secondary ear reconstruction with cartilage grafts covered by axial, random and free flaps of temporoparietal fascia. *Plast Reconstr Surg* 1983;72:141–152.

52. Fox JW, Edgerton MT. The fan flap: an adjunct to ear reconstruction. *Plast Reconstr Surg* 1976;58:663–667.

53. Tegtmeier RE, Gooding RA. The use of a fascial flap in ear reconstruction. *Plast Reconstr Surg* 1977;60:406–411.

54. Schuknecht HF. Congenital aural atresia. *Laryngoscope* 1989;99:908–917.

55. Jahrsdoerfer RA. Congenital atresia of the ear. *Laryngoscope* 1978;88[Suppl 13]:1–48.

56. Carlsson P, Häkansson BO, Rosenhall U, et al. A speech-to-noise ratio test with the bone-anchored hearing aid: a comparative study. *Otolaryngol Head Neck Surg* 1986;94:421–426.

57. Toufexis A. An eary tale. *Time,* Nov 6, 1995:60.

58. Rodriguez A, Cao YL, Ibarra C, et al. Characteristics of cartilage engineered from human pediatric auricular cartilage. *Plast Reconstr Surg* 1999;103:1111–1119.

59. Arevalo-Silva CA, Cao Y, Vacanti M, et al. Influence of growth factors on tissue engineered pediatric elastic cartilage. *Arch Otolaryngol Head Neck Surg* 2000;126:1234–1238.

60. Arevalo-Silva CA, Eavey RD, Cao Y, et al. Internal support of tissue-engineered cartilage. *Arch Otolaryngol Head Neck Surg* 2000;126:1448–1452.

61. Saim AB, Cao Y, Weng Y, et al. Engineering autogenous cartilage in the shape of a helix using an injectable hydrogel scaffold. *Laryngoscope* 2000;110:1694–1697.

CHAPTER 46

Acquired Deformities of the Auricle

Mack L. Cheney and Tessa A. Hadlock

PRINCIPLES

Reconstruction of the auricle poses many challenges for the reconstructive surgeon. The goals of reconstruction are to achieve normal appearance and sensation of the structure. It should be symmetric with the contralateral ear in size, shape, and orientation; it should be in proper relation to the periauricular skin and scalp; and the postauricular sulcus should be preserved. However, the intricate anatomy of the auricle makes these goals quite difficult to attain. The auricle's complex, three-dimensional convolutions are supplied by limited and inconsistent vascularization, and the ratio of cartilage to skin is high. In addition to the inherently complex anatomy of the "typical" ear, there exists a wide degree of variation among individuals (1–3).

The presence of supple and well-vascularized skin is essential for success in auricular reconstruction. Cutaneous resurfacing is often necessary in the management of acquired auricular deformities, because auricular injuries are often combination injuries to the skin and underlying cartilage. In this situation, the scar tissue that affects the skin must be excised and replaced to allow for adequate three-dimensional reconstruction. The reconstruction of auricular defects after oncologic surgery requires special consideration because reconstructive plans are influenced by the nature of the excisional defect, the presence or absence of an irradiated field, and the need for careful clinical monitoring of the area.

Although auricular reconstruction poses unique challenges to the surgeon, many of the principles of reconstruction of other areas of the head and neck also apply to the auricular region. Anatomic landmarks such as the vermilion border, eyebrow, nasal alar margin, and ear constitute free margins due to the discontinuity of skin borders surrounding these structures. Because such margins offer little or no resistance to tension created by surgical procedures in adjacent soft tissue, the immediate and delayed consequences of tissue manipulation must be anticipated. The helix of the ear does not have the same cosmetic importance as other free margins of the face, because slight asymmetries are not always noticeable or can be camouflaged by changes in hairstyling. On the other hand, auricular cartilage is very supple and soft tissue contraction forces will tend to distort the ear if attention is not paid to primary closure and to local tissue tension.

Reconstruction in the auricular area must take into account hair-bearing scalp in the proximity to avoid placing hair-bearing skin over the auricle. The hairline above the site of the proposed reconstruction is usually high enough to avoid interfering with accurate positioning of the ear. The exception to this is when placing hair-bearing skin is necessary to achieve normal height with respect to the contralateral ear.

ANALYSIS OF THE AURICLE

Analysis of the dimensions and proportions of the external ear are important for planning reconstructive procedures (4). Leonardo da Vinci first noted that the vertical height of the ear is approximately equal to the distance between the lateral orbital rim and the root of the helix at the level of the brow. Ear width is approximately 55% of its length, the helical rim protrudes 1 to 2.5 cm from the skull, and the angle of the protrusion from the skull averages 25 to 30 degrees. The vertical axis of the ear is inclined posteriorly at an angle of approximately 20 degrees from the vertical. When planning the reconstruction, however, it is most important to use the contralateral side as a template because individual variation is the rule rather than the exception in anatomic auricular features and location (5) (Table 46.1).

TABLE 46.1 *Average length and width of the normal auricles*

Age (years)	Male Length (mm)	Male Width (mm)	Female Length (mm)	Female Width (mm)
1	50.0	31.5	46.8	29.1
6	55.3	33.4	53.5	32.5
18	63.5	35.3	59.0	32.5

Adapted from Farkas LG. Growth of normal and reconstructed auricles. In: Tanzer RC, Edgerton MT, eds. *Symposium on reconstruction of the auricle.* St. Louis: Mosby, 1974.

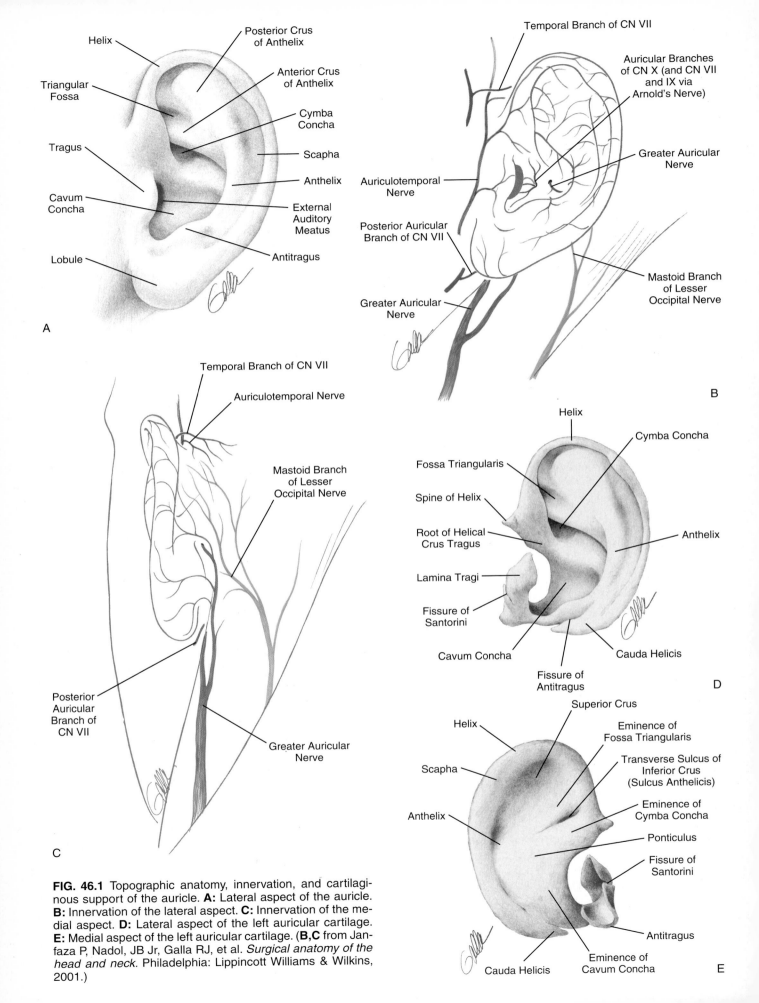

FIG. 46.1 Topographic anatomy, innervation, and cartilaginous support of the auricle. **A:** Lateral aspect of the auricle. **B:** Innervation of the lateral aspect. **C:** Innervation of the medial aspect. **D:** Lateral aspect of the left auricular cartilage. **E:** Medial aspect of the left auricular cartilage. (**B,C** from Janfaza P, Nadol, JB Jr, Galla RJ, et al. *Surgical anatomy of the head and neck.* Philadelphia: Lippincott Williams & Wilkins, 2001.)

ANATOMY AND EMBRYOLOGY

Anatomic landmarks of the auricle are important when considering reconstructive options (7). Topographic landmarks of the auricle are illustrated in Fig. 46.1. The cartilaginous framework of the auricle must be thought of in terms of three-dimensional components. The cartilaginous units, starting medially, are the conchal complex, the anthelical and antitragal complex, and the helical and lobular complex.

Embryologically, the auricle arises from the first (mandibular) and second (hyoid) arches. The helix appears in these arches during the sixth week of gestation. The anterior hillocks give rise to the tragus, the root of the helix, and the superior helix, whereas the posterior hillocks become the anthelix, tragus, and lobule.

The arterial supply to the auricle is derived from branches of the superficial temporal artery and the postauricular artery, both of which arise from the external carotid artery. The venous drainage is via the postauricular vein into the external jugular system, with additional support from the superficial temporal and retromandibular veins.

The auricle is innervated by the great auricular nerve (C2–3), auriculotemporal nerve (V3), lesser occipital nerve, and greater branch of the vagus nerve (Arnold's nerve).

USE OF COSTAL CARTILAGE AS A FRAMEWORK FOR AURICULAR RECONSTRUCTION

By fashioning a new auricle or portions of it from autogenous costal cartilage, the surgeon can avoid the use of auricular prostheses or alloplastic implants. Prostheses pose a problem with adherence to the skin, and patients tend to prefer reconstructions that utilize autogenous materials. Additionally, alloplastic implants have been shown in many reports to exhibit an unacceptably high extrusion and infection rate. Although autogenous tissue reconstructions are preferable, the ribs become more brittle and ossified with age, so reconstruction utilizing costal cartilage must be carefully considered in patients more than age 50 years.

The cartilaginous components of the sixth, seventh, and eighth ribs provide the raw material for the creation of the framework. The synchondrosis between the sixth and seventh ribs serves as the body of the framework, whereas the helix is fashioned from the eighth rib. As with the techniques used in microtia repair, determination of the appropriate size and individual shape of the framework is taken from a pattern of the contralateral auricle. The cartilage framework is stabilized and properly positioned based on preoperative measurements. A temporoparietal fascial flap is commonly used to cover the cartilage framework to ensure viability and to accept a split-thickness skin graft.

TEMPOROPARIETAL FASCIAL FLAP

In the cover of the cartilaginous framework in auricular reconstruction, the tissue used should be thin, vascular, hairless, and capable of accepting skin grafts of a good color match. The temporoparietal fascial flap (9–14) satisfies these requirements, with the added advantages that the anatomy of the flap is well known to the head and neck surgeon (15,16), a large quantity of tissue (14 by 12 cm) can be harvested, it can be rotated to cover a wide range of auricular defects, and the flap may be transferred to the contralateral auricular region using microvascular techniques (17).

The temporoparietal fascia, also known as the superficial temporal fascia, is continuous with the superficial musculoaponeurotic system, as well as the galea (Fig. 46.2). It lies deep to the skin and subcutaneous tissue to which it is firmly bound (particularly in the area of the temporal line). This fascia should not be confused with the fascial layer surrounding the temporalis muscle proper. The temporoparietal fascia attaches to the zygomatic arch, whereas the temporalis muscular fascia passes deep through the arch to insert on the coronoid process of the mandible. Measuring on average 2 to 3 mm in thickness over the parietal area, the temporoparietal fascia is highly vascular, with an abundant and consistent supply from the superficial temporal artery and vein.

In harvesting the flap, care must be taken to keep the hair follicles and subcutaneous fat on the lateral aspect of the flap under direct vision. Careful avoidance of the hair follicles prevents the iatrogenic complication of alopecia. The medial plane of flap elevation is over the temporalis muscular fascia in the loose connective tissue separating the temporoparietal fascia from the muscular fascia.

Once the vascular pedicle has been identified and protected, the elevation can proceed anteriorly to the edge of the hair-bearing scalp, thus protecting the frontal branch of the facial nerve. The posterior margin of the flap should capture the posterior branch of the superficial temporal artery and vein and can be back cut to the vascular pedicle to facilitate flap rotation.

SYSTEMATIC APPROACH TO AURICULAR RECONSTRUCTION BASED ON ANATOMIC LOCATION

Most acquired auricular deformities are partial defects. This section considers the techniques most useful for repairing specific acquired defects of the auricle based upon anatomic location (19).

Preauricular Defects

The most common preauricular defects occur secondary to excision of cutaneous lesions located in this area. The function of the facial nerve should be carefully examined prior to the removal of lesions in this location and monitored intraoperatively. Surgical options for the repair of preauricular defects include preauricular rotation flaps, VY advancement flaps, and simple cheek advancement flaps (Fig. 46.3). With careful planning, the resultant scar can be placed within the preauricular crease with minimal deformity.

FIG. 46.2 Anatomy of the temporoparietal flap. (From Cheney ML. *Facial surgery: plastic and reconstructive.* Baltimore: Williams & Wilkins, 1997.)

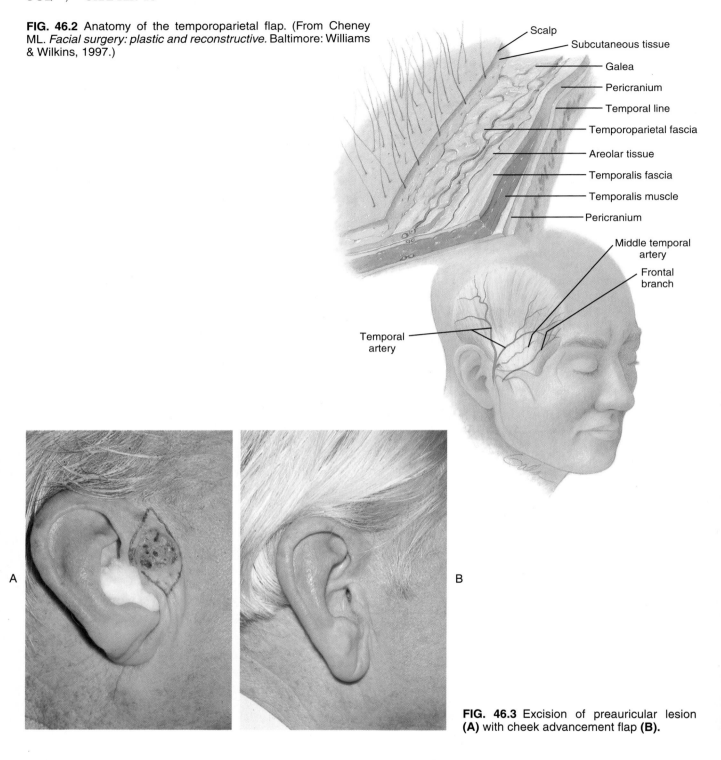

Scalp
Subcutaneous tissue
Galea
Pericranium
Temporal line
Temporoparietal fascia
Areolar tissue
Temporalis fascia
Temporalis muscle
Pericranium
Middle temporal artery
Frontal branch
Temporal artery

A

B

FIG. 46.3 Excision of preauricular lesion **(A)** with cheek advancement flap **(B)**.

Defects of the Conchal Bowl and Root of the Helix

Seen either secondary to cutaneous lesions or after otologic surgery, defects of the conchal bowl or root of the helix can be reconstructed with a helical advancement flap (Fig. 46.4).

In cases in which there is skin loss of the conchal bowl, repair is most successful with skin grafts, as they provides adequate coverage while also allowing for careful monitoring of the area (Fig. 46.5).

Upper Third Defects

Although the upper third of the auricle can be concealed by hair, it is functionally important in the wearing of eyeglasses. Several surgical options are available for the correction of upper third defects; primary closure, helical advancement flaps, and autogenous cartilage framework with temporoparietal fascial coverage. Both primary closure and helical advancement flaps are reserved for smaller, less complicated auricular

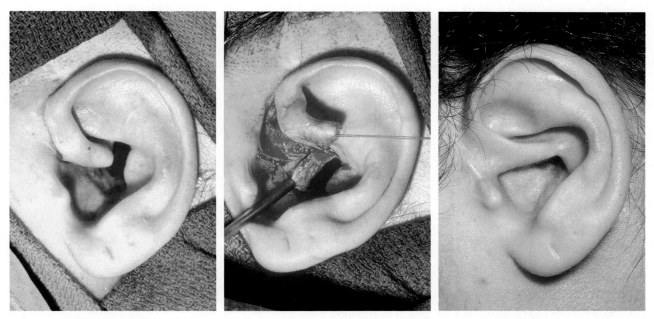

FIG. 46.4 Helical advancement flap to repair a defect of the conchal bowl following multiple otologic procedures for chronic otitis media.

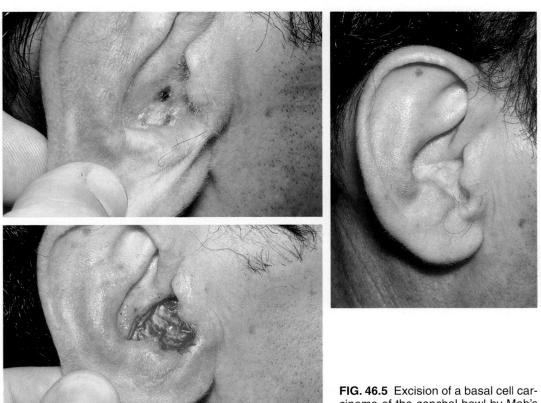

FIG. 46.5 Excision of a basal cell carcinoma of the conchal bowl by Moh's technique followed by repair with split-thickness skin graft.

defects. The helical advancement flap is preferred over primary closure when the defect is limited to the helix. Primary closure is ordinarily used when the defect extends from the helical rim into the body of the auricle. Reconstruction using a temporoparietal fascial flap with autogenous cartilage framework is indicated in cases where large composite portions of the upper third of the auricle have been removed (Fig. 46.6). Lateral skin defects of the upper and middle third of the auricle can be closed with simple rotation advancement flaps (Fig. 46.7). This technique (20) is preferred over skin grafts or

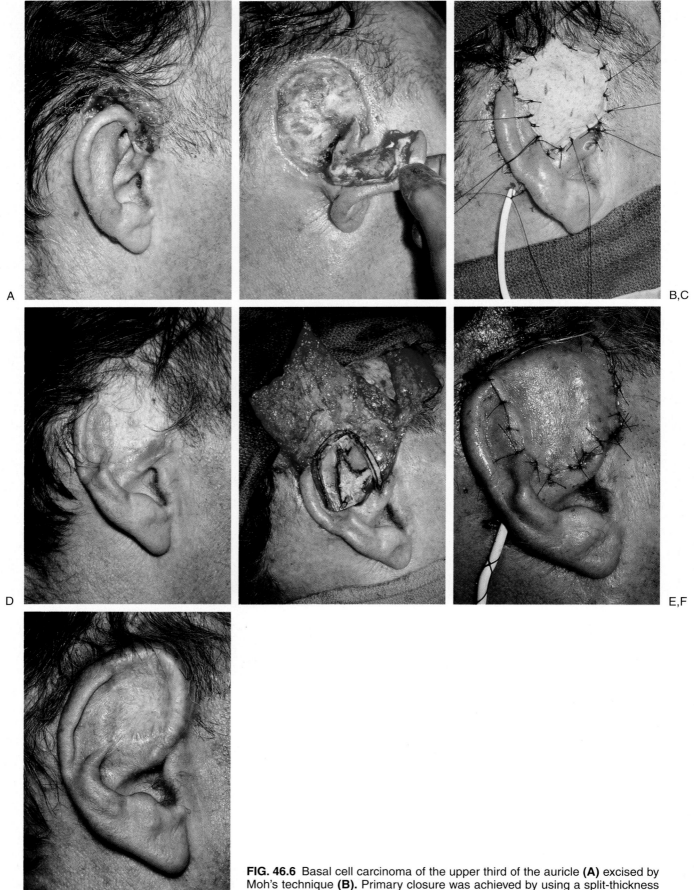

FIG. 46.6 Basal cell carcinoma of the upper third of the auricle **(A)** excised by Moh's technique **(B)**. Primary closure was achieved by using a split-thickness skin graft **(C, D)** followed by a secondary temporoparietal fascial flap **(E–F)** and split-thickness skin graft **(G)** reconstruction 6 months later.

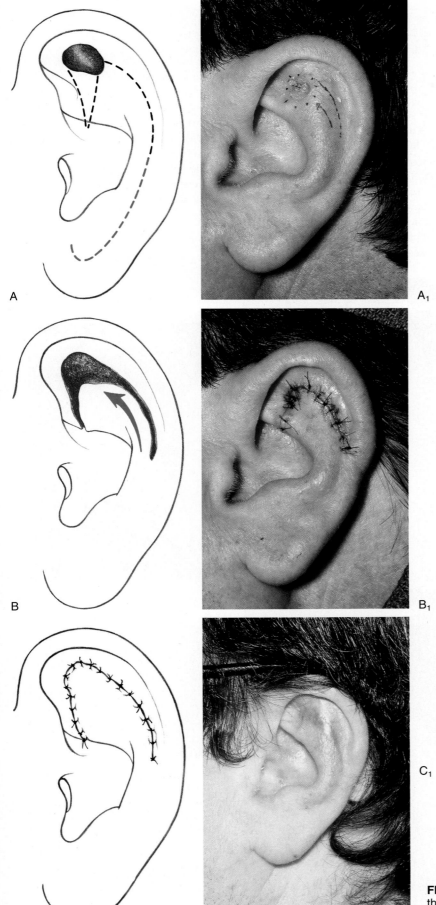

FIG. 46.7 Primary repair of a surgical defect of the triangular fossa **(A, A₁)** using an advancement flap **(B, B₁, C, C₁)**.

primary closure because skin color is well matched, the alteration of free margins of the upper auricle is not affected, and the incisions are well hidden in the scapha.

Middle Third Defects

The absence of the middle third of the auricle is a very noticeable auricular deformity. Major defects of the middle third of the auricle necessitate the use of cartilage grafting techniques to obtain adequate structural support. Simple defects can be closed primarily with satisfactory results, but larger and more complex defects require reconstruction techniques that incorporate lateral and medial skin coverage with interposed cartilage to ensure structural support within the skin flaps (see Laceration and Avulsion Injuries).

Lower Third Defects

When reconstructing the lower one-third of the ear and lobule, the repair must include cartilage grafting techniques to provide the support necessary to ensure long-term results. A versatile technique for reconstruction of the lobule is to use conchal cartilage in a two-stage procedure. The cartilage is embedded in a pocket below the auricle. Six weeks later, the cartilage and overlying skin are elevated and the postlobular area is skin grafted (Fig. 46.8). This technique provides good skin color match, results in minimal local edema, produces a naturally shaped and textured earlobe, and allows proper lobule positioning.

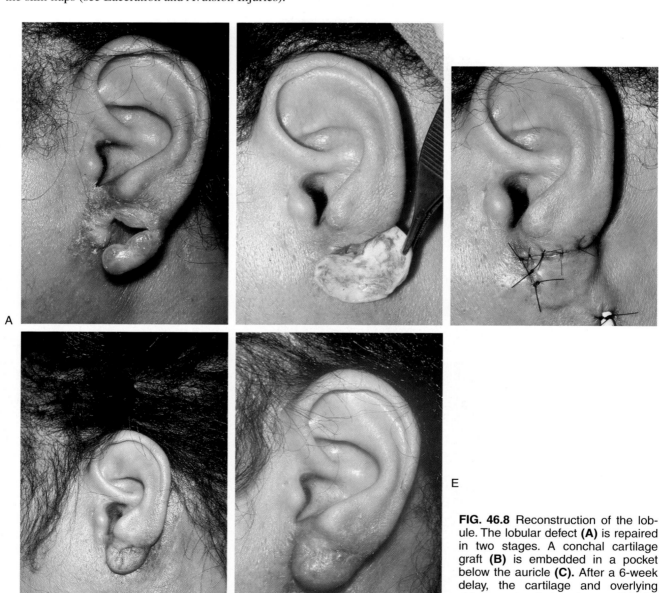

A   B, C   E   D

FIG. 46.8 Reconstruction of the lobule. The lobular defect **(A)** is repaired in two stages. A conchal cartilage graft **(B)** is embedded in a pocket below the auricle **(C)**. After a 6-week delay, the cartilage and overlying skin are elevated and a postlobular crease created with split-thickness skin graft **(D). E:** Postoperative result at 6 months.

Full-Thickness Defects

To be reliable, a full-thickness graft must bring with it its own vascularity (21–23). This is particularly true in the repair of full-thickness auricular defects where the vascularity of the recipient site is limited. A reliable technique is the use of the postauricular myocutaneous flap. This flap has many advantages: a dependable vascular supply, good skin color match, and locally available tissue. Based on the postauricular artery and vein, it uses as its component parts of the postauricular skin and postauricular muscle. It can be elevated, folded upon itself, and used to reconstruct full-thickness defects of the upper and middle auricle (Fig. 46.9).

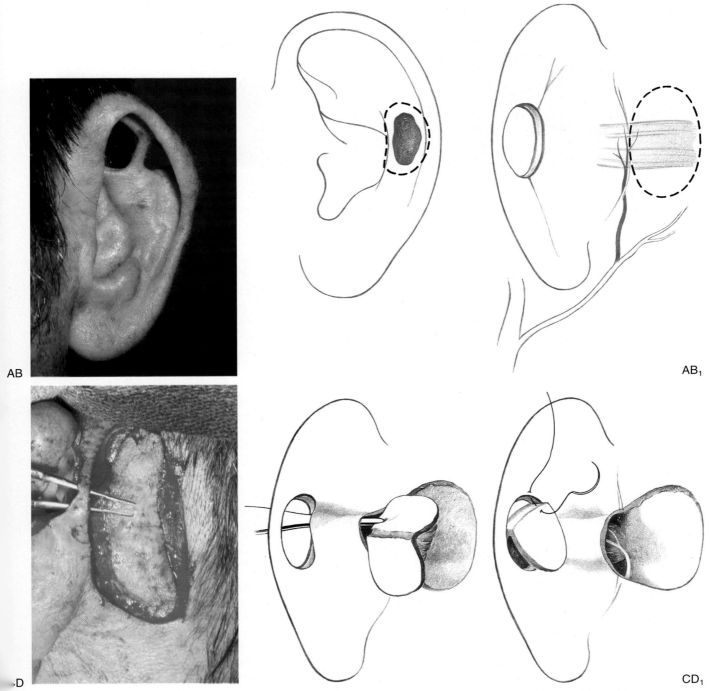

FIG. 46.9 Postauricular myocutaneous flap for full-thickness repair of the auricle. After excision of the defect **(A₁, A, B)** a postauricular myocutaneous flap is outlined **(B₁)**, elevated **(C₁, C, D)**, rotated into the defect **(D₁)**, and sutured into place **(E₁, E)**. The postoperative appearance is shown in **(F)**.

Continued

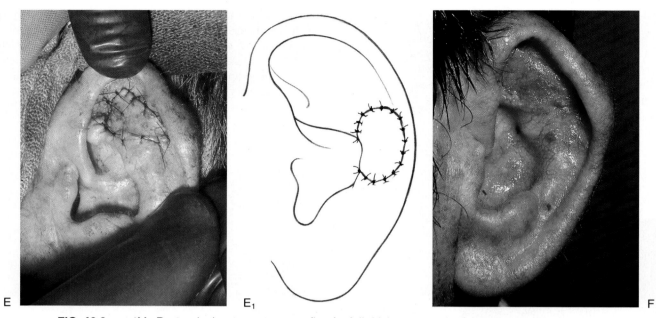

FIG. 46.9, cont'd. Postauricular myocutaneous flap for full-thickness repair of the auricle. After excision of the defect (**A₁, A, B**) a postauricular myocutaneous flap is outlined (**B₁**), elevated (**C₁, C, D**), rotated into the defect (**D₁**), and sutured into place (**E₁, E**). The postoperative appearance is shown in (**F**).

REPAIR OF AURICULAR INJURIES CATEGORIZED BY TYPE OF TRAUMA

The most common forms of auricular trauma are laceration and avulsion injuries, auricular hematomas, animal and human bites, auricular burns, and iatrogenic defects. Because each defect is unique, the surgeon must draw upon a broad understanding of available reconstructive techniques to customize the repair.

Laceration and Avulsion Injuries

Acutely traumatized ears should be managed with minimal debridement after thorough cleansing of the auricle (24). The tissue must be handled carefully and care taken to align cartilage edges. In complex and severe injuries, the reattachment should progress in an orderly fashion, starting from known landmarks and free margins.

In 1972 Baudet et al. (25) proposed a simple technique for repair of avulsions of the auricle. Like many of the successful techniques for auricular reattachment, this is a two-stage technique (26). The advantages of the Baudet technique include maintenance of the integrity of the cartilage and high success rates (Fig. 46.10). The technique requires the careful debridement of the avulsed segment and preservation of the segment in an ice slush until the patient can be taken to the operating room. The postauricular skin over the mastoid is removed to create a vascular bed over the temporal and mastoid area. The medial surface of the avulsed segment is deepithelialized. Because cartilage is a barrier to reestablishment of a vascular supply, the auricular cartilage is fenestrated. These fenestrations should be positioned to avoid damage to important structural landmarks of the anterior auricle. The avulsed segment is placed upon the newly created postauricular bed and reattached to the auricle. Suction drainage is applied to promote adherence of the flap to the vascular bed and facilitate revascularization. A second stage is required for elevation and creation of a postauricular sulcus.

In selected cases, microvascular replantation (27) of avulsed auricular segments can be accomplished. It is important to carefully inspect all avulsed auricular segments under magnification in an attempt to identify acceptable vessels for reanastomosis. In most cases, vessels are not identified or are not in acceptable condition for microvascular anastomosis. However, when vessels are present and viable, this technique can result in impressive results with minimal auricular distortion and a high resistance to secondary soft tissue and cartilage infection (Fig. 46.11).

Auricular Hematomas

Auricular hematomas are common in busy emergency rooms, particularly in areas of the country where wrestling is a popular sport (28,29). The treatment for this clinical problem is local incision and drainage with compression dressings (Fig. 46.12). The wound is thoroughly irrigated, and hemostasis is obtained with bipolar cautery. The wound is then reapproximated with a mattress suture, and clear Silastic sheeting is used as a bolster so that the affected area can be monitored. The bolster is left in place for 7 to 10 days.

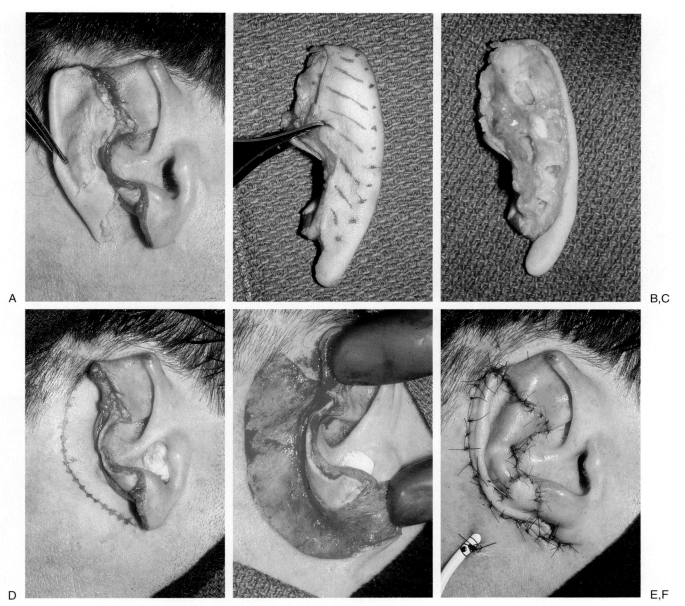

FIG. 46.10 The Baudet repair of avulsion injuries of the auricle. The avulsed segment **(A)** is deepithelialized on the medial surface **(B, C).** The cartilage is fenestrated to allow vascular ingrowth **(C).** The postauricular skin is excised **(D)** to create a vascular bed **(E).** The avulsed segment is reattached to the auricle and suction drainage applied **(F).** A second stage is required for elevation of the auricle and recreation of a postauricular sulcus.

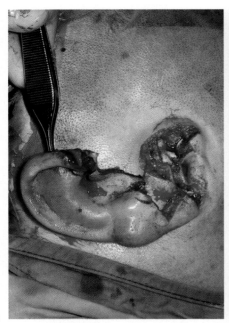
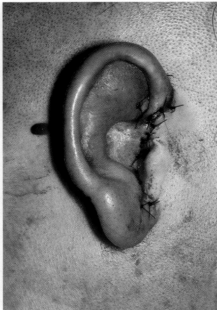
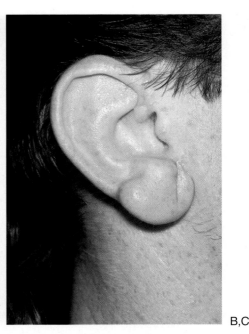

A

B,C

FIG. 46.11 A: Auricular avulsion injury presents 12 hours after original injury. Local debridement techniques utilized to identify a viable vascular pedicle. **B:** At completion of microvascular anastomosis, soft tissue was debrided, antibiotic irrigation was used, and the skin margins were reapproximated. **C:** Appearance of the auricle 6 weeks after the original injury.

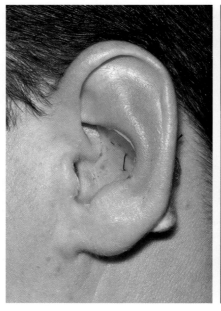
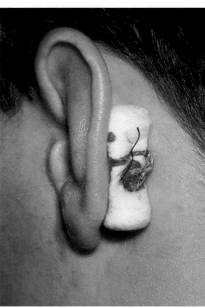

FIG. 46.12 After drainage of an auricular hematoma, the skin is reapproximated to the cartilage framework with a mattress suture and clear Silastic sheeting is used as a stent.

Human and Animal Bites

Human bites to the auricle constitute a difficult management problem. The technique of reconstruction is dictated by the size and location of the defect, as well as the time elapsed between injury and medical attention. For cookie-bite injuries of the middle and upper third, two-stage postauricular flaps yield most optimal cosmetic results (Fig. 46.13). Unlike the other flaps used to repair such defects, this flap incorporates cartilage into the reconstruction. The flap is placed in apposition to the anterior auricular skin during the first stage. The second stage of reconstruction requires placement of autogenous septal cartilage, division of the postauricular flap, and draping of the postauricular flap over the medial surface of the ear and is performed 2 to 3 weeks after the initial procedure. The postauricular flap is then divided after a period of 3 weeks, and skin is used to cover the postauricular area. A bolster dressing can be used but must be carefully monitored because ischemic changes can occur. Results have been satisfactory when using this technique for reconstruction of the helix and scapha.

More extensive auricular loss requires the use of a temporoparietal fascial flap in addition to autogenous costal cartilage framework (Fig. 46.14). A skin graft is placed over the temporoparietal fascia after the cartilage graft has been positioned. Postoperative edema may persist for up to 1 year.

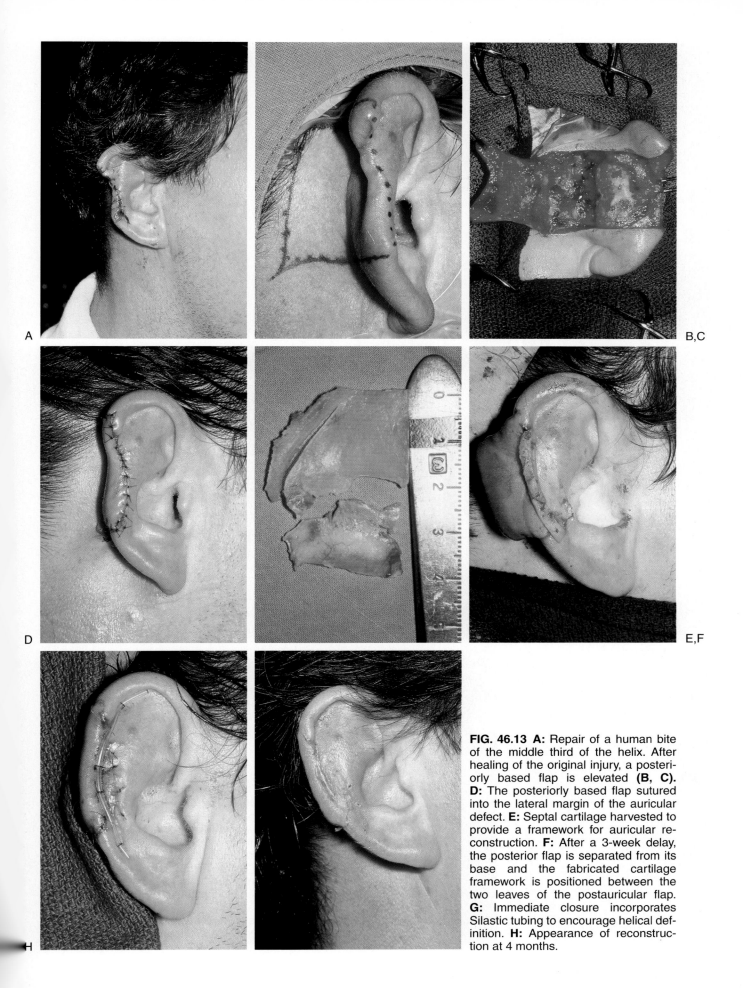

FIG. 46.13 A: Repair of a human bite of the middle third of the helix. After healing of the original injury, a posteriorly based flap is elevated **(B, C).** **D:** The posteriorly based flap sutured into the lateral margin of the auricular defect. **E:** Septal cartilage harvested to provide a framework for auricular reconstruction. **F:** After a 3-week delay, the posterior flap is separated from its base and the fabricated cartilage framework is positioned between the two leaves of the postauricular flap. **G:** Immediate closure incorporates Silastic tubing to encourage helical definition. **H:** Appearance of reconstruction at 4 months.

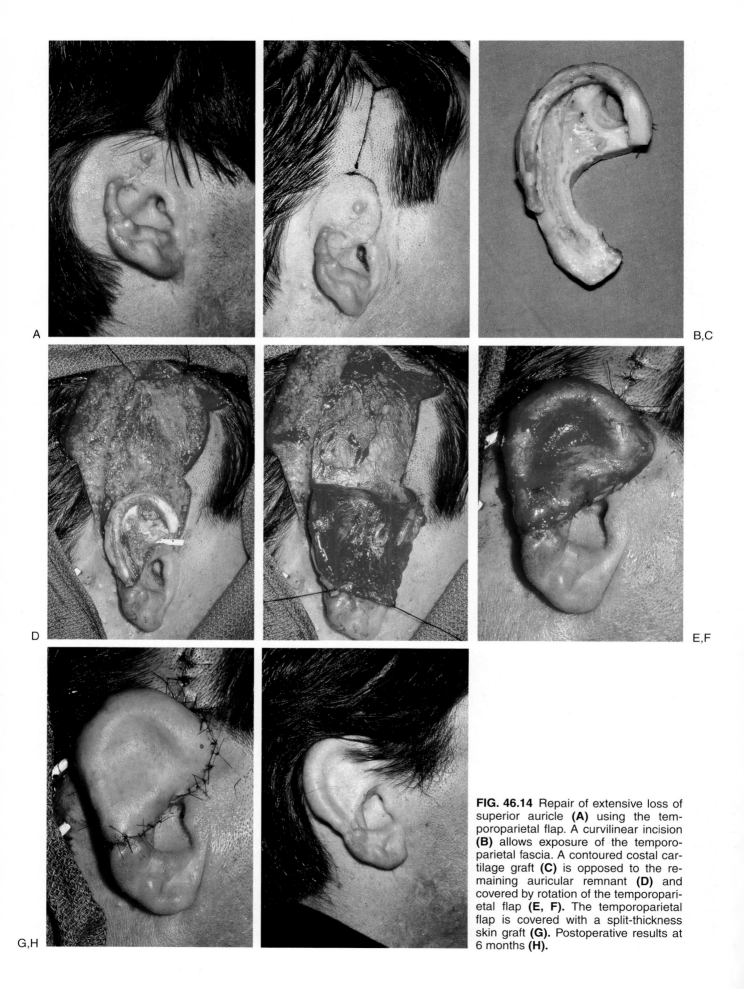

FIG. 46.14 Repair of extensive loss of superior auricle **(A)** using the temporoparietal flap. A curvilinear incision **(B)** allows exposure of the temporoparietal fascia. A contoured costal cartilage graft **(C)** is opposed to the remaining auricular remnant **(D)** and covered by rotation of the temporoparietal flap **(E, F).** The temporoparietal flap is covered with a split-thickness skin graft **(G).** Postoperative results at 6 months **(H).**

Auricular Burns

Burns of the auricle most commonly involve the upper third. The most successful is with a conchal bowl transposition flap (30). The composite flap can be rotated on the narrow anterior soft tissue pedicle based at the root of the helix. The composite pedicled tissue, from the concha, can be rotated superiorly and used to reconstruct full-thickness defects of the upper third of the auricle (Fig. 46.15).

Auricular Keloids

Auricular keloids are common sequelae of trauma to the lobule in susceptible individuals. The most common inciting event is ear piercing; however, they can arise from a variety of other manipulations, including elective procedures around the ear, such as otoplasty and face-lift incisions. A variety of techniques have been used in management of keloids, including laser excision, injection of interferon, simple excision, and steroid injections. Accepted treatment begins with intralesional injections of triamcinolone acetonide suspension 40 mg/ml (Kenalog 40) given 2 weeks apart for a total of four to five sessions. The effect of the treatment is evaluated every 2 weeks, and when a response is shown, surgery is planned.

Atraumatic surgical excision within the margins of the keloid tissue is performed followed by intraoperative intralesional injections of Kenalog 40 (Fig. 46.16). Postoperatively, the patient is monitored carefully for any evidence of reformation of the keloid. At 3 to 4 weeks, a booster-dose of

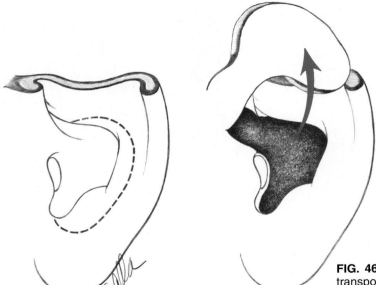

FIG. 46.15 A conchal composite flap of cartilage and skin is transposed to repair the upper third of the auricle. The remaining nonepithelialized surfaces at the newly created helical rim and conchal bowl are covered with split-thickness skin graft.

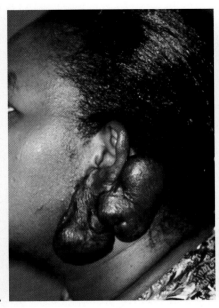

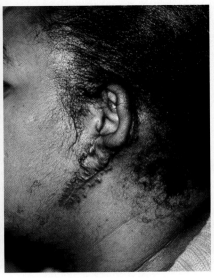

FIG. 46.16 Massive keloids of the auricle **(A)** successfully managed by preoperative and intraoperative injections of steroids, excision, and primary closure **(B)**.

Kenalog 40 is given. Patients are then monitored monthly for any evidence of recurrence. If there is evidence of keloid reformation in the postoperative period, Kenalog 40 treatments are reinstituted. Low-dose radiation therapy is held in reserve for intractable keloid formation (Table 46.2).

Other Acquired Auricular Defects

Pixie Ear

A common acquired auricular deformity is that of "pixie ear," seen after face-lift surgery. As a general rule, this can be corrected effectively by using a mini–face-lift incision around the lobule with advancement of the facial skin to release the lobular defect (Fig. 46.17).

TABLE 46.2 *Management of auricular keloids*

Steroid injection, intralesional: Kenalog 40 weekly × 6 weeks
Intralesional injection at surgery
Excision within margins
Intralesional injections starting 3 weeks postoperatively
For recurrence: repeat and consider low-dose radiation therapy

Adapted from Farrior RT, Stambaugh KI. Keloids and hyperplastic scars. In: Thomas JR, Holt GR, eds. *Facial scars.* St. Louis: Mosby, 1989;211–228.

Skin Loss

To replace large areas of skin loss of the auricle, the skin must be thin, pliable, a good color and texture match, and of good vascularity and elasticity to firmly adhere to the auricular cartilage.

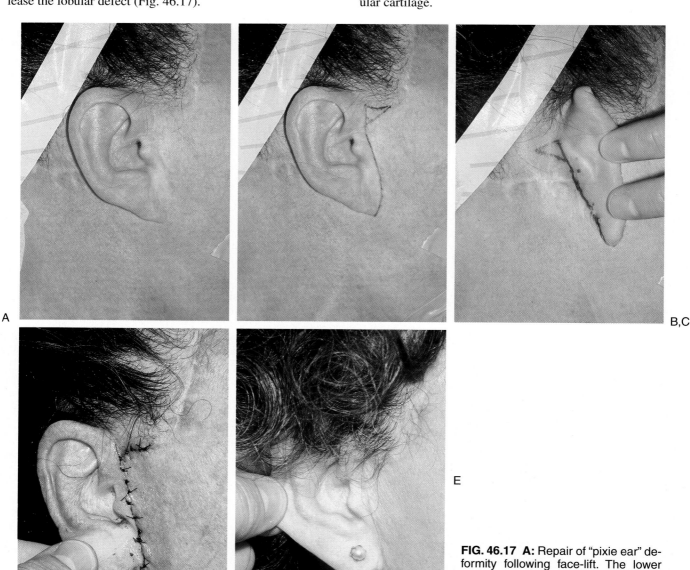

FIG. 46.17 A: Repair of "pixie ear" deformity following face-lift. The lower auricle is released using both anterior **(B)** and postauricular **(C)** incisions and advancement of facial skin **(D). E:** Postoperative appearance at 6 months.

When autogenous auricular cartilage can be preserved, the tissue used for coverage must drape over the cartilage with minimal tension so that cartilage distortion is limited. The temporoparietal fascial flap with a split-thickness skin graft is best for this purpose (Fig. 46.18).

CHRONIC OSTEOMYELITIS OF THE TEMPORAL BONE

Chronic osteomyelitis of the temporal bone typically presents with a history of chronic drainage, progressive loss of temporal bone architecture, and chronic pain syndrome (Chapter 17). Although many therapeutic options exist for the treatment of this problem, aggressive temporal bone debridement with immediate soft tissue coverage with pedi-

cled or microvascular flaps provides early neovascularization of the area and has proven to be very successful in arresting the progress of this disease (Fig. 46.19). The temporoparietal fascial flap, with its rich vascular supply and proximity to this area, has proven a viable option when resurfacing of a marginally vascular external auditory canal is desired.

RECONSTRUCTION AFTER AURICULECTOMY

On occasion, large lesions of the auricle that do not involve the temporal bone necessitate complete removal of the ear. Several options are available for reconstruction, including the use of a cervical bilobed cutaneous flap that can be rotated over the temporal bone and designed to preserve the

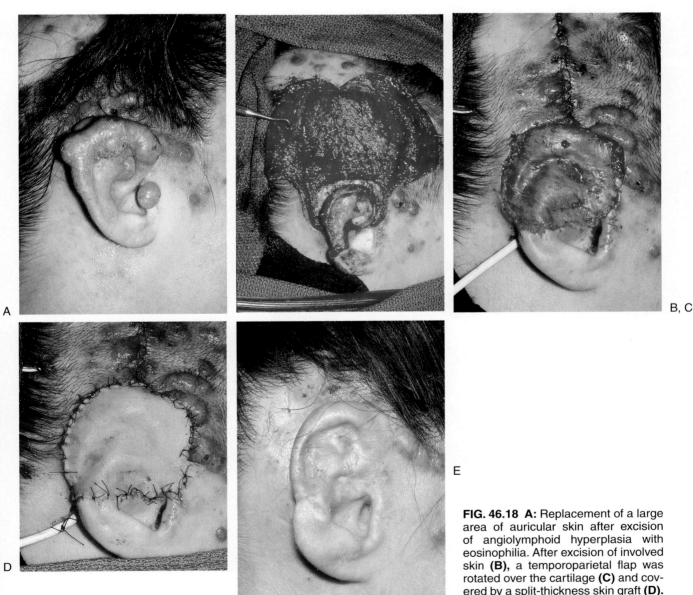

A

B, C

D

E

FIG. 46.18 A: Replacement of a large area of auricular skin after excision of angiolymphoid hyperplasia with eosinophilia. After excision of involved skin **(B)**, a temporoparietal flap was rotated over the cartilage **(C)** and covered by a split-thickness skin graft **(D)**. **E:** Postoperative appearance after 12 months.

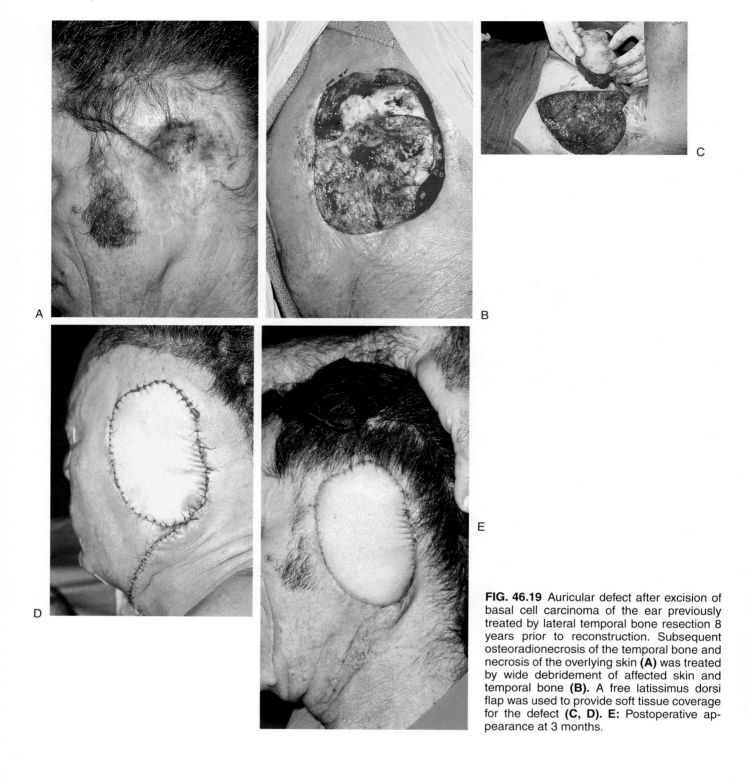

FIG. 46.19 Auricular defect after excision of basal cell carcinoma of the ear previously treated by lateral temporal bone resection 8 years prior to reconstruction. Subsequent osteoradionecrosis of the temporal bone and necrosis of the overlying skin **(A)** was treated by wide debridement of affected skin and temporal bone **(B).** A free latissimus dorsi flap was used to provide soft tissue coverage for the defect **(C, D). E:** Postoperative appearance at 3 months.

external auditory canal (Fig. 46.20) (32). Additional options include chest rotation flaps and microvascular tissue transfer. In many of these cases, the primary goal is to preserve the function of the external auditory canal in sound transmission rather than to recreate the auricle. In selected pa-

tients, after a sufficient disease-free interval, complete auricular reconstruction with a costal cartilage framework, temporoparietal fascial flap, and skin graft could also be considered.

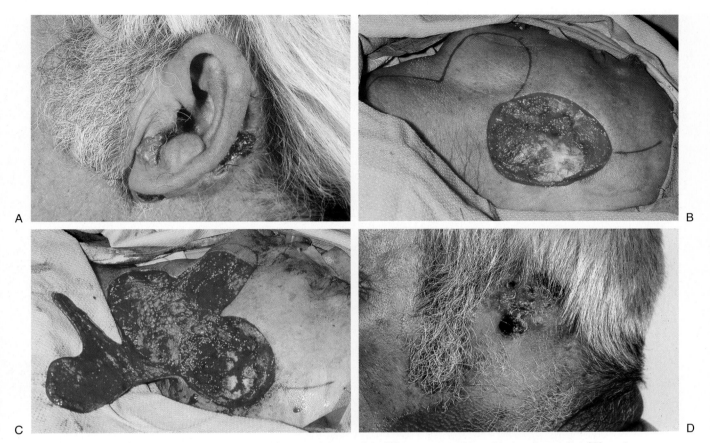

FIG. 46.20 Extensive basal cell carcinoma of the auricle **(A)** was treated by wide local excision **(B)** and repaired primarily by a bilobed rotation flap **(B, C)**, with maintenance of the external auditory canal **(D)**. An auricular prosthesis was placed 6 weeks after surgery.

REFERENCES

1. Tanzer RC, Bellucci RJ, Converse JM, et al. Deformities of the auricle. In: Converse JM, ed. *Reconstructive plastic surgery,* 2nd ed, vol 3. Philadelphia: WB Saunders, 1977:1671–1773.
2. Herberhold C, ed. Reconstruction of the auriculum. *Facial Plast Surg Monograph* 1988;5:385–460.
3. Werrda H. Plastic surgery of the ear. In: Kerr AG, ed. *Scott Brown's otolaryngology,* 5th ed, vol 3. London: Butterworths, 1987:185–202.
4. Tolleth H. Artistic anatomy, dimensions, and proportions of the external ear. *Clin Plast Surg* 1978;5:337–345.
5. Adamson JE, Horton CE, Crawford HH. The growth pattern of the external ear. *Plast Reconstr Surg* 1965;36:466–470.
6. Farkas LG. Growth of normal and reconstructed auricles. In: Tanzer RC, Edgerton MT, eds. *Symposium on reconstruction of the auricle.* St. Louis: Mosby, 1974.
7. Allison GR. Anatomy of the external ear. *Clin Plast Surg* 1978;5: 419–422.
8. Janfaza P, Nadol, JB Jr, Galla RJ, et al. *Surgical anatomy of the head and neck.* Philadelphia: Lippincott Williams & Wilkins, 2001.
9. Rose EH, Norris MS. The versatile temporoparietal fascial flap: adaptability to a variety of composite defects. *Plast Reconstr Surg* 1990;85: 224–232.
10. Brent B, Upton J, Acland RD, et al. Experience with the temporoparietal fascial free flap. *Plast Reconstr Surg* 1985;76:177–188.
11. Smith RA. The free fascial scalp flap. *Plast Reconstr Surg* 1980;66: 204–209.
12. Tegtmeier RE, Gooding RA. The use of a fascial flap in ear reconstruction. *Plast Reconstr Surg* 1977;60:406–411.
13. Horowitz JH, Persing JA, Nichter LS, et al. Galeal-pericranial flaps in head and neck reconstruction. Anatomy and application. *Am J Surg* 1984;148:489–497.
14. Jenkins AM, Finucan T. Primary nonmicrosurgical reconstruction following ear avulsion using the temporoparietal fascial island flap. *Plast Reconstr Surg* 1989;83:148–152.
15. Marty F, Montandon D, Gumener R, et al. Subcutaneous tissue in the scalp: anatomical, physiological, and clinical study. *Ann Plast Surg* 1986;16:368–376.
16. Abul-Hassan HS, Von Drasek Ascher G, Acland RD. Surgical anatomy and blood supply of the fascial layers of the temporal region. *Plast Reconstr Surg* 1986;77:17–28.
17. Hing DN, Buncke HJ, Alpert BS. Use of the temporoparietal free fascial flap in the upper extremity. *Plast Reconstr Surg* 1988;81:534–544.
18. Cheney ML. *Facial surgery: plastic and reconstructive.* Baltimore: Williams & Wilkins, 1997.
19. Brent B. The acquired auricular deformity. A systematic approach to its analysis and reconstruction. *Plast Reconstr Surg* 1977;59:475–485.
20. Ramirez OM, Heckler FR. Reconstruction of nonmarginal defects of the ear with chondrocutaneous advancement flaps. *Plast Reconstr Surg* 1989;84:32–40.
21. Elsahy NI. Ear reconstruction with a flap from the medial surface of the auricle. *Ann Plast Surg* 1985;14:169–179.
22. Renard A. Postauricular flap based on a dermal pedicle for ear reconstruction. *Plast Reconstr Surg* 1981;68:159–165.
23. Krespi YP, Ries WR, Shugar JMA, et al. Auricular reconstruction with postauricular myocutaneous flap. *Otolaryngol Head Neck Surg* 1983;91:193–196.
24. Mladick R. Salvage of the ear in acute trauma. *Clin Plast Surg* 1978;5: 427–435.
25. Baudet J, Tramond P, Goumain A. A propos d'un procédé original de réimplantation d'un pavillon de l'oreille totalement séparé. *Ann Chir Plast* 1972;17:67–72.

26. Mladick RA, Horton CE, Adamson JE, et al. The pocket principle: a new technique for the reattachment of a severed ear part. *Plast Reconstr Surg* 1971;48:219–223.

27. Mutimer KL, Banis JC, Upton J. Microsurgical reattachment of totally amputated ears. *Plast Reconstr Surg* 1987;79:535–541.

28. Giffin CS. The wrestler's ear (acute auricular hematoma). *Arch Otolaryngol* 1985;111:161–164.

29. Schuller DE, Dankle SD, Strauss RH. A technique to treat wrestlers' auricular hematoma without interrupting training or competition. *Arch Otolaryngol Head Neck Surg* 1989;115:202–206.

30. Donelan MB. Conchal transposition flap for postburn ear deformities. *Plast Reconstr Surg* 1989;83:641–654.

31. Farrior RT, Stambaugh KI. Keloids and hyperplastic scars. In: Thomas JR, Holt GR, eds. *Facial scars.* St. Louis: Mosby, 1989:211–228.

32. Songcharoen S, Smith RA, Jabaley ME. Tumors of the external ear and reconstruction of defects. *Clin Plast Surg* 1978;5:447–457.

Index